FOURTH EDITION

INTEGRATIVE THERAPIES
IN REHABILITATION

Evidence for Efficacy in Therapy,
Prevention, and Wellness

FOURTH EDITION

INTEGRATIVE THERAPIES
IN REHABILITATION

Evidence for Efficacy in Therapy, Prevention, and Wellness

Edited by

Carol M. Davis, DPT, EdD, MS, FAPTA
Professor Emerita
Department of Physical Therapy
University of Miami, Miller School of Medicine
Miami, Florida

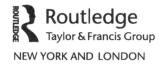

Routledge
Taylor & Francis Group

NEW YORK AND LONDON

First published in 2017 by SLACK Incorporated

Published 2024 by Routledge
605 Third Avenue, New York, NY 10017
4 Park Square, Milton Park, Abingdon, Oxon OX14 4RN

Routledge is an imprint of the Taylor & Francis Group, an informa business

Library of Congress Cataloging-in-Publication Data

Names: Davis, Carol M., editor.
Title: Integrative therapies in rehabilitation : evidence for efficacy in
    therapy, prevention, and wellness / edited by Carol M. Davis.
Other titles: Complementary therapies in rehabilitation.
Description: Fourth edition. | Thorofare, NJ : SLACK Incorporated, [2017] |
    Preceded by Complementary therapies in rehabilitation : evidence for
    efficacy in therapy, prevention, and wellness / edited by Carol M. Davis.
    3rd ed. 2009. | Includes bibliographical references and index.
Identifiers: LCCN 2016013714 (print) | ISBN
    9781630910433 (alk. paper)
Subjects: | MESH: Rehabilitation--methods | Complementary Therapies--methods
    | Holistic Health
Classification: LCC R733 (print) | NLM WB 320 | DDC
    615.5--dc23
LC record available at http://lccn.loc.gov/2016013714

ISBN: 9781630910433 (hbk)
ISBN: 9781003524625 (ebk)

DOI:10.4324/9781003524625

Dedication

- To John Bond, cherished colleague and friend in publishing since 1990. I am grateful for your support, wise advice, and friendship, and for your willingness to take a chance on this book from the very beginning, even though I showed the outline to you on a restaurant napkin.

- To James L. Oschman, PhD, soulful scientist, colleague, and friend. Your productive mind and writing about the science of energy medicine made it possible for me to make sense of my practice of John F. Barnes myofascial release, and opened up the world of subtle energy for me to explore.

Contents

ACKNOWLEDGMENTS

In this fourth edition, I am grateful to the following people for their support:

- To my authors, once more, for updating your material with the latest evidence. Your contributions make this book timely and interesting.

- To my friend and colleague, John F. Barnes, PT. You intuited much of the information about fascia that science is now validating 40 years later. Thank you for your courage to stay the course, and thank you for continuing to teach your John F. Barnes myofascial release approach for the benefit of all of us who practice this healing therapy, and for the benefit of our patients. Your gifts to healing are unparalleled in our time.

- To Tony Schiavo, my outstanding editor, who has been right beside me from the beginning of this issue editing and giving your expertise, support, and friendship. I love our conversations about energy and life.

- To my other friends at SLACK Incorporated, including Brien Cummings, Acquisitions Editor, who got this project started before Tony Schiavo joined us; Michelle Gatt and her marketing team; April Billick, Managing Editor, for the art; and Emily Densten, Project Editor. The SLACK team is an author's dream, and I am eternally grateful for our wonderful creative relationship.

- To Dr. Jordyn Rice, my DPT student at the University of Miami who helped me sort through all of my articles and bring order to chaos. Kind of.

- To Dr. Neva Kirk-Sanchez, my chair at the University of Miami Department of Physical Therapy, for her support, encouragement, and friendship over the last 26 years.

- To my family and friends who listen to me go on and on about fascia and the majestic vibrating extracellular matrix: my sister Susan Doughty, my brother Bill Doughty, and my dear friends Meryl Cohen, Jamiss Sebert, Patricia Calhoun, and Tara Carrington. I feel blessed beyond measure to have you all in my life.

ABOUT THE EDITOR

Carol M. Davis, DPT, EdD, MS, FAPTA, received her undergraduate degree in biology from Lycoming College, Williamsport, Pennsylvania, an MS with certificate in physical therapy from Case Western Reserve University, Cleveland, Ohio, a Doctorate in Humanistic Studies (psychology and philosophy; EdD) from the School of Education at Boston University, Boston, Massachusetts, and a clinical doctorate in physical therapy (DPT) from Mass General Institute of Health Professions, Boston, Massachussetts.

As a faculty member at the University of Miami School of Medicine, Miami Florida, Dr. Davis served as Clinical Assistant Professor with Family and Internal Medicine from 1983 to 1985, during which time she coordinated the Fellowship in Clinical Geriatrics. She served as Professor and Vice Chair of the Department of Physical Therapy from 1987 to 2009. She retired from her position in 2015 with the University of Miami Miller School of Medicine as Professor Emerita in the Department of Physical Therapy. Additionally, she has held the positions of Clinical Staff and Clinical Instructor at Massachusetts General Hospital, Boston, Massachusetts, Assistant Professor at the University of Alabama in Birmingham, and Assistant Professor and Co-Chair *ad interim* of physical therapy at Sargent College of Boston University.

She is an internationally recognized speaker and consultant in teaching and developing curriculum in attitudes and values, ethics, geriatrics, and complementary therapies in rehabilitation. Dr. Davis authored the book *Patient Practitioner Interaction: An Experiential Manual for Developing the Art of Health Care*, now in its sixth edition, and she coauthored the text *Therapeutic Interaction in Nursing* with Dr. Christine Williams. These texts were published by SLACK Incorporated.

Today, Dr. Davis is an active guest lecturer on the structure and function of fascia, teaches the John F. Barnes myofascial release approach nationally and internationally, and practices physical therapy and J.F. Barnes myofascial release 2 days per week in Miami, Florida. She has studied the John F. Barnes myofascial release approach since 1989 and uses it regularly as a complement to her physical therapy treatments. In 2003, she was awarded the Catherine Worthingham Fellow award for a lifetime of outstanding service to the profession by the American Physical Therapy Association.

CONTRIBUTING AUTHORS

Brent Anderson, PhD, PT, OCS, PMA-CPT (Chapter 15), a licensed Physical Therapist and Orthopedic Certified Specialist, is a leading authority in performing arts medicine, Pilates for Rehabilitation, and Pain Management Through Movement and Spine Health. He lectures widely at national and international symposia and consults with physical therapy companies, universities, and other educational bodies throughout the world. In addition, he owns and operates one of the most comprehensive Pilates conditioning and physical therapy centers, which has become a model for many other Pilates studios worldwide. Brent is the founder of Polestar Pilates Education, which currently operates in more than 40 countries and 12 languages.

Brent received his degree in Physical Therapy at the University of California, San Francisco in 1989, and his PhD in Physical Therapy at the University of Miami in 2005. He currently serves as adjunct faculty at the University of Miami, Miami, Florida Department of Physical Therapy. His doctoral thesis explored the impact of Pilates rehabilitation on chronic low back pain using psychoemotional wellness and quality of life measures. Brent has been a member of the American Physical Therapy Association since 1987 and he formerly served as President of the Performing Arts Special Interest Group in the Orthopedic Section. He is also a longtime member of the International Association for Dance Medicine and Science and the Pilates Method Alliance.

Ellen Zambo Anderson, PT, PhD, GCS (Chapter 20) received a Physical Therapy degree from West Virginia University, Morgantown, West Virginia, a master's degree in Movement Sciences from Columbia University, New York, New York, and a PhD in Health Sciences from Rutgers, The State University of New Jersey, New Brunswick, New Jersey. She is an Associate Professor of Physical Therapy in the Department of Rehabilitation and Movement Sciences at Rutgers, School of Health Related Professions. Dr. Anderson has co-written a book, *Complementary Therapies for Physical Therapy*, and has presented nationally on incorporating complementary therapies into a physical therapy plan of care. She is also the primary author of the *Special Olympics Young Athletes,* an inclusive sports-play program for children ages 2 to 8. Dr. Anderson is interested in the use of physical activity and mind-body medicine for addressing physical and mental health diagnoses and promoting healthy lifestyles.

John F. Barnes, PT (Chapter 6) graduated in physical therapy from the University of Pennsylvania, Philadelphia, Pennsylvania in 1960. He is President and Director of the Myofascial Release Treatment Centers and National Myofascial Release Seminars located in Malvern, Pennsylvania, and Sedona, Arizona, where he and his staff treat people referred from all over the world when medicine, surgery, and traditional therapies have failed. John Barnes has educated more than 100,000 people in his workshop series over the past 40 years across the United States and Canada. He is the author of 2 books: *Myofascial Release* and *Healing Ancient Wounds: The Renegade's Wisdom*.

Jennifer M. Bottomley, PhD, MS, PT (Chapters 11, 12, 17) has a bachelor's degree in Physical Therapy from the University of Wisconsin, Madison and an advanced master's degree in Physical Therapy from the MGH Institute of Health Professionals in Boston, Massachussetts. She has a combined intercollegiate doctoral degree in Gerontology (University of Massachusetts, Amherst) and Health Science and Service Administration (Union Institute, Cincinnati, Ohio) and a second PhD from The Union Institute in Health Service Administration, Legislation, and Policy Management with a specialty in Gerontology.

Dr. Bottomley has practiced since 1974 in acute care, home care, outpatient clinics, nursing homes, and long-term care facilities. Currently, she is an academic and clinical educator in Geriatric Physical Therapy Internationally and throughout the United States. Jennifer is an Associate Professor at Simmons College in Boston, Massachussetts teaching the Neuromuscular courses and serves as an Adjunct Professor at the MGH Institute in Boston, Massachussetts. She serves as a consultant on several federal advisory boards, including an appointment to the White House Advisory Panel for Health Care Reform. She practices clinically in the Boston area in homeless shelters on a pro bono basis coordinating rehabilitation services for the *Committee to End Elder Homelessness/HEARTH* in Boston and serves on the Board of Directors for HEARTH. Jennifer serves as the current President for International PhysioTherapists working with Older People (IPTOP), a geriatric specialty group of the World Confederation for Physical Therapy (WCPT). She is currently serving on an interdisciplinary AARP panel addressing Elder Isolation—Identification and Interventions. She has been recognized by many awards and recently (2011) received the Lucy Blair Service Award from the American Physical Therapy Association (APTA) and has given the Maley lecture. She received an International Service award from WCPT in 2015.

Judith E. Deutsch, PT, PhD, FAPTA (Chapter 10) received her BA in Human Biology from Stanford University, Stanford, California, her MS in Physical Therapy from University of Southern California, Los Angeles, California and her PhD in Pathokinesiology from New York University, New York, New York. She completed a post-doctoral fellowship in rehabilitation research at University of Medicine and Dentistry of New Jersey, Newark, New Jersey. Dr. Deutsch is Professor and Director of the Research in Virtual Environments and Rehabilitation Sciences (Rivers) in the doctoral programs in Physical Therapy at Rutgers University, Newark, New Jersey. Her scholarship and teaching include neuro rehabilitation, motor learning, evidence-based practice and knowledge-to-action. She develops and tests virtual environments for rehabilitation. Previously she studied the outcomes of physical therapists practicing Structural Integration. She is coauthor with Ellen Zambo Anderson of *Complementary Therapies for Physical Therapy.*

Jan Dommerholt, PT, DPT, MPS, DAAPM (Chapter 19) graduated from the Interstudy Academy of Physiotherapy in Arnhem, the Netherlands, in 1986. After moving to the United States, he completed a combined master's degree in Biomechanical Trauma and Health Care Administration from Lynn University, Boca Raton, Florida and a doctorate of Physical Therapy from the University of St. Augustine for Health Sciences, St. Augustine, Florida. Currently, he is a PhD candidate at Aalborg University in Denmark. He is President of Myopain Seminars and Bethesda Physiocare in Bethesda, Maryland, and CEO of PhysioFitness in Rockville, Maryland. He is the editor of 4 textbooks, and author of close to 60 book chapters and nearly 100 articles.

Barbara Funk, MS, OTR, CHT (Chapter 9) graduated with a master's degree in Occupational Therapy from Boston University, Boston, Massachusetts in 1979. She is a Senior Occupational Therapist and Coordinator of the Cancer Rehabilitation Program at the Rehabilitation Institute of Michigan, Detroit, Michigan. She has been practicing occupational therapy for 37 years expanding her knowledge base and skills in several different areas including certification in hand therapy, training in lymphedema management (Klose and Norton Miller), John F. Barnes myofascial release, and craniosacral therapy. Her daily practice of classical yoga, influencing body, mind, emotions, and energy, is the wellspring for vitality and service.

Mary Lou Galantino, PT, MS, PhD (Chapter 18) is a Distinguished Professor at Stockton University, Galloway, New Jersey and Adjunct Scholar at the University of Pennsylvania, Philadelphia, Pennsylvania, where she conducts research on integrative medicine and chronic diseases. She is the Holistic Health Minor Coordinator at Stockton and collaborates with the Department of Family Medicine and Community Health at Penn as an Associate Professor. From 2002 to 2004 Dr. Galantino was an NIH-NCCAM (National Center for Complementary and Integrative Health) post-doctoral fellow at Penn and has enjoyed a 30 year clinical, research, and training career. She has extensive experience with cancer and HIV populations and has been an advocate locally and nationally for rehabilitation services since the early 1980s through her oncology rehabilitation training at MD Anderson University of Texas Cancer System, Houston, Texas. Dr. Galantino serves on the Advisory Board of the Cancer Support Community in Wilmington, Delaware.

She received Health Resources and Services Administration government grants to service HIV patients in Texas and New Jersey and established community based rehabilitation interventions for people living with chronic disease locally and through her Fulbright in South Africa in 2014. She is a co-investigator on an American Physical Therapy Association Oncology Grant exploring the benefit of yoga for distal sensory neuropathy and is presently completing an HIV disability study in concert with colleagues from Rutgers University in New Brunswick, New Jersey and the University of Witwatersrand in Johannesburg, South Africa. Her training in yoga led her to investigate management of joint pain for breast cancer survivors using yoga and t'ai chi.

As a facilitator of learning in the classroom and clinic, she engages participants and patients in clinical question inquiries to procure the latest evidence based assessment and integrative approaches to rehabilitation. Dr. Galantino enjoys bringing together teams of experts to solve difficult clinical cases. Through the Interprofessional Education initiative in Stockton's School of Health Sciences she is excited to extend collaboration across the campus, in local and global clinical settings. She views healing as an ongoing collaborative process and recognizes opportunities that emerge in the relationship of practitioner-patient. This reciprocal relationship is an iterative all inspiring experience as holistic ideas evolve and manifest in meaningful ways.

Deborah A. Giaquinto-Wahl, MSPT (Chapter 8) received her bachelor's degree in Physiology at the University of California, Davis in 1986. She then went on to become a certified Athletic Trainer and the assistant trainer at the Sacramento City College. Returning to graduate school she received her master's degree in Physical Therapy at the University of Miami in Florida in 1990. Debbie directed her post-graduate studies in manual therapy and happened upon craniosacral therapy 10 years ago and has utilized it ever since. Debbie serves as a teaching assistant for craniosacral courses through the Upledger Institute in Palm Beach Gardens, Florida, and utilizes these techniques daily in her practice near Annapolis, Maryland.

Janet Kahn, PhD, MT (Chapter 7), a Research Assistant Professor in Psychiatry and Research Affiliate in the Department of Rehabilitation and Movement Sciences at the University of Vermont, Burlington, Vermont, is a massage therapist who specializes in treating people with chronic pain. A research scientist and advocate of research on massage, Dr. Kahn has served as President of the Massage Therapy Association Foundation (1996-2000) and Director of the Massage Therapy Research Consortium (2003-2008). Seeing that research alone would not secure for integrative health care professions such as massage the recognition due, Dr. Kahn entered the world of policy, serving first as Executive Director of the Integrative Healthcare Policy Consortium (2005-2011) and currently as Senior Policy Advisor to the Academic Consortium for Integrative Medicine and Health. In 2011, President Obama appointed her to the National Advisory Group on Prevention, Health Promotion, and Integrative and Public Health, where she still serves. With Dr. William Collinge, and funding from the National Institutes of Health, Dr. Kahn has created 2 programs bringing the power of touch to American households. Touch Caring and Cancer teaches family members of people with cancer how to offer safe massage to alleviate symptoms of cancer and its treatments. Mission Reconnect, available as a mobile app, offers veterans and their partners training in partner massage and 11 other mind-body skills. Dr. Kahn lives in Burlington, Vermont, where she breathes clean air and enjoys the beauty of Lake Champlain and the Green Mountains.

Kevin R. Kunkel, PhD, MSPT, MLD-CDT (Chapter 9) has a history including athletics and scholastics. Through the guidance of his parents, Dr. Kunkel pursued areas of interest that were most familiar to him. Kevin's father, Bill Kunkel, played professional baseball as a pitcher with the New York Yankees and served as a Major League Umpire. His mother, Maxine Kunkel, served as a 10th grade Biology teacher. He matriculated to Stanford University in California and participated in 2 College World Series as a pitcher while completing a bachelor of science in Biology. After graduation he followed the path into professional baseball like his father and older brother, Jeffrey Kunkel. Following baseball, Dr. Kunkel, followed his sister's career path and went on to receive a master's degree in Physical Therapy in 1990. He then received a doctor of philosophy in Physical Therapy in 2010 again at the University of Miami in Florida with the support of his wife, Susan Kunkel.

Dr. Kunkel began practice as a physical therapist in 1991 and then developed an outpatient clinic, The Flagler Institute for Rehabilitation. Always willing to pursue unique challenges, Dr. Kunkel became one of the few Physical Therapists in the State of Florida to be certified in the treatment of lymphedema in 1999. He is proud of his involvement in providing rehabilitation to oncology patients. Years of clinical experience allowed Dr. Kunkel to pursue research focusing on lymphedema and he now presents nationally on the topic. His years of clinical experience in this unique field have provided Dr. Kunkel with an opportunity to share this information with the newest generation of Physical Therapists. He has been an Assistant Professor at Nova Southeastern University, Ft. Lauderdale, Florida and an adjunct Professor at The Miller School of Medicine at The University of Miami.

Patrick J. LaRiccia, MD, MSCE (Chapter 18) is Board Certified in Internal Medicine and a Pennsylvania licensed acupuncturist. Currently, he is research director for the Won Sook Chung Foundation in Moorestown, New Jersey; on the medical staffs of Penn-Presbyterian Medical Center in the division of General Internal Medicine and the Hospital of the University of Pennsylvania in the department of Physical Medicine and Rehabilitation in Philadelphia, Pennsylvania; maintains a private practice of medical acupuncture; and is adjunct scholar at the Center of Clinical Epidemiology and Biostatistics at the Perlman School of Medicine at the University of Pennsylvania. He is primarily involved in clinical research related to complementary/alternative medicine. He is a past president of the New York Society of Acupuncture for Physicians and Dentists and the Acupuncture Society of Pennsylvania. He has received an award for acupuncture research and an award for his contribution to acupuncture in Pennsylvania.

Lynn B. Littman, MA, MAc, LAc, DiplAc (Chapter 18) is an acupuncturist in private practice who is licensed in Pennsylvania and nationally board certified in Acupuncture by the National Certification Commission for Acupuncture and Oriental Medicine. She is also a tenured Assistant Professor in the Department of Biology at the Community College of Philadelphia in Pennsylvania. She has earned a master of arts degree in Biology from Temple University, Philadelphia, Pennsylvania and worked as a Clinical Research Administrator on projects in Cardiology, Oncology, Neuroscience, Rheumatology, Infectious Disease, and Women's Health. In 2012, she coauthored *A Short Guide to Peer-Reviewed, Medline-Indexed Journals in Complementary/Alternative Medicine in Holistic Nursing Practice.*

Teresa M. Miller, PT, PhD, GCFP (Chapter 14) is currently an Associate Professor in the Doctor of Physical Therapy (DPT) Program at the State University of New York (SUNY) Downstate Medical Center, Brooklyn, New York. Dr. Miller was initially exposed to the Feldenkrais Method by 2 physical therapy faculty members while completing her bachelors of science in Physical Therapy at Downstate from 1979 to 1981. In 1986, while working at a large teaching hospital, she became part of a physical therapy study group, which included 2 members trained in the Feldenkrais Method who mentored her over the next 9 years—Harold Rosenthal, PT and Steven Frieder, PT, PhD. In 1993, Dr. Miller completed an MS Program in School Psychology at St. John's University, Jamaica, New York and joined the physical therapy faculty at SUNY Downstate. In 1999, she completed the East Coast Feldenkrais Training Program and became Guild Certified in the Feldenkrais Method. In 2007, Dr. Miller completed her PhD in Physical Therapy from Temple University in Philadelphia, Pennsylvania. Her dissertation was on Decision Making Processes of Physical Therapists and Feldenkrais Practitioners. As part of her teaching and clinical practice, Dr. Miller integrates evidence-based practice in physical therapy, neurophysiology, motor control and motor learning, systems theory, mindfulness, visual and motor imagery, and concepts from the Feldenkrais Method. She runs a small private practice on Long Island.

Sangeeta Singg, PhD, ACN (Chapter 16) received her masters of arts in Sociology from Mississippi State University, Stakville Mississippi and masters of science and PhD in Psychology from Texas A & M University—Commerce, Commerce, Texas. Currently a professor of psychology at the Angelo State University, San Angelo, Texas, she started the graduate counseling psychology program and served as Director until 2011. She is a licensed psychologist in the State of Texas and has practiced and taught counseling psychology for over 35 years. She is also certified as an Applied Clinical Nutritionist and a Purification and Weight Loss Coach. Her research interests and publications are in the areas of counseling psychology, student personal responsibility, health psychology, childhood sexual abuse, self-esteem, post-traumatic stress disorder, depression, color preference and color therapy, memory, alternative methods of healing, grief, suicide, and Reiki. She has served as the President of the Psychological Association of Greater West Texas since 2010 and on the Board of Directors of American Heart Association, Tom Green County Division for the last 32 years, 4 of these years as the Board President.

Kerri Sowers, PT, DPT, NCS (Chapter 18) is an Assistant Professor of Health Science at Stockton University in Galloway, New Jersey. She obtained her DPT from Stockton University and is currently working toward her PhD in Physical Therapy at Nova Southeastern University, Fort Lauderdale, Florida. She continues to focus on neurological clinical practice at Atlanticare Regional Medical Center, an acute care setting which is a Level II Trauma Center and Comprehensive Stroke Center. She is a Fédération Equestre Internationale (international level) Classifier for Paraequestrian sport and serves on the United States Equestrian Federation Adaptive Sports Committee. Her research interests are understanding the effect of exercise on stress, fatigue, and quality of life in patients diagnosed with Primary Immunodeficiency Disease, and analysis of balance and movement patterns in paraequestrian athletes.

James Stephens, PT, PhD, GCFP (Chapter 14) was originally trained as a biologist. While earning his PhD in neuroscience, he participated in a workshop with Moshé Feldenkrais that galvanized his interest in pursuing study of this method. With no Feldenkrais training on the horizon, he studied physical therapy at Hahnemann University, Philadelphia, Pennsylvania where he earned a degree in 1983. He earned his Feldenkrais certification in the Toronto (1987) training. Jim worked for 10 years in physical therapy practices at Temple University Hospital, Philadelphia, Pennsylvania and Moss Rehab Hospital in Philadelphia, Pennsylvania. Following that, Jim has worked in outpatient physical therapy settings, done home care, and is currently on the staff of the LIFE program at the University of Pennsylvania, a multi/inter-disciplinary program serving the needs of the frail elderly population of West Philadelphia. Throughout all of his physical therapy practice and settings he has integrated Feldenkrais Method into physical therapy treatment with his patients. He has also maintained a private Feldenkrais practice through to the present time. In 1994, Jim began his academic career as full time faculty in physical therapy programs first at Widener University, Chester, Pennsylvania then at Temple University. During this time, he began a research program investigating outcomes of Feldenkrais interventions with different groups of people. This has so far resulted in more than 50 peer-reviewed papers, journal articles, abstracts, and presentations. Jim is a member of the American Physical Therapy Association neurology and geriatrics sections where he has served as a reviewer. He has served as a mentor for many students and practitioners researching the Feldenkrais Method and is a member of the research committee of the Feldenkrais Educational Foundation of North America (FEFNA). He continues teaching an online course in Motor Learning and Control through the Temple University Physical Therapy program.

Matthew J. Taylor, PT, PhD, RYT (Chapter 13) created Dynamic Systems Rehabilitation of Scottsdale, Arizona. The clinic is based on a fusion of classical yoga therapeutic principles and his doctoral work in modern transformation learning and creativity theory. He is a 1981 United States Army/ Baylor University, San Antonio, Texas graduate. From 1990 to 2003 he owned a private practice with a medically oriented gym that grew from a staff of 2 to 17 over 15 years in a town of 3500 people. His doctoral work investigated a yoga-based back school. He is past president of the board of directors of the International Association of Yoga Therapists and initiated their professional standards process and research conferences. In addition to a busy clinical practice, he leads continuing education workshops for health care and yoga professionals. Widely published on integrative rehabilitation from a clinical perspective, his practice has also been featured numerous times for its integrative organizational model. He recently edited the textbook, *Fostering Creativity In Rehabilitation*. He is also an expert legal witness for yoga injury cases and directs www.smartsafeyoga.com.

FOREWORD

Please join me in congratulating Carol Davis, DPT, EdD, MS, FAPTA on the fourth edition of an impressive tour de force in amassing and culling through the latest scientific evidence for the efficacy of therapeutic modalities, such as T'ai Chi and yoga therapeutics, that were and still are considered by some to be in the realm of pseudoscience. (The scientific community is traditionally a conservative lot—and for good reason, as this attitude keeps us honest and careful about what we claim to be truth in explaining nature). However, the scientific evidence in support of these integrative therapies continues to grow and evolve dynamically in response to advances in knowledge and to the public's frustration with health care practices that tend to overutilize drugs and underutilize skilled, hands-on approaches.

The fourth edition of this text has a subtle yet significant change in title from *Complementary Therapies in Rehabilitation* to *Integrative Therapies in Rehabilitation*. This change in wording reflects a recent paradigm shift in medicine, and parallels the development of major centers and institutes in high-ranking medical schools across the country. Specifically, the healing approaches discussed in the major sections of the fourth edition, including body work, mind/body work, and energy work, are now perceived more as an integral part of the whole body healing process. In fact, the Academic Consortium for Integrative Medicine & Health claims that, "Integrative medicine and health reaffirms the importance of the relationship between the practitioner and patient, focuses on the whole person, is informed by evidence, and makes use of all appropriate therapeutic and lifestyle approaches, health care, and disciplines to achieve optimal health and healing."[1]

While some critics of integrative medicine claim that it has become the currently preferred term for nonscience-based medicine, I applaud Carol Davis and her esteemed group of coauthors for taking one small step forward in this controversial area of health care. May *Integrative Therapies in Rehabilitation* provide impetus for the much-needed health care reform that cuts costs, addresses the tremendous growth in the aging population and the prevalence of chronic disabling conditions, and includes the healing of the whole person in the provision of health and rehabilitative care.

Carolee Winstein, PhD, PT, FAPTA
Professor, Biokinesiology and Physical Therapy
University of Southern California
Los Angeles, California

REFERENCE

1. Introduction. Academic Consortium for Integrative Medicine & Health website. www.imconsortium.org/about/about-us.cfm. Accessed April 21, 2016.

I

Introduction

Introduction to
the Fourth Edition

Carol M. Davis, DPT, EdD, MS, FAPTA

"What? A fourth edition? That's great! Who would have thought?"

I never know quite how to respond to folks who offer this as a compliment that this text, *Complementary Therapies in Rehabilitation*, has survived for this long in a professional world that, in the past, seemed skeptical of any therapies not based on Western science and can be downright hostile about even considering holistic approaches. But the fact remains that, not only are the therapies introduced in this text in the 1998 first edition surviving in rehabilitation, it is difficult to find clinics nowadays that do not integrate holistic therapies with standardized treatments. And to acknowledge this increased acceptance, you will notice a change in the title in this fourth edition from *Complementary Therapies* to *Integrative Therapies*. Approaches that feature elements of mind-body interaction and holistic energy flow, such as T'ai Chi, yoga, Pilates, myofascial release, dry needling, and manual lymph drainage, are now commonly found as a part of many—if not most—rehabilitation programs in the West.

Why is this so? Simply because, as centuries of outcomes reveal, they work. They facilitate the healing process above and beyond strengthening, mobilization, and endurance exercises; and patients are asking for them. The Internet has raised the bar in communicating health outcomes around the world. Thus, more health care curricula are including coursework in these therapies as a part of entry-level education. Text books that stress evidence of efficacy are welcomed as necessary for curriculum objectives. This is such a book.

But more than that, my publisher, my fellow authors, and I hope to inspire scholarly interest in something larger than the concrete world of mechanistic therapies, standard therapies based on Newtonian physics. For holistic integrative therapies introduce the importance of the effects of quantum physics, or the vibration of subtle energy, on cellular response and feelings of well-being. When this happens, our practice takes on a fuller, richer depth of purpose.

Most of us who are clinicians have experiences that we cannot fully describe in Western Newtonian terms. For example, clinical intuition works in ways that defy intellect. Sometimes it seems as if we "take a journey into the invisible" with certain patients, and we come out changed by the impact of this invisible that is upon us.[1] These patients remain in our memories, not simply because something we did contributed to a positive outcome for them. Indeed, often the reverse is

Davis CM.
Integrative Therapies in Rehabilitation: Evidence for Efficacy in Therapy,
Prevention, and Wellness, Fourth Edition (pp 3-4).
© 2017 Taylor & Francis Group.

true. We remember those patients who, in their dying, brought us closer to what it means truly to live a life of meaning. In the words of scientist Stephen Buhner, "Our contact with that meaning, often at crucial times in our lives, teaches us a great deal about what it means to be a human being, gives us hope to go on, and often, more than anything, gives us a deep and abiding sense that we are not alone."[1]

Integrative therapies, therapies that emerge out of recognition of the power and influence of invisible subtle energy on cells, broaden a health care practitioner's options to help restore his or her patients to homeostasis, balance, and healing. Many of these therapies are, as indicated, centuries old.

The effect of subtle energy, or vibration, on cellular response—collagen, nerve, cardiac, DNA—are being investigated by Western science from multiple approaches with very compelling results. This text offers an up-to-date view of the efficacy of many therapies used in rehabilitation today that Western science once ignored and viewed as superficial to standard of care.

Like the editions before it, this fourth edition begins with a review of the latest science designed to shed light on the specific mechanism of action of holistic therapies. With each new edition, chapters—particularly the science chapters—have been updated with more current references and a new chapter (Chapter 4) that explores the latest relevant investigations into how subtle energy is impacting health and healing has been added. As a result of my scholarly work since the publication of the last edition of this text, I have come to realize the central role that the living extracellular fascial matrix has on the spread of subtle energy and, thus, communication to all cells, which is an integral part of each of these holistic therapies. Likewise, as we slowly come to understand that the physics of our body tissue that we learned about in kinesiology class is totally based on solid-state physics, we recognize that the science of biotensegrity, which emphasizes the physics of soft tissue, will rewrite all the kinesiology texts in the near future. There are no solids in our bodies. Even bones are crystallized fascia. "Fascia and the Extracellular Matrix: Latest Science Discoveries That Forecast the Importance of This Tissue to Health and Healing" is the title of the new science chapter of this edition. Further, some chapters have been phased out in this fourth edition, and a new chapter titled "Dry Needling" (Chapter 19) by internationally recognized expert Dr. Jan Dommerholt has been added by reviewer request.

As we enter the second half of this second decade in this new century, it will be interesting to see how this mystery of quantum events, of measuring what we cannot see, unfolds before the publication of the next edition of this text. Surely, we will come to know more about the nature of consciousness and of the importance of intention and beliefs of the therapist and patient on our outcomes. What prevails as ever true is that we cannot stop the forward trajectory of the research into the "touch of the invisible" on all of us.

REFERENCE

1.   Buhner SH. Reclaiming the invisible. *Altern Ther Health Med.* 2007;13(2):16-19.

1

Energy Techniques as a Way of Returning Healing to Health Care

Carol M. Davis, DPT, EdD, MS, FAPTA

Some days, it gets very frustrating for me to treat patients in this new century. Doesn't it for you? I mean, I came into physical therapy in the 1960s to help people with movement problems to heal, to get better. When I first began my career, I loved the challenge of healing each new patient and trying out all of the skills I had learned. I loved finding out that what I had learned actually produced positive outcomes! I spent a lot time with my patients; I helped them to get better, and they thanked me for it! I was very happy and felt fulfilled, and so I thanked them as well! I had found a career that would serve me well and one that I could serve in proudly.

What happened to those days? What happened to health care as the previous century ended and the new one began? Gradually, we were all being asked to see more patients in less time. As proficient as I was with my interviews, treatments, and home programs, I still lagged behind by the end of the day. Very behind. Further, the people in charge expected something different from me than what I was prepared to give. I was called into my superior's office one day and told the following:

> Look, Carol, you're just not carrying your load here. We have a certain amount of units we need to fulfill to break even with the current capitation and reimbursement system, and you've got to be more efficient. We don't want you to give up your wonderful rapport with patients, but just be aware of the time you're spending and speed it up a little. Actually, speed it up a lot. Oh, and remember, get their insurance coverage right away, because if they're Universal, we have to get approval before you even talk to them. So don't waste a session you're not going to get paid for.

The economics of health care had taken over. Service shape shifted into business, and a sea of change overtook my profession. Reluctantly, I seized an opportunity to go back to teaching full-time. I never got the hang of speeding up the process of listening to people's stories. I was not inefficient; in fact, I actually developed clinical mastery over 25 years of practice. However, what was being asked of me, my colleagues, and my students—of all of us—was to stop being health care professionals devoted to being worthy of the trust that people in need placed in us, and to start earning enough money for our practices to stay alive. Meanwhile, while our calling seemed to abandon us, I read in the paper that many of those responsible for reimbursing us for our services were pocketing huge

Davis CM.
Integrative Therapies in Rehabilitation: Evidence for Efficacy in Therapy, Prevention, and Wellness, Fourth Edition (pp 5-12).
© 2017 Taylor & Francis Group.

sums of money (a large share of which was rightfully ours) paid by the public to ensure that the service we provided was adequately reimbursed. This is what was happening during the late 1900s and what is currently happening during the early 21st century.

What exactly are the differences between a professional and a person in business who provides a needed service? Put simply, the hallmark of a profession—whether it's medicine, law, or theology—is to help people solve a particular problem or prevent a problem from happening. We are educated with a body of knowledge and the art of being present with clients and patients with that knowledge, to have the capacity to decide if, indeed, we are qualified to help them. We are trained to listen carefully as the patient describes his or her problem, and then we name or diagnose it. Professionals have what it takes to develop and execute a sufficient and up-to-date treatment plan for the problem with the skills we learned as our craft. We have what it takes to decide how long people should be in our care to experience benefits and to teach them the treatment process so that they can eventually take care of themselves. We have the knowledge and virtue to charge a just and reasonable amount for our services. In other words, our aim in service is not to use our patients for our economic gain, but rather to charge fairly for the service we provide.

This is the foundation of all of the professions—the moral bedrock. Inherent in the description of what we do that distinguishes us from those in business to provide a service are the following 2 factors: the person who comes to us has a problem that he or she cannot seem to solve without our help and the critical element in solving this problem hangs on the relationship we establish with that person as we assist in solving the problem. I maintain that individuals in medicine and health care have allowed every one of those processes to be taken away from us. It feels as if we have given up our power to a different purpose. I believe that that purpose was intended to force us to become more fiscally accountable, as the percentage of the annual gross national product in the United States that was going to health care was curving upward like a hockey stick at the turn of the century. We needed to find a way to reign in the costs.

I am convinced that we have thrown the baby out with the bathwater. In our attempts to control cost, and yet still stay alive as a profession to be able to see patients and help them, we've sold our souls to the unit, to the demand of quantity over quality. How will we ever pull ourselves out of this deep rut in which we find ourselves? How can we get back on track and help the pendulum to swing back to the middle, into balance? No one in health care is happy with the way it is now except for those who are profiting.

How Can We Tip the Pendulum to Swing Back to a Spirit of Healing in Rehabilitation?

There is a real and fundamental need for a shift in health care away from the business emphasis and back to sincere, professional helping and healing. But how can we tip the pendulum so that this shift occurs soon? My belief is that all of us who practice health care can relate to what we call, for want of a safe word, a "sixth sense." You can't practice health care for long without experiencing a kind of clinical intuition that is not seated in our left brains, but rather comes from deep inside of us and very often emerges at the most opportune moments and in a way that we cannot even understand, let alone try to describe to someone else. It's a shared mystery that we all acknowledge, for which we are very grateful but also keep somewhat private. For this is an applied science we practice, and this right-brained intuition is universally seen as nonscientific and certainly not based in fact. Yet most of us who have been around long enough learn to trust it and even find ourselves quieting down and going inside to ask that voice for help, especially when we are stumped with what to do next.

I don't know about you, but sometimes I sure would like to claim that the brilliance that comes from this sixth sense is really mine, but deep in my heart I know that the information of clinical intuition comes from somewhere and something beyond me. Some may claim it as "forgotten knowledge" learned long ago and filed away for just this moment when we need it. But most of us realize that there is a transcendent quality to this awareness and feel humbly grateful for it, for it never leads us astray and we and our patients benefit from it enormously.

While I carefully listen to my patient as he or she tells me his or her story, I realize that the more I am able to move out of my left brain and into a deep listening (even if I only have 10 minutes to listen), the better my response is going to be. In short, I believe that the process of finding our way out of this health care fiasco is through this inner core of our practice. The way out lies not in our rational left brains alone. We can't use logic and rationality alone to figure out how to move our-selves to a new place in our professions. The way out, I maintain, is once again—each and every time—to become present to our patients from our hearts and to emphasize the mind-body connection with each of them. This does not mean that we should ignore the specialized knowledge that we worked so hard to attain. By no means. The storehouse of knowledge remains at the ready for when we need it to make sense out of what we are experiencing. But when we listen solely from our rational left brains and our hearts are not in the listening, our patients feel as if they are being treated like problems, like depersonalized sources of information. When we listen from our hearts as well, we become more efficient and more personally involved. We "get it" sooner, and we recognize what questions we must ask to get the priorities of this particular patient right, to weed out the chaff and focus in on the kernels that will be critical to our being effective. When we practice by incorporating mind and body in our therapy, we stimulate the whole of the patient to be engaged in the healing process. Then health care becomes what it is meant to be—a process of individualized care for the purpose of healing.

I practice outpatient physical therapy, and I have studied a manual complementary therapy known as *myofascial release*, as taught by John F. Barnes, PT, that helps me tremendously when treating musculoskeletal and neuromuscular problems with movement effectively. When I relax and go inside, as I have learned, I believe that I gain access to the universal energy that is all around us. In my mind, I actually picture this source energy that we cannot see flowing into my body through my head and up from the floor through the bottoms of my feet. (Of course, no one can see energy any more than we can see velocity. What we see is the product or the work that the energy does in the form of heat, pressure, or vibration.) I state an inner intention that this healing energy that is available to us all will flow through me and out of my hands and into my patient to release any blockages to flow, to bring about the highest good. I sit at the head of my patient while he or she is lying supine, I place my hands under his or her occiput, and I go inside and just wait. Eventually I will pick up a rhythmic movement under my hands that feels a little like a balloon filling up and then deflating slightly over and over again, approximately 6 or 8 times a minute. This, I've learned, is the cranial rhythm. When I first was invited to experience the cranial rhythm by Barnes in 1989, I doubted that I would feel anything. But when I finally felt it, I experienced a movement different than I'd ever imagined and so I realized that I could not be making this experience up. In other words, when I quieted myself and brought the focus of my attention to down inside my body and let go of my left brain's need to understand this experience, I was able to discern this gentle cyclic rhythm of flow.

After a few minutes, I scan the person's body/mind and I listen to my sixth sense for any information about where to start with my myofascial release that might differ from where my left brain perceived the problems to be while I was previously carrying out my interview, postural, functional, and movement examination.

CASE EXAMPLE

Mrs. R. was an 82-year-old retired social worker who had received physical therapy for the past 10 years for a kyphoscoliosis, osteoporosis, and osteoarthritis. She walked with a rolling walker and a twinkle in her eye. She was very motivated to keep active, as she realized that sitting still would be the death of her. Her kyphosis was measured with my goniometer at a 30-degree angle at its peak at about T5 when she first presented to me. Mrs. R. had lost several inches in height, and her pain ranged between 4 out of 10 (on good days) and 8 out of 10 (on bad days). In spite of this, the patient walked with her walker for 1 hour each day. She came to me because her pain was lingering in the range of 8 out of 10 every day, she felt that her legs were becoming weaker, and it was becoming difficult for her to perform certain tasks around her home, such as doing dishes, taking walks, and cleaning the house. Mrs. R. wondered whether I knew of some exercises that would help strengthen her legs. She had been told that nothing could be done for her kyphosis. She had had a plate inserted at the lumbosacral junction years earlier, followed later with Harrington rod surgery. The rods eventually became too painful to bear, so she had them removed 2 years later. The surgical scar went from her occiput to her sacrum.

I told the patient that I believed that I could help her with exercises for her legs, back, and arms. I thought that I might also be able to help her to straighten up a little more. At least I was willing to see if the total of that kyphotic curve was bony, or if some of it was soft tissue and therefore amenable to release. I was anxious to release the tight anterior fascia around her rectus abdominus, iliopsoas, and diaphragm.

Mrs. R. was a little skeptical at first, but she agreed to let me try. She informed me that she had been a hospital social worker, had been married to a physician, and that her son-in-law was chief of a division at the National Institutes of Health. She also said that no other physical therapist had ever told her about fascia or releases; they simply taught her how to perform a few good exercises and sent her on her way. Now and again, she was able to receive some heat and some paraffin for her arthritis in her hands, but never any releases of any sort.

I completed my examination of her posture and balance, and then I asked her to lie supine on the treatment table with pillows. I sat at her head, and I instructed her to bring her attention to her breathing. As Mrs. R. breathed normally, I asked her to scan her body and tell me what she felt. She said that she felt my hands on her head moving slightly, and that it felt good. She felt nothing else, except for the pain in her back. I moved one hand to her sternum, gently tractioning toward her chin, and I gave traction at the occiput with my other hand for about 5 minutes, achieving some release and lifting. I released her pectorals for another 5 minutes and then went to her diaphragm. As I placed one hand on top of her abdomen just below her rib cage and the other under her back to do a transverse plane release, she said, "Oh, I feel the heat coming out of your hands. It feels like I have a hot pack on." I invited the patient to assist me by maintaining her attention on breathing so that her stomach inflated before her upper chest, and to just relax and stay focused inside her body rather than on her thoughts. I invited her to go on a vacation in her mind. (I find that this helps patients to get out of the left brain "work" mode and get into their bodies.)

Then I released Mrs. R.'s iliopsoas bilaterally, my fingers pressing down gently on that strap muscle that tightens up to keep us forward flexed at the hips, and I asked her to turn over on her stomach. I placed my hands on either side of her kyphotic curve, took the slack out, placed a slight tension toward her pelvic rim, and I just waited. Soon the fascia under my hands began to feel like it was "melting" like soft butter, and a rather dramatic releases began to occur. I followed the release to the fascial barrier as the melting feeling abruptly stopped, and then I patiently waited at the barrier for the next release. Sweat was beading under my eyes and I felt heat under my hands, but I was not working hard. A lot of energy was being released from the fascia around the patient's stuck rib cage. Soon she said, "Oh! I can feel myself getting taller! I'm straightening out under your hands. My feet are moving farther down on the table. I can feel myself letting go and getting taller."

I finished up with some work on Mrs. R.'s cervical area and her thorax in rotation and extension as she sat on the side of the table. Then I gave her some exercises for pelvic mobility, back and shoulder extension, cervical rotation, and straight leg raises with ankle cuff weights. As she stood up at the side of the table she said, "I feel so different. I have never felt like this before after physical therapy. I feel energized, and light and taller." She later declared to everyone in the office while walking out of the treatment room with her walker, "Look at me! Just look at me! I'm taller. I feel like I could walk forever!"

Mrs. R. later told me that the feeling of being taller translated functionally in her daily life to being able to reach items that were placed higher in her kitchen cupboards and to being able to see herself in the mirror. I wanted to take a systematic look at what exactly was happening with Mrs. R. that resulted in outcomes that surprised her so dramatically, so I decided to do a case study with her. My students and I took before and after photos of the patient with my Polaroid grid camera. We also measured her height, her performance on the Timed Up and Go test, her balance standing on one foot, her forward reach, her vital capacity, her pain level, and her quality of life with an instrument called the *36-Item Short Form Health Survey*. After 2 weeks of treatment involving a total of 3 45-minute sessions of myofascial release followed by 15 minutes of exercise, we noted positive changes in most measures. For instance, the patient's pain was reduced to 2 or 3 out of 10, which was very bearable for her. We videotaped an interview with her at the conclusion of 2 weeks, and her report of the improvements she experienced focused on what she felt with the energy work, both during the releases on the treatment table and for up to 48 hours after the releases.

I would have hoped for—even expected—eventual positive changes in most measures with exercise alone, but perhaps not in height and posture. My question was, "What part did the myofascial release (the energy work) play on our positive outcome?" I don't know for sure. Mrs. R. served as her own control, having experienced physical therapy without energy work for years. Were our outcomes simply a result of the positive rapport we developed? I imagine that the way we are with our patients, not just what we do, has a lot to do with our outcomes. I suspect that we will come to discover that even our interactions can, in part, be analyzed to be helpful by way of our positive expectations, our compassion for our patients that may translate into bioenergetic forces that assist with healing. Science is moving rapidly forward in documenting the effects of intention, compassion, and empathy in interpersonal exchanges.

The most dramatic of all of the factors that we tested for change in Mrs. R. was her exit interview, during which she described the effect of the myofascial release on her energy level and her perception of how she felt at home following treatment as compared with years of physical therapy without myofascial release. After 2 to 3 days, gravity would again seem to take over, and she could feel herself shrinking, but her pain level maintained at a 2 to 3 out of 10 and she was able to walk more comfortably and function around her house without having to lie down in the morning and afternoon.

Although Mrs. R. tells quite a dramatic story, her positive outcomes parallel those of all of the patients I have treated with myofascial release in our faculty practice. In fact, at the same time that I was treating Mrs. R., I was also treating another older woman with a remarkably similar kyphoscoliosis who walked with a rolling walker. She had not had the surgeries that Mrs. R. had had, but she had experienced several years of traditional physical therapy. My students and I repeated the single case design with her and got similar results. Once again, as we videotaped her exit interview, she remarked that the differences she felt with physical therapy that included myofascial release was a feeling of being able to stand taller and feeling more energy. Functionally, that meant that she could stand at the sink and wash her dishes without having to lean on her elbows to hold herself up so that she could breathe. This positive effect, again, lasted 2 days or so.

What does this have to do with the crisis in health care, and how we find our way out of this rut we are in?

ENERGY MEDICINE AS A WAY OUT OF THE CRISIS IN HEALTH CARE

I believe that we are all surrounded not just by air, but also by a healing energy field that is available to all of us if we let it in. David Bohm[1] first wrote about this in the 1930s. Science is confirming that people are like crystals, made up of a vibrating matrix of life that is capable of resonating with the energy of the earth, like the crystals in a radio receiver. In his book *Energy Medicine—The Scientific Basis*, James Oschman[2] goes into great detail while describing the properties of the living matrix, and central to the vibrational energetic function in the body/mind is the connective tissue, the fascia. The interface between mind and matter is a topic that is no longer ignored in medical science, and research is revealing the importance of the communication between the electromagnetic field that surrounds us and the cell membrane, the nucleus of the cell, and the DNA within that nucleus.[3] As Barnes[4] wrote in his book on myofascial release, fascia surrounds every cell in the body, extending into each cell, forming a cytoskeleton. It is responsible for our ability to maintain vertical posture in gravity.[5] Fascia determines our shape and architecture, and some believe that it acts as the "copper wire"—the conduction mechanism to transmit bioenergy—the ch'i of our body/minds, the flow that is responsible, in part, for homeostasis, for self regulation, for our ability to stay in remarkable balance, to heal ourselves and maintain our healing state as our natural state.[2,6] Every cell in our body/mind is encased in this conducting tissue made up of collagen, elastin, and a central, more fluid polysaccharide layer. It is more accurate to visualize each cell embedded in the fascia, like shells in the wax of a candle, than it is to visualize fascia simply surrounding each cell. Oschman reported the following[2]:

> ....gravity, pressure, tension, muscle pull, each movement on our bodies causes the crystalline lattice of the connective tissue (fascia) to generate bioelectronic signals that are precisely characteristic of those tensions, compressions and movements. Thus, the connective tissue fabric is a semiconducting communication network that can carry the bioelectronic signals between every part of the body and every other part.

Perhaps the fascia serves as the pathways for body energy, or ch'i. Perhaps the fascia forms the elusive meridians described in traditional Chinese medicine. Western science has been slow to accept the concept of meridians because they cannot be dissected out in cadavers, but neither can a major part of the distal lymphatic system, also responsible for life-sustaining flow. Even though we cannot "see" the air traffic route a plane takes from Miami to Frankfurt, I hope that the captain has filed a flight plan nonetheless, accurately reporting the coordinates he or she intends to take.

The fluid nervous system, described so artfully by Candace Pert in *Molecules of Emotion*,[6] also contributes to this flow of communication. The 3 types of natural chemicals that make up this communication system include the (1) neurotransmitters (serotonin, dopamine, norepinephrine, acetylcholine, histamine, glycine, gamma-aminobutyric acid, and many more), (2) steroids (cortisol, testosterone, estrogen, progesterone), and (3) peptides (the largest category, which regulates life processes with secretions such as insulin and growth hormone, helps to regulate the emotions with the endorphins and includes many other peptides that are not yet named). When we add the flows of nerve stimulation, blood, and lymph to bioenergetic and neurochemical flows, we can begin to see how important "keeping the channels open" is to the healthy functioning of the body/mind. We hypothesize that if fascial restrictions close channels, flow would be interrupted and dysfunction and disease can result. We know that multiple sclerosis results from the interrupted flow of nerve stimuli due to a degeneration of the myelin sheath. Parkinson's disease results from an inadequate amount of, and therefore diminished flow of, dopamine. Immune system functioning is very dependent on the emotions, as is being described by the science of psychoneuroimmunology and psychoendocrineimmunology.[6] Aerobic exercise has been shown to positively effect the secretion of neurotransmitters that help prevent mood disorders and depression.[7] Fascial tightness is responsible for myalgias, diminished lung function, trigger points, carpal tunnel syndrome, and a whole host of musculoskeletal disorders.[5] Envision what would happen if the fascia surrounding the vital organs of the chest or pelvis become tightened. Diminished flow of and to cardiac, lung, gastrointestinal, and pelvic organs would severely disrupt the balance of the body/mind needed for optimum function and could contribute to many of the pain syndromes and organ dysfunction of chronic illness.

What we have yet to learn from science, however, is the exact mechanism of healing action that results from this flow of ch'i, energetic, and chemical communication. We do know the various causes of connective tissue dysfunction: trauma, scarring, infection, dehydration, habitual postures, repetitive motion injuries, and quite possibly the wear and tear of daily life in gravity along with the postures that attend our varying emotions as we struggle through life.

It becomes clear that whatever we can do as health care professionals to assist with energy flow very likely will be facilitative to our goals of treatment, wellness, and prevention, as all of these events are continuous with balance and self-regulation. As manual therapists, what science has demonstrated is that, when we are calm and centered, removed from functioning in our left brains and focusing our attention into our bodies, we can open ourselves up to receive the vibrations from the earth's energy.[2] These electromagnetic signals from the core of the earth are thought to be picked up by the pineal gland and melatonin cells (magnetite-bearing tissue in the brain), conducted over the fascia perineural system throughout our body/mind, amplified somewhere in the body up to 1000 times, and finally projected out through our hands and into the body/minds of our patients.[2] This is termed *Schumann resonance* after the scientist who explored the connection of our brainwaves with the energy of the earth.[8] Through the process of entrainment, the therapist who is calm and centered, intending to bring about the highest good, can transmit this energy to patients, as described by Zimmerman[9] in his studies of therapeutic touch practitioners. If the patient is also in the right state to receive this energy, the entrainment can extend to him or her. How this results in healing is still in question. We believe that the vibration of the energy affects the system positively in 2 ways. With the pressure of our hands in gravity over the fascial tensegrity system, a piezoelectric effect takes place wherein mechanical pressure is converted to chemical energy, and the polysaccharide layer between the collagen and elastin of the fascia changes from a stiffer gel into a more fluid soluble state, "releasing" the structure of the tightened fascia in such a way that results in what may be a more permanent release than what we see with traditional stretching of soft tissue. A tensegrity system, described first by Buckminster Fuller, is characterized by "a continuous network (tendons, ligaments, fascia) supported by a discontinuous set of compressive elements."[2] In his work with tensegrity, Heidemann[10] provides a conceptual link between the structural systems and the energy-information systems described previously. Further, Oschman stated the following[2]:

> The body as a whole and the various parts, including the interiors of all cells and nuclei, can be visualized as tensegrity systems…Mechanical energy flows away from a site of impact through the tensegrous living matrix. The more flexible and balanced the network (the better the tensional integrity), the more readily it absorbs shocks and converts them to information rather than damage.

Flexible and well-organized fascia and myofascial relationships enhance performance and reduce the incidence of injuries.[2]

But the architecture of the fascial matrix in this biotensegrity system turns out to be much more than just a structure that disperses pressure throughout the system. The science of subtle energy is revealing how this piezoelectric structure facilitates the physiological function of electron and photon transfer of information into the cells by way of the biotensegrity cytoskeleton in the exterior of the cells in the fascial matrix, into the interior of the cellular cytoskeleton through the cell membrane. The physiology of this system is yielding critical information in the study of the development of neoplasms.[11]

Even more impressive, the contribution of the tensegrity system to optimum function is, in part, due to the fact that the entire system is a vibratory continuum. When a tendon on a model of the system is plucked, the entire system vibrates. Molecules do not have to be touching to receive the vibratory stimulus from our hands on the surface.

RETURNING HEALING TO HEALTH CARE

If we are all surrounded by a healing energy field as Oschman,[2] and before him physicists such as Bohm,[1] maintained, if we are a living tensegrous system that vibrates continuously, and if we as health professionals have the capacity to assist our patients through energy medicine techniques to maintain the connection with the healing energy surrounding us to prevent the disruption of the flows that ensure self-regulation and the natural state of wellness, then our role as healers becomes clear. The crisis in health care becomes obsolete. What patients require from us is to assist them in opening up to the vibrations, the connections that contribute to energy flow. We do that by including as a part of our treatments complementary and alternative therapies to enhance the flow of ch'i and restore balance and wellness. We also strive to foster relationships with each patient characterized by rapport, empathy, active listening, and a true desire that he or she be able to open up to the energy that is available to him or her to heal him- or herself. Finally, and perhaps most importantly, practitioners must practice those techniques that keep their channels open and flowing as well.

This is the future of health care that restores the healing process to our medical profession. It is not only possible, but probable, that these changes will occur rapidly, for they have already begun. There is good science to support this dream of what can be. Once again, patients will be served by us in ways that make us excited to be involved in the healing process and grateful for each day and each interaction. Vibration is the key phenomenon to watch develop in this new science. We must be aware of the power of our thoughts in vibrating reality to us. The intention of the health care practitioner must be carefully focused on the most optimum outcome available for each patient.

Larry Dossey asked in a 2002 editorial, "Can the thoughts and intentions of health-care professionals affect their patients physically, nonlocally, at a distance? Should they be considered as factors in the therapeutic relationship that develops between a health-care professional and her client?"[12] Indeed, we need not be certified in a complementary therapy to support the holistic healing of our patients. Simply providing quality care with the intention that our patients heal and be able to open up to receive the healing energy vibration that surrounds us all is what is required for the new, healing health care. What a pleasure it will be to practice in the coming years of this century.

REFERENCES

1. Bohm D. *Wholeness and the Implicate Order.* London, United Kingdom: Routledge and Kegan Paul; 1980.
2. Oschman JL. *Energy Medicine: The Scientific Basis.* 2nd ed. New York, New York: Elsevier; 2016.
3. Rosch PJ. Bioelectromagnetic and subtle energy medicine: the interface between mind and matter. *Ann N Y Acad Sci.* 2009;1172:297-311.
4. Barnes JF. *Myofascial Release: The Search for Excellence: A Comprehensive Evaluatory and Treatment Approach.* Paoli, PA: Rehabilitation Services, Inc; 1990.
5. Simons DG, Travell JG, Simons LS. *Myofascial Pain and Dysfunction: The Trigger Point Manual, vol 1.* 2nd ed. Baltimore, MD: Lippincott Williams & Wilkins; 1998.
6. Pert CB. *Molecules of Emotion: Why You Feel the Way You Feel.* New York, NY: Simon & Schuster; 1997
7. LaPerrier A, Antoni M, Fletcher MA, Schneiderman N. Exercise and health maintenance in HIV. In: Galantino ML, ed. *Clinical Assessment and Treatment of HIV/Rehabilitation of a Chronic Illness.* Thorofare, NJ: SLACK Incorporated; 1992: 65-76.
8. Konig HL. ELF and VLF signal properties: physical characteristics. In: Persinger MA, ed. *ELF and VLF Electromagnetic Field Effects.* New York, NY: Plenum Press; 1974: 9-34.
9. Zimmerman J. Laying-on-of-hands healing and therapeutic touch: a testable theory. BEMI currents. *Journal of the Bio-Electro-Magnetic Institute.* 1990;24:8-17.
10. Heidemann SR. A new twist on integrins and the cytoskeleton. *Science.* 1993;260(5111):1080-1081.
11. Tadeo I, Berbegale AP, Escudero LM, Alvaro T, Noguera R. Biotensegrity of the extracellular matrix: physiology dynamic mechanical balance and implications' in oncology and mechanotherapy. *Front Oncol.* 2014;4:39.
12. Dossey L. The dark side of consciousness and the therapeutic relationship. *Altern Ther Health Med.* 2002;8(6):12-16,118-121.

II

The Science That Supports Complementary Therapies

Psychoneuroimmunology
The Bridge to the Coexistence of Two Paradigms

Carol M. Davis, DPT, EdD, MS, FAPTA

In 1971, Wallace and colleagues[1] published the results of research that seemed to point toward a mind-body link and coined the term *relaxation response.*[2] Around the same time, Robert Ader and Nicholas Cohen[3] were researching the phenomenon of anticipatory nausea resulting from the effects of chemotherapy on patients. Ader's patients were becoming sick just thinking about chemotherapy drugs long before taking them. The authors were aware of research published in 1928 that focused on Ivan Pavlov's dogs salivating to the sound of a bell,[4] and that was really all that they were looking for in their current research—a laboratory model to confirm that similar conditioning was what was also happening to their patients. They gave rats cyclophosphamide along with saccharin-sweetened water. Then, when researchers took away the chemotherapy and gave the sweetened water alone, they waited to see whether the rats vomited. When they did, they indeed had their laboratory model of "learning" by conditioning that seemed to be occurring in Ader's patients.

Ader realized, however, that the chemotherapy not only caused nausea in his patients, but also depressed their immune systems, lowering their resistance to infectious disease. What he did not anticipate is that the rats developed nausea and learned by conditioning to depress their immune systems when they were given the sweetened water alone. This biochemical result seemed to provide powerful evidence, using reductionistic research methods, that the mind and the body are not able to be separated.[5] Somehow, the mind, which is still thought to reside in the nervous system, "told" the immune system to become suppressed in the absence of a chemotherapeutic immunosuppressive agent.

Interestingly, Ader and Cohen[3] pointed out that the effects on conditioning were observed and reported as early as 1895 by Mackenzie,[6] who provoked an allergic response in a patient with asthma by showing the patient an artificial rose. Later, Osler repeated this observation. But science had no theory that would substantiate such a response, for the mind "had no influence on the body." Anyone can see, however, how valuable a contribution these authors made to science by publishing their results, no matter what the prevailing theory of science would accept or reject.

Subsequent research over the past 20 years has demonstrated, again with rigorous science, that there is a continuous dialogue between the mind and the nervous and immune systems, suggesting that emotions can affect the immune system in both positive and negative ways. With their results,

Davis CM.
Integrative Therapies in Rehabilitation: Evidence for Efficacy in Therapy,
Prevention, and Wellness, Fourth Edition (pp 15-25).
© 2017 Taylor & Francis Group.

Ader and Cohen[3] coined the term *psychoneuroimmunology* (PNI) to describe a new basic science of mind-body medicine, health care, and research. In this term, *psycho* means from the mind or psyche, *neuro* means via the brain or neurons, and *immunology* means to the immune system.

The following 2 pathways of communication have been identified between the mind and the body: the autonomic nervous system (sympathetic and parasympathetic) and the nonadrenergic noncholinergic nerves. Felten et al[7] maintained that these pathways innervate bone marrow, thymus, spleen, and mucosal surfaces where immune cells develop, mature, and encounter foreign substances. "Each [of the 2 nerve systems] communicates with the immune cells directly through the release of chemical messages which range from adrenaline, noradrenaline, and acetylcholine to small proteins called neuropeptides…and cause an inflammatory or anti-inflammatory effect on the immune system," they wrote.[7]

This foundational challenge to Cartesian separatist thought paved the way for reductionistic methods to be used to verify holistic principles. The beginning of an important bridge was formed, which may span the seemingly uncrossable void to link reductionism and holism into coexistence.

APPLICATION OF PSYCHONEUROIMMUNOLOGY

With regard to the initial studies that tested the application of PNI to patient care, *The New England Journal of Medicine* reported in a 1991 study that rates of both respiratory infection and clinical colds rise in a dose-response manner with the increase in degree of psychological stress.[8] In 1989, David Spiegel, a psychiatrist at Stanford Medical School, and colleagues[9] published their research that concluded that individuals with breast cancer who were randomly placed in weekly support groups lived markedly longer than control patients assigned only to regular care. These studies have been followed by countless more,[3] and now research departments in the nation's major medical centers that are investigating hypotheses based on the science of PNI compete successfully for National Institutes of Health (NIH) grants. Among the most important to rehabilitation is the research that investigates the effects of massage[10] and exercise[11] on the immune systems of those with chronic and fatal diseases, such as HIV and AIDS.

At the encouragement of Thomas Richard Harkin, who served as a United States Senator from Iowa from 1985 to 2015 and in the United States House of Representatives from 1975 to 1985, a congressional mandate created the NIH Office of Alternative Medicine in 1992 to investigate and approve proposals for research on alternative methods of healing. Although roadblocks and criticisms from the prevailing science bias against alternative approaches made the initial 2 years of this office quite difficult,[12] the office finally seems to be establishing itself. Scientists at the NIH did not want to add possible "legitimacy by association" to researchers who had no formal education in reductionistic methods. They felt that practitioners of holistic approaches were using their association with the NIH to promote illegitimate research, but in the end they realized that they had no choice but to accept the congressional mandate.[12] The Office of Alternative Medicine was later renamed to the National Center for Complementary and Alternative Medicine. It is currently known as the National Center for Complementary and Integrative Health.

In spite of the fact that proposals seldom could be reviewed for the usual NIH standards of the quality of the principle investigator's "track record," nor for "scientific merit," in 1996 the office awarded selected research centers a total of $9,744,535 in grant funds. In a rather critical 1996 article from the *New York Times*, the following institutions were listed as recipients[12]:

1. The University of Virginia School of Nursing, Charlottesville, Virginia (use of magnets to relieve pain)

2. Kessler Institute for Rehabilitation, West Orange, New Jersey (use of Chinese herbs with neurological problems including stroke)

3. Columbia University, New York, New York (Chinese medicine and women's health)

4. University of Texas Health Science Center at Houston, Houston, Texas (alternative cancer therapies)

5. Beth Israel Hospital, Boston, Massachusetts (conventional therapy for low back pain vs acupuncture and massage)

6. Minneapolis Medical Research Foundation, Minneapolis, Minnesota (alternative therapies for addiction)

7. Bastyr University, Seattle, Washington (survey of 1500 to 2000 people with AIDS to determine alternative therapy use and results)

8. University of Maryland School of Medicine, Baltimore, Maryland (alternative medicine effects on bone and muscle pain)

9. University of California-Davis, Davis, California (survey alternative practitioners, including Native Americans, on use of therapies to treat patients with asthma)

10. Stanford University, Stanford, California (alternative therapies, such as massage and the use of support groups, to enhance the quality of life of older people)

Interactions between the mind or psyche and the neural and immune systems have been shown to have relevance in a broad range of diseases, such as cancer and arthritis; viral infections, such as HIV; and other autoimmune diseases. However, knowledge of just how these systems interact is still not conclusive.

Perhaps the most monumental breakthrough in science is the research from the Human Genome Project that shattered conventional belief that genes control the majority of cellular function in humans. Genetic determinism has been replaced by the updated knowledge that the power to control our lives and our cellular functions rests in the mind of each person. Our perceptions, our beliefs, and our misperceptions are constantly sending vibrational messages to our cells.[13]

A 1995 *Science & Medicine* article by Black[14] revealed how the brain and the immune system interact via hormones, neurotransmitters, and cytokines traveling through blood and nerves. This bidirectional chemical communication is regulated by corticotropin-releasing factor, which is stimulated by thoughts and emotions or immune activation to affect the hypothalamic-pituitary-adrenal axis. Stress, in particular, compromises immunity. Stressful life events have been linked with susceptibility to infection, reactivation of herpes virus, and cancer and HIV progression. Effects on depression and on other clinical aspects are also under study.[15]

The positive effects of exercise, massage, therapeutic touch, and manual therapies on the immune system securely places both alternative therapies and PNI research in rehabilitation.[10,11] These therapies are listed among the "alternative therapies" in what is commonly referred to as the NIH "Chantilly Report"[15] and are placed in categories as follows:

1. Mind-body interventions: psychotherapy, support groups, meditation, imagery, hypnosis, biofeedback, dance and music therapies, art therapy, prayer, and mental healing

2. Bioelectromagnetic application to medicine:

   a. Thermal applications of nonionizing radiation: radio frequency (RF) hyperthermia, laser and RF surgery, and RF diathermy

   b. Nonthermal applications of nonionizing radiation for bone repair: nerve stimulation and wound healing

3. Alternative systems of medical practice (70% to 90% of all health care worldwide): popular health care, community-based health care, professionalized health care, traditional Asian medicine (including acupuncture, Ayurveda), homeopathy, anthroposophical extended medicine (elements of naturopathy plus homeopathy), and naturopathic medicine

4. Manual healing methods: touch and manipulation, osteopathy, chiropractic, massage therapy, and biofield therapeutics (healing touch, therapeutic touch, and specific human energy nexus therapy)

5. Pharmacological and biological treatments (drugs and vaccines not yet accepted in mainstream medicine): antineoplastons, cartilage products, ethylenediaminetetraacetic acid), immunoaugmentive therapy, 714-X (also known as trimethylbicyclonitramineoheptane chloride), Coley's toxins, MTH-68/H, neural therapy, apitherapy, iscador, and biologically guided chemotherapy

6. Herbal medicine (folk remedies that rely on botanical knowledge of the effects of herbs on the body)[16]

7. Diet and nutrition in the prevention and treatment of chronic disease: perhaps the best-known example is Dean Ornish's program for reversing heart disease that emphasizes nutrition, yoga, meditation, guided imagery or visualization, and exercise

INTEGRATION OF REDUCTIONISM WITH HOLISM

It appears from the most recent literature that holistic practices, reductionistic medicine, and health care finally are coming together. While many holistic practices do lend themselves to verification with reductionistic methods, others clearly do not. Meanwhile, the public and health care professionals are continuing to explore the benefits of complementary and alternative therapies. Most important, because of the reductionistic results revealed by PNI, biomedical research is finding it more difficult to ignore the mind-body connection.

While research is being conducted and these 2 explanatory paradigms struggle to coexist, many nurses and physical and occupational therapists are using various complementary therapies in their practices and are experiencing what they and their patients describe as success, even when traditional approaches, such as exercise and mobilization, have not helped. This text was created to help reveal the variety of efforts in this area. The chapters in this text may make it more difficult for those who would dismiss complementary therapies out-of-hand as nonscientific and not appropriate for professionals to use because the results cannot be duplicated in controlled studies.

The accepted belief among holistic practitioners with regard to interrater reliability is that holistic methods have the intention to affect not just one system, but all body systems, by influencing the patient's vital life force in a positive way through the manipulation of the body's energy system. In spite of numerous studies, the very existence of body energy is still questioned by most reductionists.[17] However, holistic practitioners believe that once the bioelectromagnetic field is altered by one therapist, another therapist with his or her own energy field will not be able to locate the same energy field response from the patient, as it has already been affected by the first researcher.[18]

That does not mean that we should ignore the need to understand and test alternative approaches to help make them complementary in rehabilitation. The most common complaints of those who chose "nonconventional" therapies in a 1993 study by Eisenberg et al[19] were chronic conditions often treated in outpatient physical therapy departments, such as musculoskeletal pain, headache, arthritis, and back pain. Patients also reported insomnia, depression, and anxiety, all of which often accompany chronic musculoskeletal conditions.

Just as Mackenzie[6] reported the inexplicable finding of his patient's allergic response to an artificial rose in 1895, practitioners must continually document and publish systematic observations of methods, clinical decision making, the patient's descriptions of the effects of treatment, and subsequent outcomes when alternative and complementary therapies are used.

PROFESSIONALS BEST SUITED TO TRANSFORM ALTERNATIVE THERAPIES INTO COMPLEMENTARY THERAPIES

Clearly, doctorally and postdoctorally prepared scientists, rehabilitation professionals, psychologists, physicians, and exercise physiologists are the most adequately prepared individuals to conduct the scientific studies that will make the biggest impact in allowing us to offer the greatest number of safe and tested alternatives to the greatest number of patients at the most reasonable cost. We will then be working toward a truly sustainable health care system.[2] However, many postbaccalaureate-prepared health professional clinicians and teachers also have the appropriate educational background suited to conduct systematic studies and tests, to prepare in-depth case studies, and to contribute to a central data bank designed to report the outcomes and adequacy of those therapies not easily explored by controlled reductionist research.

Likewise, most professional-level health practitioners are well educated in the theoretical foundations and the art of treatment, and can rather easily expand their knowledge and art to take alternative therapies and make them complementary for their work. For example, psychologists, art and music therapists, ministers, priests, and rabbis are well-positioned to apply selected appropriate mind-body interventions listed in the NIH Chantilly Report.[15] Physical therapists, occupational therapists, nurses, and massage therapists, are—or should be—well-educated to perform alternative massage methods. As this text illustrates, physical therapists can rather easily extend their traditional education in touch and exercise to incorporate the approaches of therapeutic touch and other touch therapies, such as Jin Shin Do, Rolfing, Qi gong, and the Rosen Method. They often have the interest and desire to complete the years of training required to become certified Feldenkrais and Alexander practitioners. Indeed, many have done this, and many others have completed necessary training to use the Trager approach, T'ai Chi, and so on, in their treatment approach.

Some physical therapists have also extended their professional education to be qualified to conduct research on alternative therapies.[20] For example, Steven Wolf, PhD, PT, FAPTA, from Emory University in Atlanta, Georgia was awarded a National Institute on Aging FICSIT (Frailty and Injuries: Cooperative Studies of Intervention Techniques) grant to study the effects of T'ai Chi on balance in older people.[20] As the authors of this text revealed, even more physical and occupational therapists have studied specific alternative approaches to make them complementary to their practice. Mind-body approaches, such as yoga, T'ai Chi, and those aspects of traditional Chinese medicine, such as acupuncture, acupressure, polarity, reflexology, and Touch for Health, that are proposed to "balance" the vital energy and assist in pain control and in the prevention of disease are all being practiced by physical and occupational therapists.

Exercise, proper diet and nutrition, herbal medicine, and improved medications that mimic the body's own immune system defenses have become the foundation of the treatment plans that turn what once were rapidly fatal diseases, such as AIDS, into chronic diseases with which one can live many years.[11] Physical therapists seem best prepared to prescribe exercise for ill persons whose diseases have affected many systems. In contrast, exercise physiologists and sports medicine personnel have entered the exercise area with an emphasis on exercise prescription for prevention and wellness.

THERAPEUTIC PRESENCE: HOLISTIC PRINCIPLES IN ACTION

Embracing a new theory of care that is diametrically opposed to the system that we are trying to reform carries many risks. For example, believing that all illness is a metaphor and that we are all 100% in control of our health is as absurd as believing that we are passive victims of germs and our genetic heritage and that there is nothing we can do except follow our physician's orders.[21] Even before being validated, even against the advice of some medical scientists, alternative therapies are routinely being integrated with conventional therapies as complementary to facilitate healing, and the valuable aspects of holism cited previously are being applied universally in health care. If people have consistently reported that a treatment is working to help relieve their symptoms over a long period of time, then this outcome measure of personal anecdote should be considered one type of evidence of efficacy, regardless of whether the treatment fits the qualifications of accepted research design.[22]

Just as this text illustrates, based on the teachings of such ancient practices as traditional Chinese and Ayurvedic medicine and on the recordings kept by more recent systems of thought, such as homeopathy and naturopathy, the alternative approaches based on holism are being applied with increasing frequency as complementary to conventional practice.

Holistic Application of Traditional and Complementary Treatments

PNI has helped to show that healing is facilitated not only by the alternative approach itself, but also by way of the principles of therapeutic presence or the holistic nature of how health professionals are with their patients. The characteristics of one who uses oneself as a therapeutic agent with the patient reflect the philosophy of holism.[23] Cancer surgeon and holistic physician Bernie Siegel[24] continually points out just how important the doctor-patient relationship is to one's recovery from cancer.

John Carmody, a marathon athlete recovering from leg surgery for his incurable multiple myeloma, wrote in the journal *Second Opinion*[25] that the first of his 2 postoperative physical therapists responded to his fatigue from surgery and 2 crushed lumbar vertebrae with great insensitivity, saying, "You just have to push through the pain…it's mainly a question of your will to get better." He goes into rather lengthy detail documenting the physical therapist's callousness and indifference to him, not only to his weakness, but also to his fear of never being able to walk again. For example, her response to his request for help in positioning his hands and feet to get up off the bed to use his walker was, "It doesn't matter. Just get on with it. Push off the bed and start walking." Finally, he responded to her continual insinuations that he was a rather clumsy coward with an outburst, an attack on her to "back off," accusing her of patronizing him and showing a severe lack of sympathy for his unique situation as a patient. Carmody was an athlete with pain from his treatment for incurable cancer, but more than that, he was a productive writer and a person able and willing to benefit from needed instruction. Yet, she never seemed to relate to those unique characteristics in him. She treated him as if he were a "thing," a noncompliant complainer.

When this therapist was replaced by a second clinician, Carmody's perceptions of the first therapist's insensitivity and nastiness were confirmed. His second physical therapist acknowledged his pain and instructed him to breathe through it as a way to assist in relaxation and pain control. She took the time to show him where he should place his hands to take his weight as he rose from the bed to begin walking with the walker. She spoke to him gently and encouragingly, and she conveyed optimism, telling him that she knew he could do this, it would just take time. This gentle and personal approach got him over his hopeless hump and soon he progressed, first to using crutches and, eventually, to a welcome discharge home.

As he exercised at home, he heard the voice of his second physical therapist encouraging him and, as he felt stronger, he started swimming and tackled other challenges to increase his strength and function. She had facilitated hope, and he was motivated to recover because she had spoken to him, connected with him in his uniqueness, believed in him, and encouraged him by her very presence.[25] The positive effects of compassion on the patient's healing response illustrate PNI, no matter whether the employed treatment is traditional or complementary.

What are the roots of compassion? What allows some of us to be able to extend ourselves to our fellow humans who happen to be our patients on certain days but not on others? What forces interfere with the capacity to respond to our patients with sympathy or empathy? And why is it important to be able to be therapeutically present? Isn't just satisfying our contract to "teach and fix" enough?[26]

Therapeutic presence is the capacity to, at the very least, sympathize with patients or enter into "fellow feeling" and interact from the space of genuinely shared emotion.[27] This demands that professionals feel with their patients and respond to them in a way that acknowledges the "feeling with"—the interconnection.[28] Biomedical ethicists suggest that our moral obligation as health care professionals mandates that patients, as people, should never feel dehumanized or treated as "things" separate from the human race.[29] According to our codes of ethics and the writings of medical ethicists, we are morally obliged to act in certain ways that reflect what it means to be professional, to respond to fellow human beings who place trust in us because of their vulnerability in times of need.[29,30]

Part of medical and health care education should therefore be devoted to developing self-awareness of the behaviors that we bring with us into our professional education that interfere with communicating interest in and rapport with our patients. These behaviors are based on the appropriate values and attitudes of the mature healing professional so that competent practitioners can know how to display morally responsible caring to patients, even on days when their lives are out of balance and stressful. Patients deserve to be responded to with not only proficient knowledge, but also well-advised care and compassion suited to the uniqueness of each person and his or her problem.[23,29,30]

CROSSING OVER INTO EMPATHY—HOLISTIC INTEGRATION

Therapeutic presence describes a connection with patients that is based on the principles of holism, of interconnectedness, that makes an uncomfortable wall, a separateness, impossible. In contrast to sympathy, empathy is a unique interaction that actually involves the experience of "crossing over" into a "shared moment of meaning" that is deeply felt and makes it impossible not to experience the impact of one's actions on the patient, both negative and positive.[26,31] Anyone, a health care professional or a patient, who has experienced the emotional "at-oneness" felt with the crossing-over moment in empathy, where one is so identified with the other that, for a brief millisecond, you forget that the other is separate from you, has experienced the interconnectedness of holism.[26] Sympathy is not, as many would believe, harmful for patients.[27,28] Indeed, it is encouraging and helpful for patients to feel as if a health care professional has walked with them on their journey for a while and that the feelings shared were more than simply acknowledged, they were "fellow feelings" resulting from a strong bond or connection. Pity is harmful in that it is sympathy with a feeling of being worthier than the person pitied, and so it distances the patient with a "poor you" attitude that again depersonalizes the patient.[26,28]

Therapeutic presence, or using oneself to make a warm and encouraging connection with the patient, is based on the important acknowledgments that the mind and feelings of the patient are inseparably linked with the patient's physical body and that the patient's feelings, emotions, and beliefs are just as critical in his or her recovery as exercise, medications, and rest.[23]

Carmody comments from the patient's perspective[25]:

> [R]easonable patients—the majority—know full well that medicine is fallible, uncertain, and very human. What healers risk in meeting their patients as their equals in humanity is little compared to what they stand to gain. For both the efficacy of their treatments and their growth as human beings, health care professionals will be wise to take down as many barriers as they can, give away as many distancing privileges as possible. [Health professionals] who have been sustaining me are alike in their ability to create a sense of "we." We patients and healers are sharing a joint venture, even a joint (somewhat macabre) adventure. This sharing can make us free. I feel free to ask about any problem and express any emotion, positive or negative. They, I hope, feel free to speak truthfully, to be playful or somber as the moment dictates. In a word, we have all become friends, and also joint apprentices to a basal truth: All of us are simply people. Our lives are short. None of us has ever seen God, let alone been mistaken for God.

This interconnectedness stands in sharp contrast to the rigid boundaries of allopathic medicine where health care workers are taught to work "on" patients. I am not suggesting to dissolve the important boundaries that must exist between patient and therapist to ensure therapeutic objectivity. Many have written on miscommunications that can be harmful to therapist/patient effectiveness when helper/helpee boundaries are ignored.[26] Patients should never feel obligated to help their practitioners, nor, as Carmody felt, should they feel as if their helpers are concerned only with the physical—with their leg, blood count, or urine output.[25] Patients have the right to believe that their health care practitioner is concerned about them as unique human beings with special rights, patients' rights, always acknowledging the inextricable interaction of mind and body. The meaning that a patient attributes to his or her experience of illness or injury has very much to do with his or her history and very personal hopes for the future. To ignore this in patient care is to ignore the uniqueness of the person and risk the necessary cooperation of the patient in the goals that are set for care. To ignore this is to fail to maximize the positive effects of the mind on the body.

Patients need professionals to be clearly worthy of their trust, both in the knowledge and skill they bring to their problem as well as in the relationship that is formed.[30] What Carmody asks for, and what holism suggests, is that the professional recognize the importance of patient autonomy. Autonomy is the moral responsibility that professionals do everything possible so that the patient can remain in charge of his or her own problem. With this in mind, the most relevant perspective, for both patient and professional, is to acknowledge that they both need each other, not only to fulfill their unique missions, but also to grow, develop, and change. In this way, patients take on a more equal status in the interaction, practitioners consult with them at every choice point, and practitioners always follow the moral tenets of informed consent. This important moral attitude serves to lift self-esteem and to help patients to feel autonomous and like adults in a culture that can be very unfamiliar and frightening. This preservation of one's self-esteem can be an important mind-body advantage in the healing process of the patient and in preserving the quality of the moments that practitioners spend with their patients.

APPLYING HOLISTIC PRINCIPLES IN HEALTH CARE

Whether employing traditional or complementary therapies, *The Heart of Healing*[2] suggests that there are several ways in which medicine and health care can change to reflect therapeutic presence, the compassionate use of oneself as a partner to the patient in the process of examination and treatment, which actualizes the finest ideals of holistic practice. What is suggested is that health care should reflect the following changes:

1. *A commitment to treat people, not diseases.* Instead of asking, "What is wrong with this person, and how can it be fixed?" we will ask, "Who is this [unique] person, and how can he or she be helped to achieve maximum health?" Depending on the nature of the problem, once evaluated carefully, patients might be better served by a psychotherapist, a physical therapist, a bodyworker, or biofeedback for chronic headache.

2. *A reassessment of the appropriate use of technology.* Twenty-eight percent of the $70 billion spent by Medicare[2] in 1985 went to people during their last year of life, with 30% of that $70 billion being spent during their last month of life alone.

3. *A new openness to complementary therapies.* The survey published by Eisenberg and associates[19] seemed to show that patients who were educated carefully chose the benefits and risks of trying "nonconventional" therapies. Unfortunately, an editorial published in the same 1993 issue of *The New England Journal of Medicine*[32] deprecated many of the alternative treatments that Americans had chosen. "Many of the relaxation techniques, massage therapies, special diets, and self-help groups could be considered to be lifestyle choices more than therapeutic interventions," the editorial stated. Other therapies were singled out as being "patently unscientific," including chiropractic, herbal medicine, homeopathy, and acupuncture—although the editorial

did grant that such therapies are sometimes recommended by, or even delivered by, physicians.[19] At the very least, since the mid 1980s, research in PNI has strongly concluded that lifestyle choices are therapeutic interventions.

4. *A new view of prevention.* Even though more Americans are exercising and are quitting smoking than ever before, prevention still lags behind in insurance reimbursement and in money for health care. Money for infant, child, and maternal health programs for the poor dropped steadily in the 1980s. This drop in funding has led to higher rates of prematurity and related developmental disorders, such as cerebral palsy and mental retardation. The savings gained in cutting money for prenatal programs is dwarfed by the costs of caring for premature babies.[2]

The new health care system should be directed toward not only preventing disease and integrating alternative approaches that help the body to heal itself, but also preventing social conditions that foster disease and poor health among the whole, the world community.

INTEGRATIVE MEDICINE

No system of medicine or health care has all of the answers. Conventional or Western medicine and health care do some things very well. "But conventional medicine manages crises so well that it tends to treat every condition as if it were a crisis."[33] Andrew Weil,[33] a graduate of Harvard Medical School, has developed a new medical school residency curriculum at the University of Arizona, Tuscon, Arizona that teaches what he terms *integrative medicine*. He maintains that if we would apply allopathic medicine only to crisis cases, then money would be saved and harm would not be done to the body's own ability to heal in the attempt to eliminate symptoms of a disease. He suggests the following[33]:

> Allopathic medicine and health care are appropriate for approximately 10% to 20% of all health problems, and that for the other 80% to 90%, where there is no emergency and where there is no need for strong measures, there is time to experiment with other methods, alternative therapies that are cheaper, safer, and ultimately more effective because they work with the body's healing mechanisms rather than working against them.

Weil's new 2-year fellowship for family and internal medicine physicians has the main goal to "emphasize the body's own healing system and healing potential so that doctors and patients will work from the premise that people can get better, that the body can heal itself, and that we should explore all available methods and ideas out there that can facilitate the process."[33] The fellowship begins with a course in the philosophy of science, "to train doctors to know what science is, what are its appropriate uses, and how to interpret scientific research."[33] The next didactic area of study is the history of medicine, including traditional Chinese and Ayurvedic medicine, placing a great emphasis on mind-body interactions. Fellows will also be instructed on the spirituality of medicine, emphasizing experiences of death and dying, and the birthing process. Finally, they will be required to master the universally useful approaches of interactive guided imagery, successful for stress-related illness, and the techniques of 2 of the following 3 alternative health care systems: (1) osteopathic manipulation, (2) medical acupuncture, and (3) homeopathy.

Eventually, nurses and other practitioners will be invited into the program; the long-term goal is to develop an integrative medical clinic devoted to patient care and research on patient outcomes. Patients will be matched for age and condition, one will be followed by the conventional medical clinic and the other by the integrative medical clinic. In this way, Weil hopes to collect the data that will start to turn around the resistance for funding of alternative therapies and therapy for prevention from insurance agencies and other funding sources. Fellows were accepted in June 1996 at the University of Arizona, Tucson.[33]

Because health care and medicine occupy a central place in our culture, Weil hopes that the changes in the care of people will spill over into other social systems and professions, and that the principles of holism will begin to be viewed as preferable to the current linear and fragmented way in which we interact with one another in society and in the world.[33,34]

CONCLUSION

Healing and medical care were once synonymous in medicine, even in the United States, but are no longer.[2] The focus of medicine and health care in the 20th century has been on correct diagnosis of symptoms and on curing symptoms with the one best "magic bullet" available. High technology and reductionistic science have served us well in crisis medicine and in the cure of infectious disease. As we come to the final years of the 20th century, and to the end of the first millennium of the common era, we may remember that one of the definitions of millennium is "a thousand years of peace and prosperity."[35] Current information, indeed, much more now than the wake-up call of the data from Eisenberg et al's 1993 study,[19] has forecasted that consumers will find a way to be served by a health care system that returns the emphasis of care to the whole body's ability to heal itself, even as they receive the benefits of allopathic medicine.[12] Weil[33] comments that this is one of the true benefits of capitalism. Neither consumers nor providers in business are bound by an ideology. Where the market goes, business goes. And consumers are helping to drive a rapidly changing health care system "market."[33]

What seems necessary is a form of medicine and health care that combines the best of allopathic medical care and holistic treatment. And this moment is being facilitated by the increase in the reporting of rigorous research in holistic and complementary therapies, and the increase in the reporting of meaningful case study research and clinical practice outcomes from those who are recognizing the importance of utilizing holistic practices over the attempts to "fix" people by following the protocols of the randomized trial research route.[36]

This text is offered as support for part of the beginning of this paradigmatic shift. The shift is indeed occurring, with or without cooperation, and it would be in their best interest for health care practitioners, researchers, and teachers to be aware of how this shift is affecting their practice, and what research and credentialing methods are needed to help ensure the safety of patients.

When people are ready to acknowledge that it is far more important to link who we are in health care and what we do with healing and service with doing the good for fellow members of our community rather than with just being part of a business whose job is to correctly diagnose a disease based on symptoms and then treat that disease alone, we will begin moving into our rightful place in society as health care professionals.[2] When medical scientists agree to be flexible about what constitutes acceptable rigor or merit in research and minimize their suspicion of alternative approaches because these approaches appear to allow the body to heal itself by influencing all systems for the good (thus, these approaches fail to fit the criteria of rigorous science),[37] we will see an even greater advancement of a health care system that more adequately meets the needs of citizens at less cost.

What is being asked for—and demanded by many—is health care based on the principles of holism that emphasize healing over curing, and that is safe, that is supported by systematic research whenever possible, and that is less costly and toxic. This new health care will bring to the world the safest, most cost effective, and most flexible system possible both for prevention and healing. What it means to help someone, really help a person, will then become clear to many of us for the first time.

REFERENCES

1. Wallace RK, Benson H, Wilson AF. A wakeful hypometabolic physiologic state. *Am J Physiol.* 1971;221(3):795-799.
2. Institute of Noetic Sciences, Poole W. *The Heart of Healing.* Atlanta, GA: Turner Publications, Inc; 1993.
3. Ader R, Cohen N. The influence of conditioning on immune responses. In: Ader R, Felten DL, Cohen N, eds. *Psychoneuroimmunology.* 2nd ed. San Diego, CA: Academic Press; 1991:611-646.
4. Pavlov IP. *Lectures on Conditioned Reflexes.* New York, NY: Liveright; 1928.
5. Ader R, Cohen N, Felten D. Psychoneuroimmunology: interactions between the nervous system and the immune system. *Lancet.* 1995;345(8942):99-103.

6. Mackenzie JN. The production of so-called "nose cold" by means of an artificial rose. *Am J Med Sci*. 1895;91:45-57.

7. Felten SY, Felten DL, Olschowka JA. Nonadrenergic and peptide innervation of lymphoid organs. *Chem Immunol*. 1992;52:25-48.

8. Cohen S, Tyrrell DA, Smith AP. Psychological stress and susceptibility to the common cold. *N Engl J Med*. 1991;325(9):606-612.

9. Spiegel D, Bloom JR, Kraemer HC, Gotteil E. Effect of psychosocial treatment in survival of patients with metastatic breast cancer. *Lancet*. 1989;2(8668):888-891.

10. Galantino ML, McCormack GL. Pain management. In: Galantino ML. *Clinical Assessment and Treatment of HIV/Rehabilitation of a Chronic Illness*. Thorofare, NJ: SLACK Incorporated; 1992: 104-114.

11. LaPerriere A, Antoni M, Fletcher MA, Schneiderman N. Exercise and health maintenance in HIV. In: Galantino ML. *Clinical Assessment and Treatment of HIV/Rehabilitation of a Chronic Illness*. Thorofare, NJ: SLACK Incorporated; 1992:65-76.

12. Kolata G. In quests outside mainstream, medical projects rewrite the rules. *New York Times National*. 1996; CXLV(50,462):A1,14.

13. Watters E. DNA is not destiny: the new science of epigenetics. *Discover*. http://discovermagazine.com/2006/nov/cover. Published November 22, 2006. Accessed January 25, 2016.

14. Black PH. Psychoneuroimmunology: brain and immunity. *Science & Medicine*. 1995;2(6):16-25.

15. Alternative Medicine: Expanding Medical Horizons. Report to the NIH on Alternative Medical Systems of Practices in the United States. Pittsburgh, PA: US Government Printing Office, Superintendent of Documents; 1992.

16. Benzie IFF, Wachtel-Galor S, eds. *Herbal Medicine: Biomolecular and Clinical Aspects*. 2nd ed. Boca Raton, FL: CRC Press; 2011.

17. Rubik B. Energy medicine and the unifying concept of information. *Altern Ther Health Med*. 1995;1(1):34-39.

18. Hanten WP, Dawson DD, Jwata M, et al. Craniosacral rhythm: examination of interexaminer and intraexaminer reliability of palpation and relationships between the rhythm and cardiac and respiratory rates of the subject and examiner. *Phys Ther*. 1996;76(5):S5.

19. Eisenberg DM, Kessler RC, Foster C, Norlock FE, Calkins DR, Delbanco TL. Unconventional medicine in the United States. Prevalence, costs, and patterns of use. *N Engl J Med*. 1993;328(4):246-252.

20. Reynolds J. Profiles in alternatives. *PT Magazine*. 1994;2(9):52-59.

21. Borysenko J. The best medicine. *New Age Journal*. 1990;47:102-103.

22. Cassidy CM. Social and Cultural factors in medicine. In: Micozzie MC, ed. *Fundamentals of Complementary and Alternative Medicine*. 5th ed. St. Louis, MO: Elsevier Saunders; 2015: 41-67.

23. Davis CM. *Patient Practitioner Interaction: An Experiential Manual for Developing the Art of Health Care*. 2nd ed. Thorofare, NJ: SLACK Incorporated; 1994.

24. Siegel BS. *Love, Medicine & Miracles. Lessons Learned About Self-Healing From a Surgeon's Experience With Exceptional Patients*. New York, NY: Harper & Row; 1986.

25. Carmody J. The case: bad care, good care, and spiritual preservation. *Second Opinion*. 1994;20(1):35-39.

26. Davis CM. What is empathy and can empathy be taught? *Phys Ther*. 1990;70(11):707-715.

27. Schleler M. *The Nature of Sympathy*. Hamden, CT: Anchor Books; 1970.

28. Wyschogrod E. Empathy and sympathy as tactile encounter. *J Med Philos*. 1981;6(1):25-43.

29. May WF. *The Physician as Healer/Images of the Healer in Medical Ethics*. Philadelphia, PA: Westminster Press; 1983.

30. Pellegrino ED. What is a profession? *J Allied Health*. 1983;12(3):168-176.

31. Stein E. *On the Problem of Empathy*. 2nd ed. The Hague, Netherlands: Martinus Nijhoff/Dr. W Junk; 1970.

32. Campion EW. Why unconventional medicine? *N Engl J Med*. 1993;328(4):282-283.

33. Weil A. The body's healing systems/the future of medical education. *J Alt Comp Ther*. 1995;1(1):305-309.

34. Han T. Humanities in medical education: between reduction and integration. *Korean J Med Educ*. 2015;27(3):163-165.

35. *Webster's II/New Riverside Dictionary*. Boston, MA: Houghton Mifflin Co; 1984.

36. van Haselen R. Closing the gap between research and practice: is it the key to increasing the impact of CAM research? *Complement Ther Med*. 2015;23(4):635-636.

37. Harris SR. How should treatments be critiqued for scientific merit? *Phys Ther*. 1996;76(2):175-181.

3

Quantum Physics and Systems Theory
The Science Behind Complementary and Alternative Therapies

Carol M. Davis, DPT, EdD, MS, FAPTA

Complementary and alternative therapies, also referred to as *holistic therapies* or *energy medicine*, are becoming more commonly researched in refereed journals since the establishment of the National Institutes of Health (NIH) National Center for Complementary and Integrative Health (formerly known as the Office of Alternative Medicine and, later, the National Center for Complementary and Alternative Medicine) and its awarding of grants. Few would disagree with the fact that more and more patients and clients are turning to holistic therapies as an adjunct to allopathic therapies. A 1998 *Journal of the American Medical Association* study by Astin[1] reported increased use of alternative therapies because patients felt that this approach to healing was more consistent with their ideas about health and the body. But credible published research on the effectiveness of holistic therapies lags behind public acceptance, largely because these therapies and their mechanisms of action do not lend themselves for study by way of the gold standard of medical research—the randomized controlled trial. As a result, one may hear the opinion that complementary and alternative therapies should not be used because they are not science based, that is, they have not been proven to be effective according to the rules of medical science.

Most assuredly, when we stray from the reductionist model for verifying efficacy, we open ourselves to criticism and accusation of exploitation of patients and unscientific, or even unsafe, practice. This chapter will review the current controversy over the use of complementary and alternative therapies as illustrated in the debate over noncontact therapeutic touch in another 1998 *Journal of the American Medical Association* article.[2] This chapter focuses on an explanation of the scientific theories behind holistic, energy-based therapies, specifically quantum physics and systems theory. Mind/body health central to the function of complementary therapies, will be described through the works of current scientists, and then citations of research that found clinical efficacy of the use of complementary therapies will follow. The chapter concludes with recognizing this paradigm shift in the foundations of medical science, from reductionism to holism, as a vehicle for the possible return of the concept of healing to health care, a service profession that is more commonly referred to now as an industry or business and, as such, has been largely criticized of late to be profit oriented and competitive.

Davis CM.
Integrative Therapies in Rehabilitation: Evidence for Efficacy in Therapy, Prevention, and Wellness, Fourth Edition (pp 27-34).
© 2017 Taylor & Francis Group.

STRUGGLE FOR LEGITIMACY:
THE CONTROVERSIAL THERAPEUTIC TOUCH ARTICLE

In 1998, the American media exploited the controversy over complementary therapies by highlighting the results of a sixth grader's science fair project that was rewritten by her parents and submitted to and subsequently published in the *Journal of the American Medical Association*.[2] The article "launched an assault" on the alternative healing practice of noncontact therapeutic touch (TT).[3] It concluded that the failure of 21 experienced TT practitioners to detect the energy field of the investigator (the sixth grader who hovered her hands over one of the practitioner's hands) must mean that the beneficial claims of TT are groundless, that further professional use of this therapy would be unjustified, and that patients or clients should "refuse to pay" for this therapy. The article was later deemed to have serious methodological flaws.[3,4] Leskowitz[3] published a full analysis of this critique; in summary, judgment surrounding this article was centered on the fact that the journal's peer-review process apparently was altered. Not only was there was no primary physician input, but several methodological flaws were cited. The authors' objectivity should have been questioned by virtue of their membership in the controversial organization, Quackwatch. Further, the article claims logically inconsistent conclusions, and the only logical conclusion that can be drawn from the experimental method was that the purported energy field of the experimenter's hand could not be detected accurately by those sitting behind a screen exposing their hands to the test. No clinical treatments were given; thus, to conclude that TT is an ineffective therapeutic process because a purported mechanism of action was not found to be accurate is a huge leap. For example, aspirin was used for decades successfully, with its mechanism of action only becoming understood in the 1970s. No mention was made of the possible effect of the mother's admitted skepticism on the energy field of the young experimenter. (Ambient electromagnetic fields are thought to be easily inhibited by several factors,[5-7] especially the intention of the participant.) An incomplete statistical analysis was offered (less than 50% of the correct answers were reported, so study results could not have been truly random) and a perfunctory literature review dismissing more than 800 documented studies on TT claiming inadequate validity, but failing to set standards for validity, round out the criticism of this controversial article.[3]

It is becoming clearer that attacks against holistic approaches simply because they do not lend themselves to proof of efficacy by the randomized controlled trial no longer carry blind acceptance from the community of professionals. That is not to say that holistic approaches should be exempt from careful study. The threat of patient exploitation is increased when there are unsubstantiated claims of patient benefit for new therapies; however, most holistic therapies are not new. They have been practiced as mainstream in other parts of the world for centuries and are now making their way into Western medicine as the limitations of traditional health care in the West, especially for those with chronic illnesses and pain, become more frustrating for patients and practitioners alike.

PARADIGM SHIFT: REDUCTIONISM ENHANCED BY HOLISM

Chapter 1 describes the emergence of the science of mind/body medicine and health care, a more holistic view than that of reductionism. In truth, science never stands still. The current perspective that many in Western medical science tenaciously hold onto—the reductionist approach to the search for scientific truth, or cause and effect (instituted in the 17th Century by French philosopher René Descartes and later perfected by the great mathematician Sir Isaac Newton) alone—is inadequate to explain some of the most compelling exceptions to current scientific theory. In the 1600s, science was inhibited by the prevailing view that illness and disease were the result of a capricious and punitive God. In an attempt to perfect the study of cause and effect, Descartes declared that only that which could be perceived (the physical or material) would be studied, and the nonmaterial or ephemeral would fall under the purview of the church. Eventually this view led to the linear reductionistic model of science where that which is being studied is reduced to its smallest unit (ideally a molecule), and the structure that it may influence is reduced to its smallest unit (ideally a single cell type or even a part of the cell, such as a receptor) to try to eliminate the effects on the outcome of the research of interfering variables or chance. Efforts then concentrated on perfecting our ways of perceiving that which exists in solid form, from the microscope and stethoscope to the tremendous advances in medical technology of the 20th century. At the same time, with this linear and reductionistic theoretical framework, there has been an unsuccessful shift toward finding the "magic bullet" to cure disease. The pharmaceutical industry has dominated health care, and its research and development efforts have helped to drive up the cost of health care. With these and other events occurring over the past 20 years, we ended the 20th century with a crisis in health care, with private insurance corporations making major medical care decisions with profit for stock holders and CEOs foremost and managed competition coming under more intense criticism for patient abuse and neglect. The profession of medicine has never been under more intense disfavor.[8]

Studying the macroscopic—the material world only—and ignoring nonmaterial reality, such as motivation, consciousness, and the role of the transcendence or faith in illness, fails to explain the profound effects of the invisible, the nonmaterial, or what we cannot perceive. Important exceptions to theories that lie outside the explanatory power of Newtonian physics currently are accumulating and can no longer be tossed aside as interesting outliers. For example, reports and studies reveal that the spontaneous remission of space-inhabiting tumors,[9] extrasensory perception, clinical intuition,[10] the power of prayer to help people heal,[11] and the impact of loving touch on premature infants[12] are extremely important and relevant examples of events that Newtonian physics and Cartesian logic cannot explain. The search for truth, for plausible explanations of what is happening in these instances recorded in studies of health care and healing, can no longer rely on the validity of the "scientific facts" generated largely by the randomized controlled trial and grounded in traditional Newtonian physics.[13]

HOLISTIC APPROACHES AND BODY ENERGY: THE IMPORTANCE OF FLOW

Holistic approaches, or complementary and alternative therapies, have in common what the World Health Organization refers to as, "...care wherein people are viewed in totality within a wide ecological spectrum and which emphasizes the view that ill health or disease is brought about by an imbalance, or disequilibrium, of a person in his or her total ecological system and not only by the causative agent and pathogenic evolution."[14]

In holistic health, the totality of the person is often referred to as incorporating not just the body, but also the following 4 quadrants of need and function: (1) the physical (body and movement), (2) intellectual (brain and mind), (3) emotional (feelings), and (4) spiritual (desire to know the nature of self, purpose for living, questions relating to the transcendent aspect of life). Complementary and alternative therapies focus on impacting all 4 quadrants of meaning and function and emphasize the scientifically validated link between the mind and body.[5,15-19] In contrast to reducing the variables, or finding the magic bullet, these therapies are administered to impact the whole of the person in an effort to help a client or patient recover from illness and/or injury and stay healthy by facilitating the person's flow of natural energy, or ch'i. Holistic theory, the foundation for medicine and health care practiced in most areas of the world outside of the West, suggests that ch'i is responsible for health and homeostasis when it is free flowing and balanced. In other words, a human's natural state is to be "healed," and the body/mind can, and does, heal itself continuously. The evidence that people heal themselves continually is the foundation of the rationale for the double-blind, placebo-controlled clinical trial. Blocks to a person's ch'i interfere with his or her health and render the body/mind vulnerable to succumbing to pathogens, or biochemical imbalance. These blocks to the flow of natural energy can occur from disruptions in each of the 4 quadrants of need and function. In sum, rather than "fixing" the ill or injured individual, facilitating self-healing is the goal of holistic practice.

CONTROVERSY OF CH'I

The concept of the body emitting an energy (ch'i) has been accepted in traditional Chinese medicine for centuries. In the West, however, it is controversial, in part because it has been impossible to identify the structure of the pathways of the energy flow, referred to as *meridians*. Likewise, it has been difficult to measure "whole-body" energy, in contrast to the measurement of energy produced by the work of various body organs, such as muscle energy (electromyography), cardiac energy (electrocardiogram), and brain energy (electroencephalogram). But the work of Valerie Hunt[20] seems to be moving the scientific community toward the acceptance of recording body energy—or more accurately, the body/mind—in valid and reliable ways. Hunt has succeeded in constructing an experimental environment that successfully filters out interfering energy from the earth's core and surroundings. It is accepted in Western medicine that many lymph channels cannot be isolated, yet the flow of lymph is not questioned. Like airline travel routes that exist on a map but cannot be "seen," meridians have been charted on the map of the human by the Chinese and have been used successfully in the manipulation of body energy using acupuncture and acupressure for the health and healing of people for centuries. Recently, a consensus conference at the NIH on the published research on acupuncture issued a recommendation that body energy, as described in the research as ch'i, be studied more diligently.[21]

SCIENTIFIC FOUNDATIONS OF COMPLEMENTARY THERAPIES

How can clinicians explain the documented positive outcomes and what they observe is happening with patients when holistic therapies are applied? If traditional Newtonian physics fall short in offering theoretical explanations, where can we turn for a more comprehensive approach to the description of reality? The current view is that the results from holistic therapies are more adequately explained by Albert Einstein's quantum physics and by systems theory from the biological sciences.

To explain, one must start with the basic structure of all matter, seen and unseen. Atoms are often referred to as the *building blocks* of all that we know as real. The periodic table of the chemical elements categorizes all discovered atoms according to their atomic weight, or the number of electrons they have revolving around the nucleus. Newtonian physics states that what is real is solid and is made up of atoms joining together to form molecules that, in turn, form solid discrete bits of matter with clearly differentiated boundaries. What is real is thus relegated solely to matter that we can perceive with our senses. But quantum physics, developed by Einstein, Max Planck, Niels Bohr, David Bohm, and others, tells us that just because we cannot perceive a part of all that is real (the nonmaterial, the nonlocal, the invisible) does not mean that it does not exist and is not present, interacting in meaningful ways with what we do perceive.

Atoms make very strange building blocks, for the relative space between the nucleus and the orbiting electrons is very vast. The power of the electron charge seems to make it "feel" very dense. It was the behavior of the electron rather than the entire atom that interested quantum physicists. Einstein, Planck, Bohr, Bohm, and others were interested not just in the atom and molecule, but also in the function of the subatomic particles that make up the atom, specifically of electrons (what their properties were and how electrons interacted to form substances).

Most uniquely, quantum physics takes into account the role of the nonmaterial, especially consciousness, in the physical world.[22] In traditional materialistic theory, the invisible consciousness of the examiner is considered to be separate from any part of what is being examined, whereas in holistic theory, grounded in quantum physics, this separation is not thought to exist. That which is being examined is affected by the examiner in ways that cannot be perceived directly. Foundational to mainstream traditional "objective" science is the theory that the knower and the known are thought to exist in completely separate domains; the boundaries of solid mass clearly separate matter into discrete parts. However, electrons and subatomic particles do not appear to be composed solely of solid matter. Electrons behave as if they are solid particles under certain circumstances, but they disappear into invisible waves under other circumstances. Also, electrons are observed to take instantaneous jumps from one atomic orbit to another in some experiments, with no intervening time and no journey through space—an impossible feat for a solid particle.[23] Quantum physics maintains that the behavior of subatomic particles has everything to do with the qualities of solid matter, as they form the building blocks of matter. However, quantum physics has experimentally shown that there is no such thing as "solid" matter, only what *appears* to be solid based on our brain's interpretation.

The Copenhagen interpretation of quantum physics maintains that there is no such thing as strict causality because precise predictions for individual subatomic particles are impossible. There is no such thing as locality, for once 2 or more subatomic particles have interacted, they are instantaneously connected, even across astronomical distances. Further, what is done to one is immediately reflected in the other, faster than any communication over distance could account for. Finally, if all subatomic particles are connected nonlocally, then any view that holds that particles can be reduced or separated and isolated is untenable.[23] Not all physicists accept the Copenhagen interpretation as valid, but several experiments in the 1980s produced results that confirmed these predictions consistently.[6,24,25]

These results, however, do not invalidate materialism altogether. In the everyday world of macroscopic objects, the mechanistic theories of Newtonian physics are approximately correct, which is why much of health care has been able to rely on it so successfully. At the fundamental, subatomic level, there is a totally different world view that incorporates both macroscopic and microscopic realities, where the traditional laws of space and time do not apply. Many physicists now argue that the nature of reality is that it is composed primarily not of discrete physical particles, but of probability waves that are a function of intelligence alone.[24] Thus, the world is made up of wave/particles, and our brains interpret the vibration of the particles (1044 times/second) as solid, much in the same way that our brains translate 24 still frames/second into the motion of a movie, the individual notes and rests of a symphony into the melody, and the flash of red, blue, and green electrons on a special screen as a moving television picture. From the quantum perspective, the "perception of our brains" creates the sharp edges of the world we see. However, as anyone who is color blind will tell us, we each see the world as it is displayed on our individual retinas and interpreted by our individual perceptions, even though we share common cultural agreements about what constitutes, for example, the green of grass or the blue of sky.

SYSTEMS THEORY

Holistic theory holds that the whole is always more than the sum of its parts. Quantum physics, with its wave/particle nature of electrons, makes this possible. Everything that is known about reality is an inextricable part of a larger system, from the smallest part of the universe, the electrons of the atoms of the DNA of, for example, the mitochondria, which is part of the system of the cell, which is part of the system of the blood, which is part of the circulatory system, which is part of the body/mind of the person, who is part of a family system, which is part of the community, which is located in a city, which is located in a state, which is located in a country, which is located in a hemisphere, which is located in an ecology system on the planet, and the planet is part of the solar system, which is part of the cosmos, and so on. Nothing that is made up of molecules with shared electrons can be isolated from that with which it interrelates. One cannot truly know the nature of water by studying hydrogen or oxygen alone. One must study what happens when the electrons of 2 hydrogen atoms and 1 oxygen atom interrelate, share orbits, and interact with each other to form the larger system of water. To reduce the water to its 1 oxygen atom and then experiment with that oxygen atom and conclude that the outcome of the experiment impacted water would be a false conclusion.

Holism holds that the same is true for humans. We cannot reduce a person to one cell or one system alone, study the impact of a variable on the part of the system, and then truly know how the entire system was affected without collecting data on the outcome to the entire system. This has proven to be too difficult, as there are so many systems and so many variables. Therefore, science has simply adopted reductionism as its best attempt to determine cause and effect, and has acted as if the human can be separated into parts to be studied. The difficulties of this stretch of the imagination can be profoundly experienced, for example, in the various toxic side effects of medications.

Holistic therapies use whatever the human being offers in the moment of therapy as the focus of attention (eg, pain, headache, fascial restrictions, fatigue, malaligned posture). By way of the manipulation of the client's and the practitioner's energy, these therapies attempt to influence the whole of the person by unblocking energy that is blocked or imbalanced and therefore restoring length to soft tissue and homeostasis. For example, the myofascial release practitioner attempts to lengthen tight fascia and balance the craniosacral rhythm, the noncontact therapeutic touch practitioner balances the energy flow around the body, and the Feldenkrais practitioner attempts to help the person analyze and feel alternatives to habitual ways of moving, thus providing a greater choice of efficient posture and movement and opening up the mind to consider movement and position in space in a totally new way. We do not yet know how this takes place nor do we know how to measure the mechanism of action between the practitioner and client or patient. Current science is attempting to craft a new paradigm for energy medicine, in part by measuring the energy output from the hands of healers and describing the effects of that energy[26] through careful examination of what happens to ch'i during the administration of therapy[20] and of the nature of electron interaction and how electrons interrelate with each other.[26-30] The research cited here is just a small portion of what can be found in the literature and is offered as a starting point for the reader who is interested in this area of inquiry.

RESEARCH EVIDENCE

A review of the literature and reading the chapters in this text reveal that there has been a quantum leap in researching the effectiveness of complementary and alternative therapies during the past 15 years. Several universities and health centers are currently competing for funding from the National Center for Complementary and Integrative Health for research on such topics as the efficacy of therapeutic touch and manual therapies, massage, acupuncture, and magnets, to name a few. Psychoneuroimmunology is an established research unit at many medical universities, and the outcomes of this research have dramatically impacted many areas, such as the treatment of patients with AIDS. Substantial bodies of evidence exist, for example, on biofeedback, acupuncture, and the use of botanicals. T'ai Chi as a treatment modality is receiving a lot of attention among those interested in falls prevention.[7] Much of this research is published in European languages, such as French and German, but the August 1999 issue of *Physical Medicine and Rehabilitation Clinics in North America* was devoted to reporting the evidence on the use of holistic therapies.[31] Several other texts have been published,[32-36] including the book *Complementary and Alternative Medicine: An Evidence-Based Approach*,[36] which was written by the former director of the Office of Alternative Medicine and summarizes much of the research up until 1999. Several journals (both peer reviewed and non–peer reviewed) report various levels of research in complementary and alternative therapies, including *Advances in Mind-Body Medicine* (Fetzer Institute), *Subtle Energies & Energy Medicine* (International Society for the Study of Subtle Energies and Energy Medicine), *The Journal of Alternative and Complementary Medicine* (Mary Ann Liebert, Inc, publishers), *Alternative Therapies in Health and Medicine* (Innovision Communications), *Noetic Sciences Review* (Institute for Noetic Sciences), and the *Journal of Consciousness Studies: Controversies in Science & the Humanities* (Imprint Academic of the United Kingdom).

CONCLUSION

This chapter began with the report of a rather contentious episode in the history of the development of medical science wherein a poorly written research article in a major medical journal came up with less than well-founded conclusions criticizing one complementary therapy. Holistic approaches are unique and do not lend themselves to the randomized controlled trial for proof of efficacy. In 1997, the Council on Science and Public Health (formerly known as the Council on Scientific Affairs) of the American Medical Association suggested that "physicians should evaluate the scientific perspectives of unconventional theories for treatment and practice, looking particularly at potential utility, safety, and efficacy of these modalities."[37] Whereas reductionistic theory is based on traditional linear, competitive views of reality that stress exclusion and win-lose strategies, holistic theory is circular and oriented toward inclusion and win-win strategies. Although noncontact therapeutic touch has resulted in positive outcomes for thousands, as documented in the literature, it should not necessarily take the place of traditional forms of therapy, some of which have been shown to be efficacious by traditional science. Nontraditional, holistic therapies are being investigated as they are being practiced, with the hope that once they are shown to be helpful they will be accepted as complementary to traditional forms of therapy. In this way, complementary and alternative therapies will help expand the current medical science paradigm to include the manifestations of quantum physics-energy medicine. Perhaps, then, in the West there can be a return to a focus on what helps patients to heal, rather than on dividing up treatment times into appropriate units for billing purposes and referring to this as "therapy."

Holistic therapies, based on quantum physics and systems theory, emphasize evaluation and treatment of the whole person and application of whatever treatment modalities that help people to return to their natural state of healing, facilitated by enhancing the flow of body energy, or ch'i. Perhaps in the 21st century, observations will be refined to be able to more clearly explain the positive benefits of healing energy, even as it is manifested in careful listening and nurturing touch. For now, one can practice holistically even with empathic listening skills. The growing body of evidence in holistic complementary and alternative therapies represents the growing edge of the science of health care. Further, the subtle but powerful shift to a new paradigm of medical science that incorporates both traditional Newtonian physics and quantum physics will undoubtedly yield rich rewards for patients and practitioners alike. This text is an attempt to help stimulate that positive change.

REFERENCES

1. Astin JA. Why patients use alternative medicine: results of a national study. *JAMA*. 1998;279(19):1548-1553.
2. Rosa L, Rosa E, Sarner L, Barrett S. A close look at therapeutic touch. *JAMA*. 1998;279(13):1005-1010.
3. Leskowitz E. Un-debunking therapeutic touch. *Altern Ther Health Med*. 1998;4(4):101-102.
4. Achterberg J. Clearing the air in the therapeutic touch controversy. *Altern Ther Health Med*. 1998;4(4):100-101.
5. Pert CB. *Molecules of Emotion: Why You Feel the Way You Feel*. New York, NY: Simon & Schuster; 1997.
6. Rarity JG, Tapster PR. Experimental violation of Bell's inequality based on phase and momentum. *Phys Rev Lett*. 1990;64(21):2495.
7. Wolf SL, Barnhart HX, Ellison GL, Coogler CE. The effect of Tai Chi Quan and computerized balance training on postural stability in older subjects. Atlanta FICSIT Group. Frailty and Injuries: Cooperative Studies on Intervention Techniques. *Phys Ther*. 1997;77(4):371-381.
8. Lipton BH, Bhaerman S. *Spontaneous Evolution: Our Positive Future and a Way to Get There From Here*. Carslbad, CA: Hay House, Inc; 2010.
9. Chopra D. *Quantum Healing: Exploring the Frontiers of Mind/Body Medicine*. New York, NY: Bantam Books; 1989.
10. Schulz ML. *Awakening Intuition: Using Your Mind-Body Network for Insight and Healing*. New York, NY: Harmony Books; 1998.
11. Dossey L. *Healing Words: The Power of Prayer and the Practice of Medicine*. San Francisco, CA: HarperCollins; 1993.
12. Field T, Schanberg S, Scafidi F, et al. Tactile/kinesthetic stimulation effects on preterm neonates. *Pediatrics*. 1986;77(5):154-158.

13. Han T. Humanities in medical education: between reduction and integration [article in Korean]. *Korean J Med Educ.* 2015;27(3):163-165.
14. World Health Organization. *Traditional Medicine.* Washington, DC: WHO Publications; 1978.
15. Ader R, Cohen N. The influence of conditioning on immune response. In: Ader R, Felten DL, Cohen N, eds. *Psychoneuroimmunology.* 2nd ed. San Diego, CA: Academic Press; 1991:611.
16. Pert CB, Ruff MR, Weber RJ, Herkenham M. Neuropeptides and their receptors: a psychosomatic network. *J Immunol.* 1985;135(2 Suppl):820s-826s.
17. Pert CB. Healing ourselves and society. Presentation to the Elmwood Symposium (unpublished). Boston, MA; 1989.
18. Pert CB. The wisdom of the receptors: neuropeptides, the emotions, and bodymind. 1986. *Adv Mind Body Med.* 2002;18(1):30-35.
19. Wallace RK, Benson H, Wilson AF. A wakeful hypometabolic physiological state. *Am J Physiol.* 1971;221(3):795-799.
20. Hunt VV. *Infinite Mind: The Science of the Human Vibrations of Consciousness.* Malibu, CA: Malibu Publishing Co; 1989.
21. National Institutes of Health. Acupuncture consensus statement and literature review. *The Integrative Medicine Consult.* 1999;1(3):23.
22. Stapp HP. *Mind, Matter and Quantum Mechanics.* New York, NY: Springer-Verlag Berlin Heidelberg; 1994.
23. Sharman HM. Maharishi Ayurveda. In: Micozzi MS, ed. *Fundamentals of Complementary and Alternative Medicine.* New York, NY: Churchill Livingstone; 1996: 244.
24. Aspect A, Grangier P, Roger G. Experimental tests of realistic local theories via Bell's theorem. *Phys Rev Lett.* 1981;47(7):460.
25. Aspect A. Bell's inequality test: more ideal than ever. *Nature.* 1999;398:188-190.
26. Rubik B. Energy medicine and the unifying concept of information. *Altern Ther Health Med.* 1995;1(1):34-39.
27. de Quincey C. Old roots of a new science: historical review. *Noetic Sciences Review.* 1993;Winter:30.
28. Schwartz GE, Russek LG. Dynamical energy systems and modern physics: fostering the science and spirit of complementary and alternative medicine. *Altern Ther Health Med.* 1997;3(3):46-56.
29. Walleczek J. Bioelectromagnetics and the question of "subtle energies." *Noetic Sciences Review.* 1993;Winter:33.
30. Denner SS. The science of energy therapies and contemplative practice: a conceptual review and the application of zero balancing. *Holist Nurs Pract.* 2009;23(6):315-334.
31. Schulman RA, Cohen AC, Harmon RL. Complementary therapies—physical medicine and rehabilitation. *Phys Med Rehabil Clinics of NA.* 1999;10:3.
32. Davis CM. *Complementary Therapies in Rehabilitation: Holistic Approaches for Prevention and Wellness.* Thorofare NJ: SLACK Incorporated; 1997.
33. Horstman J. *Arthritis Foundation's Guide to Alternative Therapies.* Atlanta, GA: Arthritis Foundation; 1999.
34. Micozzi MS. Characteristics of complementary and alternative medicine. In: MS Micozzi, ed. *Fundamentals of Complementary and Alternative Medicine.* New York, NY: Churchill Livingstone; 1996:5.
35. Micozzi MS, ed. *Current Review of Complementary Medicine.* Philadelphia, PA: Current Medicine Group; 1999.
36. Spencer JW, Jacobs JJ. *Complementary and Alternative Medicine: An Evidence-Based Approach.* St. Louis, MO: Mosby; 1999.
37. Dickey NW. Foreword. In: Spencer JW, Jacobs JJ, eds. *Complementary and Alternative Medicine: An Evidence-Based Approach.* St. Louis, MO: Mosby; 1995.

4

Advances in the Science of Energy Medicine
Vibration, Photons, and the Zero Point Field

Carol M. Davis, DPT, EdD, MS, FAPTA

This is a time of paradox in medical care in that 2 different things can both be true: Medical pharmaceutical and holistic care are both important. Many of us have faced frightening critical illness, either firsthand or through the experience of a loved one, but through the miracles of chemotherapy and/or surgery have survived that life-threatening event and moved on to live healthy lives. We are so grateful for the medical research in cancer and infectious diseases that has allowed loved ones who would have died even just 10 years ago to live. Likewise, more and more people are taking responsibility for their own health by quitting smoking, eating fewer trans fats, and getting more regular exercise. These are wonderful signs indicating that modern medicine is helping us to live in more healthy ways.

It is also true, however, to say that today's health care professionals practice *disease management* more than *health care.* Although many health care insurance plans reimburse for an annual physical examination, it is still far easier to obtain third-party reimbursement for therapy related to treating disease than it is for fostering health and healing.

It is also true that many health professionals are not happy with the way politics and business has co-opted the profession that they spent many years preparing for simply to serve. Service has too often yielded to business and profit, and there is great unhappiness, and a deep desire for meaningful change.

Patients and clients are growing more discontented with a health care system that emphasizes the idea that good health is elusive, not a natural state of balance, and the pathway to long life and happiness lies in pharmacology. Medicine and surgery have both saved lives and also let the public down repeatedly, and thousands of people die each year of the side effects of medication, iatrogenic diseases caught while being hospitalized, and medical malpractice.

With this growing backdrop, as people read and become more informed, they are claiming health as a natural state, realizing that the body/mind is meant to be healthy, and maintaining life-long health involves a process of unifying mind, body, and spirit. Energy medicine practices, or

Davis CM.
Integrative Therapies in Rehabilitation: Evidence for Efficacy in Therapy, Prevention, and Wellness, Fourth Edition (pp 35-42).
© 2017 Taylor & Francis Group.

complementary therapies, are now commonly viewed as healthier alternatives to pharmacology and traditional medicine, particularly for chronic illness.

Yet, medical establishment leaders and government-supported medical researchers are slow to embrace energy-based therapies. Some of the reasons for this are undoubtedly political. Furthermore, the research on energy-based therapies often must wander from the gold-standard randomized controlled trial because energy is a very elusive subject to pin down. Traditional medical science then rejects energy-based therapies as unproven. You can only measure energy by the work it does, indirectly. It does not lend itself to validation and reliability measures that are the hallmark of reductionism. How do you research something that you cannot measure? Many scientists still say that you cannot, so they dismiss bioenergetic therapies and the hypotheses that they are based on as pseudoscience all the while acknowledging the limitations of traditional medicine.

But the train has left the station. People are turning to energy-based therapies over traditional health care in ever-increasing numbers because of their positive effects. And more and more young scientists are publishing their hypotheses about the mechanisms of action of bioenergy therapies, based in an unfolding discovery of quantum physics, the physics of subatomic particles, and how they affect us and the world we live in. We are living in a major paradigm shift regarding our understanding of how the universe really "works" and the reality of what we perceive with our 5 senses.

MYSTERY OF PHOTONS

Quantum physics is a mystery. It is difficult to read and understand, even by the most talented of scientists. Yet we are learning more and more that the mysteries of this world of invisible waves have a major impact on the world we perceive as solid.[1]

Adult learning theory states that adults must be able to integrate new ideas with what they already know if they are going to keep, and use, new information. Information that conflicts sharply with what is already held to be true, and thus forces a reevaluation of the old material, is integrated more slowly. Information that has little conceptual overlap with what is already known is acquired slowly.

Quantum physics asks us to believe in forces that are too small to see, hear, feel, or touch directly, but quantum physicists are, in greater numbers, writing and speaking about how they have determined that our universe really works and how quantum events, particularly the action of subatomic photons (little packets of light) are affecting our body/minds every moment of every day. This new information is difficult to integrate because it diverges sharply with what we believe to be true from what we see and experience in the real world. Yet, science reminds us that the evidence is now incontrovertible that this real world as we know it constitutes only 4% of all that is. Ninety-six percent of all that is is "dark" to us, dark or unseeable energy and matter.[2,3] How do we access it if it is dark? How do we discover what effects this 96% of all that is has on us as human beings and on the world as we know it? That discovery is happening now in wondrous ways as the new science unfolds.

UNFOLDING AWARENESS OF
WHAT CONSTITUTES THE "NEW SCIENCE"

The new science, sometimes referred to as *noetic science*, is becoming more refined as each year passes in this new century. In the first edition of *Complementary Therapies in Rehabilitation*, published in 1997, we presented the science of *psychoneuroimmunology*, or mind/body science, as a key feature of the new science, science that was diverging from traditional Newtonian physics, which emphasized reductionism and the measurement of parts of a whole to determine cause and effect.[4] Spurred on by the outbreak of HIV and the recognition that exercise as a treatment had a measurable positive effect on both body and mind, on both the immune system and on mental state, such as depression, psychoneuroimmunology bridged the body/mind dichotomy that had been practiced in reductionistic science and medicine since the 1600s. With this work and the discoveries of National

Institutes of Health researcher Candace Pert,[5] we recognized that the mind and body are inseparable parts of one whole, the mind is not simply found in the cranium but rather is located throughout the entire body in various communication systems that inform each and every cell of what is happening to the whole, and emotions and thought (ie, activities of the mind) have a direct effect on all of the cells of the body. The details of how that cell-to-cell transmission takes place remained mysterious, but we knew from Pert's work that the molecules of emotion were being transmitted, in part, by endocrine, neurotransmitter and neuropeptide molecules, and perhaps other unknown messengers.

In the second edition of this text, published in 2004, we introduced quantum physics and systems theory as the sciences that offered more of a sound theoretical base to the understanding of what might underlie the mechanism of action of energy-based, holistic complementary therapies. We went into as much detail as we could based on our understanding of the relevance of electron and subatomic particle action to the physiology of mind and body, and the importance of recognizing that the whole is more than the sum of all the parts.

In the third edition of *Complementary Therapies in Rehabilitation*, published in 2009, many more advances were made in bringing the knowledge of how the universe really "works" to the understanding of possible mechanisms of action in health and healing, illness, and disease, and how complementary therapies that impact people in all areas of need and function (physically, intellectually, emotionally, spiritually, and socially) really work.[6] The new science, science that is holistic rather than reductionistic and based on enfolding Newtonian physics into quantum physics, is undergoing a wave of new discoveries that relate directly to the health of people and the health of the earth and the entire universe. Our hypothesis in that edition of the role of photons in contributing to the needed extra energy of the cells has been confirmed by the work of Gerald Pollack at the University of Washington.[7]

So, in this fourth edition, we offer the latest science in each of the chapters, along with an up-to-date review of the latest research on fascia. Biotensegrity and mechanotransduction offer us new insights into how the flow of subatomic particles and vibration (electrons and photons) impact the physiology of our cells on a moment-to-moment basis.

NEW SCIENCE AND HOW IT RELATES TO THE OLD SCIENCE

Cellular biologist Bruce Lipton[8] summarized the path from reductionism to holism in the following way: to understand nature and the human experience, we must transcend the "parts" aspect that was focused upon in reductionism (to understand the whole, divide it into as many small parts as possible, and study all of the parts, thus helping you to understand the whole) and look more toward the integration and coordination of all parts of the universe, both material and immaterial, into a larger whole. This revisioning of conventional science to a new or noetic science will, as Lipton believes, "rescue us from extinction."[8]

Lipton states that conventional or traditional science can be seen as hierarchical, with basic scientific theories supporting or giving foundation to upper level knowledge (Figure 4-1). At the base of all traditional scientific understanding is *mathematics*, the laws of which are absolute, certain, and indisputable. Built upon our understanding of math is *physics* and built upon physics are the laws of *chemistry*. The laws and science of chemistry support the next tier, *biology*, and biology supports the final top layer, *energetic psychology*.

The new science is expanding our understanding on all 5 of these levels. For example, our growing understanding of the laws of mathematics is enhanced by the disciplines of fractal geometry and chaos theory. *Fractal geometry* informs us that all that we can see and know in the physical universe is derived from the integration and interconnectivity of all the parts, often turned back on themselves in common patterns that repeat over and over from the branching of tributaries of a river, to the branching of veins in a leaf, and capillaries in a section of living tissue. Most importantly, in the larger view, cooperation and harmony seem to trump the old dictum of survival of the fittest as the predominant descriptor of how the universe organizes itself. *Chaos theory* proves that ultimately,

Figure 4-1. Traditional scientific understanding.

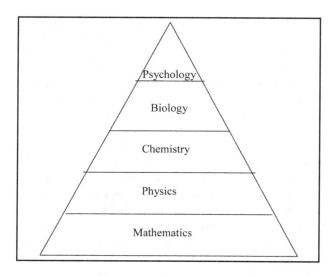

if one waits long enough, there is underlying order in even the most chaotic of events, and, more importantly, small changes have a huge impact in nature when we take a longer, larger view. To prematurely interrupt a process as it unfolds to its order, even for the noblest of reasons, can result in the kind of devastation that we are experiencing in the growing disaster of the warming of the atmosphere, the steady decline in colonies of honeybees, the extinction of so many species of plants and animals that sustain a balanced and ordered planet. We acted as if the earth were a "thing," ours to manipulate for our own advancement, not as if the earth were a balanced living entity that would suffer globally from our manipulations.

The changes in our understanding of *physics* emerge out of our mounting awareness of the nature of mind, or consciousness, as nonlocal. Books on the nature of consciousness, such as *The Law of Attraction: The Basics of the Teachings of Abraham*[9] and *The Secret*,[10] have caught the attention of those who are both excited and terrified to contemplate that we may actually be able to affect, even to create, what happens to us day to day by what we pay attention to, what we think about, and what we observe. Consciousness studies unfold the concept that thought is, indeed, matter in wave form and that the universe is made up of far more than the 4% of matter that we can experience with our 5 senses. People are beginning to consider what Albert Einstein, Max Planck, Niels Bohr, David Bohm, and Werner Heisenberg wrote about in the first half of the 20th century as having practical validity in their lives—that the universe is not a bunch of solid physical parts, but is instead an entanglement of vibrating energy waves, a small portion of which our senses interpret as hard matter, and that the observer of all of this actually creates what is observed out of wave form. Of late, exciting theory has been offered regarding the invisible energy field that surrounds us, and how our interaction with this field at the quantum level affects our health and our vibrational balance.

The third level, *chemistry,* is expanding its theoretical base by focusing on the true nature of solid matter (ie, the atoms that are made up of nuclei and spinning subatomic electrons and other particles, such as photons). These subatomic particles are not solid at all, but rather are made up of vibrating strings or immaterial energy vortices, such as quarks. As such, vibrational chemistry concerns itself with "the role of vibration in creating atomic bonds and driving molecular interactions."[8] We know that chemical reactions that occur regularly in our bodies can be influenced by vibration, be it from free radical action from the food we eat the vibration of our cell phones, or our thoughts. The idea that *how* we think about the food we eat can actually affect how our body digests that food is the stuff of vibrational chemistry.

The new *biology* rejects the theory that, if we fully understand all of the parts, down to the smallest cells, then the whole will be made clear. Noetic biology posits that all that is physical is energetically entangled with and influenced by the vibrational space that surrounds us, the zero point field.

In addition, the new biology endorses James Lovelock's hypothesis that "the Earth and the biosphere represent a single living and breathing entity known as Gaia."[11] Noetic biology also endorses the science of *epigenetics,* the recognition that underlying the genetic code of the DNA is another force that is influenced by vibration, thought, and perception of the environment, among others, and, in fact, vibration actually dictates the "on-off" function of the genes. In other words, perception and consciousness (bioenergetic vibrations) trump genetic determinism.[12]

Finally, *energetic psychology* focuses on the idea that our perceptions control our lives; that the life we experience evolves from the vibration of thought and the meanings we give to our thoughts and perceptions. Physiochemical processes are placed in a wider context of the role of energy fields and how our subconscious gets programmed by our thoughts. The focus then lifts from stopping with a pharmaceutical management of body chemistry and analytical analysis of repeatedly going over "what went wrong in our lives," to teaching people how to evaluate the nature of their thinking, and then, in the moment, choose thoughts that are more resonant with relief, with decreased resistance and with gratitude. The attention shifts from emphasizing the negative to helping people describe and create experiences for themselves and for their children that enhance joy and appreciation. With the choice to change a thought comes a change in the entire body chemistry and mood. Practicing hope and optimism results in a happier, less stressful, and longer life.[13]

BIOENERGETICS: THE NEW SCIENCE OF HEALING

Bioenergetics has been called the "new science of healing."[14] We now know that we are vibrating, bioenergetic beings, but in our mechanistic tradition we have treated illness as a chemical imbalance that is resolved by altering body chemistry to restore balance. As a result, we have searched for remedy almost exclusively in the use of pharmaceuticals to alter natural chemistry, or surgery to repair and replace diseased or damaged "parts" without a diligent effort to understand the concomitant effects of either practice on the whole of us—the physical, intellectual, emotional, and spiritual aspects.

PARADIGM SHIFT: CHEMICAL TO VIBRATIONAL OR BIOENERGETIC

What if all illnesses were perceived not as a chemical imbalance primarily, but as a *vibrational imbalance,* resulting from an alteration in the natural healthy frequency of the vibration of cells that then upsets the chemical balance and harmony in our living systems? How would this change our view of meaningful interventions for pain and illness?

In his 2003 article, James Oschman, both a new scientist and an excellent reviewer of new science, stated the following[15]:

> From observing the successes of many different kinds of energy therapists, I have come to the radical conclusion that there is only one kind of problem that arises in the human body, one way to diagnose that problem, and one way of treating it. The common denominator is energy. All of those conditions we refer to as diseases stem from an energetic imbalance located somewhere in our body. And all of our successful treatments come from correcting that imbalance...The common denominator to all chronic disease is inflammation, caused by free radicals which are fundamentally electronic and energetic in nature.

He continues by saying that energy therapists have one intention—to affect the imbalance in energy, to affect the "local density of electric polarization, and this affects inflammation,"[15] whether by manual therapies, cold laser therapy, or pulsed electromagnetic field therapy.

Inflammation, the production of free radicals, is responsible for the body's ability to heal itself. These unstable molecules lack one or more electrons, and to restore electrical balance the molecule must steal an electron from another molecule, thus destroying bacteria, viruses, and cellular debris. Problems arise when free radicals persist after they have done their clean-up job, turning acute inflammation into chronic disease, and when free radicals attack normal cells, proteins, DNA, and lipids. The body needs an antioxidant defense to scavenge the free radicals and render them harmless, and then to restore damaged molecules.[16-18]

Electromagnetic healing devices, such as low-level laser and pulsed electromagnetic field therapy, introduce electrons into the system, the ultimate antioxidants. And the energy field that is emitted from the hands of skilled holistic manual therapists may be accomplishing the same effect.[15]

POSSIBLE INTERACTION OF THE BODY/MIND WITH THE SURROUNDING ZERO POINT FIELD

Mark Comings,[19] a new science theoretical physicist and engineer, has long been studying the nature of what we know as energy, and how living systems engage with energy. In his 2007 article, Comings suggested the following[19]:

> Nobel Prize physiologist and bio-physicist A.V. Hill, and later, physiologist D.R. Wilkie, proved that the amount of energy that is needed to drive muscle contraction exceeds the amount of energy produced by the mitochondria. Where does that extra energy come from? Researchers do not yet know. One path of discovery would be to investigate other chemical processes within the body that might be contributing to this energy. Another, perhaps "deeper," path would be to ponder the possible contribution of energy from the space that surrounds us, from the quantum vacuum state or the zero point field, that is not a vacuum at all, but is filled with energy.

So-called "empty" space is enormously full of energy. In her 2006 article, Elizabeth Rauscher said, "The actual situation appears to be that the fundamental nature of so-called empty space is enormously energetic. It is, in fact, a very energy dense medium filled with radiant potential to degrees that far exceed, by many orders of magnitude, the energies constituting matter."[20] This subtle energy matrix that surrounds us, which we move about in, much like the water that surrounds swimming fish, influences our physiological and biological systems in ways that are just beginning to be understood. It all has to do with the science of bioenergetics and vibration.

We know that living organisms are literally efflorescing with biophotons that are being understood more and more as being fundamental to their functioning. Even in the darkest of dark environments, living organisms give off light, photons, from within. Comings offers this[19]:

> Looking at life in the context of the "quantum plenum," or energetic space that surrounds us, we can say that because space is also itself radiating an enormously intense flux of vacuum photons, they must be pervading and thus somehow influencing living systems in fundamental ways that are not yet comprehended. Perhaps all this work going on in biophotonics needs to be contextualized within the pre-existing radiant flux of vacuum photons…or what I would prefer to call "plenum photons"…a large flux of which characterize the nature of space at a fundamental level.

We are on the threshold of a quantum shift in understanding how the body/mind interacts with low-frequency electromagnetic activity in the atmosphere, which encompasses everything and may influence how we think and function. Rauscher stated the following[20]:

> I started out as a skeptic about the concept that such low intensity and low frequency fields could affect humans and animals so profoundly. Magnetic and electromagnetic fields emitted from the earth are fundamentally related to life, which evolved on this planet. Certain frequencies affect brain waves of humans, and canines, one of which is one of the main frequencies that is emitted by photon interactions with the upper atmosphere…around 9.4 Hz…the brain wave frequency of a relaxed state of mind.

ROLE OF FASCIA IN QUANTUM COMMUNICATION

Oschman emphasized the importance of the fascia in healthy functioning of the mind/body. He maintained that biological communication systems (nervous system, circulatory system, endocrine system, immune system) do not adequately explain what we observe in outcomes, particularly the speed with which a human can respond to various stimuli. He suggested that there is a high-speed, body-wide energetic communication system that includes not only the nervous, circulatory, and immune systems, but also all of the other systems in the body. In his 2009 article, he called this energetic system the "living matrix" and suggested that it is made up of the crystal lattice of fascial cells that surround each and every cell in the body/mind.[21] Fascia, rather than being an insulator, has been found to be a superconductor of energy.

Oschman views intuition as, "an emergent property of a very sophisticated semiconducting liquid crystal matrix that is capable of storing and processing a vast amount of subliminal or non neural information..." including how to hit a baseball. He maintains that "since research has shown it is impossible to hit a baseball..."[22] that is, because there is just not enough time between the instant a pitcher releases a ball and the moment it crosses the plate for a hitter to spot it, react to it, and swing the bat in time to meet it, some other kind of link between sensation and action must exist. Oschman suggested that this link can be found in the primordial matrix of consciousness within and around cells, the fascial semiconductor matrix. We must rely on intuition to hit the ball.[23]

Consciousness, intuition, a split second response to sensation that exceeds the speed of 20 meters/second of the nervous system, result from subatomic particle communication along the fascial matrix.[22]

From a quantum view of the function of photons in human physiology, it might be suggested that health at a basic, vibrational level results from balance, resonance, and homeostasis perpetuated by the transmission of energy from the DNA by way of invisible photons.[24] Illness then may result from imbalance, loss of communication from the photons, and loss of healthy vibration as a result of blockage in photon communication brought on by blocks in the photon pathways, the fascia.

Fascial restrictions resulting from a solidifying of the ground substance in fascia that is dehydrated has lost the ability to conduct photons because of lack of hydration, much like wood sap dehydrated turns into resin, and resin dehydrated under pressure turns into amber. Manual therapists practicing energy-based myofascial release thus rehydrate the fascia by releasing the restrictions by way of the piezoelectric effect, which normalizes the vibrational communication system and eliminates pain and imbalance as the flattened fascial cells (and the cells that they surround) "plump up" and vibrate for their own healing.[23]

Fascia is the tissue that composes the living crystal matrix that serves as the container of the mind. Pert's research on neuropeptides revealed that the molecules of emotion and their receptors can be found everywhere in the body, on every kind of cell.[5] They are not confined to the nervous system. As mentioned previously, the mind is not in the brain. Mind is a whole-body phenomenon. The subconscious can be found in the entire body. At the moment of physical or emotional impact, energy gets trapped in the fascia which then dehydrates and causes a restriction. Fascial restrictions can be caused by absorption of energy in auto accidents and by absorption of energy in deep fear and grief as a result of scars and inflammation, habitual postures, repetitive motion injuries, and the simple wear and tear of life in gravity over the years. This energy stays trapped in the fascia until it is released by manual energy–based myofascial release. Once the energy is freed from the tissue, other energy-based therapies can assist the healthy vibrational flow, restoring health and healing, reducing pain, restoring balance to all flows: endocrine, breath, blood, lymph, neurotransmitter, neuropeptides, hormone, and steroids.

According to a peer-reviewed journal article on energy medicine[25]:

> A normal cell has an electrical potential of about 90 millivolts. An inflamed cell has a potential of about 120 mv and a cell in a state of degeneration may drop to 30 mv. By entraining the electrical fields of the cells within its range to the magnetic pulses emitted by a pulsed electromagnetic machine, cells can be brought back into a healthy range.

Perhaps one day, instead of relying on pharmaceuticals to change the chemistry in our body-minds for rebalancing, we will find a way to use vibrations that resonate with the natural vibrations of the DNA in our cells, and thus empower our cells to heal. With stem cell transplants and vibrational interventions from devices, such as low-volt laser and pulsed electromagnetic devices, as well as the healing power of bioenergetic transmission from the hands of those therapists whose intention is to boost natural healing energy, we may be able to offer health and healing in ways that minimize negative side effects and return to a more natural state of balance, homeostasis, and self-regulation that is confirmed and supported by the healing energy that is all around us.[25] That is something worth hoping for.

REFERENCES

1. Cifra M, Fields JZ, Ashkan F. Electromagnetic cellular interactions. *Prog Biophys Mol Biol.* 2011;105(3):223-246.
2. Reiss AG, Strolger LG, Tonry J, et al. Type 1a supernova discoveries at z1 from the Hubble Space Telescope: evidence for past deceleration and constraints on dark energy evolution. *Astrophysical Journal.* 2004;607:665-687.
3. Boyd RS. "Dark energy" still baffles astronomers. *Miami Herald.* September 27, 2007:7a.
4. Davis CM. *Complementary Therapies in Rehabilitation: Holistic Approaches for Prevention and Wellness.* Thorofare, NJ: SLACK Incorporated; 1997.
5. Pert CB. *Molecules of Emotion: Why You Feel the Way You Feel.* New York, NY: Simon & Schuster; 1997.
6. Davis CM. *Complementary Therapies in Rehabilitation: Evidence for Efficacy in Therapy, Prevention, and Wellness.* 3rd ed. Thorofare, NJ: SLACK Incorporated; 2009.
7. Pollack EH. *Cells, Gels and the Engines of Life.* Seattle, WA: Ebner & Sons; 2001.
8. Lipton B. Toward a new noetic science: embracing the immaterial universe. *Shift.* 2006;9:8-12.
9. Hicks J, Hicks E. *The Law of Attraction: The Basics of the Teachings of Abraham.* Carlsbad, CA: Hay House; 2006.
10. Byrne R. *The Secret.* New York, NY: Atria Books; 2006.
11. Lovelock J. *The Ages of Gaia: A Biography of Our Living Earth.* New York, NY: WW Norton, 1988.
12. Jaenisch R, Bird A. Epigenetic regulation of gene expression: how the genome integrates intrinsic and environmental signals. *Nat Genet.* 2003;33(Suppl):245-254.
13. Scioli A, Chamberlin CM, Samor CM, et al. A prospective study of hope, optimism and health. *Psychol Rep.* 1997;81(3 Pt 1):723-733.
14. Smith K. Bioenergetics: the new science of healing. *IONS Shift.* 2006;10:11-13,34.
15. Oschman, J. Breakthrough in subtle energies and energy medicine. *Bridges ISSSEEM Magazine.* 2003;14(4):1,5-9.
16. Challem J. *The Inflammation Syndrome: The Complete Nutritional Program to Prevent and Reverse.* Hoboken, NJ: John Wiley & Sons, Inc; 2003.
17. Gallin JI, Snyderman R, Fearon DT, Haynes BF, Nathan C, eds. *Inflammation: Basic Principles and Clinical Correlates.* 3rd ed. Philadelphia, PA: Lippincott Williams and Wilkins; 1999.
18. Ingber DE. Mechanobiology and diseases of mechanotransduction. *Ann Med.* 2003;35(8):564-577.
19. Comings M. The quantum plenum: the hidden key to life, energetics and sentience. *Bridges ISSSEEM Magazine.* 2007;17(1):4-13,20.
20. Rauscher E. Science, mysticism, and the new tomorrow. *Bridges ISSSEEM Magazine.* 2006;17(1):1,14-19.
21. Oschman JL. Charge transfer in the living matrix. *J Bodyw Mov Ther.* 2009;13(3):215-228.
22. Slater-Hammel AT, Stumpner RL. Batting reaction time. *Research Quarterly.* 1950;21:353-356.
23. Oschman JL. The intelligent body. *Bridges, ISSSEEM magazine.* 2005;16(1):11-13.
24. Prasad A, Rossi C, Lamponi S, Pospisal P, Foletti A. New perspective in cell communication: potential role of ultra-weak photon emission. *J Photochem Photobiol B.* 2014;139:47-53.
25. Feinstein D, Eden D. Six pillars of energy medicine: clinical strengths of a complementary paradigm. *Altern Ther Health Med.* 2008;14(1):44-54.

Fascia and the
Extracellular Matrix
Latest Science Discoveries That
Forecast the Importance of
This Tissue to Health and Healing

Carol M. Davis, DPT, EdD, MS, FAPTA

It has been said that science evolves...one death at a time. What is implied here is that new discoveries in science that push up against long-established theories will be, at best, ignored, and, at most, attacked vigorously as lacking merit, and the proponents are often publicly shamed and ostracized. Because it proves challenging to discard theories that deepen our understanding of science, especially those that admit more "outliers" to the accepted explanatory bell curve as more and more members of the scientifically elite die off, new theories start to gain traction and make their way into serious contemplation. In sum, theories that guide our investigations will be expanded and built upon to admit more of the outliers that were previously not able to be explained by the prevailing thought.

Each of the science chapters in this text's first 3 editions have introduced cutting-edge ideas that have not yet become fully embraced by the medical scientific community. This chapter is no exception. It summarizes some of the latest research about the living fascial matrix that exists in human beings. Here is what I have come to realize after 25 years of studying this fascinating tissue: we cannot view what it means to be a functioning human being without a close examination of, and respect for, the tissue that "holds the space" for all the trillions of cells within the fascial matrix, the extracellular environment of all living cells that exists as one continuous tissue from the top of our heads to the bottom of our feet.

We have paid the consequences since the 1600s for our ideas of what it means to be a functioning human being because the only way to discover what was under the skin during the time of René Descartes and Leonardo Da Vinci was to cut open a cadaver, the casing of what once was human, with a knife. Those cuts destroyed the hologram of the living, functioning mass of cells, organs, and tissues that together formed what it meant to be whole, to function in an integrated way as a whole human being. And we adopted the scientific view of *mechanistic reductionism* as a way to understand the parts and how they might all work together. By decree that we could fully understand the function of a human being by examining all of the parts, like a machine, we lost total track of

Davis CM.
Integrative Therapies in Rehabilitation: Evidence for Efficacy in Therapy,
Prevention, and Wellness, Fourth Edition (pp 43-53).
© 2017 Taylor & Francis Group.

the pathway of the force that constitutes the "more" in the more adequate scientific understanding of how systems work, that "the whole is always more than the sum of the parts." That integrated pathway of forces that unite all of the systems to work in harmony is now recognized by many as the living, vibrating fascial matrix.

The science of cellular physiology has long been frozen in an outdated biological model of biochemistry. A more accurate description of cellular dynamics is now known to be grounded in the effects of energy, of subatomic waves or vibrations, and in biochemistry. In other words, the 96% of "all that is" (dark matter and dark energy)[1] has been identified as the foundation of human cellular function, hidden underneath the 4% of tangible matter that biology admits as "real."[1] The 4% of matter that can be appreciated and known with our 5 senses is the materialistic world of Isaac Newton and Descartes. The science of Albert Einstein, Max Planck, and Niels Bohr, the quantum science of subatomic particles and waves, has been influencing our cells from the very origin of life. We simply have not had the tools, nor perhaps the desire, to discover how.[2,3] Human beings are living vibrational translators. Each of our 5 exteroceptive sensors functions by translating sound, light, heat and pressure, odors, and taste into recognizable information. The total of our sensory apparatus is a living translator of vibration, including our proprioceptors, our pressure and pain receptors, arguably even our intuitive sense.[4] Vibrations generate responses along the nervous system and are also transmitted throughout the fascial environment of every cell. The transmission of these subatomic vibrations takes place along with the "flows" of the body (blood, lymph, neurotransmitters, neuropeptides, steroids, hormones, air).[5] Subatomic vibrations of mechanical energy, electrons, and photons effect change as they are transmitted along the cytoskeleton of fascia outside of the cells and within the cells down to the DNA of the nucleus of the cells, directly impacting cellular action.[6,7] These vibrations stimulate the linking of amino acids with functioning proteins and impact chromosomes for the excitation and inhibition of our genes, our DNA.[7] This chapter describes some of what the new science has discovered about the impact of subtle energy or subatomic vibrations on cellular function, and describes what we have discovered about a large component of the pathway of those vibrations—the extracellular matrix, the living, vibrating fascial web.

If they had happened only a few years ago, many of these discoveries would have been viewed as either miraculous or outlandishly untrue. But improved technological measurement and courageous scientists, authors, and publishers have forged ahead to inform us of the discoveries of the way human beings actually function down to the cellular level.

Fascia: What Is It Really?

A common mistaken view of fascia that emerged from cadaver dissection was that fascia is that white cottony, filmy stuff that holds us together, a kind of packing that surrounds the main organs and functional components of the body.[8] It was seen as almost inert, a kind of soft yet tough plastic wrap material to be discarded so that the important "stuff" (ie, nerves, blood vessels, muscles) could be viewed without distortion. Nothing could have been further from the truth, however, as, on closer inspection, all cells are actually embedded within a spider web fascial network, and cells cannot function without their fascial interconnection. A more thorough examination of muscle, for example, reveals that the myofibrils of fascia are critical to the functioning of muscle cells. There is no such thing as a muscle, but rather a myofascial tissue. The same can be said for all cells of the body.[8]

All of our 35 to 100 trillion cells[9] are embedded within the extracellular matrix (ECM) of fascia, and require this environmental matrix to exist and to function. It is fascia that allows the human organism to function as a whole rather than just as a collection of parts.[10] In sum, it might be said that the ECM is to the cells as air is to living beings.

TYPES OF FASCIA

Many texts divide fascia into 3 main categories: (1) superficial (the layer just below the dermis), (2) deep (surrounding and infusing muscle, bone, blood vessels, and organs), and (3) visceral (the deepest and toughest layer, the dura). In 2009, Langevin and Huijing[11] suggested that we be more precise in our description of the fascia, and listed 12 different forms according to function and location. The International Fascia Research Congress, which has been held every 2 years since 2007, has served as transmitters of the latest basic science and clinical research on fascia. Much of that research has been collected in 2 basic texts: *Fascia: The Tensional Network of the Human Body: The Science and Clinical Applications in Manual and Movement Therapy*[12] and *Fascial Dysfunction: Manual Therapy Approaches.*[13]

COMPOSITION OF FASCIA: THE EXTRACELLULAR MATRIX

All fascia, or the ECM, is composed of 4 main components: (1) strong fibers of *collagen*, (2) stretchy *elastin* fibers, (3) various *colloidal gels* or glues (polysaccharide type II gel ground substances), and (4) various concentrations of *water*.[8] Other cells are also present, such as myofibrils in the muscle, glial cells in the brain, and Golgi tendon organs in the tendon, depending on the function of the fascia that is being examined. In addition, there are 12 different types of collagen, depending on the requirement of the tissue. But all of the body's cells are embedded within some form of this ECM, and this environment is absolutely necessary for life. The fascial matrix allows the cells to receive messages, communicate with one another, receive nutrition, excrete waste, and vibrate for optimum function.[14]

Contrary to common belief, the "brain" of the cell is not the nucleus, as was assumed for many years, but the cell membrane, which is the portal between the vital extracellular fascia conduction system and the cytoplasm. Cells can continue to exist and function long after enucleation, but they cannot function without the cellular membrane, the portal for life-giving vibrations.[15]

FASCIA AS A SENSORY ORGAN, AN ORGAN OF COMMUNICATION

The fascial matrix is now known to be one of our richest and arguably the largest of our sensory organs. Fascia contains 10 times more sensory nerve endings than muscle.[16] Our proprioceptors, touch receptors, Golgi tendon organs, Pacini and Ruffini receptors, and free nerve endings all lie within the fascial matrix. Taking all of the nerve endings found in fascia, the amount of sensory receptors may even surpass the receptors of the retina, which is always believed to be the richest sensory organ in the body.[17] Finally, Schleip asserts that, "…fascia provides definitely our most important perceptual organ."[18] Schleip also said that fascia's responsiveness to sensory input may have implications in how fascia responds to various manual therapies that are able to minimize painful fascial restrictions. However, another prevailing view is related to the effects of pressure and shear on the colloidal nature of the tissue and the subsequent alteration in the water content of the ECM.[19]

EXTRACELLULAR MATRIX GROUND SUBSTANCE: KEY TO RELEASING FASCIAL RESTRICTIONS

Fascia at birth is an open-flowing web-like system with no restrictions or areas of dehydration or congealing, no "roping up" of the web strands or plating together of the tissue. However, soon after birth, being exposed to living in the constant pulling down of gravity, the trauma of falling off beds, chairs, tricycles, and slides, and being hit with flying toys and balls will cause fascia to congeal and dehydrate, to toughen up to protect sensitive structures. This dehydration of fascia also occurs as scar tissue accumulates from thwarted inflammation, and from simply not drinking adequate amounts of water. As a result, over the years we begin to develop these interruptions in the beautiful web that we call "fascial restrictions," and we can spot the postural pulls of fascial rope as curvatures of the spine and other postural malalignments. But the structural pulls are only part of the problem. When the ECM congeals and hardens, the embedded cells can no longer respire, communicate, or receive life-giving nutrients. The body loses homeostasis and becomes vulnerable to infection and imbalance of the flows that keep us healthy (breath, blood, endocrine, lymph, digestive, and steroid flows that maintain physical and emotional well-being).

The ground substance gel or "glues" of the ECM have been studied in depth, and they hold key characteristics that facilitate the various important functions that fascia plays, including both structural and vibrational. The gels consist of proteoglycans (PGs) and glycosaminoglycans (GAGs) that have been found to be Type II gels (of 3 types of gel). All gels undergo phase transition, or the ability to change form from solid to liquid to gel. Gelatin is a Type I gel. According to Marsland and Brown,[20] Type I gels, such as gelatin desserts, decrease in volume during setting and become more firm or gelled with cooling. Type II gels (PGs and GAGs of the ground substance) increase in volume during setting and the temperature must increase before it becomes less solid and more gel-like.[21] In other words, pressure on fascia, along with the infrared energy from the hands during manual therapy, will cause the ground substance of a fascial restriction to become less stiff, more in solution. And when shear or stretch accompanies the pressure as in manual therapies, Pollack[22] and Meltzer and Standley[23] have reported that fascial tissue will not only "melt" and stretch out or elongate, but given sufficient time (ie, 3 to 5 minutes) the colloidal nature of the tissue will release electrons and cytokines. These cytokines, or messenger molecules, include interleukin-8 (anti-inflammatory), interleukin-3 (red blood cell formation), and interleukin-1B (nitric oxide or vasodilator).[23] In addition, Fernández-Pérez and associates[24] at the University of Granada, Spain, have documented major immunological modulation with sustained pressure and shear manual therapy, termed *myofascial induction*; this is similar to the sustained myofascial release as taught by John F. Barnes, PT (see Chapter 6 of this book). Increased lymphocyte count was observed at 20 minutes following the application of this style of pressure, shear, and longer length of time (4 to 10 minutes).

ROLE OF WATER IN THE FUNCTION OF THE EXTRACELLULAR MATRIX

Finally, Pollack's work in *Cells, Gels and the Engines of Life* more clearly describes the effect of crystallized water in the ground substance activity.[25] Most people think of water as also able to undergo phase transition from ice to liquid to steam with increasing temperature (as in Type II gels), but Pollack describes a fourth phase of water, crystal water or H_3O_2. Water transforms from H_2O to H_3O_2 when it enters our bodies. Crystals, whether liquid or solid, include properties such as the ability to store energy, transmit energy, and store memory. The crystalline nature of H_3O_2 water adds to the colloidal properties of the ECM, facilitating the matrix as a conductor of electrons and subatomic vibrations or communication signals among all cells. Fascia that has been dehydrated and compressed will rehydrate with pressure and shear, facilitating an in-flow of crystallized water into the tissue and increasing the fluidity of the tissue and the ability to send out messenger molecules.[20,25]

The time factor here is critical for effectiveness in elongating shortened dehydrated fascia or fascial restrictions that, with the strength of 2000 lb/in^2 can cause extreme pressure on pain sensitive structures.[2] Fascial restrictions pull posture critically out of line, generating such pathologies as scoliosis, herniated discs, spinal cysts, osteophytes, osteoarthritic changes, and temporomandibular joint pain. Barnes[26] maintains that most manual therapies do not achieve a maximum effect as they are administered too rapidly, and are injurious to the tissue, causing further inflammation by damaging cellular structures, tearing at the cross links that form in the matrix rather than more gently melting the gel, and facilitating the positive messenger cell action and positive immunological actions.

It is widely accepted that all disease begins with inflammation. The significance of the time factor with manual therapies decreasing the negative effects of inflammation cannot be overstated. James Oschman affirmed the following[27]:

> It is widely accepted that the best prevention [to chronic inflammation in cells] is the regular consumption of antioxidants such as …NSAIDs, vitamins C and E, dietary antioxidants such as turmeric and so on. The most recent research, however, shows that while these molecules are highly effective in vitro, they are much less potent than we would like them to be in the living organism. From what we know about the inflammatory barricade, there is an obvious explanation for this. The inflammatory barrier the body establishes around a site of injury is designed to prevent leakage of free radicals into the surrounding healthy tissues. The barricade also slows the entry of circulating antioxidants. The essential medical issue becomes, "What do we do about this?"

The positive influence from sustained-release myofascial release becomes obvious. Not only is tissue able to be repaired and fascial restrictions reduced, but because of the bioconductivity of the fascial web cells can once again breathe and receive subatomic vibrations necessary to homeostasis, and the body can heal itself. As science progresses, we glimpse a more precise view of how subtle energy impacts cellular function, coursing through the fascial ECM as mechanical pressure, hormones, neurotransmitters, oxygen, nutrients, steroids, and cellular information to each of the cells. Cells require these vibrations for optimum function. And in the words of Harvard vascular biologist Donald Ingber, "…it is becoming increasingly clear that epigenetic factors, particularly mechanical and structural cues that influence cell behavior, have a central role in embryogenesis and tissue physiology, as well as in a wide variety of diseases."[28]

FASCIA AS A CONDUCTOR OF BIOENERGY: THE IMPORTANCE OF BIOTENSEGRITY AND MECHANOTRANSDUCTION

Most current research on fascia steers clear of the implications of fascia as a semiconductor of subatomic vibrations at quantum speed from cell to cell. Oschman has said, "To leave energetic considerations out of medicine is to leave life out of medicine."[10]

Our bodies and our cells are structurally constructed as tensegrity systems, an architectural system where bones float in a fascial network of balanced tension, which serve 2 critical purposes. First, biotensegrity systems are able to withstand and transmit forces throughout the fascial web, minimizing damage to the whole. Second, the tensegrity systems also act as subatomic superconductors, facilitating the flow of the vibrational energy, information, throughout the entire body, penetrating the cell membrane and flowing into the cytoplasm and nucleus of the cell. Perhaps the most wellknown tensegrity system is Buckminster Fuller's geodesic dome, a structure of continuous flexible material or wires intersecting a discontinuous set of more solid compression elements or struts.[29] It turns out that on the macro level, the entire body structures of most living things, for example, mammals, are composed of tensegrity systems where the bones form the discontinuous struts and the tendons and ligaments act as a continuous tensional system.[2] This system explains how the bodies of living things can absorb impacts without major damage, as the energetic forces are dispersed throughout the system within the ECM. Mechanical energy moves away from the point of impact. The more flexible the fascial matrix is, the more efficiently the body disperses this energy. However, the current understanding is that this energy, with perhaps associated emotions, is captured within the tissue that is designed to support and protect, and can develop into pockets of fascial restrictions dehydrating the ECM, causing pressure and pain. Until these energy "cysts" are located and released, often with accompanying emotions, they become layered and roped over time, and can pull on solid structures, such as bones and vertebral discs, and generate severe pain syndromes that are diagnosed as herniated discs, ovarian cysts, fibroid tumors, and even neoplasms.[26,30]

BIOTENSEGRITY STRUCTURES EXTEND INTO THE CELL NUCLEUS

The biotensegrity system does not end outside the cell membrane. Within each cell is a cytoskeleton composed of filaments, tubes, and fibers that serves not only as a structural support for the cell, but also as a conduction system of vibration for communication from the ECM, through the cell membrane by way of integrins, into the cytoplasm and into the nucleus down to the actual DNA of the genes and chromosomes of the cell, directly impacting cellular function. This cellular cytoskeleton "presents as a 3D meshwork of protein filaments that are submerged in the liquid phase of the cytosol. The main components of the submembrane cytoskeleton…are the actin filaments and the protein crosslinking them…[A]ctin-binding proteins act in the role of links and control the organization of actin into a structure resembling a network gel."[31] In other words, this intercellular cytoskeleton web structure strongly resembles the living fascial matrix web outside the cell, but its components are not the components of fascia (ie, collagen, elastin, Type II gel) but are actually composed of protein and actin filaments. Thus, we have 2 webs of biotensegrity tissue intricately linked and immaculately designed for protection and for the flow of vital elements and information for optimum physiological function and homeostasis.

BIOCOMMUNICATION FUNCTION OF THE CYTOSKELETON OUTSIDE AND INSIDE THE CELL

Cellular mechanotransduction is the mechanism whereby cells convert mechanical signals into biochemical responses. Several elements have been shown to play a critical part in this process. Again, in the words of Donald Ingber[30]:

> Analysis of cellular mechanotransduction…has focused on identification of critical mechanosensitive molecules and cellular components. Stretch-activated ion channels, caveolae, integrins, cadherins, growth factor receptors, myosin motors, cytoskeletal filaments, nuclei, extracellular matrix, and numerous other structures and signaling molecules have all been shown to contribute to the mechanotransduction response.

As the ligand, or mechanical force signal, flows through the ECM, thousands of signal receivers on the cell membrane vibrationally "tune" to receive stimuli.[5] As the stimulus and receptor tune to each other, much like a tuning fork, transmembrane-linking molecules called *integrins* funnel the signal into the cytoplasm where it is received and acted upon to produce amino acid chains for function. If the amino acid is not available, the signal is transmitted into the nucleus where it stimulates messenger RNA to be copied from the double helix DNA, which migrates out into the cytoplasm to construct the amino acid chain for function.[15]

This discovery has tremendous implications. The biotensegrity system composed of the colloidal ECM of fascia in combination with the cytoskeleton actually transmits the mechanical energy of the pressure of a manual therapist's hands throughout the web that extends down into the body, into the nucleus of the cell. Cellular biology and epigenetics have shown that the common belief that the boundaries between skin, cellular environment, cell interior, and nucleus with genetic material are separate and impermeable and can no longer be perpetuated. Thus, any person who manually touches the skin of a living being comes in contact with a continuous interconnected fascial web and cytoskeleton of tissue that extends into the nucleus of the cell down to the actual genes. Oschman puts it this way: "…when you touch a human body, you are touching a continuously interconnected system, composed of virtually all of the molecules in the body, linked together in an intricate web work."[2(p.48)]

The crystalline lattice of the fascial web generates bioelectronic signals in response to mechanical forces throughout the body. This intricate system of the whole is designed to facilitate cellular homeostasis through physiological integration. Communication within living systems takes place by way of both chemical and bioenergetic languages. Communication can no longer be understood as a function of the nervous system and the neurotransmitters alone. This living system enables every cell to receive instantaneous information on the activities of all other cells in every part of the body. Unlike nerves, only the fascial web is in contact with all cells of the body. Biochemistry charts reactions that take place within solution. With the discovery of biotensegrity and the cytoskeleton, solid-state biochemistry has advanced. There are messages that travel through the matrix and messages that travel in the matrix itself, as by electronic conduction of vibration of subatomic particle.[32] The process of piezoelectricity, or flow of electrons from mechanical pressure in the biotensegrity system, is largely responsible for this communication.[32]

THE BODY'S ENERGIES

When scientific discoveries are made that cannot be linked logically to existing theory, very often these hypotheses are discarded. The concept of body energy has been well established since the early 1900s when it was discovered that various cells and organs emit an energy field that can be measured on the skin, such as cardiac (electrocardiogram), muscle (electromyography), and brain (electroencephalogram) energies. Concepts of life energy flow and healing energy vibration have surfaced from time to time and have been discarded as impossible.[32] Now, however, technology is advancing to the point where we can actually measure energy flow and identify the effects of energy on cells and on the genes within cells.[7]

Feinstein and Eden[33] hypothesize that several energy fields work together in governing fundamental biological processes. They maintain that the types of energy most pertinent to the function of the human organism include (1) *electrical energies*, (2) *electromagnetic energies*, and (3) *subtle energies*.

Electrical energy is the moving of electrons and protons. Each cell in the body has an outer positive electrical charge and a negative inner charge, which oscillate in the process of membrane exchange. Neurological impulses move along nerve cells with this energy, and it is a comparatively slow-moving energy flow. Likewise, the mechanical energy that moves with pressure in the surface of the body by way of the piezoelectric effect throughout the biotensegrity system is an example of electrical energy flow.

Electromagnetic energy waves fall along a spectrum that extends from radio waves, to microwaves, to infrared light, to visible light, to ultraviolet light, to x-rays, to gamma rays. Electromagnetic energy travels in waves (eg, light from the sun, infrared energy from a person's hands) but is absorbed by matter as a photon particle. Feinstein and Eden,[33] Oschman,[2] and many others now suggest that the energy field surrounding the body, first identified by Harold Burr[34] at Yale in the 1930s, is an *electromagnetic biofield,* which coordinates the various chemical actions of the body's trillions of cells as "decisively as a magnetic field aligns metal filings." The biochemical paradigm is simply too slow to be effective in this coordination across the entire body. This biofield of electromagnetic energy is hypothesized to hold a blueprint for the healthy functioning of all the cells where biological information is "'broadcast' to genes, neurons and other governing mechanisms."[40(p.45)] Feinstein and Eden discuss cellular biologist Bruce Lipton's work[15] in the following passage[34]:

> Hundreds upon hundreds of scientific studies over the past 50 years have revealed that "every facet of biological regulation" is profoundly affected by "invisible forces" of the electromagnetic spectrum. He explains that specific patterns of "electromagnetic radiation" regulate DNA, RNA, and protein synthesis, alter protein shape and function, and control gene regulation, cell division, cell differentiation, morphogenesis (the process by which cells assemble into organs and tissues), hormone secretion, nerve growth and function, "essentially the fundamental processes that contribute to the unfolding of life." But, he

laments, "though these research studies have been published in some of the most respected mainstream biomedical journals, their revolutionary findings have not been incorporated into our medical school curricula."

Subtle energies cannot be detected directly, but their effects can be measured. These energies are vibrational and flow within the living fascial matrix as the energies of memory, feelings, and thoughts.[35] Science has the technology to measure the influence of thoughts on genetic expression, and the influence of meditation on the growth and length of the telomere of the genes in the DNA.[32]

EFFECTS OF SUBTLE ENERGY AND ELECTROMAGNETIC ENERGY ON CELL FUNCTION

The science of epigenetics is evolving rapidly and informing us about the influence of subtle energies on the physiology of our cells in remarkable ways. *Epigenetics* is the science that describes the effects of subtle energy or the vibration of thought on cellular nerve processing in the brain, and on the cellular expression of our DNA. Outdated science theory dictated that the genes we were born with were the only forces at work to develop cellular expression. For example, if 90% of the men in a family died before the age of 45 years, it felt like a death sentence to any male children in that family. We now know, at first from differences that were observed with identical twins, that a variation in gene expression was occurring, but we did not know what was causing the variation. Why did one twin have Alzheimer's disease and the other one did not, although they had identical genes? The answer was revealed in the recently advanced science of mapping our genes and watching their expression as we grow and develop. We now know that only approximately 2% to 10% of our total complement of genes actually dictates cell activity. Ninety percent to ninety-eight percent of our genes are controlling the remainder by way of "on/off" switches[15]; that 90% to 98% responds to the conscious and subconscious thoughts and beliefs that we hold. If those male children born into that family believed that they were doomed to die at a young age, then their physiology would most often cooperate. But when we introduce contrary thoughts to the prevailing belief, and when people examine and alter the negative subconscious thoughts that they hold, we now know that they hold the key to changing genetic expression.

We now have data to show that the vibration of positive thoughts and the vibration of a peaceful, meditative mind can literally change brain function and the expression of DNA.[36] Herein lies one of the keys of what we formerly described as "unexplainable miracles," and the prevailing theory has been modified to admit the outliers. Ricard and colleagues discuss the neuroscience of meditation[36]:

> Compared with novices, expert meditators' brain activity diminished in anxiety-related regions—the insular cortex and the amygdala—in the period preceding the painful stimulus…Other tests in our lab have shown that meditation training increases one's ability to better control and buffer basic physiological responses—inflammation or levels of a stress hormone—to a socially stressful task such as giving a public speech or doing mental arithmetic in front of a harsh jury.

Finally, a recent study with Kaiser Permanente Colorado members was designed to assess 1-year outcomes in patients with chronic pain and chronic illness, or stress-related illness practicing mindfulness-based stress reduction activities.[37] Measuring functional status, pain, self-efficacy, depression, anxiety, somatization, psychological distress, work productivity, and changes in health services utilization, significant improvements were recorded in self-reported mental and physical pain, including joint and back pain, and in psychological symptoms and self-efficacy. Significant decreases were observed in visits to primary care, specialty care, emergency departments, and hospital admissions over the year. Thus, the mindfulness-based stress relief program was associated not only with improvements in patient-centered outcomes over 1 year, but also in reductions in health services utilization up to 18 months.[37]

Finally, telomeres, the protective caps at the end of chromosomes, have been associated with cellular and organismal longevity. Shortened telomere length has been associated with chronic stress and depression. Researchers studying the effects of meditation on slowing cellular aging have found that some forms of meditation seem to have a positive effect on preserving telomere length. Positive states of vibration from meditation seem to affect the DNA health and longevity.[38]

CONCLUSION

Terry Tempest Williams has spoken about the process of transitioning into a new consciousness in this way[39]:

> I think we will look back at this time in history as a time of great transition. I think about a particular bridge in the Penobscot area of Maine. When we would drive from Bucksport to Belfast, we had to cross this bridge. For years we would cross this rickety, rusted green bridge, and every time we crossed it, we would hold our breath and think, "I hope we make it across." [A]nd then some time down the line, we noticed a new bridge was being built. We were still driving on the old bridge, but I was mindful each time we crossed the old bridge, of the beauty and the design, and at times, the precariousness of this new bridge that was under construction. I kept thinking, "I hope we make it to the new bridge before the old bridge falls down." And then, one miraculous day, the new bridge was built and we were driving across it. The old bridge was no longer in use.

In 10 years when the next edition of this text is published, what will we accept as common knowledge? How will our prevailing theories about how the universe really "works" be added to and built upon to admit the pesky outliers, exceptions to the rule? One of my most exciting moments as a clinician unfolded in the 44th year of my practice when, as a John F. Barnes myofascial release physical therapist, I was treating a well-known oncology researcher at the University who had suffered from recurrent spinal cysts. Using sustained-release myofascial release and exercise, she and I, together with her constant home releases and exercising, were able to minimize her discomfort and get rid of her spinal cysts that had recurred over a period of several years. Remember: a cyst is a fluid-filled ball surrounded by fascia that develops to protect sensitive structures from noxious stimuli. By using the principles of pressure and shear, elongating the fascia, and melting the ground substance gel, we were able to give her tissue more room, more space, so that the soft tissue could move without restriction.

One day as she lay supine on my table, as I was elongating her leg into adduction and internal rotation, reaching up into her iliotibial band, pelvis, and low back with my sustained release, I asked this renowned National Institutes of Health oncology researcher, "Janice, (pseudonym) do you believe that our cells talk to one another?" She replied, "Of course, everyone knows that." And then I asked, "Do you believe that some cancers might result from a problem in communication between cells and their neighbors?" When she responded, "Yes, I believe that may be so," I knew that science was moving forward. New bridges are being built.

So, stay tuned! I wonder what the science chapter in the fifth edition of *Integrative Therapies in Rehabilitation* will explore. I am very excited to discover it. I hope you are too.

REFERENCES

1. Moskowitz C. What's 96% of the universe made of? Astronomers don't know. www.space.com/11642-dark-matter-dark-energy-4-percent-universe-panek.html. Published May 12, 2011. Accessed January 29, 2016.
2. Oschman JL. *Energy Medicine: The Scientific Basis*. 2nd ed. New York, NY: Elsevier; 2016.
3. Lipton BH, Bhaerman S. *Spontaneous Evolution: Our Positive Future and a Way to Get There From Here*. Carlsbad, CA: Hay House; 2009.
4. Waldman M, Newberg A. Intuition, wisdom and the brain. *Science of Mind*. 2015;88(5):94.
5. Pert CB. *Molecules of Emotion: Why You Feel the Way You Feel*. New York, NY: Simon & Schuster; 1997.

6. Ingber DE. Cellular mechanotransduction: putting all the pieces together again. *FASEB J.* 2006;20(7):811-827.

7. Church D. *The Genie in Your Genes: Epigenetic Medicine and the New Biology of Intention.* Santa Rosa, CA: Elite; 2007.

8. Van den Berg, F. Extracellular matrix. In: Schleip R, Findley FW, Chaitow L, Huijing P, eds. *Fascia—The Tensional Network of the Human Body.* Edinburgh, Scotland: Churchill Livingstone; 2012: 165-170

9. Bianconi E, Piovesan A, Facchin F, et al. An estimation of the number of cells in the human body. *Ann Hum Biol.* 2013;40(6):463-471.

10. Oschman JL. *The Living Matrix.* www.thelivingmatrixmovie.com. Presented March 14,15, 2009. Accessed January 29, 2016.

11. Langevin HM, Huijing PA. Communicating about fascia: history, pitfalls, and recommendations. *Int J Ther Massage Bodywork.* 2009;2(4):3-8.

12. Schleip R, Findley TW, Chaitow L, Huijing P, eds. *Fascia: The Tensional Network of the Human Body: The Science and Clinical Applications in Manual and Movement Therapy.* Edinburgh, Scotland: Churchill Livingstone; 2012.

13. Chaitow L, ed. *Fascial Dysfunction: Manual Therapy Approaches.* United Kingdom: Handspring Publishing; 2014.

14. Lee RP. The living matrix: a model for the primary respiratory mechanism. *Explore (NY).* 2008;4(6):374-378.

15. Lipton B. *The Biology of Belief: Unleashing the Power of Consciousness, Matter, & Miracles.* Santa Rosa, CA; Elite Books; 2005.

16. Van de Wal J. The architecture of the connective tissue in the musculoskeletal system: an often overlooked functional parameter as to proprioception in the locomotor apparatus. In: Huijing PA, Hollander P, Findley T, Schleip R, eds. *Fascia Research II: Basic Science and Implications for Conventional and Complementary Health Care.* Munich, Germany: Elsevier GmbH; 2009: 21-35.

17. Mitchell JH, Schmidt RF. Cardiovascular reflex control by afferent fibers from skeletal muscle receptors. *Compr Physiol.* 2011;suppl 8:623-658.

18. Schleip R. Fascial plasticity—a new neurobiological explanation: Part 1. *J Bodyw Mov Ther.* 2003;7(1):11-19.

19. Meert GF. Fluid dynamics in fascial tissues. In: Schleip R, Findley T, Chaitow L, Huijing P, eds. *Fascia: The Tensional Network of the Human Body: The Science and Clinical Applications in Manual and Movement Therapy.* Edinburgh, Scotland: Churchill Livingstone; 2012: 176-181.

20. Marsland DA, Brown DES. The effects of pressure on sol-gel equilibria with special reference to myosin and other protoplasmic gels. *Journal of Cellular and Comparative Physiology.* 1942;20(3):295–305.

21. Freundlich H. Some recent work on gels. *J Phys Chem.* 1937;41(7):901–910.

22. Pollack GH. *Cells, Gels and the Engines of Life.* Seattle, WA: Ebner and Sons; 2001.

23. Meltzer KR, Standley PR. Modeled repetitive motion strain and indirect osteopathic manipulative techniques in regulation of human fibroblast proliferation and interleukin secretion. *J Am Osteopath Assoc.* 2007;107(12):527-536.

24. Fernández-Pérez AM, Peralta-Ramírez MI, Pilat A, Moreno-Lorenzo C, Villaverde-Gutiérrez C, Arroyo-Morales M. Can myofascial techniques modify immunological parameters? *J Altern Complement Med.* 2013;19(1):24-28.

25. Pollack GH. Phase transition: a mechanism for action. *Cells, Gels and the Engines of Life.* Seattle, WA: Ebner and Sons; 2001:126-129.

26. Barnes JF. Myofascial release: the missing link in traditional treatment. In: Davis CM, ed. *Complementary Therapies in Rehabilitation: Evidence for Efficacy in Therapy, Prevention, and Wellness.* 3rd ed. Thorofare, NJ: Slack Incorporated; 2009: 89-109.

27. Oschman JL. Foreword. In: Davis CM, ed. *Complementary Therapies in Rehabilitation: Evidence for Efficacy in Therapy, Prevention, and Wellness.* 3rd ed. Thorofare, NJ: Slack Incorporated; 2009:xix-xxi.

28. Ingber DE. Cellular mechanotransduction: putting all the pieces together again. *FASEB J.* 2006;20(7):811-827.

29. Robbie KL. Tensional forces in the human body. *Orthopaedic Review.* 1977;6:45-48.

30. Nelson CM, Bissell MJ. Of extracellular matrix, scaffolds, and signaling: tissue architecture regulates development, homeostasis and cancer. *Annu Rev Cell Dev Biol.* 2006;22:287-309.

31. Shkylar TF, Toropova OA, Safronov AP, Pollack GH, Blyakhman FA. Mechanical characteristics of synthetic polyelectrolyte gel as a physical model of the cytoskeleton [Article in Russian]. *Biofizika.* 2011;56(1):78-84.

32. McCraty R, Atkinson M, Tomasino D. *Modulation of DNA conformation by heart-focused intention.* HeartMath Research Center, Institute of HeartMath, Publication No. 03-008. Boulder Creek, CA, 2003. www.aipro.info/drive/File/224.pdf

33. Feinstein D, Eden D. Six pillars of energy medicine: clinical strengths of a complementary paradigm. *Altern Ther Health Med.* 2008;14(1):44-54.

34. Burn HS. *The Fields of Life: Our Link with the Universe.* New York, NY: Ballantine Books; 1973.

35. Tiller WA. What are subtle energies? *J Sci Explor.* 1993;7(3):293-304.

36. Ricard M, Lutz A, Davidson RJ. Neuroscience reveals the secrets of meditation's benefits. *Scientific American.* http://www.scientificamerican.com/article/neuroscience-reveals-the-secrets-of-meditation-s-benefits/ November 1, 2014. Accessed January 29, 2016.

37. McCubbin T, Dimidjian S, Kempe K, et al. Mindfulness-based stress reduction in an integrated care delivery system: one-year impacts on patient-centered outcomes and health care utilization. *Perm J.* 2014;18(4):4-9.

38. Epel E, Daubenmier J, Moskowitz, JT, Folkman S, Blackburn E. Can meditation slow rate of cellular aging? Cognitive stress, mindfulness, and telomeres. *Ann N Y Acad Sci.* 2009;1172:34-53.

39. Fredericksen D. Ground truthing. Devon Frederickson interviews Terry Tempest Williams. *Guernica.* Published August 1, 2013. Accessed January 29, 2016. www.guernicamag.com/interviews/ground-truthing/.

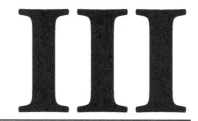

Body Work

6

Myofascial Release
The Missing Link in
Traditional Treatment

John F. Barnes, PT

The John F. Barnes myofascial release (JFB MFR) approach is a whole-body, sustained-pressure, hands-on approach for the evaluation and treatment of the human structure. Its focus is on the living crystal matrix fascial system. Physical trauma, inflammatory or infectious processes, structural imbalances from dental malocclusions, osseous restrictions, leg-length discrepancy, and pelvic rotation may all create inappropriate fascial strain.

First, a word of clarification. Several forms of myofascial release manual therapy are administered to patients and reported in the literature. Most, if not all, have value. This chapter refers solely to the holistic practice of sustained-pressure and whole-body myofascial release developed and taught by Barnes.

Some characteristics that all manual therapies share are obvious: the therapist uses his or her hands to examine and evaluate tissue and then manipulates the tissue to bring about changes at the cellular level that lead to a therapeutic benefit. The manual therapies that are most similar to the JFB MFR approach seem to be osteopathic soft-tissue myofascial release, physical therapy myofascial release, soft tissue mobilization, deep connective tissue massage, and Rolfing. But none of these manual therapies contains the full measure of principles and practices of the JFB MFR approach that are described here and that have been observed to contribute to whole-body healing and reduction in pain.[1]

The JFB MFR approach uniquely consists of the following principles and practices:

- Examination and evaluation of fascial restrictions in the entire body by way of patient history, standing posture evaluation, and palpation of tissue

- Recognition that symptoms may occur far distant from the offending fascial restrictions, and a willingness to examine and treat the whole body at each treatment session

- Centered and mindful focused hand placement over the restrictions using the skin as a tool to softly reach down into the matrix of fascia, and then opening the hands to stretch out the restricted area

- Maintaining constant sustained pressure and shear for 3 to 5 minutes or longer at the fascial barrier with soft hands, following the release and unwinding of the tissue as the ground substance "melts," the elastin stretches out and the dehydrated fascia absorbs fluid and assumes its more appropriate functional length

Davis CM.
Integrative Therapies in Rehabilitation: Evidence for Efficacy in Therapy, Prevention, and Wellness, Fourth Edition (pp 57-74).
© 2017 Taylor & Francis Group.

In contrast, most other forms of myofascial release identify the symptomatic tissue and involve applying rapid, forceful movements to tear at the cross links that form in restricted fascia, or applying pressure directly over the painful area for approximately 30 seconds.

FASCIAL RESTRICTIONS

Fascia, an embryologic tissue, reorganizes along the lines of tension imposed on the body, adding support to misalignment and contracting to protect the individual from further trauma (real or imagined). This has the potential to alter organ and tissue physiology significantly. Fascial strains can slowly tighten, causing the body to lose its physiologic adaptive capacity. Over time, the tightness spreads like a pull in a sweater or stocking. Flexibility and spontaneity of movement are lost, setting the body up for more trauma, pain, and limitation of movement. These powerful fascial restrictions begin to pull the body out of its 3-dimensional alignment with the vertical gravitational axis, causing biomechanically inefficient, high energy-consuming movement and posture.

A detailed description of the myofascial element by Janet G. Travell[2] has taught us that there is no such thing as the muscle we have identified in traditional anatomy and physiology. A smooth fascial sheath surrounds every muscle of the body, every muscular fascicle is surrounded by fascia, every fibril is surrounded by fascia, and every microfibril down to the cellular level is surrounded by fascia. Therefore, it is the fascia that ultimately determines the length and function of its muscular component, and muscle becomes an inseparable component of fascia. The implications of this important fact have been largely ignored in Western and traditional health care.

FASCIA

The fascia is a tough connective tissue that spreads throughout the body in a 3-dimensional web from the head to the feet functionally, without interruption. It has been estimated that if every structure of the body except the fascia were removed, the body would retain its shape. As described by Scott[3] and Oschman,[4] the fascia serves a major purpose in that it permits the body to retain its normal shape and thus maintain the vital organs in their correct positions. It also allows the body to resist mechanical stresses, both internally and externally. Fascia has maintained its general structure and purposes over the millennia. These functions are evident in the earliest stages of multicelled organisms, in which 2 or more cells were able to stay in contact, communicate, and resist the forces of the environment through the connective tissue.[3]

Fascia covers the muscles, bones, nerves, organs, and vessels down to the cellular level. Therefore, malfunction of the system due to trauma, poor posture, or inflammation can bind down the fascia, resulting in abnormal pressure on any or all of these body components. It is through that process that this binding down, or restriction, may result in many of the poor or temporary results achieved by conventional medical, dental, and therapeutic treatments.[5]

As Travell[2] has explained, restrictions of the fascia can create pain or malfunction throughout the body, sometimes with bizarre side effects and seemingly unrelated symptoms that do not always follow dermatome zones. It is thought that an extremely high percentage of people suffering with pain and/or loss of motion may have fascial restriction problems. Most of these conditions go undiagnosed, however, as many of the standard tests, such as radiographs, myelograms, computed tomography scans, and electromyograms, do not show the fascia. If we cannot see it, we cannot look for restriction with our eyes.

Touching patients with skilled hands, however, can be one of the most potent ways of locating fascial restrictions and effecting positive change. Touching patients through mobilization, massage, and various forms of exercise and movement therapy, coupled with the gentle, refined touch of the JFB MFR approach and the sophisticated movement therapy known as *myofascial unwinding*, creates a sensorimotor interplay. This experience of contact and movement is the very experience we need to reprogram our biocomputer, the mind-body, the basis for learning any new skill. Those practicing the JFB MFR approach use the skin and fascia as a handle or lever to create new options for enhanced function and movement of every structure of the body. The JFB MFR approach helps to remove the straitjacket of pressure caused by restricted fascia, eliminating symptoms, such as stiffness, pain, and spasm. Then, through its influence on the neuromuscular and skeletal systems, it creates the opportunity for patients to "learn" new enhanced movement patterns. Both manipulation and sustained JFB MFR are highly effective treatments when they are accomplished with skilled hands and trained minds. They are designed to be used together to enhance the total effect. Joint manipulation is specific, attempting to improve the motion and function of a particular joint. The JFB MFR approach, however, is a whole-body approach designed to discover and rectify the fascial restrictions that may have caused the effect or symptoms.

DISCOVERING FASCIAL RESTRICTIONS

The skin has many ways of perceiving the universe. There was a time when it was considered the largest organ of the body, covering approximately 18 square feet and weighing approximately 8 pounds (ie, 6% to 8% of one's total body weight).[6,7] It has approximately 640,000 sensory receptors that are connected to the spinal cord by more than 500,000 nerve fibers. The tactile fibers vary from 7 to 135/cm^2.[6-8] The tactile surface of the skin is the interface between not only the body and our world, but also the mind's thought process and our physical existence.[8] This is also the interface by which therapists can facilitate incredible changes in the patient through the amazing plasticity of the central nervous system and the brain. Embryologically, both the skin and the nervous system are produced by ectoderm. When considering the connection of mind and body, we might question whether the skin is the outer surface of the brain or whether the brain is the deepest layer of the skin.[8,9]

Recent discoveries have revealed that there is, indeed, a much larger sensory organ in the body than the skin. According to Robert Schleip,[10] the total surface area of the fascial web or network "possesses a ten times higher quantity of sensory nerve receptors" than the myofascia. Further, with the combination of embedded proprioceptors and unmyelinated free nerve endings found throughout the entire fascial web, fascia may possibly have more sensory receptors than the retina of the eye, once considered the most important sensory receptor. But in terms of surface area, it is clear now that the skin in combination with the entire fascial web is a huge sensory organ that is available for us to use to modify perceived sensation, including pain and pressure.

Touch by itself can be powerfully therapeutic.[6] It can also serve as a powerful diagnostic tool by itself and through its role in proprioception. Of all of the senses, the proprioceptive sense is generally the least understood by most people; thus, it is seldom consciously used. However, when this sense is developed through the awareness and use of the more holistic right brain rather than the logical left-brain "knowing," proprioceptive input opens up vistas of untapped intuitive potential for clinicians in both evaluation and treatment. The development of our proprioceptive sense also allows us to detect the quality and quantity of the often unnoticed very fine motion that is inherent in our bodies. As this approach is developed and refined, it is discovered that when we quiet our mind and body and gently touch the patient with both hands on the dorsum of his or her feet, for example, our proprioceptive senses help us in our evaluation by feeding us information as if our hands were moving like a mirror image to the patient's movement, thus detecting the subtle motions occurring in the patient's body that we cannot see or feel any other way. This activity, when practiced and honed, allows us to discover fascial restrictions and feel when they release. The informed touch of the JFB MFR approach also allows us to feel the motion that will take the patients' bodies into the 3-dimensional position necessary for more total structural release or, as for many, for bringing disassociated memories to a conscious level, as will be discussed later in this chapter.

John F. Barnes Myofascial Release: The Blending of Current and Emerging Explanatory Paradigms

A *paradigm* is a theoretical model that provides a way of describing, believing, and understanding what we consider to be real.[11] A paradigm shift changes our models of reality, our concepts and logic, and can create anxiety, fear, and anger in those persons deeply entrenched in the status quo. For others, it represents an opportunity for growth. Fear paralyzes some, while it provides the stimulus and motivation to move to higher and deeper levels of understanding, awareness, and achievement for others. The current paradigm or theory upon which Western medicine is based (reductionism) is becoming less and less adequate, as it fails to explain such common phenomena as spontaneous remission of tumors, how the mind and emotions affect the physiology of the body, extrasensory perception, and other observed and documented occurrences.

The current paradigm that drives medicine, health care therapy, and research springs from the centuries-old "either/or" logic of Aristotle. In it, everything is isolated, individual, and separate. There is no "middle ground" or shades of gray. This kind of thinking makes one theory wrong because another is right, or one person wrong because another is right.[12] Such thinking is exclusionary; it does not acknowledge connectedness among individuals or allow for the possibility of the coexistence of explanatory models.

Based on the logic of Aristotle, the universe, as perceived by Isaac Newton and René Descartes, is a giant machine that functions precisely, logically, sequentially, and correctly. This model of classic physics, which is the basis of our current paradigm, is informed by reductionistic research, which carefully allows for only one correct solution to a problem. In the field of medical science, theories based on this model and its research have reduced human illness to the "biochemistry of disease," completely losing sight of the fact that the disease or dysfunction is part of a whole person. It is obvious that this model "has reached its limits and has crossed into absurdity."[4,12] The emerging explanatory paradigm (holism) places priority on describing connectedness, relativity, complexity, multiple possibilities, and a nonlinear mind-body unity. The practice of the JFB MFR approach has to do with wholeness, connectedness (connective tissue), the wave-and-particle theory of atoms, and the subatomic realm of quantum physics.

Both systems theory and quantum physics, in part, describe the awareness and facilitation of interwoven, nonlinear systems in the universe where the whole is greater than, and makes sense of, the parts.[4,13] This theory contrasts reductionism, where the parts make sense of the whole because the whole is nothing more than the total of all the parts.[4,12] This paradigm shift requires a change of perspective and represents a "breakthrough in science. It connects living biological systems to physics and shows nature to be much more than just mechanical. The whole universe is alive and participating."[12]

Fascial Web as an Energetic Communication System

The neurobiological explanation of communication is the old, traditional perspective that all cells function as a result of impulses from the brain and the nervous system. That is a linear, reductionist point of view, which was proven to be an inadequate method to understand the human being back in the 1920s by Max Planck, the father of quantum physics.[14] Of course, nerves are an essential aspect of human function, but the function of the fascia and of all of the body's cells are dependent on far more than nerves.[4] Every nerve and blood vessel of our body is embedded within the fascial system and, when restricted, these cells are totally controlled by it.[4]

In *The Extracellular Matrix and Ground Regulation: Basis for a Holistic Biological Medicine*,[15] Alfred Pischinger, one of Germany's leading scientists, stated that there is no nerve or blood vessel that touches any one of the 100 trillion cells in your body. Nerve conduction is too slow to explain the instantaneous action of every cell throughout your body. Our primary body communication system is frequencies of light that travel through the fluidity of our fascial system; the ground substance, which is the environment of every cell of our body.[4]

As a JFB MFR therapist, it is helpful to move away from the fragmented, linear, reductionist mode of thinking into a more global, felt sense of our environment and our world. As we begin to understand the beauty of the fractal nature of ourselves and our universe, we will have more accuracy and enhanced ability to help others.

Traditionally, medical education teaches that emotions are totally separate from the structure of the body. The body is essentially a machine, and when a part breaks down it is to be medicated, surgically altered, or have some form of therapy directed at it and it alone. For years, this Cartesian viewpoint or model has been accepted as true, and patients were treated accordingly, even though logic and our experience tells us that it could not be true.

The JFB MFR approach is a logical expansion of the very roots of the health professions. It incorporates quantum theory and systems theory into practice, but it does not necessitate the dismantling of traditional health care or physical therapy. Rather, the JFB MFR approach represents a powerfully effective addition of a series of concepts and techniques that enhance and mesh with our traditional medical, dental, and therapeutic training.

CLOSE EXAMINATION OF THE ANATOMY AND PHYSIOLOGY OF FASCIA

The fascia is generally classified as superficial (lying directly below the dermis), deep (surrounding and infusing with muscle, bone, nerves, blood vessels, and organs to the cellular level), or deepest (the dura of the craniosacral system, encasing the central nervous system and the brain). However, one of the most erroneous concepts throughout the literature is the idea that fascia is simply a plastic wrap–like tissue surrounding organs. On the contrary, the fascial web not only surrounds all tissue, but all cells are embedded within fascia. Fascia forms the immediate environment of every one of the body's 50 to 75 trillion cells.

At the cellular level, fascia creates the interstitial spaces. It has extremely important functions in support, protection, separation, cellular respiration, elimination, metabolism, and fluid and lymphatic flow. It can have a profound influence on cellular health and the immune system. Therefore, trauma or malfunction of the fascia can cause poor cellular efficiency, necrosis, disease, pain, and dysfunction throughout the body.[4,16]

MOLECULAR STRUCTURE OF FASCIA

Connective tissue is composed of collagen, elastin, and the polysaccharide gel complex, or ground substance.[4,17] These form a 3-dimensional, interdependent system of strength, support, elasticity, and cushion.

Collagen is a protein consisting of 3 polypeptide chains that line up to form fibrils in such a way as to ensure that there are no weak points that could give way under tension. Collagen fibers thus contribute strength to fascial tissue and guard against overextension.

Elastin, another protein, is intrinsically rubber-like. Its fibers are laid down in parallel with an excess length of collagen fibers in places where elasticity is required, such as skin and arteries. This combination absorbs tensile forces. Tendons, specialized for pulling, mainly contain these elastocollagenous fibers.

The polysaccharide gel complex, mainly composed of hyaluronic acid and proteoglycans, fills the spaces between fibers. Hyaluronic acid is a highly viscous substance that lubricates the collagen, elastin, and muscle fibers, allowing them to slide over each other with minimal friction. Proteoglycans are peptide chains that form the gel of the ground substance. This gel is extremely hydrophilic, allowing it to absorb the compressive forces of movement. Cartilage, which acts as a shock absorber, contains much water-rich gel.

As long as the forces are not too great, the gel of the ground substance is designed to absorb shock and disperse it throughout the body. If fascia is restricted at the time of trauma, the forces cannot be dispersed properly and areas of the body are then subjected to an intolerable impact, resulting in injury. Injurious forces do not have to be enormous; a person who lacks sufficient "give" can be severely injured by minor forces.[4,5,18]

Realizing this, we can explain the sports and performance injuries that recur despite extensive therapy, strengthening, and flexibility programs. An athlete with fascial restrictions will not efficiently absorb the shocks of continued activity. Thus, the body absorbs too much pressure in too small an area, and the body keeps "breaking down" during performance. This same effect takes place over time from the microtrauma of discrepancies of leg length due to weight bearing on a continuously torsioned pelvis. Each step sends imbalanced forces throughout the body, which then tries to compensate through muscular spasm and fascial restrictions, ultimately producing symptoms.

The JFB MFR techniques are performed to reduce these symptoms of pain, spasm, and malalignment. In addition to increasing range of motion, the enormous pressure of the fascial restrictions is eliminated from pain-sensitive structures, alleviating symptoms, restoring the normal quantity and quality of motion, and restoring the body's ability to absorb shock without compensatory injury.

Physiological Responses Unique to J.F. Barnes Sustained Myofascial Release

The art of the JFB MFR approach is finding the restrictions that are unique to each individual, and then using sustained pressure of 5 minutes or longer, which eventually elicits the following important phenomena: piezoelectricity, mechanotransduction, phase transition, chaos theory, and, ultimately, resonance. These are the key components explaining the effectiveness of sustained JFB MFR, and are described in part by James Oschman[18] in his chapter, "Fascia as a body-wide communication system," in the book *Fascia: The Tensional Network of the Human Body: The Science and Clinical Applications in Manual and Movement Therapy.*

Piezoelectricity

Piezoelectricity is a Greek word that means pressure electricity. It is a well-known fact that each of our cells is crystalline in nature. When you place pressure into a crystal it creates a bioelectrical flow.[19] The sustained pressure of JFB MFR, coupled with the critical time element (5 minutes or longer per restriction), creates and sustains a bioelectrical flow in our body, which leads into mechanotransduction.

Mechanotransduction

Mechanotransduction is a process whereby physical force generates cellular biochemical responses in the ways that previously were attributed only to biochemistry and genetic action on cells.[19] The internal tensegrity structure within the nucleus of the cell, the cytoskeleton, responds to pressure from the extracellular matrix or the fascial environment outside the cell, by way of communicating forces over the web of tissue into the nucleus. When the microenvironment alters the cell shape, the nucleus responds, and there is current research that shows that this may be the genesis of malignancies.[20]

Importantly, Meltzer and associates[21] and Cao and associates[22] have found that sustained-release myofascial release can produce interleukin-8, our body's own natural anti-inflammatory agent. Research has shown that inflammation is an important part of the healing process; however, when inflammation has been thwarted it tends to solidify the ground substance of the fascial system, which should be fluid. This then blocks healing and over time tends to continue to solidify into crushing restrictions that produce the symptoms that many of your patients come to you to treat.

Phase Transition

When piezoelectricity and mechanotransduction dovetail together, phase transition takes place, like when ice transforms into water. A similar occurrence happens in our bodies. The solidified or dehydrated ground substance of fascia, with sustained pressure, becomes more fluid, allowing the tissue to rehydrate and to glide, taking crushing pressure off of pain-sensitive structures.[23,24]

Chaos Theory

Everything in traditional medicine and therapy insists upon order and control. However, true growth and healing cannot occur in a controlled, orderly way. Systems theory states that nature goes through continuous periods of order, chaos, order, chaos, etc. It is in the chaotic phase that reorganization occurs.[25] As a result of reorganization, the system then returns to a higher level of order. For phrase transition to occur, it appears that a period of molecular chaos is required for the ice to transform into water, or, in our body/mind, for the solidified ground substance of the fascial system to transform into a more viscous/fluid state.

Resonance

Oschman[24] reports several studies on the vibration and biomagnetic energy that human beings emit. When one human touches another human, their vibratory rates can be quite different on the molecular level; however, this author hypothesizes that with sustained pressure at the fascial restriction, the vibratory rates of the 2 will become identical, creating resonance. Resonance is the very essence of the JFB MFR approach. This resonance is what the author calls a *release* and it occurs locally, but it also vibrates distantly throughout the living crystal matrix of fascia in the cranial area and throughout the body. Resonance, unfortunately, does not occur in the same way in other forms of manual therapy because these other forms of therapy are too quick, hence providing only temporary results. This is why it is so important to learn the "art" of locating all of the fascial restrictions that are totally unique to each individual in any one moment in time.

FUNCTIONS OF FASCIA

The fascia, as mentioned earlier, is particularly significant in supporting and providing cohesion to the body structures; thus, its functions are varied and complex. Functional, biomechanically efficient movements depend on intact, properly distributed fascia. Fascia creates a plexus to support and stabilize, thus enhancing the body's postural balance. Appropriately, loose fascia permits movement between adjacent structures, which are free of friction due to the presence of bursal sacs. In addition, loose tissue contains a fluid that serves as a transport medium for cellular elements of other tissues, blood, and lymph. In this manner, fascia also supports a nutritive function.[26]

Fat is stored in the superficial fascia. This layer also provides a covering that helps conserve body heat. The deep fascia is an ensheathing layer. It maintains physiologic limb contour and enhances venous and lymphatic circulation. In combination with intermuscular septa and interosseous membranes, the deep fascia provides additional surface area for muscle attachment.[4,27]

Structurally, the planes in connective tissue allow the passage of infectious and inflammatory processes. The presence in the tissue of histiocytes, however, offers a defense against bacteria. These phagocytes also remove debris and foreign matter from fascia. In addition, connective tissue neutralizes or detoxifies both endogenous (produced under physiologic conditions) and exogenous (introduced from outside the body) toxins. Finally, its fibroplastic qualities permit fascia to assist in healing injuries by depositing collagenous fibers via scar tissue.[27]

In addition to the structural function of fascia, research by Langevin[27] at the University of Vermont, Burlington, Vermont, by Ingber[19] at Harvard University, Cambridge, Massachusetts, and by Schleip[10] from Germany, has clarified the role of fascia as a whole-body communication network. Fascial cells, responsive to mechanical forces, seem to generate 3 categories of signals: (1) electrical, (2) cellular, and (3) tissue remodeling.[19] Ingber's work reveals that mechanical distortion of fascial cells profoundly affects the cells' behavior that can "switch cells between distinct gene programs (eg, growth, differentiation, and apoptosis)." As stated earlier, by way of tensegrity and solid-state mechanochemistry, fascial cells may "mediate mechanotranduction and facilitate integration of chemical and physical signals that are responsible for control of cell behavior."[19]

FUNCTION OF THE MICROTUBULES OF FASCIA

Much of what I have learned over the years has first appeared to me in flashes of insight or intuitive hunches that later were substantiated by scientific discovery. As I was treating patients several years ago, for instance, I became more and more aware of visuals that were flowing through me. I experienced a felt sense of the visual, sometimes coupled with emotion and then usually followed by an intellectual understanding. As I was treating a patient one day, I started to see the fascial system, even at its tiniest of levels, as tiny little tubes with a hollow core. Within the hollow core was fluid, through which consciousness flowed as vibrations of light.

Over the years while treating people from all over the world, as I centered myself and engaged the individual's myofascial release barrier, more and more images, sensations, and understandings about the reality of the human structure and experience began to dawn on me. It continued to deepen over the years with each experience. Interestingly, one day a book mysteriously showed up on my desk, and to this day I do not know where it came from. It was titled *Shadows of the Mind: A Search for the Missing Science of Consciousness* by Roger Penrose.[28] Penrose is considered to be one of the world's leading mathematical physicists; he often publishes with a colleague, Dr. Stuart Hameroff, a physician, deeply involved in anesthesia research and the effects of anesthesia on consciousness. As I skimmed through the book, his phraseology began to catch my attention. He wrote about how he had determined where consciousness enters the physicality and he described it as "entering in microtubules with a hollow core through which water flowed with frequencies of light flowing through it as fluid intelligence."[29]

Penrose, with his expertise in quantum physics, delved into microbiology of brain cells where he examined cytoskeletons and microtubules, minute substructures lying deep within the brains neurons. He argued that microtubules—not neurons—may indeed be the basic units of the brain, which, if nothing else, would dramatically increase the brain's computational power. Furthermore, he contended that, in consciousness, some kind of global quantum state must take place across larger areas of the brain and that it is within the microtubules that these collective quantum effects are most likely to take place. This led to the following question: are microtubules quantum computers? I'll quote their theory from 2 other articles:[30,31]

> The interiors of neurons and glia cells are functionally organized by webs of protein polymers—the cytoskeleton, the major components are microtubules, actin and intermediate filaments. Microtubules are self-assembling hollow cylinders, whose walls are crystalline lattices. Some evidence links the neuronal cytoskeleton to cognitive functions and theoretical models suggest that interactive microtubule subunits function as molecular automata capable of nanosecond scale computation.

Over the years, I had seen that instead of the fascia functioning as an insulator as we were taught, it was actually like a fiber optic cable capable of carrying enormous amounts of information, consciousness, and energy throughout the fluidity of the fascial system.

And this: A controversial 20-year-old theory of consciousness published in Physics of Life Reviews claims that consciousness derives from deeper level, finer scale activities inside brain neurons.[32-34]

The recent discovery of quantum vibrations in microtubules inside brain neurons corroborates this theory, according to review authors Stuart Hameroff and Sir Roger Penrose. They suggest that EEG rhythms (brain waves) also derive from deeper level microtubule vibrations, and that from a practical standpoint, treating brain microtubule vibrations could benefit a host of mental, neurological, and cognitive conditions.[35]

The theory, called "orchestrated objective reduction" ("Orch OR"), was first put forward in the mid-1990s by eminent mathematical physicist Sir Roger Penrose, FRS, Mathematical Institute and Wadham College, University of Oxford, and prominent anesthesiologist Stuart Hameroff, MD, Anesthesiology, Psychology, and Center for Consciousness Studies, The University of Arizona, Tucson. They suggested that quantum vibrational computations in microtubules were "orchestrated" ("Orch") by synaptic inputs and memory stored in microtubules, and termed by Penrose "objective reduction" ("OR"), hence "Orch OR." Microtubules are major components of the cell structural skeleton.[35]

An important new facet of the theory is introduced. Microtubule quantum vibrations (eg, in megahertz) appear to interfere and produce much slower EEG "beat frequencies." Despite a century of clinical use, the underlying origins of EEG rhythms have remained a mystery. Clinical trials of brief brain stimulation aimed at microtubule resonances with megahertz mechanical vibrations using transcranial ultrasound have shown reported improvements in mood, and may prove useful against Alzheimer's disease and brain injury in the future.

Lead author Stuart Hameroff concludes, "Orch OR" is the most rigorous, comprehensive and successfully-tested theory of consciousness ever put forth. From a practical standpoint, treating brain microtubule vibrations could benefit a host of mental, neurological, and cognitive conditions."[34]

MYOFASCIAL RELEASE EFFECT ON COLLAGEN

Collagen comes from the ancient Greek word that means "glue-producer." The feeling that one perceives during myofascial release treatment is rather like stretching glue. The therapist follows this sensation with sensitive hands as it twists and turns, barrier through barrier, until an increased range of motion is accomplished.

A therapist cannot mechanically overstretch the collagenous aspect of the fascia. Although we are as yet unable to prove it, the improvements seen after myofascial release are probably due to a stretching of the elastic component, a shearing of the cross-links that can develop at the nodal points of the fascia, and a change in the viscosity of the ground substance from a more solid to a gel state. The work of Gerald Pollack and associates[35] confirms that the infrared energy from the therapist's hands and the piezoelectric response of the colloidal ground substance of the fascia, with sustained pressure, literally melts the ground substance. This change in viscosity increases the production of hyaluronic acid and increases the glide of the fascial tissue. Also observed regularly is what appears to be a positive effect on the spindle cells, the Golgi tendon organs of the musculotendinous component, and the tone of the peripheral, autonomic, and central nervous systems.[4,5]

Thus, to separate fascia from its influence on muscle and their influence on each other is impossible. In other words, we have been evaluating and treating an illusion. Anatomical and scientific reality demand that we consider both muscle and fascia as inexorably linked as one. Understanding their integrated characteristics, we use this more accurate information to inform our evaluation and treatment. My experience has shown that medicine, modalities, muscle energy techniques, mobilization, manipulation, temporomandibular joint appliances, massage, and flexibility and exercise programs affect *only* the muscular and elastic components of the fascial system. Only the JFB MFR approach, with its emphasis on using bioenergy and the piezoelectric effect that occurs as we sustain the release, barrier after barrier, affects the total fascial system. This is why it is important to add this form of myofascial release techniques to our current treatment regimens. Otherwise, we are only treating part of the problem and part of the patient.

Symptoms May Present Distant to Restrictions

Due to the ubiquitous nature of the whole-body fascial web, patients have been known to experience distant symptoms far from the origin of the offending fascial restriction rope or plate. Occipital headaches, upper cervical pain and dysfunction, and temporomandibular pain and malfunction might actually result from fascial restrictions in the pelvic area, pulling down all the way up the spine and into the head, face, and neck. In addition, it is this author's belief that, during trauma, or with the development of a structural imbalance, a proprioceptive memory pattern of pain is established in the central nervous system. Beyond the localized pain response from injured nerves, these reflex patterns remain to perpetuate the pain during and beyond the healing of the injured tissue, similar to the experience of phantom limb pain. Also in operation is the psychosomatic mode of adaptation, which is part of Hans Selye's general adaptation syndrome.[36]

Once fascia has tightened and is creating symptoms distant from the injury, all of the appropriate, traditional localized treatments will produce poor or temporary results because the imbalance and excessive pressure from the myofascial tightness remain untreated.

Application of
J.F. Barnes Sustained-Release Myofascial Release

When the location of the fascial restriction is determined, gentle pressure and slight shear are applied in its direction. It is hypothesized that this has the effect of pulling the elastocollagenous fibers straight. When hand or palm pressure is first applied and sinking into the elastocollagenous complex, the elastic component is engaged, resulting in a "springy" feel. The elastic component is slowly stretched until the hands stop at what feels like a firm barrier. This is the collagenous component. This barrier cannot be forced; it is too strong. Instead, the therapist continues to apply gentle sustained pressure, and soon the firm barrier will yield to the previous melting or springy feel as it stretches further. This yielding phenomenon is related to viscous flow; that is, a low load (gentle pressure) applied slowly will allow a viscous medium to flow to a greater extent than a high load (quickly applied pressure).[4] The viscosity of the ground substance has an effect on the collagen, since it is believed that the viscous medium that makes up the ground substance controls the ease with which collagen fibers rearrange themselves.[37] As this rearranging occurs, the collagenous barrier releases, producing a change in tissue length.[4]

It is important to keep in mind the properties of fascial tissue. Viscoelasticity "causes it to resist a suddenly applied force over time. Creep is the progressive deformation of soft tissues due to constant low loading over time. Hysteresis is the property whereby the work done in deforming a material causes heat and hence energy loss."[37] The therapist follows the motion of the tissue, barrier to barrier, until freedom is felt. The Arndt-Schultz law also explains how the gentle, sustained pressure of myofascial release can produce such consistent changes and improvements. The law states that there is a therapeutic window of effectiveness, where weak stimuli increase physiologic activity while very strong stimuli from the same source can inhibit or abolish activity.[38]

The development of one's tactile and proprioceptive senses enhances the "feel" necessary for the successful completion of these techniques. We were all born with the ability to feel the releases and the direction in which the tissue seems to move from barrier to barrier. When first learning myofascial release, students perform the techniques mechanically. With a little practice, however, they discover the feel and move to a more artful or higher level of achievement.

No prior knowledge of mobilization or manipulation is required to learn the concept and techniques of the JFB MFR approach. The procedures should be combined with neuromuscular technique (muscle energy), joint mobilization, and manipulation by skilled practitioners. However, since it is usually fascial restrictions that created the osseous restrictions in the first place, releasing the fascia first is often the desired order of treatment.

The biomechanical, bioelectrical, and neurophysiological effects of the JFB MFR approach represent an evolutionary leap for our professions and our patients. This is a total approach, incorporating a physiologic system that, when included with traditional therapy, medicine, or dentistry, acts as a catalyst and yields impressive, clinically reproducible results.[1,5]

MYOFASCIAL CRANIAL TECHNIQUES

The application of myofascial release to the cranium is most effective when light pressure is used. Once you have learned to "read the body," more pressure may be indicated at times. Practitioners are taught to start lightly on the mechanical level. Through time and experience, their awareness and sensitivity increases to the point where treatment on the head or body flows in a dynamic fashion.[5]

MYOFASCIAL UNWINDING: THE BODY REMEMBERS

To ask how the mind communicates with the body or how the body communicates with the mind assumes that the 2 are separate entities. The research of Popper and Eccles[25] confirms this. My research and experience with myofascia have shown that they seem to respond as a single unit or 2 sides of the same coin. Mind and body act as if they are different aspects of the same spectrum, immutably joined, inseparable, connected, influencing, and intercommunicating constantly. The JFB MFR techniques and myofascial unwinding seem to allow for the complete communication of mind with body and body with mind, which is necessary for healing. The body remembers everything that ever happened to it, and research by Hameroff[39] indicates that the theory of quantum coherence points toward the storing of meaningful memory in the microtubules, cylindrical protein polymers that we find in the fascia of cells. Mind-body awareness and healing are often linked to the concept of *state-dependent memory*, learning, and behavior, also called *déjà vu*.[36] We have all experienced this when, for example, a certain smell or the sound of a particular piece of music creates a flashback phenomenon, producing a visual, sensorimotor replay of a past event or an important episode in our lives with such vividness that it is as if it were happening at that moment. Based on the work of Hameroff and colleagues and my own experience, I would like to expand this theory to include position-dependent memory, learning, and behavior, with the structural position being the missing component in Selye's state-dependent theory as it is currently described.[40]

My experience has shown that during periods of trauma, people form subconscious indelible imprints of the experience that have high levels of emotional content. The body can hold information below the conscious level, as a protective mechanism, so that memories tend to become dissociated or amnesiac. This is called *memory dissociation*, or reversible amnesia. The memories are state (or position) dependent and can therefore be retrieved when the person is in a particular state (or position). This information is not available in the normal conscious state, and the body's protective mechanisms keep us away from the positions that our mind-body awareness construes as painful or traumatic.

It has been demonstrated consistently that when a myofascial release technique takes the tissue to a significant position or when myofascial unwinding allows a body part to assume a significant position 3-dimensionally in space, the tissue not only changes and improves, but memories, associated emotional states, and belief systems also rise to the conscious level. This awareness, through the positional reproduction of a past event or trauma, allows the individual to grasp the previously hidden information that may be creating or maintaining symptoms or behavior that deter improvement. With the repressed and stored information now at the conscious level, the individual is in a position to learn which holding or bracing patterns have been impeding progress and why. The release of the tissue with its stored emotions and hidden information creates an environment for change.

EVIDENCE OF EFFICACY FOR MYOFASCIAL RELEASE

This chapter refers only to the unique practice of the JFB MFR approach, but the literature is replete with articles on the efficacy of "myofascial release." A review of the methods of the treatment administration rarely is sufficiently detailed to know exactly how the manual therapy was administered. Several articles actually cite the work of Barnes as foundational to their treatment, but actually are revealed to be manual therapy that may or may not be sustained, and in every case except 4,[41-44] show application over the symptomatic area alone, without reference to whole-body examination or evaluation before treatment.

Nonetheless, there is a paucity of published studies on myofascial release in particular, very likely due in part because you cannot blind subjects who are receiving manual therapy in double-blind trials. Subjects know when they are touched. (One can, however, blind the pre- and post-test evaluators and compare results from an experimental group with a control group.) Also, as soon as the therapist touches the client or patient with the intent to offer myofascial release, the energy of the system is affected by that touch, and the therapist and subject lock into an energetic cybernetic system between themselves, making interrater reliability very difficult to reproduce.[45] Having said that, a review of the current published and abstract literature reveals the start of a collection of evidence.

Ajimsha and colleagues[45] published a recent systematic review of randomized trials on the effectiveness of myofascial release as reported in the literature. They define myofascial release according to some of the criteria established by Barnes as "a form of manual therapy that involves the application of a low load, long duration stretch to the myofascial complex, intended to restore optimal length, etc."[45] No mention is made, however, of the holistic examination of each patient for restrictions far away from the symptoms.

Only 19 of the 133 studies identified in their search of the Cochrane Library, MEDLINE, CINAHL, Academic Search Premier, and PEDro Database fit the eligibility criteria. Those studies looked at the effectiveness of myofascial release on hamstring tightness, pelvic rotation, subacute low back pain and plantar fasciitis in healthy subjects following high-intensity exercise, nonspecific cervical and lumbar pain, temporomandibular joint disorders, fibromyalgia, tension headache, breast cancer, venous insufficiency, lateral epicondylitis, and plantar heel pain.

Nine studies indicated that MFR may be better than no treatment or sham treatment and 7 studies demonstrated that MFR plus a traditional treatment is more effective than no treatment. One study found that use of proprioceptive neuromuscular facilitation, a neuromuscular muscle energy technique, was superior to MFR for reducing hamstring tightness.

The authors concluded that much of the difficulty in analyzing these studies revolved around the incomplete description of the type of MFR being used, the experience level of the therapist, and the comfort of the patient with the therapist (which they described as being the subjective component of the design). Comfort between patient and therapist is critical for positive outcomes, they maintain. Their final conclusion was, "Although the quality of the RCT [randomized controlled trial] studies varied greatly, the result of the studies was encouraging, particularly with the recently published studies."[45]

The *Journal of Alternative and Complementary Medicine* published an article in 2013[46] responding to the question of whether the in vitro results of Paul Standley and associates reporting on cytokine stimulation from sustained myofascial release might be measured in vivo.

In their 2013 study, Fernández-Pérez et al[46] randomly assigned 39 healthy men to experimental or control groups. Each person in the experimental group underwent 3 predetermined myofascial release treatments while those in the control group remained in a resting position for the same amount of time. Venous blood was collected before and immediately following treatment. Change in counts of T lymphocytes (T cells) CD3, CD4, CD8, B lymphocyte CD19, and natural killer cells were examined between baseline and 20 minutes post-intervention. At baseline, experimental and control subjects did not differ significantly in any of the immunological markers and natural killer cells.

The myofascial release techniques applied to all healthy subjects included the suboccipital release for 4 minutes, compression of the 4th ventricle over the occipital area for 6 minutes, and anterior cervical fascia (thoracic inlet) release over the posterior neck and anterior pectoral areas for 10 minutes. These techniques are among the many taught by JFB MFR therapy courses.

Researchers found no significant time x group interaction effects on the T lymphocyte and natural killer cell counts; however, a higher CD19 count in the experimental group post-intervention ($P = .001$) was measured. This is a strong indicator that sustained myofascial release has a positive effect of the modulation of the immune system, and further argues for the effect of energy flow, or subatomic particle transmission throughout the fascial web, a point of controversy among myofascial release researchers and therapists.[46]

Cubick and colleagues[42] published a case report using the JFB MFR approach with a female patient with complications of rheumatoid arthritis (RA) and collagenous colitis. This patient had cervical and systemic pain, fatigue, and explosive diarrhea as a result of RA and collagenous colitis that were occurring even though the patient had been receiving infliximab infusions for several months. She underwent 6 treatments of JFB MFR from 3 therapists (1 experienced, 2 students) for 45 minutes/session over the course of 2 weeks. This case study was focused not only on whether the JFB MFR approach might reduce existing symptoms of pain, fatigue, and increase range of motion and quality of life during the treatment sessions, but also on how long any relief of symptoms might continue following the discontinuation of therapy.

Researchers reported that the JFB MFR approach aided in decreasing the patient's pain and fatigue and improving the quality of her life during the 2 weeks of treatment as measured by pre- and post-testing; these positive effects remained for up to 7 weeks following the last treatment. The return of her symptoms as recorded in her 8-week follow-up post-test results were attributed by the patient to a stressful weekend related to the recent death of her husband. The authors of this study point out that the JFB MFR approach seemed to have longer-lasting results than traditional massage and manual therapies.[43]

Abstracts of 2 presentations at a national scientific session in 2001 were published in *Physical Therapy*. Bezner and colleagues[47] from Southwest Texas State University examined the effects of myofascial release techniques on pulmonary function measures. Forty women and 18 men (mean age, 26 years) with no pathology were randomly assigned to a control group or an experimental group. The experimental group (n = 30) received myofascial release to the shoulder, chest, and abdomen for 10 minutes, while the control group (n = 28) received therapeutic light touch to the same areas for the same amount of time. Pre- and post-pulmonary function measures were recorded prior to treatment, immediately following, and 1 week following treatment. Forced vital capacity, forced expiratory volume in 1 second, slow vital capacity, inspiratory volume, and expiratory reserve volume measures were compared by t-test. Researchers found no differences between the 2 groups. One might argue that, in the absence of pathology, myofascial release techniques would not affect already sufficiently lengthened fascia.

Kegerreis and colleagues[48] from the University of Indianapolis examined the immediate and cumulative effects of a transverse plane myofascial release on the respiratory diaphragm. Thirty subjects from a community hospital chronic pain and rehabilitation program were randomly assigned to a treatment or a control group. All individuals received one session of energy-based myofascial release to the diaphragm lying supine. All of the patients were evaluated for changes in heart rate, respiratory rate, blood pressure, rib cage expansion, and forced vital capacity 5 to 10 minutes post-treatment. Sixteen of the subjects were examined after 4 treatment sessions for the cumulative effect. Control group subjects received light touch only, with no attempt to "follow the release as it progressed through fascial barriers" as was done with experimental group subjects. Multianalysis of variance and post hoc multivariant tests were used on individual dependent variables." A significant immediate and cumulative effect existed in lowering respiratory rate for the treatment group ($P < .05$) using within-subjects multivariant testing. Significant differences were not detected immediately or cumulatively for heart rate, blood pressure, rib cage expansion, or forced vital capacity.[49]

The authors concluded that myofascial release may be clinically useful in lowering respiratory rate in patients with chronic pain. Variance in the results may have resulted from inconsistent rest periods following treatment at each session before measuring post-test results.

Davis[50] and her students at the University of Miami presented a paper at the June 2002 annual scientific meeting of physical therapists that examined the effects of the JFB MFR approach on the fascial restrictions limiting a golf swing. Four men who were amateur golfers (handicap greater than 10) and 2 male professional golfers (handicap less than 10) underwent data collection on the golf course and in the clinic. The professional golfers were tested one time on the driving range to establish a best-practice benchmark for each of the variables. Of particular interest was the shoulder-hip relationship in rotation in the swing, named the X-factor by golf professionals. Each of the 4 subjects was videotaped swinging a golf club, and their X-factors were measured to compare with the measures obtained from the professionals. In addition, the 4 subjects underwent pre- and post-test measures of seated (static) thoracic rotation, dynamic shoulder and hip rotation, and swing speed measures. Each subject received 30 to 45 minutes of myofascial release from the same experienced therapist based on what limitations of fascia were found in each subject on examination. Individuals were given a home program to do daily and returned 2 weeks later for follow-up. A second treatment was given based on reexamination, and the home program was modified. Post-test measures were then taken following the second treatment.

The researchers found a significant positive correlation ($R_{pre} = 0.54$, $R_{post} = 0.82$, $R_{diff} = 0.79$) between seated thoracic rotation and swing speed. Significant or near-significant differences were also obtained when comparing professional and pretreatment amateur results for seated thoracic rotation ($P = .02$) and X-factor ($P = .07$). In sum, the researchers concluded that a myofascial release treatment program appears to play a role in improving certain identified soft-tissue range of motion variables, such that amateur golfers' performance more closely approximates that of professionals'. One subject reported an inability to play more than 8 holes of golf without back pain that persisted for several years. Following one treatment, which included the use of wedges to de-rotate the ilia, he played 18 holes without pain. One year later, he reported that he continued to play 18 holes without pain, and he was continuing with his home exercise wedging "sporadically."[50]

Davis and colleagues[50] also examined the effects of myofascial release integrated with therapeutic exercise on 2 older women (patient 1, 78 years old; patient 2, 82 years old) with severe kyphoscoliosis. Each subject received 2 weeks of treatment consisting of 45 minutes of myofascial release and 15 minutes of exercises 2 or 3 times each week. Each subject walked with a rolling walker and had received exercises alone for her osteoporosis and osteoarthritis for several years previously. Thus, each served as her own control with regard to reporting any differences that she experienced with this treatment protocol compared with exercise alone. Pre- and post-test measures examined pain (Visual Analog Scale [VAS]), range of motion, strength, balance (one leg stance and forward reach), quality of life (36-Item Short Form Survey), functional mobility (Timed Up and Go test), posture (Polaroid [Waltham, MA] grid pictures in 4 positions), vital capacity, and patient exit interview on videotape.

Results were that postural changes by grid picture were evident in both patients. Both patients experienced decrease in pain (4.8/10 to 2.1/10 and 10/10 to 4/10) and an improved quality of life following the final session with 2 weeks of treatment. Patient 1 also improved in Timed Up and Go and range of motion. Patient 2 improved in vital capacity, Timed Up and Go, functional reach, and one leg stance. Most significant with regard to myofascial release was that both patients in separate exit interviews described being acutely aware of the feeling of energy and release of tight tissue under the therapist's hands during treatment, an experience that they had never felt before with physical therapy. In addition, both, unbeknownst to the other, described feeling energized and able to function with more energy and "pep" for an average of 2 days after treatment.[44]

LeBauer et al[41] reported similar results utilizing the JFB MFR approach with a female adult patient with idiopathic scoliosis. The subject, who had a double major curve with a Cobb angle of 45 degrees, following 6 weeks of 2 60-minute MFR sessions/week, reported significant decrease in pain by VAS (4.8/10 to 1.8/10) and improvement in her quality of life and pulmonary function as measured by her Scoliosis Research Society-22 Questionnaire scores (3.82 to 4.45) and her University of California, San Diego Shortness of Breath Questionnaire scores (9 to 4).

Lewit and Olsanska[42] performed a study on the reduction of myofascial pain using myofascial release as described in this chapter on abdominal scars. They described the results in 51 subjects undergoing myofascial release to abdominal scars. Treatment produced marked immediate results in 36 of the 51 cases.

In the April 2007 issue of *Journal of Bodywork and Movement Therapies*, Russell[51] reported the effects of 3 weeks of Swedish massage along with myofascial release on a 35-year-old woman with restless legs syndrome (RLS). Forty-five–minute massage treatments were given twice weekly with a space of 2 days in between sessions. The subject kept a log, recording hours of sleep; nocturnal waking; intensity and type of RLS symptoms; caffeine, alcohol, tobacco, and medication intake; and an estimate of her stress level. Frequency, intensity, and duration of symptoms were kept in the Functional Rating Index before, during, and after the study. Tingling sensations, urgency to move the legs, and sleeplessness were decreased after 2 treatments and continued to improve throughout the 3 weeks. It was conjectured that massage and myofascial release may have increased the natural release of dopamine, which has been shown to improve symptoms of RLS.

MYOFASCIAL RELEASE AND PELVIC FLOOR DYSFUNCTION

Several studies have been reported in the literature on the effectiveness of myofascial release on pelvic dysfunction in women and men. Weiss,[52] for instance, investigated the effectiveness of a manual therapy technique similar or identical to myofascial release trigger point therapy for interstitial cystitis and urinary urgency/frequency. Forty-five women and 7 men (10 of whom had interstitial cystitis and 42 who had urgency-frequency syndrome) received myofascial release manual trigger point therapy to the pelvic floor for 1 to 2 visits each week for 8 to 12 weeks. Results tabulated from a completed symptom score sheet indicated the rate of improvement. Of the patients with urgency-frequency syndrome with or without pain, 35 (83%) experienced moderate to marked improvement or complete resolution of symptoms. Seven of the 10 (70%) with interstitial cystitis reported moderate to marked improvement. Ten of the patients also underwent electromyography, and mean resting pelvic floor tension decreased from 9.73 to 3.61 microvolts. Positive results were maintained for up to 12 months as long as patients continued practicing stress reduction techniques, Kegel exercises, and other physical therapy exercises.

In a 2005 review article on chronic pelvic pain published in *Johns Hopkins Advanced Studies in Medicine*, Learman said, "It is essential to address perpetuating mechanisms of pain. Patients with myofascial pain should be referred to physical therapists specializing in pelvic floor muscle work."[49]

Peters et al[53] published, "Prevalence of Pelvic Floor Dysfunction in Patients With Interstitial Cystitis" in the July 2007 issue of the journal *Urology*. They suggest that pelvic floor dysfunction may set off an inflammatory response to the pelvic organs, and that "myofascial release may be offered as the first line of symptoms."[53]

Hartmann et al[54] published the results of a survey identifying current practice trends of physical therapists specializing in women's health in the January 2007 issue of the *Journal of Reproductive Medicine*. An Internet poll in mid-2005 directed to physical therapists treating localized, provoked vulvodynia revealed that more than 70% of participants indicated that they included myofascial release of the pelvic girdle, pelvic floor, and associated structures along with exercise, joint mobilization, and neuromuscular reeducation. Typical care was 1 hour-long session once weekly for 7 to 15 weeks.

CONCLUSION

Myofascial release techniques as taught by Barnes were developed and are performed acknowledging that the prevailing view of the body as a machine is totally incorrect, and acknowledging that the fascia cannot be separated from each and every one of our 37 trillion cells that it surrounds. This approach starts with the belief that one must release, or minimize, the negative effects of the patient's fascial restrictions to obtain and secure permanent recovery from the causes of pain, limitation of motion, and paresthesia secondary to postural or structural malalignments. Further, the fascial restrictions responsible for the patient's symptoms may be located far away from the area in pain; therefore, treating the location of the symptoms alone is insufficient for long-lasting resolution.

Fascia is not effectively accessed by traditional mechanical methods, such as joint mobilization modalities or traditional stretching methods. Fascia, instead, responds to the combination of the intentional application of endogenous bioelectromagnetic energy fields and the sustained mechanical pressure at the myofascial barrier, through the palms and fingers of the therapist's hands, to soften the molecular structure of the fascia. The gentle, sustained mechanical pressure of the therapist's hands at the myofascial barrier facilitates a yielding or release of the restrictions.[5,35] The mind seems to store memories and experiences in restricted fascia, for upon the release of restrictions, patients commonly become transported back to an injurious experience and with similar emotion, relate the experience in detail. Once the trauma is completely experienced and the fascial restrictions have given way, healing can commence. We have yet to learn the complete cellular mechanism of the healing process, but it is believed that once restrictions are removed from the fascia, body energy, blood, lymph, neurotransmitters, neuropeptides, and steroids are free to flow, restoring balance, homeostasis, and overall health to the system.[5]

Traditional Western medical theory based on the philosophies of Newton and Descartes cannot explain these observed patient experiences and outcomes. However, the emerging new explanatory theory of mind-body holism, based on the quantum theory of the behavior and characteristics of atoms and molecules, offers explanations for these and many other "unexplainable" outcomes. The science of energy medicine is rapidly helping to answer many of the questions that have eluded us for decades.

JFB MFR techniques are not offered to replace traditional physical therapy techniques, but rather to supplement and enhance them as a complementary approach in evaluating and treating patients with pain, restriction of motion, and structural symptoms. Success in the application of these techniques requires therapists to keep an open mind regarding holism and mind-body theory, and to develop themselves personally in such a way that their manual techniques and their attitudes and priorities in care reflect a centered, creative, artful attention to the patient's description of the problems and to the feedback they receive from the patient's mind-body as they apply the treatment. Touch must be applied with compassionate intention, focused awareness, and the conscious purpose to mechanically and bioenergetically release fascial restrictions and, thus, facilitate the reorganization of the mind-body neuromuscular system.

Our goals are to learn from each patient; to teach by example; and to remain attentive, creatively focused, sensitive, nonjudgmental, supportive, and compassionate in accepting the patient's story as authentic and treatable. We must then document our results in detail to start building a database from which we can publish our outcomes so that all may benefit.

The JFB MFR approach offers a beginning into a new world of evaluation and care that is intelligent, based on sound theories, humane in its holistic approach, and effective when traditional mechanistic approaches to care have failed. The organization and publication of systematic and thorough documentation of qualitative and quantitative data is encouraged so that we can share results with one another for the good of all patients.

REFERENCES

1. Matthews A, Berger J, Herring J, Kimmins E, Michael M. The uses of myofascial release in occupational and physical therapy. Unpublished student research. Omaha, NE: Creighton University; 2013.
2. Travell JG. *Myofascial Pain and Dysfunction: The Trigger Point Manual*. Baltimore, MD: Lippincott Williams & Wilkins; 1983.
3. Scott J. Molecules that keep you in shape. *New Scientist*. 1986;111:49-53.
4. Oschman JL. *Energy Medicine: The Scientific Basis*. 2nd ed. New York, New York: Elsevier; 2016.
5. Barnes JF. *Myofascial Release: The Search for Excellence: A Comprehensive Evaluatory and Treatment Approach*. Paoli, PA: MFR Seminars; 1990.
6. Montague A. *Touching: The Human Significance of the Skin*. New York, NY: Harper & Row; 1971.
7. Barnes JF. The significance of touch. *Physical Therapy Forum*. 1988;7:10.
8. Juhan D. *Job's Body*. Barrytown, NY: Station Hill Press; 1987.
9. Netter FH. *The CIBA Collection of Medical Illustrations: Nervous Systems*. West Caldwell, NJ: CIBA; 1983:197.
10. Schleip R. Fascial plasticity—a new neurobiological explanation: Part 1. *J Bodyw Mov Ther*. 2003;7(1):11-19.
11. Kuhn TS. *The Structure of Scientific Revolutions*. Chicago, IL: University of Chicago Press; 1970.
12. Kurtz R. *Body-Centered Psychotherapy: The Hakomi Method*. Ashland, OR: The Hakomi Institute; 1988.
13. Bohm D. *The Special Theory of Relativity*. Boston, MA; Addison Wesley; 1988.
14. Gribbin J. *Quantum Physics: A Beginner's Guide to the Subatomic World*. New York, NY: DK Publishing, Inc.; 2002.
15. Pischinger A. *The Extracellular Matrix and Ground Regulation: Basis for a Holistic Biological Medicine*. Heine H, Eibl I, eds. Berkeley, CA: North Atlantic Books; 2007.
16. Page LE. *Academy of Applied Osteopathy Yearbook 1952 Selected Osteopathic Papers*. Carmel, CA: The Academy of Applied Osteopathy; 1952: 85-90.
17. Hall DA. The ageing of connective tissue. *Exp Gerontol*. 1968;3(2):77-89.
18. Oschman JL. Fascia as a body-wide communication system. In: Schleip R, Findley TW, Chaitow L, Huijing PA, eds. *Fascia: The Tensional Network of the Human Body: The Science and Clinical Applications in Manual and Movement Therapy*. Edinburgh, Scotland: Elsevier; 2012.
19. Ingber DE. Cellular mechanotransduction: putting the pieces together again. *FASEB J*. 2006;20(7):811-827.
20. Nelson CM, Bissell MJ. Of extracellular matrix, scaffolds, and signaling: tissue architecture regulates development, homeostasis and cancer. *Annu Rev Cell Dev Biol*. 2006;22:287-309.
21. Meltzer KR, Cao TV, Schad JF, King H, Stoll ST, Standley PR. In vitro modeling of repetitive motion injury and myofascial release. *J. Bodyw Mov Ther*. 2010;14(2):162-171.
22. Cao TV, Hicks MR, Campbell D, Standley PR. Dosed myofascial release in three-dimensional bioengineered tendons: effects on human fibroblast hyperplasia, hypertrophy, and cytokine secretion. *J Manipulative Physiol Ther*. 2013;36(8):513-521.
23. Pollack GH. Phase transition: a mechanism for action. In: Pollack GH, ed. *Cells, Gels and the Engines of Life*. Seattle, WA: Ebner and Sons; 2001:126-129.
24. Oschman JL. *Energy Medicine in Therapeutics and Human Performance*. London: Butterworth-Heinemann; 2003.
25. Ahn AC, Tewan M, Chi-Sang P, Phillips RS. The limits of reductionism in medicine: could systems biology offer an alternative? *PLoS Med*. 2006;3(6):e208.
26. Chaitow L. *Neuro-Muscular Technique—A Practitioner's Guide to Soft Tissue Mobilization*. New York, NY: Thorsons; 1985: 13-15.
27. Langevin HM. Connective tissue: a body-wide signaling network? *Med Hypotheses*. 2006;66(6):1074-1077.
28. Penrose R. *Shadows of the Mind: A Search for the Missing Science of Consciousness*. Oxford, England: Oxford University Press; 1994.
29. Discovery of quantum vibrations in 'microtubules' inside brain neurons supports controversial theory of consciousness. *Science Daily*. January 16, 2014. Accessed January 30, 2016. www.sciencedaily.com/releases/2014/01/140116085105.htm
30. Hameroff SR. "Funda-Mentality": is the conscious mind subtly linked to a basic level of the universe? *Trends Cogn Sci*. 1998;2(4):119-124.
31. Hameroff S. Quantum computation in brain microtubules? The Penrose-Hameroff "Orch OR" model of conciousness. *The Royal Society*. 1998;356(1743). doi: 10.1098/rsta.1998.0254.
32. Hameroff S, Penrose R. Consciousness in the universe. *Physics of Life Reviews*. 2013;11(1):39-78. doi:10.1016/j.plrev.2013.08.002
33. Hameroff S, Penrose R. Reply to criticism of the 'Orch OR qubit'—'Orchestrated objective reduction' is scientifically justified. *Physics of Life Reviews*. 2014;11:104-112.
34. Hameroff S, Penrose R. Consciousness in the universe: a review of the 'Orch OR' theory. *Physics of Life Reviews*. 2014;11(1):39-78.
35. Pollack G. Presentation on crystallized water in the body. Paper presented at: Third International Fascia Research Congress, Vancouver, CA. March, 2012
36. Selye H. *The Stress of Life*. New York, NY: McGraw-Hill; 1976.

37. Twomey L, Taylor J. Flexion, creep, dysfunction and hysteresis in the lumbar vertebral columns. *Spine (Phila Pa 1976)*. 1982;7(2):116-122.
38. *Dorland's Medical Directory*. 26th ed. Philadelphia, PA: WB Saunders; 1985.
39. Hameroff SR. Quantum coherence in microtubules: a neural basis for emergent consciousness. *J Consciousness Studies*. 1994;1(1):91-118.
40. Selye H. History and present status of the stress concept. In: Goldberger L, Breznitz S, eds. *Handbook of Stress*. New York, NY: Macmillan; 1982:7-20.
41. LeBauer A, Brtalik R, Stowe K. The effect of myofascial release (MFR) on an adult with idiopathic scoliosis. *J Bodyw Mov Ther*. 2008;12(4):356-363.
42. Lewit K, Olsanska S. Clinical importance of active scars: abdominal scars as a cause of myofascial pain. *J Manipulative Physiol Ther*. 2004;27(6):399-402.
43. Cubick EE, Quezada VY, Schumer AD, Davis CM. Sustained release myofascial release as treatment for a patient with complications of rheumatoid arthritis and collagenous colitis: a case report. *Int J Ther Massage Bodywork*. 2011;4(3):1-9.
44. Davis CM, Doerger C, Eaton T, Rowland J, Sauber C. Myofascial release (Barnes method) as complementary in physical therapy for two patients with osteoporosis and kyphoscoliosis: two case studies. *J Geriatric Physical Therapy*. 2002;25(3):33.
45. Ajimsha MS, Al-Mudahka NR, Al-Madzhar JA. Effectiveness of myofascial release: Systematic review of randomized controlled trials. *J Bodyw Mov Ther*. 2015;19(1):102-112.
46. Fernández-Pérez AM, Peralta-Ramirez MI, Pilat A, Moreno-Lorenzo C, Villaverde-Gutierrez C, Arroyo-Morales M. Can myofascial techniques modify immunological parameters? *J Alt Compl Med*. 2013;19(1):24-28.
47. Bezner JR, Boucher BK, Hernandez M. The effects of myofascial release techniques on pulmonary function measures. *Phys Ther*. 2001;81(5):A46.
48. Kegerreis S, Worrell T, Perry D. The immediate and cumulative effects of a myofascial release technique on the respiratory diaphragm. *Phys Ther*. 2001;81(5):A46.
49. Learman LA. Chronic pelvic pain—part 2: an integrated management approach. *Johns Hopkins Advanced Studies in Medicine*. 2005;5(7):360-366.
50. Davis CM, Schrodter BS, Klatt R. The effects of myofascial release treatment program on the musculoskeletal restrictions limiting the golf swing [abstract]. *Phys Ther*. 2002;82(16)
51. Russell M. Massage therapy and restless legs syndrome. *J Bodywork Movement Ther*. 2007;11(2):146-150.
52. Weiss JM. Pelvic floor myofascial trigger points: manual therapy for interstitial cystitis and the urgency-frequency syndrome. *J Urol*. 2001;166(6):2226-2231.
53. Peters KM, Carrico DJ, Kalinowski SE, Ibrahim IA, Diokno AC. Prevalence of pelvic floor dysfunction in patients with interstitial cystitis. *Urology*. 2007;70(1):16-18.
54. Hartmann D, Strauhal MF, Nelson CA. Treatment of women in the United States with localized provoked vulvodynia: practice survey of women's health physical therapists. *J Reprod Med*. 2007;52(1):48-52.

7

Therapeutic Massage and Rehabilitation

Janet Kahn, PhD, MT

This chapter is focused on the contributions of therapeutic massage in the rehabilitative process. Massage plays a central role in the emerging picture of integrative health care. In recent years, the use of massage has been recommended in 2 important guidelines on the diagnosis and treatment or management of pain. In 2007, "Diagnosis and Treatment of Low Back Pain: A Joint Clinical Practice Guideline From the American College of Physicians and the American Pain Society," was published in the *Annals of Internal Medicine*.[1] In it, their final recommendation reads, "For patients who do not improve with self-care options, clinicians should consider the addition of nonpharmacologic therapy with proven benefits...for chronic or subacute low back pain, intensive interdisciplinary rehabilitation, exercise therapy, acupuncture, massage therapy, spinal manipulation, yoga..."[1] The second guideline is from The Joint Commission (formerly known as the Joint Commission on Accreditation of Health Care Organizations and the Joint Commission on Accreditation of Hospitals) and became effective on January 1, 2015.[2] It is a clarification to its earlier pain management standard, in which it had suggested that both pharmacologic and nonpharmacologic approaches to pain management might be used, but it had provided no guidance on which nonpharmacologic approaches might be most helpful and when they should be used. The Joint Commission sets and assesses compliance with standards for hospitals, nursing care centers, home care, and office-based surgery practice programs across the United States. In the context of an increasingly robust literature on nonpharmacologic approaches to pain, and an increasing problem of opioid addiction in this country, The Joint Commission was encouraged to provide more clarification. In doing so, they recognize both the mix of therapeutic approaches to pain that can be effectively used in integrative health care and the importance of patient-centeredness as a tenet of integrative health care. This update says specifically, "[T]he following examples are not exhaustive, but strategies may include the following nonpharmacologic strategies: physical modalities (for example, acupuncture therapy, chiropractic therapy, osteopathic manipulative treatment, massage therapy, and physical therapy), relaxation therapy, and cognitive behavioral therapy..."

The document's final words acknowledge the current context[2]:

> Note: Treatment strategies for pain may include pharmacologic and nonpharmacologic approaches. Strategies should reflect a [patient]-centered approach and consider the patient's current presentation, the health care provider's clinical judgment, and the risks and benefits associated with the strategies, including potential risk of dependency, addiction, and abuse.

Davis CM.
Integrative Therapies in Rehabilitation: Evidence for Efficacy in Therapy,
Prevention, and Wellness, Fourth Edition (pp 75-98).

The previously stated guidelines are responsive not only to the research literature and addiction issues, but also to public preference. Data from the 2007 National Health Interview Survey, which is conducted by the Centers for Disease Control and Prevention's National Center for Health Statistics, reveal that more than 18 million Americans received at least one massage during that year; collectively, they made over 95 million visits to massage therapists and paid over $4 billion for these treatments.[3] What value do they find that prompts this expenditure? And should the health care system itself also be valuing massage and incorporating it more frequently into rehabilitation care?

To discuss massage and rehabilitation meaningfully requires a closer look at the concept of rehabilitation. Therapeutic massage can play a meaningful role in an individual's rehabilitation from injury, illness, repetitive strain, and the like. Just as importantly, however, massage has the potential, along with many of the modalities described in this book, to rehabilitate the current culture—a culture that, in viewing people as machine-like in their employment, has created jobs that produce repetitive strain syndromes because they are not planned around the realities of human bodies; a culture that is so confused about touch that we have an epidemic of inappropriate touch and have responded to that epidemic by banning touch in schools (and in certain professions) rather than engaging in reeducation about it; a culture that teaches "physical education" in public school without imparting much, if any, information about one's body, and that includes instructions to overrule the signs from the body that an activity or position is painful and to press on anyway. This is a culture in need of rehabilitation, in need of re-understanding the opportunities and limitations of human embodiment. Massage, along with yoga and other movement therapies, can be tremendously helpful in this regard.

THINKING ABOUT THERAPEUTIC MASSAGE

It is estimated that there are between 300,000 and 350,000 massage therapists in the United States today.[4] While all offer healing through touch, there can be wide variation in their methods. Some massage therapists practice within a Western biomechanical framework of anatomy and physiology, while others practice within an energy-based Eastern view. Even with this variation, however, massage therapists share a view of the integrity of the human being. This has been beautifully stated by Deane Juhan, author of *Job's Body: A Handbook for Bodywork,* in the following passage: "The skin is no more separated from the brain than the surface of a lake is separate from its depths… the two are different locations in a continuous medium…The brain is a single functional unit, from cortex to fingertips to toes. To touch the surface is to stir the depths."[5]

When thinking about the contemporary practice of therapeutic massage in the United States, it is helpful to keep at least 2 things in mind. First, massage is an ancient healing practice (or, more accurately, an array of practices) that is newly emerging as a health care profession and struggling, with real ambivalence, to meet the demands of that status. Second, to understand massage in the 21st century in the United States, it is helpful to view it as a modality with important roots in at least 3 separate streams: (1) sports and fitness, (2) medicine, and (3) the various wellness and human potential movements of the past 5 decades.

HISTORY

In grasping the ties of massage to medicine, it is important to remember that massage is not, in and of itself, a whole system of medicine, but rather has been an integral component of virtually every form of medicine that humans have ever devised. The Asian roots of massage reach to the origins of both Chinese and Ayurvedic medicine. Massage appears in the ancient medical texts of China, Japan, and Tibet. Its use in many countries has continued uninterrupted to the present time. In its earliest recorded forms and in contemporary Asian practice, massage therapy has been used for the promotion of well-being and for treating (if not curing) the injuries and ailments that inevitably arise over the course of a lifetime.

In contrast to the Asian experience, the inclusion of therapeutic massage in Western medicine has been erratic. Both Greek and Roman practices included it. We find specific prescriptions for rubbing, friction, chest-clapping, and so forth in the writings of Hippocrates, Galen of Pergamon, and Celsus.[6] Massage was used to treat injuries, such as sprains and dislocations, and to alleviate weariness. Alexander the Great is known to have traveled with a personal *triptai* (ie, massage therapist) for just that purpose. Massage was also used to prepare athletes before competition and to help them in postgame recovery. During the Middle Ages, classical writings about the medical uses of massage were destroyed. Nonetheless, massage continued as part of folk practice and was reintroduced as a medical treatment during the Renaissance. The French surgeon Ambroise Paré (1510-1590) wrote of massage as a treatment for both postoperative healing and joint stiffness. An important figure in developing therapeutic massage as we know it today is Pehr Henrik Ling (1766-1839), who developed a system of passive and active movements he named *medical gymnastics*, later known as the *Swedish movement cure*.[7] In the 19th century, these medical gymnastics were used to treat respiratory ailments, including asthma and emphysema; gastrointestinal problems, including constipation and incontinence; and nervous conditions, such as neuralgic pain and epilepsy.

While Ling is often credited with bringing a scientific base to massage by grounding it in the study of anatomy and physiology, the Dutch physician Johann Georg Mezger (1838-1909) systematized the work by grouping all known methods into 4 categories of soft tissue manipulation (STM): (1) gliding, (2) kneading, (3) friction, and (4) percussive strokes. Mezger's enthusiastic students had much to do with the reintroduction of massage into medical settings in the late 19th and early 20th centuries.[8]

Interest in massage in the United States heightened during World War I, when Americans became aware of the rehabilitation work available for soldiers (and civilians) among the allied nations. The Reconstruction Department of the United States Army was initiated in 1918 and included both physiotherapy and occupational therapy. Mary McMillan, a prominent figure in the development of physical therapy in England and founder of physical therapy in the United States, served as chief aide at Walter Reed Hospital in Washington DC, taught special courses in war-related reconstruction at Reed College Clinic, Portland, Oregon during World War I, and was director of physiotherapy at Harvard Medical School, Cambridge, Massachusetts from 1921 to 1925, during which time she wrote her text, *Massage and Therapeutic Exercise*. McMillan defined the 5 major strokes of Western massage as effleurage, petrissage, tapotement, friction, and vibration.[8]

While massage continued to be an important part of physical therapy treatment through World War II, its use declined after that time. Increasing availability of potent pharmaceuticals and reliance on technology in the fields of both physical therapy and nursing rendered the relatively labor intensive, and therefore costly, massage a less frequently prescribed treatment throughout the late 1940s and 1950s, through to the present.

In the 1960s, renewed interest in massage came less through medicine and more through the human potential movement. The field of therapeutic massage and bodywork benefited tremendously from opportunities that arose at the Esalen Institute in Big Sur, California, and other gathering places of the human potential movement from the intermingling of bodyworkers and psychotherapists. Here, through an exploration of the links between mental and bodily ease and distress, notions of wellness were expanded and new modalities, such as Rolfing, bioenergetics, and Aston-Patterning, were developed. This deepened the exploration of the relationship between human structure and consciousness, which had begun earlier in Europe, and is likely the greatest American contribution to the field.[9] It brought attention to the relationship between practitioner and client in creating and maximizing therapeutic effects,[10,11] an aspect of healing still in need of systematic investigation, even as the terms *patient centered* and *relationship centered* are increasingly used to describe the care offered at contemporary academic health centers and hospitals.

CONTEMPORARY PRACTICE OF
THERAPEUTIC MASSAGE IN THE UNITED STATES

In this chapter, the term *therapeutic massage* refers to the vast array of massage and bodywork modalities in use today because most massage therapists are trained in, and employ, multiple approaches. Thousands of massage therapists are trained in methods, some of which are described in other chapters of this book, such as myofascial release, neuromuscular therapy, craniosacral therapy, Rolfing, Hellerwork, Reiki, polarity, reflexology, the Trager approach, classical Swedish massage, and, to a lesser extent, the Alexander technique and the Feldenkrais Method. The field encompasses work with the soft tissues of the body (muscle, fascia, ligaments), the lymphatic system (manual lymph drainage and Swedish massage), and work in which the focus is largely energetic, whether within a framework of energy meridians (eg, shiatsu, tuina) or within a more Western concept of an energy field (eg, Reiki, therapeutic touch, polarity therapy).

A single massage treatment may incorporate many kinds of strokes performed with a variety of intentions. Both the technique and the intention are important. Physically speaking, massage therapists glide, knead, tap, compress, stretch, roll, shake, vibrate, apply friction in various ways, and simply hold, quietly, while bringing our own attention and that of the client to the area that we are holding. Through these strokes, we engage not only the musculoskeletal system, but also the circulatory, lymphatic, and nervous systems. Slow, gliding strokes of Swedish massage, for instance, engage the parasympathetic nervous system and induce a generalized relaxation response at the same time that they increase the circulation of fluids and relax the muscles themselves.[10] The various forms of therapeutic or orthopedic massage are applied with a greater attention to anatomic specificity, targeting specific muscles, ligaments, or fascia in response to the practitioner's assessment of the cause of the client's pain or dysfunction.

Massage therapists take a holistic view of the client and his or her condition. Our assessment includes a thorough history to help us to understand this "incident" of injury or pain, the full story of what this client's body/mind has experienced (eg, injuries, accidents), periods of unusual emotional or physical stress, and the "usual" stresses that he or she may experience at work or home (eg, physical stresses of work [lifting or computer use], psychological stresses). Physical examination includes observation and palpation. We observe the client's posture while sitting and standing, his or her movement in walking, active and passive range of motion, and his or her physical holding patterns in both the face and the body. All of these give us strong clues about the experience of being in that body and about primary and secondary pain patterns. Once the client is on the massage table, the assessment continues as we notice, again through observation, how the person and his or her body lies on the table and whether there are areas of vasomotor reaction. Through observation and palpation we can detect myofascial restrictions, chronic holding patterns of muscular tension, scar tissue and adhesions, and skin temperature indicating areas where energy and/or blood is not flowing efficiently and/or areas of hyperthermia.

This initial assessment allows the therapist to form a preliminary view of what is happening and to create an initial treatment plan. Therapeutic massage, however, is an ongoing dance of constant treatment and assessment. More is learned as we see how the tissue, and the client as a whole, respond to each stroke.

CASE EXAMPLE

I worked with a client who was scheduled for carpal tunnel surgery. Massage was her "last ditch" attempt to avoid the upcoming surgery. As I put my hands on the area of her upper trapezius, I found a particular pattern of nonresponsiveness in the tissue that, as I have learned from my experience, is sometimes the expression of a particular reaction to caffeine. I asked her about her caffeine intake, and the client informed me that she consumed an average of 4 to 5 cups of coffee, 3 to 5 cans of cola, and a bit of chocolate virtually every day. There are clients who can tolerate a similar amount of caffeine without it causing problematic effects on their muscles, but for this individual, as for a significant percentage of people, it created extreme chronic tension in her shoulders and neck and led to nerve impingement and diminished use of her hands that mimicked carpal tunnel syndrome. A combination of myofascial work and Swedish massage on the client's neck and upper extremities, along with a significant decrease in her caffeine consumption, rendered her able to return to quilting, gardening, and computer use without surgery.

SKILLS AND MINDSET OF THE MASSAGE THERAPIST

It is of the utmost importance that the physical work of massage takes place within the context of the practitioner/client relationship. Embedded in this relationship are both the specific intention the practitioner is holding for that session and the overall view that the practitioner holds of his or her own role and the role of the client in the healing process. It also includes the quality of the rapport that is established between them.

The rehabilitation of both the client and the culture begins with the view of integrity, of body-mind unity, that the practitioner holds, as described in the previous quote from Juhan.[5] The understanding that we stir the depths when we touch the surface (the skin) applies to many levels, including the level of the neurotransmitters and the information they provide about how we are, and perhaps even at the levels of the psyche and the soul itself.[12] Awareness of our potential to touch at this depth prompts a sense of reverence that many massage therapists experience as we work, and to which clients readily respond. Tracy Walton has described it in the following way[13]:

> By touching a body, we touch every event it has experienced. For a few brief moments we hold all of a client's stories in our hands. We witness someone's experience of their own flesh, through some of the most powerful means possible; the contact of our hands, the acceptance of the body without judgment, and the occasional listening ear. With these gestures, we reach across the isolation of the human experience and hold another person's legend. In massage therapy, we show up and ask, in so many ways, what it is like to be another human being. In doing so, we build a bridge that may heal us both.

This level of inquiry is not unique to massage therapists. Acupuncturists, psychotherapists, nurses, and others sometimes also speak of *healing presence* or *therapeutic presence* as core to the effectiveness of their work. The massage therapist holds this awareness, this way of being with another, while he or she touches.

Within this overall unfolding relationship, the practitioner holds a conscious intention toward one or more of the following, which will guide the treatment: to promote relaxation or comfort, to promote increased body-mind integration through kinesthetic awareness or somatoemotional repatterning, and/or to promote physiological or structural change (eg, increased circulation, reduction of muscular or fascial hypertonicity). Table 7-1 presents many of the massage and bodywork modalities clustered under these 3 headings of intention. Although not exhaustive in scope, this framework organizes a number of the terms familiar to the public and acknowledges that many modalities can be used for more than one of the intentions listed.

Being able to work with intention, both large and small, requires a number of skills. Andrade and Clifford[14] have conceptualized what they refer to as *intelligent touch*, which they consider as being comprised of the following 5 distinct abilities:

1. Attention: Described as "the capacity to focus on the sensory information that the practitioner receives primarily, but not exclusively, through her hands."[14] This would include the ability to detect meaningful variations in tissue temperature, texture, and tension as described previously, as well as the learned ability to detect information specific to a particular modality, such as the cranial rhythm that is a source of critical information about the craniosacral system and the health of the dura.

TABLE 7-1
TAXONOMY OF THERAPEUTIC MASSAGE AND BODYWORK ORGANIZED BY INTENTION

TO PROMOTE RELAXATION OR COMFORT

- Swedish massage
- Esalen massage
- Craniosacral therapy
- Trager psychophysical integration
- Reiki
- Polarity
- Energy balancing
- Therapeutic touch

TO PROMOTE KINESTHETIC AWARENESS, NEUROMUSCULAR EFFECTIVENESS, OR SOMATOEMOTIONAL REPATTERNING

- Craniosacral therapy
- Aston-Patterning
- Rolfing
- Alexander technique
- Feldenkrais Method
- Trager psychophysical integration
- Myofascial release
- Rubenfeld synergy method
- Hellerwork
- Muscle energy techniques
- Proprioceptive neuromuscular facilitation

TO PROMOTE PHYSIOLOGICAL OR STRUCTURAL CHANGE

- Swedish massage
- Neuromuscular techniques
- Myofascial techniques
- Rolfing
- Trager psychophysical integration
- Sports massage
- Lymphatic drainage
- Reflexology
- Oriental massage
- Muscle energy techniques
- Proprioceptive neuromuscular facilitation

2. Discrimination: Described as a refinement of the ability that comes with increasing familiarity with the feel of tissue over time and the clinical implications of the variations we find.

3. Identification: Described as the ability to know what you are touching based on a thorough knowledge of anatomy and the skill in knowing the implications of what you are feeling in terms of identifying healthy and dysfunctional tissue conditions.

4. Inquiring touch: Described previously as the continual dance of treatment and assessment; the authors consider this constant inquiry to be a hallmark of a good clinician.

5. Intention: Described as an important clinical skill, with the therapist's overall intention being "to produce as close to the ideal tissue response as possible, given the constraints of the client's characteristics and the clinical setting."[14]

Effective communication is another essential skill of the massage therapist. In addition to the hands-on work of massage, we also talk. Education is an important aspect of many massage treatments and encompasses everything from a reminder to breathe when the client seems to be forgetting; to an exploration and analysis of the client's work situation from the placement of the video screen and mouse; to proper sitting, standing, and lifting postures. Client education may also include suggestions for visualization during therapy or simply information about the body/mind so that the client can work in harmony with him- or herself and attune to, and thus enhance, the treatment.

Shapiro and Schwartz[15] also offer important reflections on intention, which they refer to as the how and why of paying attention. The effects of our attention will be most beneficial, they suggest, when the attention has such "mindfulness qualities" as acceptance, nonjudgmentalism, patience, gentleness, generosity, and the like. These qualities echo the previously mentioned words that Walton used to describe what the massage therapist brings to the client: "…the contact of our hands, the acceptance of the body without judgment, and the… listening ear."[13] At its best, massage therapy offers the client a direct experience of these qualities through the presence and contact of the therapist, and encouragement to offer him or her to him- or herself.

In addressing the why of attention, Shapiro and Schwartz[15] encourage an awareness of larger contexts in which the system, or a symptom, exists. In this way, we encourage clients to reduce tension in the neck muscles, through the breath, and by other means to ease the whole body, and through the heart to ease the tension with which they regard themselves and others. Just as the neck is part of the larger body, so too are we part of a larger social body. Our ability to bring ease, a lessening of constriction, to our corner of the world will have benefit throughout.

Offering this sort of accepting attention to our clients is a form of deep intimacy. This is as true in the many forms of bodywork that are performed with the client fully clothed as it is in practices performed with the client naked and draped. Helping clients to learn to bring such nonjudgmental attention to themselves offers them a beautiful exercise in self-intimacy. This is an important aspect of our much-needed social rehabilitation.

SKILLS AND MINDSET OF THE CLIENT

The physical aspect of massage is often a part of a larger healing process. If, for instance, a massage therapist is treating someone who has frequent headaches, his or her goals will be to relieve the immediate symptoms (headache pain), to ascertain and begin to address the myofascial patterns that produce frequent headaches, and to enlist the client in his or her own long-term care. The therapist's job is to help the client to become aware of personal patterns—postural, dietary, emotional—that may contribute to the headaches. The therapist will also want to help clients to discover the physical early warning signs of an approaching headache. If, for example, the headaches are caused by chronic tension in the muscles of the neck and/or jaw, one may be able to avert a real headache by noticing slight increases in the tendency to clench the jaw, hunch the shoulders, constrict the breath, jut the chin, and so forth. By noticing and addressing these early shifts, a client can undo minor tension before it culminates in an excruciating headache. Part of the massage therapist's job, then, is to help clients to learn how to pay attention to themselves. This attunement to the self, to one's own body and emotions, and the ability to constantly and gently release tension and adjust posture, breath, and attitude toward ease is a critical step toward lasting and creative rehabilitation for the client and for the culture. It is lasting because it is a skill that can be applied again and again. It is creative because it is a skill that can be applied to new situations. If one learns attunement to address one's headaches, it can be used later to attune to an injured limb, to the holding of breath that leaves one feeling anything less than optimal, to the rush of adrenaline that follows a near miss in traffic, and so forth.

Again, Shapiro and Schwartz[15] have coined the term *intentional systemic mindfulness* to describe the gentle loving attention a person can learn to bring to him- or herself for healing and simply for good living. Self-regulation is the process through which any system, whether an organism or an organization, maintains itself as functional within changing circumstances. Feedback loops, both positive and negative, allow the system to take in and use information about itself and the environment it is in. Enhanced attention clearly will lead to more effective self-regulation, and therapeutic massage has the capacity to increase one's awareness through the educational methods just described in the hypothetical example of the client with headaches because massage can give the client the felt experience of an alternative to the usual state. This experience of newfound relaxation, absence of pain, shift in posture, and the like can be used as a homing device, providing the client with a home base in contrast to which the pain or tension can be recognized and attended to. In sum, Schwartz[16] has explained that enhanced or conscious attention leads to connection, which, in turn, leads to self-regulation followed by order and health.

Importance of Space and Other Gifts of Massage

Clients often express a sense of timelessness during a massage. In sharp contrast with much of life, massage gives us a chance to quiet our minds, tune into our bodies, and experience the subtlest of sensations. Under these circumstances, our sense of time changes. As time opens up, so does space. Muscles become longer and broader when they relax. On the cellular level, more space is created or, more accurately, found, since its potential is always there. As space opens up, so does time. We live in an era when people complain frequently about a lack of time and/or space. We experience our lives as crowded. Even when they are crowded with people and activities we love, we experience the crowding itself as discomfort, as pain. We can reestablish a sense of well-being at any moment by bringing our attention back into the body and finding/creating space there. We can do this with the help of a massage therapist, who helps to create space within our tissues. We can also do this ourselves by bringing breath directly into the tissues and creating space that way.

Space is possible, unmanifested potential. With possibility comes choice. Addiction can be viewed as the absence of choice. It is a response or a reaction to a stimulus or circumstance without conscious thought or purposeful decision about what to do. When the phone rings, we can automatically answer it immediately or we can take a moment to decide whether we want to talk on the phone at this moment. When food is put before us, we can eat it right away because it is there or we can take a moment to notice whether we are hungry and, if so, whether this is what we want to eat. We can only make these choices, however, if we notice that there is a moment, a space in time, in which to make a decision. The absence of noticing this space is reaction, much like an automatic reflex. It is easier to notice space in time when we are living in a more spacious environment within our own body. This is one of the gifts that massage can offer.

MASSAGE AND OUR MILITARY SERVICES:
A NEW REHABILITATION CRISIS

The United States is facing an unprecedented need for skill rehabilitation. Over 2.7 million men and women had served in Iraq and/or Afghanistan, and well over 1.6 million are now veterans, many in need of multiple services, including the 970,000 diagnosed with an officially recognize disability resulting from war.[17] Veterans returning from Iraq and Afghanistan experience a complex mix of physical, emotional, and spiritual injuries that remain, as the headlines tell us, inadequately addressed. In fact, some of them remain ill-defined. A recent Department of Veterans Affairs (VA) utilization report indicates that for veterans of Operation Iraqi Freedom, Operation Enduring Freedom, and Operation New Dawn (OIF/OEF/OND), "The three most frequent diagnoses of Veterans were musculoskeletal ailments (principally joint and back disorders), mental disorders, and 'Symptoms, Signs and Ill-Defined Conditions.'"[17]

Physically, many veterans return to the United States with chronic pain of diverse causes, including musculoskeletal damage incurred while carrying extremely heavy packs in challenging terrain, traumatic brain injury, spinal injuries, and phantom limb pain, among others.[18] At least 17.5% of OEF/OIF/OND veterans in treatment at the VA are diagnosed with lower back conditions within 7 years of deployment, and 17% have diagnoses in other joints.[19]

While the causes may differ and those suffering may be somewhat younger, these wars appear to be generating a military counterpart to the epidemic of chronic pain experienced in civilian society.[19] In both spheres, there is and will continue to be a critical need for nonpharmacologic approaches to managing some of this pain to stem the tide of opioid abuse and addiction already experienced by veterans, active duty military, and civilians.[20,21]

Those returning from deployment may also have depression, post-traumatic stress disorder (68.2%),[1] and other emotional and mental conditions that interfere with daily life. OEF/OIF/OND have also produced a level and frequency of spiritual trauma—or *moral injury*, as it is often called—that is impossible to ignore even while prevalence has not yet been clearly established.[22]

The body of literature on the effects of active military and veteran use of complementary and alternative medicine (CAM) is growing, and both the VA and the Department of Defense discuss it on their websites, have ongoing pilot studies of CAM interventions, and at varying levels facilitate access to integrative health care. The VA health care system, the largest integrated care system in the United States,[23] is now making certain that CAM approaches are available as treatment options for chronic pain, including chiropractic care and acupuncture.

CAM is widely accepted by veterans. A 2011 randomized controlled trial (RCT) evaluated veterans' prior use and willingness to use various types of CAM.[24] Conducted in 5 VA primary care clinics, and utilizing a sample of 401 veterans experiencing chronic noncancer pain authors examined self-reported prior use and willingness to try chiropractic care, massage therapy, herbal medicines, and acupuncture. A majority of these veterans (n = 327; 82%) reported prior use one or more CAM modalities and nearly all (n = 399; 99%) were willing to try CAM treatment for pain. Massage therapy was the most preferred option (96%), chiropractic the least preferred (75%). The authors suggested that "…CAM may have broad appeal among veterans with chronic pain." The VA and military may, as has often been the case, constitute the leading edge of testing new rehabilitative treatment—in this case, therapeutic massage.

As an emerging health care profession, therapeutic massage has a relatively small, although growing, body of scientific evaluation. The early research in particular, while invaluable in pointing out important directions of inquiry, is often of limited enduring utility due to methodological limitations, including small sample size, lack of randomization, inability to ensure reproducibility of the therapy, absence of a meaningful comparison or control group, and inadequate blinding.[25,26] In general, the quality of the research has improved in the past 20 years, but it is still hindered by relatively low funding levels. Meta-analyses are limited by heterogeneity across studies—in the massage interventions themselves, duration of individual treatments, extent of the total intervention, and the outcomes assessed.[27,28]

While some of these issues arise in the early literature of many professions, due in part to low funding levels, there are some particular design issues that arise in the massage research literature. For instance, many studies include co-interventions that make it impossible for researchers to evaluate the specific effects of massage. Others have evaluated massage delivered by individuals who were not fully trained massage therapists and/or were following treatment protocols that did not reflect common (or adequate) massage practice. In a 2006 review of trials for massage and neck pain, Haraldsson et al said, "Most studies lacked a definition, description, or rationale for massage, the massage technique or both. In some cases, it was questionable whether the massage in the study would be considered effective massage under any circumstance."[29] The field still lacks literature on best practices for particular conditions, rendering it impossible to know whether the "best" practice was tested in a trial. In addition, it should be said at the outset that few theories about the mechanism of action for the effects that we see have been tested. With those provisos in mind, and acknowledging that the quality of massage research is steadily improving, we can consider the available literature. This includes 2 recent studies that have sought to establish optimal dosing for massage.

Systematic Reviews Involving Massage Therapy

A search of MEDLINE and the Cochrane Library yielded over 170 systematic reviews that included massage research. Few were relevant to our purposes. While the authors of an important 1994 review on the clinical effectiveness of massage commented that, "the lack of scientific rigor of the studies retrieved was the most outstanding finding of the search,"[30] the evidence has improved since then. For example, a 2004 review by the same lead author said that massage has "shown a significant promise in the treatment of musculoskeletal conditions,"[31] specifically citing back pain. In addition, a 2005 review reported, "Massage seems more beneficial than sham treatment for chronic nonspecific LBP [low back pain] but effectiveness compared with other conventional therapies is inconclusive."[32] The benefits from massage that were noted by the authors included both reduction in pain and increase in function. The back pain literature will be discussed in further detail later in this chapter.

One review examined 4 studies relevant to whether therapeutic massage as an adjuvant to routine nursing care could improve critically ill patients' ability to cope with the intensive care unit (ICU) experience.[23,33] The massage interventions varied across studies from 1 to 17 minutes, and the only RCT discussed in the review included patients with quite different reasons for being in the ICU. Nonetheless, the authors concluded that massage "could be profoundly beneficial to critically ill patients on a general level."[33]

While a 1998 review of nonpharmacologic strategies for managing cancer pain yielded only one small RCT involving massage,[34] much more research has been done on massage for cancer pain since then including a 1990 nonblind RCT by Weinrich and Weinrich[35] with 2 arms: massage and conversation control. Their single outcome measure was a visual analogue scale (VAS) of pain administered at baseline, post-treatment, 1 hour post-treatment, and 2 hours post-treatment. The subjects were 28 hospitalized cancer patients (mean age, 61.5 years) paired by medication prior to randomization. The treatment was a 10-minute Swedish back rub administered by a nursing student. While the authors concluded that men had immediate short-term pain relief ($P = .01$) from massage, it should be noted that men in the treatment group indicated twice the pain level of women in the treatment group prior to receiving massage. Thus, pain intensity could easily be at least as relevant as gender in determining the effect of treatment. While this study was hardly conclusive, it suggested that massage might be an effective treatment for cancer-related pain.

Since that time, dozens of studies have been conducted evaluating massage as a treatment for symptoms of cancer, including pain, anxiety, and nausea. The largest of these, an outcome study and not an RCT, was an evaluation of pre- and post-massage data from 1290 patients with cancer receiving massage at the facilities of Memorial Sloan Kettering Cancer Center in New York, New

York.[36] Both inpatients and outpatients were included, all of whom completed pre- and post-VAS evaluations of their pain, anxiety, nausea, fatigue, and depression levels. Results were strongly positive, with reduction of all symptoms noted for both inpatients and outpatients. For the outpatients, who received somewhat longer massages, the improvements lasted through the 48-hour follow-up period of this study. A 2005 review on the topic concluded[37]:

> Conventional care for patients with cancer can safely incorporate massage therapy, although cancer patients may be at higher risk of rare adverse events. The strongest evidence for benefits of massage is for stress and anxiety reduction, although research for pain control and management of other symptoms common to patients with cancer, including pain, is promising.

A 2000 review evaluating evidence for a number of CAM modalities in relation to the end-of-life symptoms of pain, dyspnea, and nausea identified only 3 studies of massage.[38] Two were case series and the third was the previously mentioned Weinrich and Weinrich study.[35] A review focusing on CAM therapies for treating multiple sclerosis included 3 relevant RCTs—one on STM,[39] one on Feldenkrais awareness through movement,[40] and one on reflexology.[41] The variation in these treatments illustrates one of the challenges in the field. While all 3 studies were deemed methodologically weak, they do show enough promise to warrant further investigation. The first 2 studies showed treatment group improvements in reducing anxiety, stress, and depression. The reflexology group showed significant improvement in multiple sclerosis-related symptoms, including paresthesia, urinary symptoms, muscle strength, and spasticity.

A 1999 review of studies on low back pain yielded 4 RCTs, all with small sample sizes and other limitations.[27] Two of the studies included massage only as a control condition for investigations focused on other modalities, and little attention was actually given to the massage treatment. One of the studies found massage to be superior to no treatment, 2 found massage as effective as spinal manipulation, and another found massage to be inferior to spinal manipulation. These findings are fairly positive given the minimal attention paid to designing the massage intervention. Not surprisingly, the authors concluded that more research was needed.[27] Fortunately, additional research has been conducted, and these more recent and more carefully designed studies are discussed later in the chapter. Remaining reviews either were not directly relevant to rehabilitation issues or covered uses of massage only in combination treatments that did not allow a real look at the value of this modality alone.

PATTERNS OF MASSAGE USAGE

In 2002, Cherkin et al[42] conducted a survey of licensed acupuncturists, chiropractors, massage therapists, and naturopathic physicians. They gathered systematic data from practitioners in 2 states, Washington and Connecticut, for each of these 4 modalities, including information on the practitioners themselves, their clients, and the purposes for which their clients came to them for care. Washington and Connecticut are similar in that both states had statewide licensure and different in that only Washington had mandated insurance coverage for massage. This study remains the most systematic examination of American's reasons for seeking massage treatment. Information from more than 2000 visits to these massage therapists indicates that 63% of the visits were for musculoskeletal concerns, of which roughly 75% were for chronic problems and 25% were for acute issues. Within that 63% of visits for musculoskeletal pain, back pain was the largest subcategory (20%), followed by neck (17%) and shoulder (8%) complaints. The second most-common reason for visits was wellness/relaxation (19%), which, if coupled with visits for reduction of stress and/or anxiety (5%), accounted for nearly 1 in 4 visits.[43] We will examine the literature for both of these uses, as each in its own way is relevant to successful rehabilitative efforts.

Massage for Musculoskeletal Pain

Back Pain

As noted in the introduction to this chapter, we have seen significant growth in the body of research on massage for musculoskeletal pain over the last 15 years. In his 1999 systematic review of the literature on massage for back pain, Ernst[27] located only 4 clinical trials in which therapeutic massage was employed as a single therapy intervention, and each of these was considered to have serious methodological problems. The author concluded that, while there was some suggestion that therapeutic massage may be an effective treatment for low back pain, the paucity and quality of data precluded any confident estimation. More research was encouraged; and more research has been done. A 2009 review by Furlan et al[44] examined 13 RCTs.[45-57] Although it is very common for massage to be used as an adjunct to other physical treatments for pain, this review only included trials in which the effect of massage could be extracted separately.

Massage was compared with an inert therapy (sham treatment) in 2 studies, both of which found that massage was superior for pain and function on both short- and long-term follow-ups. Eight studies compared massage with other active treatments and found that massage was similar to exercises and that massage was superior to joint mobilization, relaxation therapy, physical therapy, acupuncture, and self-care education. The beneficial effects of massage in patients with chronic low back pain lasted at least 1 year after the end of the treatment.

The 2 most-rigorous studies of the 13 studies examined by Furlan et al[44] were those of Cherkin et al[42] and Preyde et al.[56] Cherkin's team randomized 232 subjects with persistent low back pain to receive massage, acupuncture, or self-care education (via booklet and video). Acupuncturists and massage therapists were given treatment parameters that provided reasonable definition to the treatments while allowing practitioners to use their best clinical judgment in treating their clients within those parameters. Massage therapists were limited to STM (eg, no energy balancing) and could not use Asian techniques that would be too similar to acupuncture. Within those limitations, they could employ a host of techniques, including Swedish, neuromuscular, and myofascial strokes. This was an important innovation in research design because, compared to more rigid protocols, it more nearly approximates the kind of patient-tailored mixed-technique massage that one might receive in many therapists' offices. Outcomes included functionality as measured by the Roland Morris Disability Scale, bothersomeness of symptoms, disability, satisfaction with care, and cost of care. In the short-term (at 10 weeks post-treatment), massage had a significant effect on symptoms ($P = .015$) and function (Roland; $P = .01$) and reduced reported use of pain medications. At 42 weeks post-treatment, massage benefits persisted and subjects showed a decrease of 30% to 45% in annual low back pain care costs than did the other groups. Thus, the massage treatment resulted in both immediate and sustained relief, surpassing the effects of both acupuncture and self-care.

While the Cherkin et al[45] study demonstrated that massage offered relief that lasted well beyond the period of treatment, it did not, however, shed any light on why this is true. Perhaps it is because the treatments designed by the practitioners actually addressed not only the symptomatic issues of pain, but also the underlying causes of it. Perhaps the pain relief was sustained because the educational suggestions regarding exercise and posture allowed the clients to stave off any subsequent episodes of low back pain. It was acknowledged that additional research would be required to shed light into that black box and to confirm the findings through replication.

The study conducted by Preyde and her team[55] also offered an important innovation. Investigators compared what they called *comprehensive massage therapy* (CMT), composed of STM and exercise, with posture education (E&E), with each of those components delivered individually, thus offering some insight into what might be contributing to the effect of therapeutic massage treatments for low back pain. They randomized a convenience sample of 98 patients with subacute low back pain to 1 of the 3 previously listed conditions or to a sham laser treatment. Subjects were given 6 sessions within a 1-month time period. The STM was a 30- to 35-minute treatment with primarily friction and trigger point massage. The education component was 15 to 20 minutes of training in specific stretching techniques. The CMT included somewhat shortened versions of each of these treatments. The CMT group had significantly better functionality and pain scores than either the E&E group or the sham laser group at post-treatment and at 1-month follow-up ($P < 0.05$); it also had better pain intensity scores than SMT group at post-treatment only. The SMT group had significantly better functionality scores than the E&E group or the sham laser group at post-treatment ($P < 0.05$). All of the CMT subjects reported that pain levels decreased in intensity from baseline to post-treatment. At follow-up, 63% of individuals in the CMT group reported no pain compared with 27% of those in the SMT group, 14% in the E&E group, and 0% in the sham laser group. By itself, the exercise and posture training offered noticeable but nonsignificant help in pain reduction and function. There were no group differences in range of motion. In summary, while both CMT and STM produced significant improvements over exercise alone and the sham laser control, the comprehensive form was stronger, particularly in producing effects that endured 1 month post-treatment.

Comparisons Between Types of Massage

Since the time of Furlan et al's review,[43] the Cherkin team has conducted another important study on massage for chronic low back pain sufferers. In the 2001 study, the massage therapy treatments often included some advanced massage techniques, including myofascial release and neuromuscular techniques, which are not part of many basic massage training programs.[45] Thus, it was not clear whether most massage therapists, graduating from a 600-hour program (a common standard for state licensure), would be likely to produce similar results and whether most consumers would have access to this massage treatment with these effects. The team addressed this question in a 2011 RCT (n = 402) with 3 arms: (1) usual care; (2) relaxation massage, which used Swedish massage techniques; and (3) focused structural massage, which used largely myofascial and neuromuscular techniques.[57] Both forms of massage were found to be statistically and clinically superior to usual care for low back pain, producing short-term reductions in symptoms and longer-term improvements in function. While there was no statistically significant difference between the results of the 2 massage protocols, the relaxation massage results were modestly superior to those of the focused structural massage. This finding surprised many of the massage therapists involved with the study, as the focused structural techniques are often thought of as more advanced and more technical.

Two of the studies in Furlan's systematic review[43] also compared different massage approaches. A 2005 study by Chatchawan et al[44] compared traditional Thai massage with Swedish massage in individuals with back pain associated with myofascial trigger points. These researchers reported that both forms of massage were comparably effective, although they had anticipated that Thai massage would be more effective for people with myofascial trigger points. Unfortunately, there was no usual care arm in this study. The 2000 Franke et al study[48] compared forms that are not commonly, if at all, used in the United States. The results of these studies, which indicate that very different forms of massage produce quite similar results, should encourage both further trials that attempt to identify a best practice in massage for specific conditions and inquiry into what produces the effects we see from massage. Is it just simple touch and attention, if the specific strokes don't matter, or is it something else?

Neck Pain

In the previously mentioned 2002 survey of massage therapists, 17% of patient visits were for relief of neck pain.[42] Systematic reviews of the literature on massage for neck pain have concluded that while results show some promise, the quality of most studies is so poor as to preclude making practice recommendations. The authors of a 2012 Cochrane Collaboration review of 15 trials, for instance, reported the following[58]:

> The results showed very low level evidence that certain massage techniques (traditional Chinese massage, classical and modified strain/counter strain technique) may have been more effective than control or placebo treatment in improving function and tenderness.

There was very low level evidence that massage may have been more beneficial than education in the short term for pain bothersomeness. Along with that, there was low level evidence that ischaemic compression and passive stretch may have been more effective in combination rather than individually for pain reduction.

Their conclusion was that, "As a stand-alone treatment, massage for MND [mechanical neck disorder] was found to provide an immediate or short-term effectiveness or both in pain and tenderness."[58]

In the largest RCT, Sherman and colleagues[59] compared massage with self-care education for the treatment of chronic neck pain. In this RCT, 64 patients with neck pain of at least 3 months duration were randomized to receive massage (up to 10 massages over 10 weeks) or a self-care book. Data were collected at 4, 10, and 26 weeks on outcomes that included dysfunction (Neck Disability Index [NDI]), a 0 to 10 symptom-bothersomeness scale, and medication usage. They found that massage recipients were more likely than the self-education subjects to experience a clinically significant improvement on the NDI (48% vs 18% of controls; relative risk [RR] = 2.7; 95% confidence interval [CI], 1.2 to 6.5) and on the bothersomeness scale (55% vs 25% of controls; RR = 2.2; 95% CI, 1.1 to 4.5) at 10 weeks (end of treatment). At 26 weeks, the difference in function remained, but at a reduced level. There was no longer a significant difference in symptom bothersomeness. While a single small study is hardly definitive, this did suggest that massage may provide some relief for those with chronic neck pain. Importantly for all concerned with overuse of pain medications, there was a difference noted between the groups in medication usage, with increased usage among the book group participants from 63% at baseline to 77% at 26 weeks, and somewhat decreased usage among the massage recipients from 56% at baseline to 53% at 10 and 26 weeks.

Dosing Studies of Massage for Pain

Neck pain and osteoarthritis (OA) of the knee have been the first areas in which massage dosing trials have been conducted. Understanding what constitutes a "dose" of massage is not quite as straightforward as it is for pharmaceuticals. In these 2 studies, doses were varied both by the number of minutes/treatment and by treatments/week. Thus, they could examine delivering the same number of minutes of massage/week in different ways, as well as see whether total minutes/week mattered more or less than minutes/treatment.

Sherman and her team followed their previously mentioned neck pain study[59] with a study in which 228 individuals with chronic nonspecific neck pain were randomized to 5 groups receiving various doses of massage (a 4-week course consisting of 30-minute visits 2 or 3 times weekly or 60-minute visits 1 to 3 times weekly) or to a wait-list control group.[60] Both pain intensity and neck-related dysfunction (NDI) were assessed at baseline and at 5 weeks.

Log-linear regression was used to assess the likelihood of clinically meaningful improvement in neck-related dysfunction (≥ 5 points on NDI) or pain intensity ($\geq 30\%$ improvement) by treatment group. Interestingly, this team found that 30-minute treatments were not significantly better than the wait-list control condition in terms of achieving a clinically meaningful improvement in neck dysfunction or pain, regardless of the frequency of treatments. In contrast, 60-minute treatments 2 and 3 times/week significantly increased the likelihood of such improvement compared with the control condition in terms of both neck dysfunction (RR = 3.41 and 4.98; $P = .04$ and .005, respectively) and pain intensity (RR = 2.30 and 2.73; $P = .007$ and .001, respectively). They found that multiple 60-minute massages/week were more effective than fewer or shorter sessions in individuals with chronic neck pain at 4 weeks. On the basis of these data, they recommend that "…clinicians recommending massage and researchers studying this therapy should ensure that patients receive a likely effective dose of treatment."[60]

Two studies examining massage for knee OA found that massage seems to be effective in reducing pain and increasing some aspects of function.[61,62] Sherman et al[61] published the first investigation in 2012. They investigated the effects of 8 weeks of massage on pain and other symptoms in adults (n = 68) with a diagnosis of knee OA and a prerandomization score of 4 to 9 on the Western

Ontario and McMaster Universities Arthritis Index (WOMAC) and pain VAS (eg, 0 = no pain, 10 = worst pain ever).[60] Subjects were randomized to massage or to a delayed intervention control. A standardized protocol of full-body Swedish massage was administered twice weekly in the first 4 weeks to build a loading dose, then once weekly for the next 4 weeks. The massage therapy group demonstrated significant improvements in the WOMAC Global Score (-21.15 ± 2.46 mm; $P < 0.0001$), stiffness (-21.60 ± 26.99 mm; $P < 0.0001$) and physical function (-20.50 ± 22.50 mm; $P < 0.0001$), and pain (-17.62 ± 31.06 mm; $P = 0.0023$) domains at 8 weeks (end of treatment) as well as decreased pain (VAS) and time to walk 50 feet ($P < 0.05$). At 16 weeks (8 weeks post-treatment), improvements seen in the massage therapy group generally persisted. The authors concluded that massage seemed to be an efficacious treatment for knee OA.[61]

They then followed up this study with a dosing trial, hoping to identify the optimal dose of massage within an 8-week treatment regimen and to further examine the durability of response.[62] They randomized 125 adults with knee OA to 1 of 4 8-week treatment schedules of a standardized Swedish massage regimen or to a usual care control regimen. Subjects in 2 of the massage treatment arms received 30-minute massages; half of the subjects received these massages once/week and half received them twice/week. Subjects in the other 2 massage treatment arms received 60-minutes massages, again, some once/week and some twice/week.

Outcomes included the WOMAC, VAS of pain, range of motion, and time to walk 50 feet, assessed at baseline, 8, 16, and 24 weeks. In this study, as in the neck pain study, the 60-minute massages proved notably more effective than the 30-minute massages. Only the 60-minute massages produced significantly superior improvement when compared with usual care. At 8 weeks, 60-minute massages were superior on the WOMAC Global scores (24.0 points; 95% CI,15.3-32.7) in the 60-minute massage groups compared with usual care (6.3 points; 95% CI, 0.1-12.8), as well as in the WOMAC subscales of pain and functionality and in the VAS of pain. No significant differences were observed in range of motion at 8 weeks, and no significant effects were seen in any outcome measure at 24 weeks compared with usual care. A dose-response curve based on WOMAC Global scores indicated increasing effect with greater total time of massage, but that plateaued at the 60-minute-per-week dose. Receiving 60-minute massages twice/week did not yield a significantly greater improvement. Thus, the authors concluded that the greater convenience of a once-weekly protocol, combined with the inherent cost savings and consistency with a typical real-world massage protocol, rendered the 60-minute-once-weekly dose to be optimal and they recommended it as a standard for future trials.

Postoperative Pain

Two studies from 2007 examined massage as a treatment for postoperative pain.[63,64] The first involved 605 male veterans (mean age, 64 years) who underwent major surgery between February 1, 2003, and January 31, 2005, at a VA hospital in either Ann Arbor, Michigan, or Indianapolis, Indiana.[63] This well-designed RCT involved 3 arms: (1) usual care, (2) usual care plus a 20-minute Swedish back massage, or (3) usual care plus 20 minutes of nonmassage attention (eg, conversation) delivered by a massage therapist. Treatment was received for up to 6 days following the operation. The massage group had significantly better outcomes than the control group on short-term pain intensity ($P = .001$), pain unpleasantness ($P < 0.001$), and anxiety ($P = .007$). Importantly, massage recipients experienced a faster rate of decrease in pain intensity ($P = .02$) during the first 4 postoperative days. The authors found this quite notable, stating the following[63]:

> Perhaps the most important observation from this study is the immediate (short-term) effects of massage on pain intensity, unpleasantness, and anxiety. These significant reductions were most pronounced on the first postoperative day. A 1-point (1-cm) reduction in the pain score (of a possible 10) on a VAS in the acute postoperative setting may sometimes require the administration of several small (eg, 1-mg) boluses of parenteral morphine,

depending on the individual. This suggests that massage may be a very potent pain reliever in some patients.

The second study on postoperative pain was a 2-armed trial with 180 subjects comparing usual care with usual care plus massage and acupuncture.[64] While this RCT also found significantly greater decreases in pain and depression among the treatment group, it is impossible to disentangle the specific effects of massage from the contributions of acupuncture or the synergistic effect of the 2 treatments.

Massage and Sleep

Sleep, while known to be an important component of recovery, rehabilitation, and health maintenance, is a challenge for many patients in a hospital setting, from preterm infants in the neonatal intensive care unit, to adults recovering from surgery, to elderly and other patients in palliative care. In a country that is witnessing increased addiction to both illicit and prescription drugs, identifying nonpharmacologic approaches to sleep enhancement would be beneficial, including—and perhaps especially—in rehabilitation. Massage has been tested as a sleep-enhancing treatment for diverse populations and has also emerged as a frequently mentioned secondary effect noticed by subjects in massage studies of other primary focus.[65-67]

One study in particular seems most relevant to the issues of rehabilitation. The 2010 study by Nerbass et al[68] involved 40 individuals who had undergone coronary artery bypass graft (CABG) surgery and were randomized to a control group or a massage intervention group immediately following discharge from the ICU (Day 0) after CABG surgery. Intervention subjects received massage administered in each of 3 successive evenings; control subjects sat in a comfortable chair each evening. Both groups received usual care and comparable quantities of dipyrone and tramadol as analgesics. Patients maintained sleep diaries and were evaluated for sleep and pain each morning via multiple instruments. Recovery from fatigue was faster for participants in the massage therapy group, particularly on Day 1 ($P = .006$) and Day 2 ($P = .028$). Sleep effectiveness was higher for individuals in this group during all 3 days ($P = .019$) when compared with participants in the control group. Authors noted that "...the results indicate that the beneficial effects of MT were not mediated by reducing pain because the number of complaints about pain was similar in both the control and MT groups."[68] They concluded, "Massage therapy is an effective technique for improving patient recovery from cardiopulmonary artery bypass graft surgery because it reduces fatigue and improves sleep."[68]

MASSAGE AND PAIN MECHANISMS

Two features of massage are important to keep in mind when we consider the issue of "mechanism of action." First, all massages are not the same and the effects of different treatments may be prompted by different mechanisms. Second, a massage treatment is a complex mix of tissue manipulation, human connection, verbal cuing for cognitive reframing, an ongoing therapeutic relationship, and a host of nonspecific effects, including both patient and practitioner expectations. Part of the power of massage may be its ability to affect a number of these simultaneously.

There are competing theories about why massage is effective in reducing pain. Field[69] has suggested that pain reduction is one result of a cascade of effects set in motion by shifts in stress hormone levels. Many of her studies report significant post-massage increases in serotonin levels and decreases in epinephrine, norepinephrine, and cortisol. However, a more recent meta-analysis by Moyer et al[70] of relevant data contradicted one aspect of Field's findings, indicating that cortisol levels were not significantly reduced. Moyer did find evidence of significant reductions in heart rate and blood pressure, which had been reported by Meek[71] and Fakouri and Jones,[72] but not by Reed and Held.[73]

Others have suggested the gate control theory of pain as an explanatory model, or that massage works as a superficial analgesic. One would not expect these explanations to account for pain relief sustained well beyond the period of treatment, which we have seen in some of the studies reviewed in this chapter. In reviewing massage effects for rehabilitative contexts, Braverman and Schulman[74] cited evidence that massage can prompt increased joint mobility, improved connective tissue pliability and mobility, and enhanced immune system function, as well as the reduction in stress hormones already cited.

More efficient use of muscles and concomitant reduction of strain and overuse through improved postural alignment is one explanation that massage therapists often offer for why massage is effective in relieving musculoskeletal pain. This explanatory model would be applicable to immediate relief and to long-term improvement. Some of the improved postural alignment is achieved through purposefully stretching the connective tissue in areas that the therapist finds to be inappropriately constricted. Connective tissue is notoriously pliable and can become "remodeled" via many forms of mechanical stress, including overuse, underuse, or unusual use (eg, repetitive motions).[75] Connective tissue change can prompt alterations in the muscle(s) with which it is associated. For instance, the shortening of muscle fibers due to immobilization has been shown to be preceded by the shortening of the associated connective tissue that responds more quickly to the lack of movement.[76]

In a very promising paper, Langevin and Sherman[77] offer a pathophysiological model of low back pain that incorporates data on tissue remodeling and on pain-related behavior. They reference literature indicating that some people in pain are afraid that movement will cause even more pain, and therefore limit their physical activity and/or alter their movements in ways that can become repetitive misuse over time.[78,79] For instance, massage therapists often see clients who have developed inefficient and painful ways of moving, frequently involving distortions that were originally employed to protect an injury that may have long since healed. Langevin and Sherman hypothesize that "...dynamic and potentially reversible plasticity of perimuscular connective tissue plays a key role in the pathophysiology of LBP as well as in the mechanism of therapies utilizing mechanical forces (eg, massage, chiropractic manipulation, acupuncture)."[77] Clearly, this hypothesis is not limited to back pain; it can also pertain to other musculoskeletal pain.

Finally, reevoking the quote from Juhan cited earlier in this chapter about the inseparability of the skin and the brain,[5] Kerr et al[80] have offered a possible explanation that is grounded in neural plasticity. They suggest that what they call *touch healing therapies* may be effective in chronic pain treatment through 4 features that jointly encourage neural plasticity, particularly the reformation of the somatosensory cortical map. These 4 features, any and all of which can be present in a massage treatment, include (1) light tactile stimulation, (2) a behaviorally relevant and relaxed context, (3) repeated sessions, and (4) directed somatosensory attention. Chronic pain is sometimes centrally maintained, meaning that it can persist even when there is no remaining damage to the tissue (thus, no present time nociception to account for the pain sensation). Cortical dysregulation has been associated with centrally maintained pain.[81-83] Studies have indicated that remodeling is possible in the somatosensory maps of adults.[84] Body maps of patients with chronic pain have shown enlargements in the areas related to the painful body regions.[85-87] Taking all of this into account, Kerr et al hypothesize that touch healing modalities "work to renormalize somatotopic maps via a therapeutic plasticity mechanism."[80]

In sum, there are a number of models that might explain *how* massage is effective when it *is* and *why* it is not effective when it *is not*. The models offered by Langevin and Sherman[77] and by Kerr and colleagues[80] are appealing in that they offer multifactorial explanations that could apply to a multidimensional form of treatment. They remain to be tested.

MASSAGE, STRESS, AND WELLNESS

Relaxation, stress relief, and anxiety reduction are primary reasons for visits to massage therapists. Dozens of small investigations, many of which were conducted at the Touch Research Institute in Miami, Florida, indicate that massage offers immediate reductions in stress and anxiety in a variety of situations. The 5 studies presented in this section, while not exhaustive, will offer some evidence of this range.

The first of these was a 1998 study by Field et al[88] that explored the possible use of massage to ease the debridement process for burn victims. Twenty-eight adult patients with burns, recruited consecutively upon admission for debridement at a burn center, were randomized to either standard care, which included physical therapy, or standard care plus massage. The massage consisted of daily administration of a 20-minute Swedish massage to face, torso, limbs, and back for 1 week. The treatment was given just prior to morning debridement. Outcomes, taken pre- and post-treatment on the first and last days of the study, included a state/trait anxiety inventory (STAI), 3 pain measures, and a number of observational measures completed by staff. The massage group was found to have significant improvements pre- to post-treatment in state anxiety, pulse, observed affect, vocalization, and signs of anxiety. Longer-term outcomes (change from first to last day) included significant decrease in anger, depression, and all 3 pain measures. Patients who received standard care showed only a decrease in pulse pre- to post-treatment, and a decrease in one pain measure from the first day to the last day. While our confidence in the findings is weakened by the investigators' use of nonblinded observers, they nonetheless highlight a potentially important avenue of inquiry and use of massage in rehabilitation. That is, massage appears to have the potential to ease patients' experience of medical treatments that, while helpful and/or necessary, are difficult to endure.

Ahles et al[89] conducted a related study in 1999 on the potential use of massage for patients undergoing autologous bone marrow transplant (BMT). Thirty-four adults scheduled for autologous BMT at a large teaching hospital were enrolled in a nonblinded randomized comparison of standard care versus standard care plus massage. In this study, massage consisted of up to 9 20-minute Swedish massages that included strokes to shoulders, neck, and head. They averaged 3 massages/week for 3 weeks. Anxiety, depression, and mood were assessed at baseline, midtreatment, and predischarge; nausea, pain, and fatigue were assessed pre- and post-massage. While the massage group demonstrated significant improvements in diastolic blood pressure, distress, nausea, and state anxiety immediately post-treatment, no significant effects were found over time.

In another study by Field et al[90] from 1996, researchers explored the potential for 2 treatments, therapeutic massage and a combination of yoga and progressive muscle relaxation—to ease depression among adolescent mothers with clinical depression. Thirty-two adolescent mothers with depression post-delivery were given 30-minute massages (standardized Swedish protocol) or relaxation therapy (yoga plus progressive muscle relaxation) twice weekly for 5 weeks. Both treatments proved effective in significantly reducing the subjects' state anxiety. However, only the massage also significantly reduced behavioral ("fidgitiness"; $P < 0.01$) and physiological (pulse and heart rate) signs of anxiety, as well as reduced depression ($P < 0.05$). Staff observational reports of behavior indicated that the massage group had improved affect ($P < 0.001$) and cooperation ($P < 0.005$). The combination of self-report, observational, and physiological data is a strength of this study, and their converging results are encouraging in suggesting that massage is beneficial in reducing anxiety and depression with this population.

A 1999 study by Hernandez-Reif et al[91] on massage for children with cystic fibrosis is representative of many studies performed at the aforementioned Touch Research Institute that measured general indicators of relaxation/stress reduction (eg, self-reports on STAI, saliva cortisol levels) and some that measured specific conditions that were under study. In this case, peak airflow was measured. While the value of the study is diminished by its small sample size (n = 20) and lack of blinding, it still offers helpful information. The massage treatment in this study was a 20-minute evening massage given by parents to their children for 30 evenings. All but one family completed this regimen, which indicates the possibility of the use of parentally administered home-based massage in pediatric applications, should the research show that it is warranted. The comparison group received 20 minutes of reading with the parents. Researchers reported a reduction in anxiety for both parents ($P < 0.05$) and children ($P < 0.05$), as well as improved mood for children ($P < 0.05$), post-massage on the first day. There was also a significant reduction in anxiety for parents and children in the massage group from day 1 to day 30 ($P < 0.05$). Importantly, they noted an increase in peak air flow for children in the massage group from day 1 to day 30 ($P < 0.05$). These data support further study, which should include more rigorous design. Data indicating a reduction of parental anxiety mirrors other studies showing benefit from giving massage, especially for parents.

Many adults, of course, experience great stress in their workplace. Hodge et al[92] investigated the potential of seated massage as an effective workplace stress reduction intervention in their 2002 study in which 100 male and female employees (aged 25 to 60 years) of a large teaching hospital were randomized to 1 of 2 groups. Individuals in the treatment group received a 20-minute massage twice weekly for 8 weeks, performed while the employees were seated, clothed, and with their shoes off. The protocol was a blend of light-to-medium–pressure circular motions to the upper body, acupressure to the face and chest, and foot reflexology. Individuals in the control group were offered a quiet room in which to take their 20-minute breaks. Outcome measures included a range of psychological, physiological, and organizational outcomes assessed via previously validated instruments. Findings revealed that subjects in the massage group had less anxiety (state $P = .009$, trait $P = .04$), were less depressed ($P = .05$), and experienced improved emotional control ($P = .05$) compared with those in the control group. Massage subjects on 12-hour shifts also experienced a decrease in sleep disturbance ($P = .02$), although there were no significant differences noted between the 2 groups on a multidimensional measure of fatigue. Further, significant improvements were noted in heart rate and blood pressure in patients in the massage group compared with patients in the control group, and in massage subjects pre- and post-treatment. Interestingly, individuals in the massage group had significant improvements in cognition scores ($P = .000$), as assessed by the Symbol Digit Modalities Test. Work satisfaction scores remained constant in the massage group, but they decreased in the control group.

The study by Hodge et al[92] is the largest and latest of 3 published studies to explore the use of massage to reduce workplace stress.[92-94] Earlier studies by Shulman and Jones[94] and Field et al[93] also indicated that seated massage is an effective tool for this widespread problem. Shulman and Jones[94] included measurements taken 2 and 3 weeks after the completion of the intervention. While the stress reduction had somewhat diminished since the end of treatment, it was still significant. Field et al[93] compared seated massage with a rest break. Interestingly, they included a measure of brainwave activity that indicated that, although subjects receiving both massage and the rest break experienced increased frontal delta power that are indicative of increased relaxation, only the massage group also showed the decreased frontal alpha and beta powers that are indicative of enhanced alertness. This runs counter to the idea some hold that subjects would emerge from massage in a relaxed, but somewhat vegetative state—perhaps "too relaxed" to return to work effectively. It suggests instead that massage induces something similar to the state of meditation—relaxed and alert. This interpretation was supported by the finding that the massage subjects were able to complete a set of math computations more quickly and more accurately than the control subjects. This finding, which will not surprise those who have come to massage via the human potential movement, suggests the need to conduct studies investigating the potential of massage to enhance various aspects of human functioning.

Numerous studies, then, indicate that massage is effective in reducing stress in children, adolescents, and adults. This seems to be true for those diagnosed with clinical depression and anxiety, as well as for healthy subjects. Data presented support the notion that this aspect of massage can be useful in easing medical procedures, workplace stress, and in-home–based pediatric applications.

REGULATION AND INFORMATION

Currently 45 states and the District of Columbia (DC) regulate massage therapy at the state-wide level through either licensure (43 states plus DC) or certification (mandatory in Indiana and Virginia and voluntary in California). This leaves 5 states unregulated by the state although some have regulation at the county or municipal level. State standards for licensure vary somewhat, but typically require a minimum of 600 hours of training from an accredited institution and passage of either a state exam or 1 of 2 nationally recognized tests: the Massage & Bodywork Licensing Examination and the National Certification Examination for Therapeutic Massage and Bodywork. Massage therapy licensure boards decide which certifications and tests to accept on a state-by-state basis. A good review of regulatory issues for therapeutic massage and other CAM professions has been provided by Eisenberg et al in a 2002 article published in the *Annals of Internal Medicine*.[95]

ACCREDITATION AND TRAINING

There is wide variety in the education of massage therapists throughout the United States, with over 300 accredited massage schools and an estimated 1440 massage training programs that are not accredited. Many of these programs are quite small, with the majority being for-profit proprietary institutions, licensed as businesses by their local jurisdictions. Most of these are accredited as vocational schools, although this is changing as more community colleges establish massage programs and more massage schools become accredited as, or affiliated with, colleges.

Coursework typically includes anatomy, physiology and pathology, massage therapy theory and technique, assessment methods, ethics, charting, professional development, and communication skills. Supervised clinical work is provided either through on-site clinics open to the public or through field placement. An increasing number of schools also require research literacy training and practice in case study design and reporting,

Historically, most massage training program accreditation has been institutional, giving little attention to specifics of the instructional program in massage. For this reason, the Commission on Massage Therapy Accreditation (COMTA) was initiated in the 1980s to provide meaningful programmatic accreditation. COMTA received official recognition by the United States Department of Education (DOE) in July 2002. To date, a total of 90 massage schools have received COMTA accreditation. DOE recognition, combined with COMTA's shift from hours-based to competency-based standards beginning in March 2003, offered a positive challenge to massage education in the United States. Sadly, thus far the challenge has not been widely taken up and there remains great inconsistency in the academic training and clinical experience of even licensed massage therapists in North America.

CONCLUSION

Massage is a therapeutic modality employed around the world and across time. The literature investigating its effects, while still somewhat modest, is improving in rigor and growing rapidly. Widespread use of therapeutic massage for both wellness and treatment of injury and/or pathology requires that more attention be given to investigations of this modality and to bringing greater coherence in training and regulation. Heterogeneity of clinical techniques requires detailed descriptions of research interventions so that clinical applicability can be clear. Research attention should be given to those applications for which consumers most often seek therapeutic massage, particularly musculoskeletal pain and injury. Future research should also seek to measure and give meaning to those outcomes that clients report as important, but for which objective measures do not yet exist. These could include particular aspects of well-being such as groundedness, centeredness, increased happiness, and comfort with oneself. The potential contributions of distinct aspects of therapeutic massage treatments should be disentangled through research, including STM, educational interventions, and the therapeutic presence and intention of the practitioner. Far from being the nuisance that placebo or nonspecific effects were once thought to be, these practitioner/client issues may be at the heart of the healing process. Finally, inquiry is also sorely needed into the mechanisms of demonstrated effects.

REFERENCES

1. Chou R, Qaseem A, Snow V, et al; Clinical Efficacy Assessment Subcommittee of the American College of Physicians; American College of Physicians; American Pain Society Low Back Pain Guidelines Panel. Diagnosis and treatment of low back pain: a joint clinical practice guideline from the American College of Physicians and the American Pain Society. *Ann Intern Med.* 2007;147(7):478-491.
2. The Joint Commission. Clarification of the pain management standard. *Joint Commission Perspectives.* https://www.jointcommission.org/assets/1/18/Clarification_of_the_Pain_Management__Standard.pdf. Published November 2014. Accessed February 4, 2016.
3. Nahin RL, Barnes PM, Stussman BJ, Bloom B. Costs of complementary and alternative medicine (CAM) and frequency of visits to CAM practitioners: United States, 2007. *Natl Health Stat Report.* 2009;(18):1-14.
4. American Massage Therapy Association. Industry. www.amtamassage.org/infocenter/economic_industry-factsheet.html. Published February 2016. Accessed April 29, 2016.
5. Juhan D. *Job's Body: A Handbook for Bodywork.* New York, NY: Station Hill Press; 1987.
6. Tappan FM, Benjamin PJ. *Tappan's Handbook of Healing Massage Techniques.* 3rd ed. Stamford, CT: Appleton and Lange; 1998.
7. Kleen EAG. *Massage and Medical Gymnastics.* New York, NY: William Wood & Co; 1921.
8. Benjamin P. *Tappan's Handbook of Healing Massage Techniques.* 5th ed. Upper Saddle River, NJ: Prentice Hall; 2009.
9. Johnson DH. *Bone, Breath & Gesture: Practices of Embodiment, Volume 1.* Berkley, CA: North Atlantic Books; 1995.
10. Downing G. *The Massage Book.* New York, NY: Random House; 1972.
11. Murphy M. *The Future of the Body: Explorations into the Further Evolution of Human Nature.* Los Angeles, CA: Jeremy P. Tarcher/Putnam Books; 1992.
12. Pert CB. *Molecules of Emotion: Why You Feel the Way You Feel.* New York, NY: Simon and Schuster; 1997.
13. Walton T. The health history of a human being. *Massage Therapy Journal.* 1999;37:70-92.
14. Andrade CK, Clifford P. *Outcome-Based Massage.* Baltimore, MD: Lippincott, Williams & Wilkins; 2001.
15. Shapiro S, Schwartz G. Intentional systemic mindfulness: an integrative model for self-regulation and health. *Adv Mind Body Med.* 2000;16(2):128-134.
16. Schwartz GE. Psychobiology and health: a new synthesis. In: Hammonds BL, Scheirer JC, eds. *Psychology and Health: Master Lecture Series.* Vol. 3. Washington, DC: American Psychological Association; 1984.
17. Watson Institute of International and Public Affairs. Costs of war. Brown University. http://watson.brown.edu/costsofwar/costs/human/veterans. Published January 2015. Accessed April 29, 2016.
18. Institute of Medicine (US) Committee on Advancing Pain Research, Care, and Education. *Relieving Pain in America: A Blueprint for Transforming Prevention, Care, Education, and Research.* Washington, DC: National Academies Press (US); 2011.
19. Haskell SG, Ning Y, Krebs E, et al. Prevalence of painful musculoskeletal conditions in female and male veterans in 7 years after return from deployment in Operation Enduring Freedom/Operation Iraqi Freedom. *Clin J Pain.* 2012;28(2):163-167.
20. Toblin RL, Quartana PJ, Riviere LA, Walper KC, Hoge CW. Chronic pain and opioid use in US soldiers after combat deployment. *JAMA Intern Med.* 2014;174(8):1400-1401.
21. Jonas WB, Schoomaker EB. Pain and opioids in the military: we must do better. *JAMA Intern Med.* 2014;174(8):1402-1403.
22. Maguen S, Litz B. Moral injury in veterans of war. *PTSD Research Quarterly.* 2012;23(1):1-3.
23. Office of Policy and Planning. US Department of Veterans Affairs. Analysis of unique veterans utilization of VA benefits & services. www.va.gov/vetdata/docs/SpecialReports/uniqueveteransMay.pdf. Published April 29, 2009. Accessed February 4, 2016.
24. Denneson LM, Corson K, Dobscha SK. Complementary and alternative medicine use among veterans with chronic noncancer pain. *Journal of Rehabilitation Research & Development.* 2011;48(9):1119-1128.
25. Field TM. Massage therapy effects. *Am Psychol.* 1998;53(12):1270-1281.
26. Cawley N. A critique of the methodology of research studies evaluating massage. *Eur J Cancer Care (Engl).* 1997;6(1):23-31.
27. Ernst E. Massage therapy for low back pain: a systematic review. *J Pain Symptom Manage.* 1999;17(1):65-69.

28. Ernst E. Abdominal massage therapy for chronic constipation: a systematic review of controlled clinical trials. *Forsch Komplementarmed.* 1999;6(3):149-151.
29. Haraldsson BG, Gross AR, Myers CD, et al. Massage for mechanical neck disorders. *Cochrane Database Syst Rev.* 2006;3:CD004871.
30. Ernst E, Fialka V. The clinical effectiveness of massage therapy—a critical review. *Forsch Komplementarmed.* 1994;1:226-232.
31. Ernst E. Musculoskeletal conditions and complementary/alternative medicine. *Best Pract Res Clin Rheumatol.* 2004;18(4):539-556.
32. van Tulder MW, Furlan AD, Gagnier JJ. Complementary and alternative therapies for low back pain. *Best Pract Res Clin Rheumatol.* 2005;19(4):639-654.
33. Hill CF. Is massage beneficial to critically ill patients in intensive care units? A critical review. *Intensive Crit Care Nurs.* 1993;9(2):116-121.
34. Sellick SM, Zaza C. Critical review of 5 non-pharmacologic strategies for managing cancer pain. *Cancer Prev Control.* 1998;2(1):7-14.
35. Weinrich SP, Weinrich MC. The effect of massage on pain in cancer patients. *Appl Nurs Res.* 1990;3(4):140-145.
36. Cassileth BR, Vickers AJ. Massage therapy for symptom control: outcome study at a major cancer center. *J Pain Symptom Manage.* 2004;28(3):244-249.
37. Corbin L. Safety and efficacy of massage therapy for patients with cancer. *Cancer Control.* 2005;12(3):158-164.
38. Pan CX, Morrison RS, Ness J, Fugh-Berman A, Leipzig RM. Complementary and alternative medicine in the management of pain, dyspnea and nausea and vomiting near the end of life: a systematic review. *J Pain Symptom Manage.* 2000;20(5):374-387.
39. Hernandez-Reif M, Field T, Theakson H. Multiple sclerosis patients benefit from massage therapy. *J Bodyw Mov Ther.* 1998;2(3):168-174.
40. Johnson SK, Frederick J, Kaufman M, Mountjoy B. A controlled investigation of bodywork in multiple sclerosis. *J Altern Complement Med.* 1999;5(3):237-243.
41. Siev Ner I, Gamus D, Lerner-Geva L, Achiron A. Reflexology treatment relieves symptoms of multiple sclerosis: a randomized controlled study. *Mult Scler.* 2003;9(4):356-361.
42. Cherkin D, Deyo RA, Sherman KJ, et al. Characteristics of visits to licensed acupuncturists, chiropractors, massage therapists and naturopathic physicians. *J Am Board Fam Pract.* 2002;15(6):463-472.
43. Furlan AD, Imamura M, Dryden T, Irvin E. Massage for low back pain: an updated systematic review within the framework of the Cochrane Back Review Group. *Spine (Phila Pa 1976).* 2009;34(16):1669-1684.
44. Chatchawan U, Thinkhamrop B, Kharmwan S, Knowles J, Eungpinichpong W. Effectiveness of traditional v Thai massage versus Swedish massage among patients with back pain associated with myofascial trigger points. *J Bodyw Mov Ther.* 2005;9(4):298-309.
45. Cherkin DC, Eisenberg D, Sherman KJ, et al. Randomized trial comparing traditional Chinese medical acupuncture, therapeutic massage, and self-care education for chronic low back pain. *Arch Intern Med.* 2001;161(8):1081-1088.
46. Farasyn A, Meeusen R, Nijs J. A pilot randomized placebo-controlled trial of roptrotherapy in patients with subacute non-specific low back pain. *J Back Musculoskeletal Rehabil.* 2007;19:111-117.
47. Field T, Hernandez-Reif M, Diego M, Fraser M. Lower back pain and sleep disturbance are reduced following massage therapy. *J Bodyw Mov Ther.* 2007;11(2):141-145.
48. Franke A, Gebauer S, Franke K, Brockow T. Acupuncture massage vs Swedish massage and individual exercise vs group exercise in low back pain sufferers—a randomized controlled clinical trial in a 2 x 2 factorial design [article in German]. *Forsch Komplementarmed Klass Naturheilkd.* 2000;7(6):286-293.
49. Geisser ME, Wiggert EA, Haig AJ, Colwell MO. A randomized controlled trial of manual therapy and specific adjuvant exercise for chronic low back pain. *Clin J Pain.* 2005;21(6):463-470.
50. Hernandez-Reif M, Field T, Krasnegor J, Theakson H. Lower back pain is reduced and range of motion increased after massage therapy. *Int J Neurosci.* 2001;106(3-4):131-145.
51. Hsieh LLC, Kuo CH, Yen MF, Chen TH. A randomized controlled clinical trial for low back pain treated by acupressure and physical therapy. *Prev Med.* 2004;39(1):168-176.
52. Hsieh LLC, Kuo CHK, Lee LH, Yen AM, Chien KL, Chen TH. Treatment of low back pain by acupressure and physical therapy: randomised controlled trial. *BMJ.* 2006;332(7543):696-700.
53. Mackawan S, Eungpinichpong W, Pantumethakul R, et al. Effects of traditional Thai massage versus joint mobilization on substance P and pain perception in patients with non-specific low back pain. *J Bodyw Mov Ther.* 2007;11(1):9-16.
54. Poole H, Glenn S, Murphy P. A randomised controlled study of reflexology for the management of chronic low back pain. *Eur J Pain.* 2007;11(8):878-887.
55. Preyde M. Effectiveness of massage therapy for subacute low-back pain: a randomized controlled trial. *CMAJ.* 2000;162(13):1815-1820.
56. Yip YB, Tse SH. The effectiveness of relaxation acupoint stimulation and acupressure with aromatic lavender essential oil for non-specific low back pain in Hong Kong: a randomised controlled trial. *Complement Ther Med.* 2004;12(1):28-37.

57. Cherkin DC, Sherman KJ, Kahn J, et al. A comparison of the effects of 2 types of massage and usual care on chronic low back pain: a randomized, controlled trial. *Ann Intern Med*. 2011;155(1):1-9.

58. Patel KC, Gross A, Graham N, et al. Massage for mechanical neck disorders. *Cochrane Database Syst Rev*. 2012;9:CD004871.

59. Sherman KJ, Cherkin DC, Hawkes RJ, Miglioretti DL, Deyo RA. Randomized trial of therapeutic massage vs. self-care book for chronic neck pain. *Alt Ther Health Med*. 2006;12(3):63.

60. Sherman KJ, Cherkin DC, Hawkes RJ, Miglioretti DL, Deyo RA. Randomized trial of therapeutic massage vs. self-care book for chronic neck pain. *Alt Ther Health Med*. 2006;12(3):63.

61. Sherman KJ, Cook AJ, Kah JR, Hawkes RE, Wellman RD, Cherkin DC. Dosing study of massage for chornic neck pain: protocol for the dose response evaluation and analysis of massage [DREAM] trial. *BMC Complementary and Alternative Medicine*. 2012;12:158.

62. Sherman KJ, Cook AJ, Wellman RD, et al. Five-week outcomes from a dosing trial of therapeutic massage for chronic neck pain. *Ann Fam Med*. 2014;12(2):112-120. doi:10.1370/afm.1602.

63. Mitchinson AR, Kim HM, Rosenberg JM, et al. Acute postoperative pain management using massage as an adjuvant therapy: a randomized trial. *Arch Surg*. 2007;142(12):1158-1167.

64. Mehling WE, Jacobs B, Acree M, et al. Symptom management with massage and acupuncture in postoperative cancer patients: a randomized controlled trial. *J Pain Symptom Manage*. 2007;33(3):258-266.

65. Underdown A, Barlow J, Chung V, Stewart-Brown S. Massage intervention for promoting mental and physical health in infants aged under six months. *Cochrane Database Syst Rev*. 2006;(4):CD005038.

66. Yeung WF, Chung KF, Poon MM, et al. Acupressure, reflexology, and auricular acupressure for insomnia: a systematic review of randomized controlled trials. *Sleep Med*. 2012;13(8):971-984.

67. Tsay SL, Rong JR, Lin PF. Acupoints massage in improving the quality of sleep and quality of life in patients with end-stage renal disease. *J Adv Nurs*. 2003;42(2):134-142.

68. Nerbass FB, Feltrim MI, Souza SA, Ykeda DS, Lorenzi-Filho G. Effects of massage therapy on sleep quality after coronary artery bypass graft surgery. *Clinics (Sao Paulo)*. 2010;65(11):1105-1110.

69. Field T. Massage therapy research. Presentation made at: First International Symposium on the Science of Touch; May 16-18, 2002; Montreal, Quebec, Canada.

70. Moyer CA, Rounds J, Hannum JW. A meta-analysis of massage therapy research. *Psychol Bull*. 2004;130(1):3-18.

71. Meek SS. Effects of slow stroke back massage on relaxation in hospice clients. *Image J Nurs Sch*. 1993;25(1):17-21.

72. Fakouri C, Jones P. Relaxation Rx: slow stroke back rub. *J Gerontol Nurs*. 1987;13(2):32-35.

73. Reed BV, Held JM. Effects of sequential connective tissue massage on autonomic nervous system of middle-aged and elderly adults. *Phys Ther*. 1988;68(8):1231-1234.

74. Braverman DL, Schulman RA. Massage techniques in rehabilitation medicine. *Phys Red Rehabil Clin N Am*. 1999;10(3):631-649.

75. Cummings GS, Tillman LJ. Remodeling of dense connective tissue in normal adult tissues. In: Currier DP, Nelson RM, eds. *Dynamics of Human Biologic Tissues: Contemporary Perspectives in Rehabilitation*. Philadelphia, PA: F.A. Davis Company; 1992:45-73.

76. Williams PE, Goldspink G. Connective tissue changes in immobilised muscle. *J Anat*. 1984;138(Pt 2):343-350.

77. Langevin HM, Sherman KJ. Pathophysiological model for chronic low back pain integrating connective tissue and nervous system mechanisms. *Med Hypotheses*. 2007;68(1):74-80.

78. Hurwitz EL, Morgenstern H, Chiao C. Effects of recreational physical activity and back exercises on low back pain and psychological distress: findings from the UCLA Low Back Pain Study. *Am J Public Health*. 2005;95(10):1817-1824.

79. Swinkels-Meewisse IE, Roelofs J, Oostendorp RA, Verbeek AL, Vlaeyen JW. Acute low back pain: pain-related fear and pain catastrophizing influence physical performance and perceived disability. *Pain*. 2006;120(1-2):36-43.

80. Kerr CE, Wasserman RH, Moore CI. Cortical dynamics as a therapeutic mechanism for touch healing. *J Altern Complement Med*. 2007;13(1):59-66.

81. Treede R, Kenshalo DR, Gracely RH, Jones AK. The cortical representation of pain. *Pain*. 1999;79(2-3):105-111.

82. Price DD. Central neural mechanisms that interrelate sensory and affective dimensions of pain. *Mol Interv*. 2002;2(6):392-403.

83. Flor H. Cortical reorganisation and chronic pain: implications for rehabilitation. *J Rehabil Med*. 2003;(41 Suppl):66-72.

84. Pascual-Leone A, Torres F. Plasticity of the sensorimotor cortex representation of the reading finger in Braille readers. *Brain*. 1993;116(Pt 1):39-52.

85. Flor H, Braun C, Elbert T, Birbaumer N. Extensive reorganization of primary somatosensory cortex in chronic back pain patients. *Neurosci Lett*. 1997;224(1):5-8.

86. Flor H, Elbert T, Knecht S, et al. Phantom-limb pain as a perceptual correlate of cortical reorganization following arm amputation. *Nature*. 1995;375(6531):482-484.

87. Maihöfner C, Handwerker HO, Neundörfer B, Birklein F. Patterns of cortical reorganization in complex regional pain syndrome. *Neurology*. 2003;61(12):1707-1715.

88. Field T, Peck M, Krugman S, et al. Burn injuries benefit from massage therapy. *J Burn Care Rehabil*. 1998;19(3):241-244.

89. Ahles TA, Tope DM, Pinkson B, et al. Massage therapy for patients undergoing autologous bone marrow transplantation. *J Pain Symptom Manage.* 1999;18(3):157-163.
90. Field T, Grizzle N, Scafidi F, Schanberg S. Massage and relaxation therapies' effects on depressed adolescent mothers. *Adolescence.* 1996;31(124): 903-911.
91. Hernandez-Reif M, Field T, Krasnegor J, Martinez E, Schwartzman M, Mavunda K. Children with cystic fibrosis benefit from massage therapy. *J Pediatr Psychol.* 1999;24(2):175-181.
92. Hodge M, Robinson C, Boehmer J, Klein S. Employee outcomes following work-site acupressure and massage. In: Rich GJ, ed. *Massage Therapy: The Evidence for Practice.* St. Louis, MO: Mosby; 2002.
93. Field T, Ironson G, Scafidi F, et al. Massage therapy reduces anxiety and enhances EEG pattern of alertness and math computations. *Int J Neurosci.* 1996;86(3-4):197-205.
94. Shulman KR, Jones GE. The effectiveness of massage therapy intervention on reducing anxiety in the workplace. *J Appl Behav Sci.* 1996;32(2):160-173.
95. Eisenberg DM, Cohen MH, Hrbek A, Grayzel J, Van Rompay MI, Cooper RA. Credentialing complementary and alternative medical providers. *Ann Intern Med.* 2002;137(12):965-973

8

Craniosacral Therapy

Deborah A. Giaquinto-Wahl, MSPT

Craniosacral therapy is a manual therapy technique that uses the craniosacral system to promote self-correction and healing within the body. This technique looks at the human body as an integrated whole. The craniosacral system includes the bones of the cranium, the sacrum, underlying meningeal membranes and all other structures that connect to the meninges, and the cerebrospinal fluid (CSF). A therapist can use the bones of the cranium and the sacrum as bony handles to access the underlying dura and release any restrictions within the system. When restrictions are released, the organism (person) functions more efficiently. Dr. John Upledger, the founder of craniosacral therapy, once phrased it as follows: "It's like removing stones from a river so flow is not impeded." The CSF has an intimate relationship with the brain and spinal cord, and is encased within the dural system. This dural system connects either directly or indirectly to every muscle, joint, tendon, and organ in our body. Therefore, one can see that a restriction within the craniosacral system can be far reaching and may show symptoms anywhere throughout the body.

The following 2 belief systems must be in place to be cohesive with Upledger's work: (1) that cranial bones connect by jointed articulations that are mobile throughout life and (2) that there is an ongoing rhythmical motion of the underlying dural membrane caused by the production and reabsorption of CSF, which is transmitted to the bones.

The history of craniosacral therapy begins in the early 19th century with the father of osteopathy, Dr. Andrew Taylor Still, who believed that the body is a self-regulating, self-correcting system that works as a unit. He also believed that the body structure is intimately related to its function. If the system is structurally out of balance, it will constantly and inherently try to seek homeostasis.

In the early 1900s, an osteopath by the name of Dr. William G. Sutherland, Still's student, was very interested in nature's design of the human skull. Similar to most Western medicine practitioners, he was taught that the bones of the human skull calcify when full growth has been reached. When Sutherland examined the skull, he realized that the cranial sutures were actually joints and, consequently, reasoned that there had to be movement between the bones. He saw that "some cranial bones were beveled like the gills of a fish, indicating articular mobility for a respiratory mechanism."[1] Using himself as a case study, and with the aid of various ingenious devices that he created, Sutherland screwed down portions of his skull, creating restrictions within himself, and then noted the changes that occurred. As a result of the magnitude of the responses that he experienced from this self-experimentation and self-correction, Sutherland concluded that freeing up the restrictions along the cranial sutures and allowing proper movement could improve overall function.[1-3] The birth of cranial osteopathy was then established.

Davis CM.
*Integrative Therapies in Rehabilitation: Evidence for Efficacy in Therapy,
Prevention, and Wellness, Fourth Edition* (pp 99-113).
© 2017 Taylor & Francis Group.

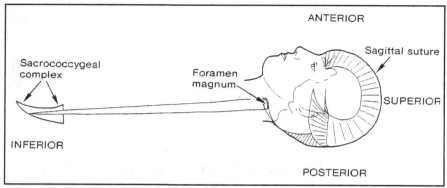

Figure 8-1. Anterior-posterior and superior-inferior axes of the dural membrane system. (Reprinted with permission from Upledger JE, Vredevoogd JD. *Craniosacral Therapy*. Seattle, WA: Eastland Press; 1983:70.)

Very few Western practitioners other than those in the osteopathic community believed that the cranial bones moved after childhood until the evolution of Upledger's work. In the early 1970s, Upledger worked with a team of physicians and researchers from Michigan State University in East Lansing, Michigan to learn the composition of the intra-articular suture material, to determine the validity of Sutherland's work with cranial manipulation, and to determine whether the cranial bones actually move.

Using electron microscopy, Upledger and his team discovered that the intra-articular suture material contained blood vessels, nerves, and connective tissue.[4-7] These findings were more conducive toward dynamic mobility vs bony fusion of the cranial bones. To determine whether cranial bones move, the Michigan State team also studied the cranial movement of live primates. By fastening antennae into the parietal bones of monkeys and through the use of radio waves, they were able to observe a rate and amplitude of movement between the cranial bones at 6 to 12 cycles/minute.[5] Meanwhile, another study published by Adams et al[8] reported findings of a rhythmic motion other than the cardiac and respiratory rate in cats at approximately 11 cycles/minute with the use of strain gauges across the parietal bones of cats. In addition, Wallace and colleagues[9] observed intracranial pulsations at a rate of 9 cycles/minute in human brain and membrane tissue with the use of ultrasound (US). Taking into account the findings of all of these studies, it now seemed realistic that Sutherland's premise of cranial manipulation held true. But what was actually causing cranial bone movement? Two theories were predominate: the stretch receptor mechanism[1] and the arachnoid granulation body theory.[2]

STRETCH RECEPTOR MECHANISM

What was previously known anatomically was that the meningeal membrane has an intimate relationship with the skull and connects at various points along the spinal canal. Referred to as the *intracranial membrane system*, it is made up of a vertical membrane system formed by the falx cerebri and falx cerebelli and continues down to form a strong, dense circle of tissue around the foramen magnum (Figure 8-1). The horizontal portion of the intracranial membrane system is created by "leaves" that run laterally off the falx cerebri superiorly and the falx cerebelli inferiorly, forming a bilayered horizontal membrane, the tentorium cerebri and the tentorium cerebelli, respectively. We also know that CSF is housed below the dura mater within the subarachnoid space and is formed within the ventricular system of the brain. Prior to the Michigan State research, Sutherland believed that the keystone of all cranial bone motion was movement at the sphenobasilar joint. He believed that there was a contraction and expansion of the ventricular system and that this tensile motion caused movement at the sphenobasilar joint,[3] an external pumping action by the brain.

Although Upledger's research confirmed the bulk of Sutherland's model, Upledger postulates that there is actually an internal pump and volume/pressure receptors that are responsible for the CSF volume changes. He theorizes that it is the CSF volume changes within the intracranial membrane system that causes the cranial bone movement. Upledger and his colleagues have posed the *pressure stat model*, explaining the craniosacral rhythm, the movement of CSF, and their relationships to the movement between the cranial bones. This model is a semi-closed hydraulic system in which CSF is constantly being produced and reabsorbed within the container of the meningeal system. Physiologically, what happens is that the CSF is produced at a rate that is twice the rate of the CSF being extracted from blood through the choroid plexus within straight sinus of the ventricle. After bathing the brain and spinal cord, it then drains at a constant rate of 1x through the arachnoid villi of the sagittal suture and is reabsorbed back into the venous system. By way of electron microscopy and cadaver dissection, pressure-sensitive receptors within the sagittal suture ground material have been located along with nerve tracks that run down to the choroid plexus of the lateral ventricles. Theoretically, these pressure receptors could signal the choroid plexus to increase production of CSF once a low threshold has been reached. When enough CSF has been produced, the meningeal membranes expand to the point of triggering stretch receptors in the sagittal suture, signaling the choroid plexus to stop production of CSF. The CSF continues to be reabsorbed through the arachnoid villi until the low threshold is reached; sense receptors in the suture will again send signals to the choroid plexus to produce CSF. This dynamic theory poses that CSF is produced at a rate twice that of the constant reabsorption, and that when an upper threshold is reached, the production is turned off by an internal homeostatic mechanism.[3]

ARACHNOID GRANULATION BODY THEORY

Another feedback mechanism that would support the rhythmic flow of CSF within the craniosacral system is one that involves the arachnoid granulation body. This body projects into the floor of the straight sinus at its angle of union with the great cerebral vein and contains a sinusoidal plexus of blood vessels that, when engorged, serves as a ball-valve mechanism. The increasing back pressure from the engorged vessels may affect the secretion of the CSF by the choroid plexus of the lateral ventricles.[3] Both the stretch receptor mechanism and the arachnoid granulation body theories support the hypothesis of the pressure stat model and its ability to be the driving force of craniosacral motion.

IMPACT OF RESTRICTIONS IN THE CRANIOSACRAL FLOW

Upledger and colleagues[3] maintain that with sufficient education and training, a skilled practitioner can locate and evaluate the quality of a person's craniosacral rhythm anywhere on the body. This rhythm is interrupted when restrictions occur. How do these restrictions occur within the system, how do these restrictions affect the patient, and what can practitioners do about it?

There are 2 types of trauma that can cause restriction in the system: direct and indirect. Direct trauma affects the structures of the cranial system, such as a bone, a suture joint, or the membrane itself. It can occur from any number of events, including a birthing injury, a direct blow from a fall or auto accident, a fracture, a surgical procedure, a tumor, or a cerebrovascular accident.

An indirect trauma eventually affects the craniosacral system, but it does not initiate there. Indirect trauma may result from repetitive motion injuries, poor sitting or standing postures, or any habits of movement or position that pull the body out of its correct anatomical alignment. An old injury elsewhere on the body may work its way back into the craniosacral system through the fascia disrupting its rhythm and flow.

The body's fascial system, as described in detail in Chapter 6, plays a large role in both direct and indirect traumas that result in restrictions to the craniosacral flow. Remember that fascia is a fibrous collagenous web of connective tissue that runs through the entire body, covering every muscle, organ, osseous structure, and cell in the body. If one uses the metaphor of a wax candle with sea- shells embedded in it, the seashells would represent every cell, organ, muscle, bone, and nerve in the body, and the wax would represent the fascia. Anatomically, fascia runs primarily in a longitudinal direction within the sagittal plane from the top of the cranium to the plantar fascia of the feet in one continuous web of connective tissue. Horizontal diaphragms or fascial planes also exist, creating compartments that facilitate integrity and stability, and allow our visceral organs to stay in place. Without these horizontal fascial planes, gravity would take over and our kidneys would drop into our pelvic bowl or our lungs would continually expand laterally and drop into the abdominal cav- ity. The horizontal fascial planes are located at the base of the occiput, the level of the hyoid bone in the throat, the thoracic inlet, the respiratory diaphragm, and the pelvic floor. The fascia of the dura surrounding the cranium and the spinal cord forms the dural sheath within which the craniosacral fluid flows and rhythm takes place.

Fascia is connected to the meningeal system through the dural sheaths as they exit the spinal column. With trauma, the fascial system can be disrupted. Since fascia is ever-present, adhesions can form and extend their influence in a multitude of patterns and directions anywhere in the body. Consequently, it is feasible that an injury to the knee could present with symptoms in the cranium, in the form of headaches or tinnitus. In either case, there is no direct line of neuromuscular or osse- ous connection to the knee itself. With this model in mind, practitioners must learn to look at the fascial system as a whole unit instead of simply focusing on the site of the symptom or injury.

An excellent clinical example of the need to explore the larger whole-body system for the cause of a particular symptom can be found in the example of Mary Clark, a United States Olympic diver, whose career came to a complete standstill due to her problems with vertigo. Clark's balance was affected so severely that she was unable to stand on the platform, let alone compete as a diver. She tried many traditional medical remedies with no results, until she was examined and treated by Upledger. He assessed Clark's craniosacral system and concluded that her vertigo was most likely stemming from an old knee injury. He palpated the lines of fascial pull, which coursed from her knee to her temporal bone, actually pulling the lateral bone of her head into an anterior torsion. The ear canal running through the temporal bone was affected, and her symptoms presented as vertigo. Releases in the fascial system allowed the temporal bone to realign and the vertigo problem was resolved.[5] Clark was able to return to diving competition, and she ultimately won the bronze medal in platform diving in the 1996 Olympic Games.

Upledger's Protocol in Evaluating and Treating the Craniosacral System

Craniosacral practitioners release fascial adhesions through diaphragm-release techniques and release membrane restrictions by mobilizing the separate bones of the cranium. The cranial bones directly adhere to the cranial membranes. Upledger has devised a 10-step sequential protocol to evaluate and treat the craniosacral system. After he assesses the craniosacral rhythm along differ- ent areas of the body, step 1 is to induce a "still point" somewhere on the patient's body.[3] Usually performed at the base of the cranium or at the level of the sacrum, a still point occurs when the practitioner intentionally manually impedes the flow of craniosacral fluid, bringing the system to a complete rest. This action balances the autonomic nervous system and enhances relaxation. While in this state of "pause," the system has a chance to self-correct and reorganize. Typically, the practi- tioner will find the cranial rhythm to be stronger and more fluid after a still point induction because such manual interference in the system forces new pathways and breaks through old restrictions.

Step 2 of Upledger's protocol addresses the horizontal fascial diaphragms located at the level of the pelvis, respiratory diaphragm, thoracic outlet (inlet), hyoid, and cranial base (better known as the *suboccipital region*). Most longitudinal fascial fibers can be accessed through these horizontal diaphragms. The practitioner is basically treating by mobilizing the tissues found between one hand on the top of the body and the other underneath in the area of the horizontal plane. For example, at the level of the pelvic diaphragm, we could be addressing not only fascial restrictions under the skin, but also problems with the lumbosacral-coccygeal complex and/or the urogenital system. Symptoms, such as urinary frequency and prostate and vaginal problems, that might be emanating from restrictions in the fascia surrounding the organs and cells in that area would be addressed.

The respiratory diaphragm located at the transition area between T12 and L1 posteriorly and just below the xyphoid process anteriorly encompasses the diaphragm muscle. Naturally, any breathing, rib excursion, esophageal, stomach, inferior vena cava, pancreas, liver, spleen, transverse colon, adrenal, and associated spinal segment problems could all benefit from the release in hypertonicity of the respiratory diaphragm.

The thoracic inlet is named for the blood, lymph, and CSF that course through this area into the thoracic cavity from the head.[1] This fascial diaphragm is located at the level of C7 to T1 posteriorly and at the clavicular/sternal manubrium level anteriorly. If this area is restricted, it can potentially back up fluid into the cranium. Between this area lies a myriad of structures that could potentially be affected by hypertonicity of the transverse fascia and, thus, reduce normal craniosacral fluid flow. The plural dome, shoulders and scapula, clavicle and first rib, arms, hyoid musculature, sternocleidomastoid, upper trapezii, scalene and platysma muscles, jugular veins, subclavian arteries and veins, and thyroid and parathyroid glands all lie within this region. One can see how a forward head with rounded shoulder posture might place severe fascial strain on these structures and cause symptoms in several locations, including a full-blown upper quadrant syndrome of neck pain, weakness in the rotator cuff muscles, subdeltoid bursitis, and paresthesias in the fingers.

The hyoid diaphragm is exactly that—above and below the hyoid. Fascial strain in this area can affect the hyoid musculature, which is important for chewing and swallowing activities. This horizontal plane is commonly compromised with a whiplash-type injury, and restrictions are associated with temporomandibular joint disease (TMJ), tinnitus, and ear infections.

The occipital cranial base is the area where the suboccipital muscles lie at the base of the skull, between the occiput, atlas, and axis vertebrae. The dural tube directly connects to the foramen magnum and to the posterior surface of the vertebral bodies of C1 and C2. Lesions are common in this area and can severely and directly compromise the craniosacral system. With a whiplash injury, the suboccipital structures get jammed together and the condyles of the occiput can be pushed forward on the superior articular facets of the atlas. This area must move freely for the atlas to rotate properly on the axis. Freeing the cranial base is also beneficial for the tissues involved with the jugular foramen. Besides freeing up back pressure from the jugular vein, the glossopharyngeal, vagus, and spinal accessory cranial nerves run through the foramen. Release here can benefit the patient neurologically.[3]

After all of the above horizontal diaphragms are released, step 3 in Upledger's protocol calls for releases of the sacrum from the lower lumbar spine and from the ilium or innominate bones. Obviously, any tissue trauma from sprains or strains of the lumbar spine and the sacroiliac joint can be addressed with this technique. Disc problems and problems with structures innervated by sacral nerve roots—the colon, rectum, gluteus, piriformis, and resulting leg-length discrepancies—can also be addressed by releasing the sacrum. The craniosacral system has a direct dural attachment to bones at the level of S2, so restrictions to it can directly have an adverse affect on the flow of the system. This can release, not only at the level of the lumbosacral spine, but also all the way up to the head and neck. The dural tube is meant to glide freely within the vertebral canal, and the occiput and sacrum are designed to move in synchrony with one another. After freeing up the sacrum, one can perform a *dural tube traction* at the sacral end.

Step 4 is a 4 tube "rock-and-glide," that, while holding both the sacral and occiput ends of the dural tube, involves rocking the tube back and forth, "flossing" the dural tube within the spinal canal. The rock-and-glide is useful for the treatment and assessment of the dural tube within the spinal canal because a trained therapist can feel between his or her hands where further craniosacral restrictions reside and can pinpoint which segments are locked up within the system. If the therapist feels that the tube is clear at the proximal end until he or she gets down to the level of T6, and then it is clear again from the distal end up to about T11/L1, then the therapist can ask him- or herself, "Is the restriction residing within the tube directly under T6? Is it just outside the dural tube in the surrounding soft tissue or joint, or is it further away somewhere in the viscera or fascia, causing a drag at the level of T6?" Once the restriction is accurately located, the therapist can use other modalities, such as joint mobilization and myofascial release, to free up these 2 levels and completely clear the dural tube from one end to the other.

In addition to using joint mobilization, muscle energy techniques, position and hold, or soft-tissue/myofascial-release techniques to free up these restrictions, Upledger reintroduced a technique first conceptualized by Sutherland called the *V-spread technique* that also incorporates a technique referred to as *direction of energy*. Both are incredibly powerful techniques for tissue healing and reorganization. The therapist simply spreads 2 fingers across the suture line or the facilitated segment that he or she wants to mobilize and, with the other hand usually on the opposite surface of the body, sets his or her intention to where he or she wants the energy to go. With compassion, energy is directed from one hand through the tissue toward the V-spread until a release is felt. Signs of a release might include heat, pulsation, and/or a softening that is perceived between the therapist's 2 fingers (Figure 8-2). Although the mechanism of action at the cellular level remains a mystery, the intentional focus of energy into the body has been scientifically determined to result from biomagnetic emanations from the practitioner's hands.[10] In the near future, scientific technology will likely advance to the point where instrumentation can quantifiably measure the results that we are seeing. However, we should not completely disregard the unexplainable; it serves us well to remember that Dr. Fritz Hoffmann created aspirin to help his father's arthritic pain in 1897. We did not have the sophistication in science until the 1970s to discern the prostaglandin response. Simply put, it worked well and Hoffmann used what worked.

After freeing up the dural tube, step 5 of Upledger's protocol focuses on addressing and correcting restrictions in the cranial bones themselves. Each bone connects to other bones and to different cranial membranes. By opening up the frontal bone anteriorly and the parietal bones superiorly, the therapist connects to the falx cerebri and the vertical membrane system. The frontal bone sits anteriorly over the cerebral cortex; therefore, decompressing this bone may have positive effects on headaches, head trauma, and frontal sinus problems. We have seen some children with cerebral palsy have an overlap of the frontal suture, and freeing it up has resulted in profound reductions in spasticity.[3] Since the horizontal plate of the frontal bone contributes to the orbit and nasal cavity, decompression here could positively affect eye pain, olfactory issues, and sinus drainage.

Step 6 is a parietal bone release. The parietal bones lie directly over the cerebral cortex. This step actually allows the practitioner to take pressure off of the brain itself. The parietal lift assists in releasing bony restrictions from the frontal, temporal, sphenoid, and occipital bones. The sagittal suture runs between the parietals, and the falx cerebri runs vertically and lies directly on the undersurface of these paired bones. By using the superior lift technique, a skilled practitioner can mobilize and release restrictions of the falx cerebri, move through the falx cerebelli, and continue caudally releasing the dural tube itself. This technique is excellent for improving fluid exchange within the ventricular system. Signs and symptoms such as headaches, sinus problems, transient ischemic attacks, memory loss, and difficulties with motor planning can be addressed with this technique. In addition, a newborn with a forceps delivery should be treated with a parietal bone release as soon as possible after birth, as the parietals are often the surface that the forceps grab onto for the extraction.

In steps 7 and 8 of Upledger's protocol, by releasing the temporal bones laterally and the sphenoid bone in the anterior-posterior directions, we address restrictions of the tentorium cerebri and tentorium cerebelli (also known as the *horizontal membrane system*). Cranial nerves III (oculomotor), IV (trochlear), and VI (abducens) run between the layers of the horizontal membrane system, and dysfunctions associated with eye movement may be addressed with these techniques.[11] Even strabismus has been corrected with this technique.[3] A skilled therapist uses the temporal bones as bony

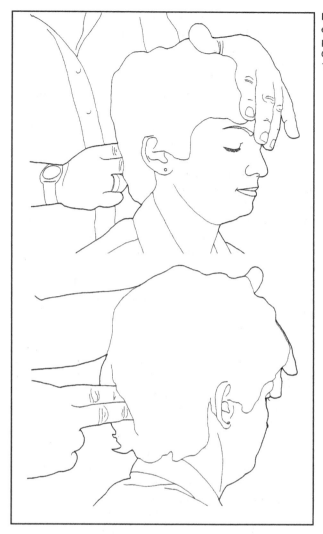

Figure 8-2. Finger placement for direction of energy release of falx cerebri. (Reprinted with permission from Upledger JE, Vredevoogd JD. *Craniosacral Therapy.* Seattle, WA: Eastland Press; 1983:73.)

handles to laterally distract the membrane. Compression of the temporals using another technique can release fascia connected to osseous and soft-tissue structures that attach to the temporal bone and mastoid process. Since the sternocleidomastoid, splenius capitis, rectus capitis, longus capitis, and temporalis muscles all attach to the temporal bones, practitioners would do well to evaluate for restrictions in the temporal bones for symptoms of neck and shoulder pain, whiplash injuries, and TMJ problems. Attention should then be brought to the mandible after the temporal bones have been cleared. (As a personal note, many times in the clinic I have found the upper cervical vertebrae of my clients to be out of alignment, and their symptoms will not completely dissipate until I release the cranial base and temporal bones.) With regard to the involvement of cranial nerves V (trigeminal; important for the muscles of mastication), VII (facial; important for facial expression and sensation of part of the tongue), and IX (glossopharyngeal; important for speech, swallowing, and the tongue), all 3 exit at the level of the brainstem and, thus, can be affected by the orientation of the temporal bones.[11,12]

The jugular foramen, just lateral to the petrous portion of the temporal bone, is an important structure, and adverse tissue tension around it can increase back pressure up into the head and sinuses. Tension here can also disrupt neural activity for the cranial nerves that run through it. The vagus nerve that innervates so many structures can go into vagotonia and cause all kinds of problems as a result of abnormal tissue tension around the jugular foramen. The auditory canal actually runs through this bone, so any problems with balance, hearing, tinnitus, and chronic ear infections may be reflective of the position of the temporal bones and their mobility. Clinically, children with autism often have a history of very severely compressed temporal bones bilaterally.[3,4] In children with dyslexia, craniosacral therapists often find the right temporal bone compressed. Finally, in children with dyscalculia (disability with respect to using mathematics), the left temporal bone is compressed.[3,5]

Step 8 is a release of the sphenoid, the final cranial bone to be released for freeing up the entire horizontal membrane system (Figure 8-3). A technique of compression and decompression is used. Sitting at the head of the supine client, the practitioner places the tips of his or her fingers gently on either side of the temple just lateral to the eyes. The initial movement is in the direction of ease, thus "unlatching the stuck door" before opening it, which is a gentle compression downward toward the surface on which the client is lying. Once fully compressed, the practitioner reverses the direction of the gentle pressure to an upward direction. Upledger maintains that 85% of all sphenoid dysfunction can be addressed with this simple technique of compression followed by decompression.[5]

Once in a while, the sphenoid, which lies behind the eyes and nose and attaches to the side of the face just lateral to the eyes, jams superior or inferior to the occipital bone. These lesions are more severe and need to be addressed independently, but much of the side-bent, torsioned, or lateral strains to the sphenoid can be addressed with the simple compression/decompression technique described above. If not, "normalizing each of the sphenobasilar dysfunctions is achieved by stabilizing the occiput and moving the sphenoid into its greatest range of motion (the named direction of dysfunction) and allowing for release,"[12] then moving into the direction of the restriction. Because the sphenoid is the only bone within the cranium that is connected to all other bones, it can be affected by many restrictions. The sphenoid, however, is typically not the source of the primary problem since the sphenobasilar joint is a synchondrosial joint having no capsule or fluid, just a cartilaginous bar between the bones. Any restriction here is often a compensatory problem stemming from fascial pull originating somewhere else in the body. Releasing the sphenoid is effective in treating such symptoms as headaches, migraines, sinusitis and allergy problems, pituitary problems, visual problems, learning dysfunctions, sacral dysfunction, coccyx compression, TMJ dysfunction, and even depression. One very interesting clinical picture is what Upledger has termed the *unhappy triad*.[5] Many times in the presence of endogenous depression, compression at vertebral level L5 to S1, the occipital cranial base, and the sphenobasilar synchrondrosis can be identified.

After all cranial bones have been released we move to step 9 of Upledger's protocol, which is balancing the mandible in relation to the cranium. A compressive then decompressive force (as done with the sphenoid) is used to release any tension at the temporomandibular joint and along the client's mandible. The therapist places each hand lengthwise along each side of the client's mandible, and uses a very gentle relaxed force to compress the mandible upward to its endpoint. Once complete, the therapist gently induces a slight downward pressure of not more than 5 g until full release has occurred. Many patients with TMJ who have been treated with this technique experience great relief.

Step 10, the final step of Upledger's protocol, is an induction of another still point, which is typically done at the patient's head. This allows his or her system to realign and integrate the work that has been done during the session.

CRANIOSACRAL THERAPY CONTRAINDICATIONS

Craniosacral therapy should not be used whenever changes in intracranial fluid pressure would be detrimental to the patient, such as in the presence of intracranial hemorrhage, an acute cerebrovascular accident, or an aneurysm.[1] It is also not recommended to induce a still point using a CV4 technique at the head of small children (under 8 years old), as a therapist could compress vulnerable structures that have not yet matured in the growing child.

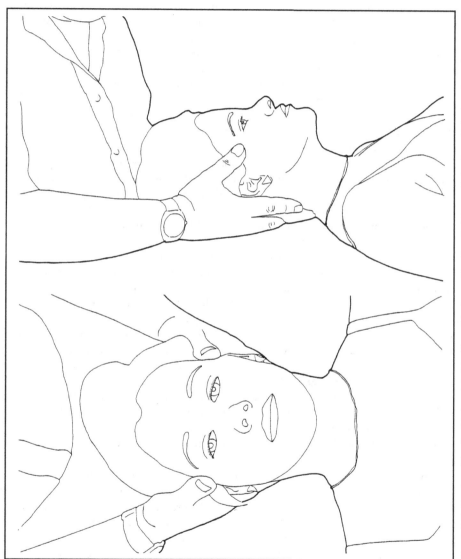

Figure 8-3. Hand position for third vault hold, sphenoid release. (Reprinted with permission from Upledger JE, Vredevoogd JD. *Craniosacral Therapy.* Seattle, WA: Eastland Press; 1983:100.)

EVIDENCE OF CRANIOSACRAL THERAPY EFFICACY

A review of the most-recent published studies renders great promise for the effectiveness of craniosacral therapy in general and the presence of the system anatomically. There were numerous studies of the pulsatile movements of the brain and spinal cord, studies that helped support the movement of CSF driven by the choroid plexus, studies that supported the mobility of cranial bones, studies that showed motion of the dural membranes by mobilizing through the cranial bones, and studies that showed a correlation between cranial mobility and sacral mobility. All of these studies and findings are in direct correlation to Sutherland's basic tenets of cranial osteopathy and Upledger's craniosacral therapy. And now, 75 later years later, modern technology and research have been able to support what clinicians have described and postulated for years.

Structurally, there is a lot of evidence that the craniosacral system exists. Early on, in the 1970s, Upledger first showed that the cranial bones moved with his research on squirrel monkeys. With radio frequency waves, he showed movement between the 2 parietal bones at a rate of 6 to 12 cycles/minute.[3] Since then, studies by Frymann,[13] Upledger and Karni,[14] Zanakis et al,[15] Lockwood and Degenhardt,[16] and Moskalenko et al[17] all have shown that there is cranial mobility.[18]

Some very exciting work from NASA has come out in support of the craniosacral concept that shows expansion of the skull correlates with expansion of the ventricles producing CSF. First, NASA researchers looked at numerous fresh cadavers (93 men and 83 women) and infused saline at 1 cycle/second (1 hertz) to expand the ventricles. They found an expansion of the skull of 0.29 mm with 15 mL of saline.[18,19] Although this movement is small, there was a direct correlation between the expansion of the ventricles and the expansion of the skull. The cranial bones expanded with the filling of the ventricles.

NASA also created a device called a pulsed phase-locked loop (PPLL) that was shown to measure the diameter of the skull in correlation with the expansion of the ventricles and an increase in intracranial pressure.[20] Wanting to measure cranial pressure in a noninvasive way, NASA then used this PPLL to see how changes in intracranial pressure affected its astronauts in an antigravity situation. The device was worn on the head of 7 patients. Each patient was measured at a 60-degree head tilt, a 30-degree head tilt, a supine position, and a 10-degree head-down tilt. The tilt positions were chosen to observe how an altered gravity vector affected intracranial pressure dynamics. Expansion distances were measured and the distance from the frontal to the occipital bone increased the most at 1.038 ± 0.207 mm in the 10-degree head-down position. NASA found that cranial diameter increased with increased intracranial pressure, and that these changes in cranial diameter pulsations were considered to be statistically significant.[20] NASA researchers said in their article that "although we have always thought of the cranial bones as rigid fixed container with constant volume, many researchers have shown the skull moves on an order of a few μm in association with the changes in intracranial pressure."[18,20]

Besides having cranial bone movement, another anatomical postulate of the cranial sacral techniques is that you can mobilize the dural membranes using the bones of the skull. Research has been performed that looked at the connection between the cranial bones and the underlying dural membranes. Kostopoulos and Keramidas[21] showed movement of the dural membrane by manually mobilizing the cranial bones in a laboratory. They attached a piezoelectric element to an embalmed cadaver along the vertical intracranial membrane, the falx cerebri. They then proceeded to do a manual frontal lift and measured the movement with an oscilloscope. They found that they were able to elongate the dural membrane by 1.44 mm by using a frontal lift and by 1.08 mm by using a parietal lift.[21] Not only did the cranial bones move, but the authors were also able to demonstrate movement of the attached intracranial membrane underneath the bone. Studies on fresh cadavers may show even more movement, and it would be prudent to perform further research in the future.

Zanakis et al have done a lot of research with cranial motion and the postulates of cranial osteopathy and craniosacral therapy. In one study, they were able to identify a possible connection between cranial suture motion and sacral motion,[22] assessing both ends of the craniosacral system at the same time. They placed infrared surface markers on the skin over the parietal bones and the frontal bones, assessing the movement between the 2 markers. While assessing the movement between the sensors, a therapist was manually palpating the sacrum, assessing the craniosacral rhythm. The practitioner would tap a sensor every time he or she felt the start of a cranial sacral impulse cycle. In this study, the researchers found a significant 92% correlation between the manual palpation of the cranial rhythm and of the movement between the cranial bone markers.[22]

With all of these anatomically based results, there are areas of craniosacral research still lacking, particularly with the ability to verify and reproduce data in relation to interrater and intrarater reliability. Rogers and colleagues[23] at the University of North Carolina at Chapel Hill published the results of a study that examined simultaneous palpation of the craniosacral rate at the head and feet of clients, examining intrarater and interrater reliability and rate comparisons. Twenty-eight adult subjects were divided in half by a curtain as they lay supine on a treatment table. One experienced craniosacral examiner was at the head and another was at the feet. The examiners' findings were recorded with the activation of a silent foot switch that was depressed when no signal was present and activated by lifting the foot at the beginning of the flexion phase of the craniosacral rhythm. Intrarater reliability measures were taken with examiner A at the head, examiner A at the feet, examiner B at the head, and examiner B at the feet. Interrater reliability measures were compared at the head and the feet. The interrater intraclass correlations (ICCs) were 0.08 at the head and 0.19 at the feet. The intrarater ICCs ranged from 0.18 to 0.30. Craniosacral rates measured at the feet and the head were not identical. The results indicate the craniosacral rhythm cannot be palpated reliably.[23] Other researchers have found similar results[24,25] and failure to demonstrate interrater reliability has led many to question its validity.[26]

One reason for the discrepancies may be explained by the phenomenon of entrainment: as soon as the energies of the client and therapist "connect," the total of the energy field shifts to incorporate the sum of the 2 energies. The scientific evidence and hypotheses surrounding the theory of entrainment are not well known, and the authors made no mention of the idea in the study and the possible effect of the examiners' energy fields on what was being measured. Another reason for differences in rate between examiners listening at the head and feet simultaneously may be that patient injury may cause differences in the CS rhythm on different areas of the same body.

Besides studying the anatomy and physiology of the craniosacral system, also important are the clinical outcomes of utilizing the treatment protocols with patients. Over the past few years, numerous studies have been conducted with various patient populations showing positive outcomes with the use of craniosacral therapy, either with craniosacral therapy alone or in conjunction with other modalities.

One study that shows great promise in the area of infertility was conducted by physical therapist Mary Ellen Kramp[27] with 10 infertile women. Many of the issues that can contribute to infertility can be traced to scar tissue, fascial restrictions, and lymphatic congestion in the pelvic region. All 10 women in the study were deemed infertile by Centers for Disease Control and Prevention standards. By definition, all 10 women were in their childbearing years and were unable to get pregnant after at least 12 consecutive months of unprotected sex with their husbands.[28] The therapist used manual therapy techniques, including craniosacral therapy, lymph drainage, visceral manipulation, and muscle energy to the pelvic area as needed per the physical therapist's evaluation. Each woman needed between 1 and 6 treatments in total. Within 3 months of the intervention, 6 of the 10 women were able to conceive and carry their babies to full term.[27] This was a small pilot study and no control group was used, so further studies would be beneficial. But it shows great promise, as these statistics bring these women to normal ranges of fertility using very cost-effective, noninvasive techniques with no side effects, and using no medications.

Another study by Mehl-Madrona et al[29] looked at combining acupuncture and craniosacral therapy. Many patients like to combine modalities and treatments in hopes of achieving the best outcomes. This is often done in clinical settings, but no evidence prior to this study has shown that combining treatments for asthma is any more effective.[29] Typically, acupuncture studies are done uncontrolled, since a double-blind control would be difficult with the nature of acupuncture and using needles. Previously, a case study involving 25 patients with asthma who were treated with acupuncture and traditional Chinese medicine showed that more than 80% improved symptomatically and became less dependent on steroids.[30] Before the study by Mehl-Madrona and colleagues, no research had been conducted supporting craniosacral therapy for asthma treatment.[29]

So, Mehl-Madrona et al decided to determine whether synergy would occur and improve patient outcomes utilizing both craniosacral therapy and acupuncture treatments for patients with asthma. Would craniosacral therapy and acupuncture be more effective together than each individual modality alone? What they found was that acupuncture, craniosacral therapy, and the combination of the 2 modalities were *all* more effective than a control group in treating asthma. They also found that it was not synergistically more effective when the 2 modalities were used in combination as compared with each individual modality alone.[29]

What was interesting and unexpected in this study was that the consistency of practitioner care did actually make a difference with patient outcomes. All patients were seen for 12 visits. Both the craniosacral therapy group and the acupuncture group were seen by the same practitioner. In the combined group, the patients were seen by 2 different practitioners, 6 times each, alternating treatments of craniosacral therapy and acupuncture, totaling 12 treatments. When compared, patient reports of anxiety were significantly and statistically less severe when the treatment practitioner was consistent. This suggests that relationships play a role in facilitating treatment effectiveness.[29]

A study by Castro-Sánchez et al[31] performed with patients with fibromyalgia also reported good results with the use of craniosacral therapy. The objective of the study was to determine the influence of craniosacral therapy on anxiety, depression, pain, sleep quality, and quality of life in 84 patients with fibromyalgia. The double-blind longitudinal study lasted over a 25-week period. Patients were randomly assigned to an intervention group or a placebo group and both were treated twice/week. The intervention group underwent 1-hour treatments using the aforementioned Upledger 10-step protocol and the placebo group received a placebo treatment of what patients thought was US on various joints, but the US was unplugged from the wall. Thirty-minute treatment times were used for the placebo group so as not to waste too much of the patients' time. Both groups maintained their regular medications and received no other treatment interventions. All subjects took a series of baseline assessment tests that included the Visual Analog Scale for pain, the 36-Item Short-Form Health Survey (SF-36) to assess quality of life, the Pittsburgh Sleep Quality Index, the Beck Depression Inventory, and the State-Trait Anxiety Inventory. All tests were given 30 minutes, 6 months, and 1 year post-treatment.

After 25 weeks and 50 treatments, those who received the craniosacral treatments showed improvement with decreased pain ($P < 0.035$) and decreased anxiety ($P < 0.029$ for state anxiety and $P < 0.042$ for trait anxiety) when compared with their baseline. No significant changes were seen in the placebo group. The craniosacral group also showed improvements in their quality of life with improved physical functions, physical role, body pain, general health, vitality, and social function. Even after 6 months, individuals in the intervention group showed a significant improvement vs their baseline in physical function ($P < 0.041$). The placebo group showed no differences (vs baseline) in any of the SF-36 questionnaire items. The groups differed significantly in physical function ($P < 0.049$) and vitality ($P < 0.050$). The 2 groups also differed significantly in sleep duration ($P < 0.039$), habitual sleep efficiency ($P < 0.047$), and sleep disturbance ($P < 0.045$) even after 6 months. The Beck Depression Inventory did show some slight differences with the cranial intervention group, but no relevant significant differences were noted with baseline or the placebo group. In conclusion, with such positive overall results, the researchers noted that "craniosacral therapy must be considered as a complementary therapy within a multidisciplinary approach for these fibromyalgia patients in conjunction with pharmaceuticals, physiotherapeutic psychological and social treatments."[31]

As one can see, these studies, along with numerous others, show support for craniosacral therapy as a treatment modality. These were only 3 patient populations, but numerous other patients can be helped with craniosacral therapy with no harmful side effects. Clinically, we have seen support in clients with attention deficit disorder and attention deficit hyperactivity disorder. When a child can go from being withdrawn and unable to communicate effectively with others to being able to sit and eat socially at the dinner table with craniosacral therapy being the only intervention, one must take notice. Patients with headaches and brain trauma are also populations that utilize the techniques. The Upledger Institute International is now conducting a study following a pilot program in support of helping former professional football players with post-concussion syndrome with the use of craniosacral therapy with some interesting results. They found an improvement of less overall pain, improved quality of life, a significant difference for symptoms associated with depression, decreased cervicogenic pain, and increased cervical range of motion.[32] The Department of Veterans Affairs is now helping veterans with post-traumatic stress disorder using craniosacral therapy with good result as well.[4] There is so much good coming out of these techniques that is hard to argue. People are healing and improving the quality of their lives with the help of craniosacral therapy.

CONCLUSION AND A PERSONAL NOTE

A review of the subtle energy techniques of craniosacral therapy has certainly expanded in the last 15 to 20 years. More researchers are finding evidence supporting that the craniosacral therapy system does exist and that its effectiveness has been proven in the clinic. In this chapter, I have described craniosacral therapy in terms of its structure, its anatomy and physiology, the basic techniques of practice, the types of clinical problems it can help, and the rationale behind how symptoms are relieved. After studying with Upledger and the Upledger Institute International, I have been able to use the basic tools with my clients and have helped many people over the years. I have brought craniosacral therapy techniques to the treatment table and integrated them into my traditional physical therapy training. I have moved from fixing my clients to being a facilitator in their healing process. As Upledger said, "it is as though we can remove some of the pebbles, some stones in their river that is impeding the flow," that is impeding their healing. I have learned that craniosacral therapy is so much more than tissue releases. It has changed the way I work with my clients. I remember in the early years I would not even speak about the techniques I was using, I would just listen to the body, use the tools in my tool box, and watch patients get better quietly without saying a word about how we were getting the results. Now, I speak freely because I know to trust my hands, to trust the techniques, and to trust what the patient's body is telling me. Mobilizing the tissues is still physical therapy, it's just that how I get there is different than what I was initially taught in school. The richness, fullness, and skill in the techniques have only expanded over the years.

Experience in practice teaches us that we are more than muscles, nerves, joints, and bones. We are whole, living human beings with aspects that are not often considered in patient care, such as energy fields, beliefs, perceptions, and emotions, and we all have spiritual connections. The trauma or disease that brings us to treatment in reality can be physical, mental, emotional, or spiritual in nature and in origin. There is really no way to separate out the aspects of ourselves that are difficult to measure from that which we can see and measure. If some part of us is out of balance, our body-mind intelligence will do what it can to re-establish homeostasis. If homeostasis cannot be achieved, according to the theories of energy medicine, disease and disharmony eventually manifest.

Upledger describes how trauma can enter the body and form what he calls *energy cysts*. Either an injury by force, trauma, or a negative experience "enter" the body and, depending on its severity and how often it is repeated, as well as the emotional state of the patient at the time of injury, the body-mind can either dissipate the trauma, "wall it off," or isolate it to minimize the problem.[3] This formation of an energy cyst decreases the patient's natural flow of body energy, "life force," or vitality. It also affects the person's craniosacral rhythm. Thus, energy cysts form the "stones in the river" impeding the craniosacral flow.

Many patients will present to the office with problems that have eluded other practitioners that they have seen and that often have been told that their symptoms are "all in their heads." It has been my experience and the experience of thousands of practitioners and patients that craniosacral therapy often unlocks those elusive symptom puzzles and thus enables us to more adequately help our patients.[3]

Is it really as simple as listening and following? You bet it is. I have seen that if I can step back and hold a supportive space for my clients, if I can get out of my own way and theirs, if I can set my own agenda aside and follow their body tissue where they need to go instead of where I think they "should" go, then the therapy session flows with much more ease and grace, and the clients and I feel much better at the end of a treatment. With trained hands, a compassionate open heart, and a listening ear, it truly is the most respectful way to be with a person.

The name of this book has changed from *Complementary Therapies* to *Integrative Therapies* because these complementary treatments are really becoming an integral part of the rehabilitation program. I am teaching this information to fourth-year medical students at the University of Maryland in College Park, Maryland. Isn't it wonderful that a medical school now gives its students an opportunity to take elective courses in integrative medicine? The University of Miami has a course in integrative medicine for its physical therapy students. All of these students will at least be familiar with this types of integrative modalities when their patients say they are receiving them. We are bridging a gap that has been a long time coming. I was given a strong foundation with my initial studies and it has truly expanded from there. The definition of *integrative* is "to bring together or incorporate (parts) into a whole." We are in 21st century health care and we have entered a new era of healing. It is time that we as clinicians read the science behind energy medicine, broaden our minds about approaches to patient care that facilitate balance and the flow of energy, and take the time for learning, practicing, and researching integrative therapies for the benefit of all.

REFERENCES

1. Magoun HI. *Osteopathy in the Cranial Field.* 2nd ed. Denver, CO: Sutherland Cranial Teaching Foundation, Cranial Academy; 1996.
2. Feely RA. *Clinical Cranial Osteopathy.* Meridian, OH: The Cranial Academy; 1988.
3. Upledger JE, Vredevoogd JD. *Craniosacral Therapy.* Seattle, WA: Eastland Press; 1983.
4. Upledger JE. *Your Inner Physician and You: CranioSacral Therapy and SomatoEmotional Release.* Berkley, CA: North Atlantic Books; 1997.
5. Upledger JE. *CranioSacral Therapy I Study Guide.* Palm Beach Gardens, FL: Upledger Institute Inc; 1997.
6. Retzlaff EW, Michael D, Roppel R, Mitchell F. Proceedings: structure of the cranial bone sutures. *J Am Osteopath Assoc.* 1976;75(6):607-608.
7. Retzlaff EW, Mitchell FR Jr, Upledger JE, Biggert T. Nerve fibers and endings in cranial sutures. *J Am Osteopath Assoc.* 1978;77:100-101.
8. Adams T, Heisey RS, Smith MC, Briner BJ. Parietal bone mobility in the anesthetized cat. *J Am Osteopath Assoc.* 1992;92(5):599-600.
9. Wallace W, Avant W, McKinney W, Thurston F. Ultrasonic measurement of intracranial pulsations at 9 cycles/min. *J Neurol.* 1975;10.
10. Oschman JL. *Energy Medicine: The Scientific Basis.* New York, NY: Churchill Livingstone; 2000.
11. Schultz RL, Feitis R. *The Endless Web: Fascial Anatomy and Physical Reality.* Berkley, CA: North Atlantic Books; 1996.
12. Kandel ER, Schwartz JH. *Principles of Neural Science.* 2nd ed. New York, NY: Elsevier; 1985.
13. Frymann VM. A study of the rhythmic motions of the living cranium. *J Am Osteopath Assoc.* 1971;70(9):928-945.
14. Upledger JE, Karni Z. Strain plethysmography and the cranial rhythm. Presented at: Proc XII International Conference on Medicine and Biology Engineering; August 19-24, 1979;. Jerusalem, Israel.
15. Zanakis MF, Cebelenski RM, Dowling D, et al. The cranial kinetogram: objective quantification of cranial mobility in man. *J Am Osteopath Assoc.* 1994;94(9):761-EOA.
16. Lockwood MD, Degenhardt BF. Cycle-to-cycle variability attributed to the primary respiratory mechanism. *J Am Osteopath Assoc.* 1998;98(1):35-36, 41-43.
17. Moskalenko IUE, Kravchenko TI, Gaidar BV, et al. The periodic mobility of the cranial bones in man [article in Russian]. *Fiziol Cheloveka.* 1999;25(1):62-70.
18. King H. (1995). Research in Support of the Cranial Concept. www.iahe.com/images/pdf/Article__-_CranioSacral_Therapy_Research.pdf

19. Ballard RE, Wilson H, Hargens AR, et al. Noninvasive measurement of intracranial volume and pressure using ultrasound. American Institute of Aeronautics and Astronautics Life Sciences and Space Medicine Conference. Book of Abstracts, pp.76-77, Houston TX, 3-6 March 1996.

20. Ueno T, Ballard RE, Macais BR, Yost WT, Hargens AR. Cranial diameter pulsation measured by non-invasive ultrasound decrease with tilt. *Aviat Space Environ Med.* 2003;74(8):882-885.

21. Kostopoulos DC, Keramidas G. Changes in elongation of falx cerebri during craniosacral therapy techniques applied on the skull of an embalmed cadaver. *Cranio.* 1992;10(1):9-12.

22. Zanakis MF, Rogers JS, Witt PL, Gross MT, Hacke JD, Genova PA. Simultaneous palpation of the craniosacral rate at the head and feet: intrarate and interrater reliability and rate comparison. *Phys Therapy.* 1997;78:1175-1185.

23. Rogers JS, Witt PL, Gross MT, Hacke JD, Genova PA. Simultaneous palpation of the craniosacral rate at the head and feet: intrarater and interrater reliability and rate comparisons. *Phys Ther.* 1997;78(11):1175-1185.

24. Hartman SE, Norton JM. Interexaminer reliability and cranial osteopathy. *The Scientific Review of Alternative Medicine.* 2002;6(1):23-34.

25. Wirth-Pattullo V, Hayes KW. Interrater reliability of the craniosacral rate measurements and their relationship with subjects' and examiners' heart and respiratory rate measurements. *Phys Ther.* 1994;74(10):908-916.

26. Nelson KE, Sergueef N, Glonek T. Recording the rate of the cranial rhythmic impulse. *J Am Osteopath Assoc.* 2006;106(6):337-341.

27. Kramp ME. Combined manual therapy techniques for the treatment of women with infertility: a case series. *J Am Osteopath Assoc.* 2012;112(10): 680-684.

28. Centers for Disease Control and Prevention. Infertility. Centers for Disease Control and Prevention web site. www.cdc.gov/nchs/fastats/fertile.htm. Updated February 6, 2015. Accessed February 5, 2016.

29. Mehl-Madrona L, Kligler B, Silverman S, Lynton H, Merrell W. The impact of acupuncture and craniosacral interventions on clinical outcomes in adults with asthma. *Explore (NY).* 2007;3(1):28-36.

30. Kleijnen J, ter Reit G, Knipschild P. Acupuncture and asthma: a review of controlled trials. *Thorax.* 1991;46(11):799-802.

31. Castro-Sánchez AM, Matarán-Peñarrocha GA, Sánchez-Labraca N, Quesada-Rubio JM, Granero-Molina J, Moreno-Lorenzo C. A randomized controlled trial investigating the effects of craniosacral therapy on pain and heart rate variability in fibromyalgia patients. *Clin Rehabil.* 2011;25(1):25-35.

32. Wetzler G, Fryer S, Roland M, Visger G. The Ricky Williams concussion project. Poster presented at: Santa Clara Valley Brain Injury Conference; February 5-7, 2015; Santa Clara, CA. www.upledger.org/img/programs/concussion-poster.pdf.

9

Complete Decongestive Therapy

Barbara Funk, MS, OTR, CHT and
Kevin R. Kunkel, PhD, MSPT, MLD-CDT

Manual lymph drainage (MLD) is one component of a comprehensive lymphedema management program termed *complete decongestive therapy* (CDT), which also includes skin care, compressive bandaging, and remedial exercise.[1] Both occupational and physical therapists receive their education from traditional training programs that include minimal background for the treatment of lymphedema disorders. However, with the higher prevalence of certified lymphedema therapists and continued research, entry-level education is offering the students of many health care programs increased exposure to lymphedema treatment.

Supplemental lymphedema training offered by specialists is needed to adequately ensure that treating therapists have the full knowledge base and manual techniques required for this management program. The Lymphology Association of North America (LANA) was established to promote the standards of care and has established a national certification for lymphedema therapists.[2] MLD provides therapists with an opportunity to facilitate the molecular and energetic flow in their patients through direct contact with the skin. Dr. Andrew Taylor Still, known as the father of osteopathy, stated, "We strike at the source of life and death when we go to the lymphatics…Thus it behooves us to handle them [the lymphatics] with wisdom and tenderness, for by and from them, a withered limb, organ, or any division of the body receives what we call reconstruction, or is builded anew."[3] Certain diseases and disorders, such as lymphedema, limit the informational streams through the energetic circuits in the living organism.[4] CDT provides the health care practitioner with the method by which to facilitate the continuous flow within the body of the lymphatic fluid, promoting self-regulation and homeostasis.

FUNCTION OF THE LYMPHATIC SYSTEM

The lymphatic system has been significantly less studied than the blood circulatory system. In fact, the former has been considered by many to be "less important, invisible, and secondary to the blood vascular system."[5] The structure and function of the lymphatic system represents the foundation of knowledge needed to apply the therapeutic techniques required in CDT. The main function of the lymphatic system is to collect protein-rich fluid within the interstitial space and transport it

Davis CM.
Integrative Therapies in Rehabilitation: Evidence for Efficacy in Therapy,
Prevention, and Wellness, Fourth Edition (pp 115-129).
© 2017 Taylor & Francis Group.

to the blood circulation.[6,7] The advancement of imaging technology allows for a deeper appreciation of the lymphatic system and has propelled it to a system of parallel importance with the blood
circulatory system.[5] "The lymphatic system constitutes a one-way transport system that operates
in conjunction with the circulatory system."[8] Anatomically, the system has 4 ongoing processes:
lymph production, lymph transport, lymph concentration, and lymph filtration.[9] The successful
completion of these activities in conjunction with the blood vascular system provides for the optimal functioning and integrity of the extracellular and intracellular environment. Damage to the
lymphatic system and/or failure of the system to successfully remove interstitial fluid can result in
infection, swelling (lymphedema), pain, dampened immune responses, and connective tissue and
fat accumulation.[6,8]

Three Basic Functions of the Lymph System

Maintain Fluid Balance in Tissues

The first function consists of removing excess fluid, bacteria, large proteins, and particulate matter away from the interstitial spaces and body tissues. The *interstitium,* which is defined as the area
between the capillary walls and the cells, "consists of a predominantly collagen fiber framework, a
gel phase of glycoaminoglycans, a salt solution and plasma proteins."[10] The removal of substances
from the interstitial spaces of high molecular weight, such as protein, is an essential function, without which death would occur within 24 hours.[11]

The extensive web of blood vessels and lymphatics travels intimately within the interstitium,
or tissue channels. It offers a route and mechanism to transmit all substances that go to and from
the cells. The environment of the lymph system at all levels, superficial to deep, is intertwined and
supported by the fascial system. John F. Barnes describes an extensive review of the fascial system in *Myofascial Release: The Search for Excellence: A Comprehensive Evaluatory and Treatment
Approach.*[12] On a cellular level, the fascia creates the interstitial spaces; on another level, it forms
layers around the muscle, influencing lymph circulation. It is through the proper functioning of this
connective tissue that many of the body's physiological processes are supported, such as humeral
and vascular profusion, lymphatic flow, bioelectric conduction,[12] and energy balance.[13] The interstitial environment, or connective tissue, is composed of collagen fibers set in proteoglycan molecules
forming the solid (gel phase) of the connective tissue and set in fluid (sol phase) where there is minimal gel.[14] The polysaccharide gel complex fills the spaces between the collagen fibers; proteoglycans
and hyaluronic acid compose the gel.[12] It has been postulated that the gel in the interstitium creates
the structure to hold interstitial fluid in place. Gel dehydration does not occur due to the electro-
static charges that cause osmosis of water into its lattice (Gibbs-Donnan Equilibrium).[9]

The fluid balance of the tissues is preserved by mutual regulation of the blood capillaries, interstitial tissues, proteolytic cells, and initial lymphatics.[15] It is a fine balance of the capillary filtration
and capillary reabsorption. Factors that can shift the equilibrium are capillary (hydrostatic) pressure, interstitial tissue pressure, and colloid osmotic pressure in the capillaries and tissue fluids
(Starling's flow mechanism).[16] The lymph minute volume generally operates at 10% of its maximum
transport capacity. This is important in maintaining homeostasis when there are shifts in the
hydrostatic and oncotic pressures. However, as we will see, this large functional reserve and safety
valve function is no longer adequate under certain circumstances, resulting in lymphedema. Under
normal conditions, the venous capillaries reabsorb 90% of the fluid, and the lymphatics reabsorb the
remaining 10%. This generates approximately 2 to 4 liters of liquid transported by the lymph system
in 24 hours and between 80 and 200 grams of protein removed.[16]

Maintain Optimum Functioning of the Immune System and Transport for Therapeutic Molecules

Through a process of lymph filtration, noxious matter (eg, bacteria, toxins, dead cells) is removed from the system. This filtering of foreign agents alerts the system to trigger through humeral and cellular support, antibodies, and lymphocytes that cause dissolution of these cells.[17] The lymphatic system also transports immune cells to injury sites and serves to deliver drugs to treat cancer and HIV that often travel in the lymphatic system. The benefit of drug delivery via the lymphatic system is that it circumvents the first pass reduction in concentration of a drug.[7]

Transport and Absorb 80% to 90% of Fat From the Intestines

The lymphatics draining the intestines absorb through the central lacteals of the villi-emulsified fat principally in the form of fatty acids. These fatty acids, or chylomicrons, are transported by the lymphatics to the thoracic duct, eventually conveyed to the blood by the left subclavian vein.[17,18] Impairment of the lymphatic system with either obstruction or damage is associated with diseases, including intestinal lymphangiectasia, Whipple's disease, and lymphoma.[19]

ORGANIZATION AND STRUCTURE OF THE LYMPHATIC SYSTEM

Creating an internal image of the vast lymphatic system facilitates our intention and direction of the treatment process. With a 3-dimensional respect and knowledge of the lymphatic structure, the therapist is best able to effectively influence the equilibrium of the system. The lymphatic system consists of organs and vessels that contain lymphoid tissue. These include the lymph vessels, lymph nodes, spleen, thymus, tonsils, and Peyer's patches (cells in the intestinal lining). Clearly, the lymph vessels and lymph nodes hold the greatest influence on lymphedema. "The lymphatic system is asymmetrical: the right side of the head and thorax and the right arm drain into the right subclavian, whereas the lymphatic vessels of the rest of the body converge at the thoracic duct, which empties at the junction of the jugular and left subclavian."[8]

Lymph Vessels

Lymph Capillaries (Initial Lymphatics)

Lymph capillaries represent the most peripheral elements of the system as a valveless network. They originate in the tissue spaces and form a web-like plexus throughout the body. Their cell walls are composed of a flat, overlapping monolayer of nonfenestrated endothelial cells. They have a diameter of 10 to 60 μm and a wall thickness of 50 to 100 nm.[8] The cells are supported by anchor filaments attached to the surrounding connective tissue and prevent the collapse of the initial lymphatic vessels when interstitial pressure increases.[8] The vessel structure allows for the absorption of fluid, large particulate matter, and proteins. It is generally felt that absorption occurs through passive conduction into the endothelial junctions. Casley-Smith and Casley-Smith[14] also describe capillary pumping action as a potential process. While they do not have valves, the initial lymphatics act as a valve by closing to stop backflow once the interstitial pressure rises.[8]

Lymph Precollectors

These vessels contain smooth muscle cells and bicuspid one-way valves. The layers of smooth muscle are capable of spontaneous contractions. However, there are areas without muscle (similar to the initial lymphatics) with a discontinuous basal lamina, and those areas act to absorb fluid instead.[8] Like the lymph capillaries, lymph precollectors also function to absorb and transport lymph from the interstitium.[16] They are the connection between the initial lymphatics and the collecting vessels.

Lymph Collectors

The lymph collectors receive lymph flow from the lymph precollectors. These vessels differ from the initial lymphatics and precollectors in that they have a continuous basal lamina and contain a secondary valve preventing retrograde flow, guaranteeing direction of fluid flow from distal to proximal or to a regional lymph node.[8] Valves are evident every 0.6 to 2.0 cm, as they are proportional to the caliber of the vessel. The segment between 2 valves is called a *lymphangion*. Lymphangion intrinsic contractions (lymphangiomotoricity) occur in normal conditions 6 to 10 times/minute and may increase to 2 to 3 times this value when stimulated during increased interstitial fluid production, activity, or MLD.[8,20] During exercise, both the amplitude and the rate of contraction increase, creating a functional reserve tenfold.

Lymph Trunks and Ducts

Lymph trunks and ducts represent the largest lymph vessels receiving lymph from the collectors. The trunks eventually empty into the ducts that return the lymph into the blood circulation at the left and right venous angles. The thoracic duct is the largest and most visible under cadaver dissection. It starts from the cisterna chyli, which receives bilateral lumbar lymphatic trunks at the level of lumber vertebrae 1 and 2. It ascends proximally to eventually discharge to the junction of the left subclavian and jugular veins.[21,22]

Lymph Nodes

Lymph nodes play an integral part in the body's defense mechanism. There are an estimated 600 to 700 nodes in the body. They receive the lymph fluid and function as a biological filtering station for noxious matter, regulate the concentration of protein in the lymph fluid, and produce lymphocytes.[17] Regions of the body drain to specific lymph node concentrations located in the cervical, axilla, inguinal, and abdominal regions. The skin areas, called *lymphotomes*, define normal drainage regions adjacent to the nodal concentrations.[23]

The lymphatic system is structurally adapted to absorb and transport lymph through intrinsic contractions. The sympathetic nervous system and the lymph volume influence the frequency rate of contractions. If lymph volume increases (such as in conditions of physical exertion or inflammation), an increase in lymph time volume would be accomplished through increased pulsation frequency and increased filling amplitude of the lymphangion. Lymph transport is also facilitated by the contraction of skeletal muscles, arterial pulsation, respiratory changes, negative pressure in the central veins, and external pressure.[16] Later in this chapter, we will address how CDT directly influences these processes.

LYMPHEDEMA

Definition and Causes

Lymphedema is defined as an abnormal accumulation of protein-rich fluid in the interstitial tissues, resulting in the swelling of a body segment, most often the extremities. Lymphedema is a disease that represents a significant health problem affecting the lives of millions of people across the globe. The World Health Organization estimates that 120 million people in 72 countries are infected with parasites, of whom 15 million have lymphatic filariasis, that 20 million people are affected by breast cancer, and that 2 to 3 million people are affected by primary lymphedema.[24]

Filarial infection (parasites) is the major cause of lymphedema in underdeveloped countries, whereas a substantial number of lymphedema cases in industrial countries result from cancer treatments. Petrek and colleagues[25] report breast cancer therapy affecting more than 400,000 women in the United States. According to the National Cancer Institute, occurrence is 50% to 70% after axillary treatment.[26]

The pathophysiology of lymphedema occurs when the lymph load (volume) exceeds its transport capacity.[27] Stagnation of fluid creates changes in the microcirculation and in the overall cellular health. Changes that may occur include chronic inflammation, increased lymphatic pressure and vasodilation, and valvular incompetence. Reactive tissue changes include the proliferation of connective tissue cells, fatty tissue deposits, fibrosis, skin thickening, skin erythema, and, in rare cases, the development of an angiosarcoma. Patients with lymphedema are often prone to repeat infections, cellulitis, erysipelas, and lymphangitis.[27] Further, reduced oxygen availability due to tissue congestion can lead to delayed wound healing.

As the girth of one's extremities and respective quadrants (ipsilateral trunk) increases, additional manifestations are noted. Reports include limitations in joint range of motion, decreased functional performance, pain, paresthesias, and weakness in the affected extremity.[28-31] Psychological morbidity is documented in several descriptive and case control studies identifying common psychological problems, such as anxiety, depression, sexual dysfunction, social avoidance, and exacerbation of existing psychological illness.[31-33]

Classification

Lymphedema is divided into 2 classifications: *primary* (idiopathic) and *secondary* (acquired). Primary lymphedema develops without obvious cause due to the malformation of the lymphatics (dysplasias). Onset may be at birth, but it most frequently develops around 17 years of age. The discovery of more than 20 genes have been linked to the development of primary lymphedema.[34] Lymphedema praecox (occurs prior to age 35 years) accounts for 83% of primary lymphedema cases, whereas lymphedema tardum (occurs after age 35 years) represents 17% of cases.[35]

The following are several of the known causes of secondary lymphedema:

- Post-cancer management (node dissection, radiation, and reconstruction)
- Significant trauma to nodes and vessels (from an accident or self-induced)
- Repeated infections, such as cellulitis
- Postsurgical procedures, such as coronary bypass
- Malignant tumor vessel blockage
- Filarial infection

Lymphedema may also develop in combination with other disorders, such as obesity, chronic venous insufficiency, lipedemia, and rheumatoid arthritis.[16]

Stages

Földi et al[36] describe 3 stages of lymphedema, from mild to severe.

- Stage I: Reversible Lymphedema
  - Accumulation of protein-rich edematous fluid
- Stage II: Spontaneously Irreversible Lymphedema
  - Protein-rich edematous fluid
  - Connective and scar tissue
- Stage III: Lymphostatic Elephantiasis
  - Protein-rich edematous fluid
  - Connective and scar tissue
  - Hardening of dermal tissues
  - Skin papillomas

In addition to these 3 stages, there is a subclinical (latent) phase that occurs with tissue alterations but is not clinically detected by circumferential measures.[37] During this time, patients describe the sensations of limb heaviness, pins/needles, and pain.[38] Early diagnosis and treatment improves the prognosis for treating lymphedema, avoiding more serious sequelae. During Stage I, pitting is evident; upon arising in the morning, swelling may not be present. During Stage II, the tissue has a spongy consistency with less pitting. During Stage III, fibrosis and hardening are noted as girth increases.

Diagnosis and Evaluation

Lymphedema is diagnosed clinically by medical history and physical examination.[39] Estimated volumetric measures are frequently used to quantify limb edema.[40] Limb volume is estimated by taking several circumferential measures at prescribed standard distances. A high correlation has been made with limb volume to the gold standard of water displacement.[41,42] Calculating volume assessments using the truncated cone method is noted by Morgan et al.[43] An optoelectronic device called a *Perometer* takes a measurement that uses a frame lifted around a dependent limb. The Perometer has been shown to be highly reliable in the measurement of limb volume.[44]

Palpation of the edematous body part for density changes is essential to determine the extent of fibrosis that develops as a result of protein accumulation Radiation therapy can also contribute to the development of radiation fibrosis and lymphedema by creating acute tissue damage, inciting an inflammatory response, connective tissue disintegration, and decreased oxygen to epithelial cells resulting in cell death.[45]

Lymphoscintigraphy, which allows the visualization of the lymphatic system, is a major diagnostic tool in the evaluation of lymphedema.[46,47] Computed tomography and magnetic resonance are additional imaging methods that may be used.[48]

As a thorough part of the evaluation and examination, indices such as the Breast Cancer and Lymphedema Symptom Experience Index are used to objectify subjective reports from the patient for baseline assessment and to track intervention progress.[49]

COMPLETE DECONGESTIVE THERAPY

History

CDT was first introduced by von Winiwarter,[50] who suggested the use of lymphatic massage and bandaging for the swollen limb. In the 1930s, Vodder was instrumental in developing a soft touch manual therapy for intact lymphatics.[13] Further, Kinmonth,[51] Kubik and Manestar,[52] and Földi et al[11] all revealed in their research a greater understanding of the anatomy, physiology, and pathophysiology of the lymphatic system. This enlarged foundation of knowledge was instrumental in the further development of a system for lymphedema management.

The Földis (Germany, 1980s) are credited with modifications to the original Vodder's manual lymph drainage technique[53] and the further extension of care creating CDT.[36] Additional variations in methods have been made by Casley-Smith and Casley-Smith,[54] Leduc and Leduc,[55] and Vodder.[56] Lerner[27] first introduced CDT in the United States in the 1980s. As one reviews the extensive international literature on lymphedema management, the nomenclature used to represent CDT may also include complex physical therapy, complex lymphedema therapy, and complex decongestive physiotherapy.

Description

This approach is noninvasive, safe, and provides the patient with the management skills needed to control his or her chronic condition. CDT is a tetrad consisting of skin care, MLD, exercise, and compression therapy. These 4 principal strategies were agreed upon by Földi, Leduc and Leduc,[55] the Vodder School (Kasseroller), and Casley-Smith et al.[57] Before engaging any person in this multimodal program, physician clearance is needed to rule out any complications that would influence the partial or full utilization of program components. However, depending on the country and even the state in which the health care professional practices, direct access allows a patient to receive intervention without a physician referral.[58] CDT should be part of a comprehensive program that offers the individual support, including medical management, nutritional guidance, psychological support, and rehabilitation. Lymphedema is a chronic disease that cannot be cured. Therefore, long-term follow-up and case management are integral components to ensure the highest levels of patient functioning over time.

Phases

The phases of lymphedema treatment as outlined by Klose and Norton[20] are as follows:

- Phase I: Treatment Phase
  - Meticulous skin and nail care
  - MLD
  - Compression bandaging
  - Remedial exercises
- Phase II: Maintenance Phase
  - Compression garments (worn during the day)
  - Bandaging (worn at night)
  - Meticulous skin and nail care
  - Remedial exercises
  - MLD as needed

Goals of Treatment

The goals of treatment include the following:

- Control lymph formation and improve drainage through existing lymphatics and collateral routes
- Eliminate fibrotic tissue (Stages II and III)
- Avoid re-accumulation of lymph fluid
- Protect against infections
- Ensure long-term maintenance for improved arm size and shape by patient
- Achieve rehabilitation goals, including pain reduction, increased range of motion, improved independence in activities of daily living, reduction of tissue and scar adhesions, normalization of postural imbalances, increased strength, and increased endurance

Components

Manual Lymph Drainage

This specific massage technique is designed to control lymph formation and improve drainage through existing vessels and collateral routes.[59] The therapist provides this manual stimulation of the lymphatic vessels by increasing the lymphangiomotoricity. Technique principles and treatment pathways have been described in detail by Vodder,[13] Földi, and Casley-Smith and Casley-Smith.[14] According to Földi et al,[36] MLD should first be applied to the contralateral quadrant of the trunk, enhancing lymphatic contractility and lymph flow through watersheds. Following truncal clearance, the root of the involved limb should be addressed, followed by the proximal to distal components.

Guides for treatment pathways are given but do not represent a fixed procedure, as each individual presents with differing tissue characteristics. The instruction in self-massage varies.[35] A major determinant is the time allowed for the intensive phase of care, which is influenced by insurance coverage, patient availability, institution policies, and severity of the condition.

MLD may also be effective as part of a treatment plan for other conditions, such as post-traumatic edema, postsurgical edema, complex regional pain syndrome, scleroderma, and chronic fatigue.[35] MLD has an extensive influence on the human constitution and life quality of the cells. Its role in decreasing sympathetic tone and stimulating the parasympathetic nervous system affects growth, recovery, and restorative tissue changes. The light, changing pressures function to decrease pain sensation and increase the lymphangiomotoricity. MLD offers immunological support by facilitating transport and deactivating pathogens. Its immediate effect is noted in its influence on the cellular environment by normalizing the function and composition of the connective tissue.

Additional rehabilitative techniques may also be beneficial for these patients. An example of this is the use of myofascial release techniques to relieve chest wall pain, fascial restrictions, and emotional holding patterns in the body.[12,60]

Features and Principles of Manual Lymph Drainage

The following features and principles of MLD are essential to its success in the treatment of pathology, which results in the increased lymphatic load[61]:

- Hand movements are used to stretch the skin in specific directions and promote variations in interstitial pressures, usually without the use of oils.

- Movements are slow, repetitive, and soporific, and usually incorporate a brief resting phase where the skin is allowed to return to its normal position.

- Pressures vary according to underlying tissues but aim to promote lymph drainage without increasing capillary filtration and hyperemia.

- Deeper or firmer movements may be incorporated when treating areas of fibrosclerosis, with compression therapy usually applied afterwards.

- The MLD sequence starts proximally and centrally, often with treatment to the neck.

- Functional and healthy regional lymph nodes are treated; for example the contralateral (opposite side) axilla and ipsilateral (same side) inguinal nodes in an upper limb lymphedema, or both axillae in lower limb lymphedema.

- Proximal areas such as contralateral and non-edematous lymph territories of lymphotomes are treated, including the midline or "watershed area" between 2 skin lymph territories.

- The ipsilateral trunk and lymphedematous limb are treated, starting proximally, often with particular attention to treating the swollen limb.

- Early in the treatment, emphasis may be on treating the anterior and posterior trunk prior to the swollen limb.

- Breathing techniques are commonly used with MLD, often combined with controlled hand pressure by the therapist, to influence drainage in the deep abdominal lymphatic vessels and nodes.

- Limb mobilization and relaxation techniques may be incorporated into the MLD treatment session.

Skin Care

Skin care includes the eradication of bacterial and fungal infections prior to initiating care and the daily application of low pH skin lotion to reduce the chances of infection. Patient education regarding the knowledge and observance of limb precautions is paramount.[62]

Compression Therapy

Compression therapy is a vital component in lymphedema management. Low-stretch compressive wraps are applied to the limb after each MLD session and worn until the following session. The compression wraps prevent the re-accumulation of evacuated fluid, limit blood capillary filtration, and improve striated muscle pump efficiency.[59] In addition, bandaging helps to soften and mobilize fibrotic tissue. These wraps provide high pressure during muscular contraction and low pressure at rest. All patients are instructed in self-bandaging techniques when practical. During the maintenance phase, adaptations to bandage techniques are created to facilitate patient independence.

At the end of the intensive phase, patients are measured and fit for elastic support garments. Limb swelling creates enlarged intercellular spaces and reduces tissue elasticity, requiring the application of elastic garments to support the limb contour.[14] Generally, the elastic garments are worn while the patient is awake during the day and short-stretch bandages are used while he or she is sleeping at night. Elastic garments need to be replaced every 4 to 6 months because they lose their compression. All patients are instructed in the proper care and donning of their garments. Alternative nonelastic compression devices are available in situations where short-stretch bandages and elastic garments are not feasible. The circaid (Medi)[63] and the Reid sleeve (Peninsula BioMedical Inc)[64] are a couple of examples of alternative wrappings.

The intermittent pneumatic pump is one of the original treatment methods used with lymphedema. The single or multiple chamber pump removes excess fluid from the interstitial spaces but does not influence protein reabsorption from the involved extremity.[55] Today, there is divided opinion on the therapeutic influence of the pneumatic pump and its role in CDT. While its adjunctive use is advocated in multiple case studies,[65-70] several authors feel that the pump is potentially dangerous and ineffective in the treatment of lymphedema.[11,14,54,71-73] Warnings include the possible formation of residual fibrotic bands at the root of limbs, increased incidence of genital edema, damage to superficial lymph vessels, and truncal edema.

Remedial Exercise

Exercise is performed while wearing the non-yielding short-stretch bandages or elastic garments. Muscular activity and exercises, both active and passive, facilitate lymph propulsion through the filling and distension of lymph vessels, hence increasing lymph flow.[59] Exercise programs are individually determined for each patient. A standard course might include passive range of motion and isotonic and isometric aspects. Specific exercise routines have been advocated by Casley-Smith in Swedborg,[74] Morgan et al,[43] Miller,[75,76] and Klose and Norton.[35] Deep breathing exercises are emphasized because they create a negative intrathoracic pressure, enhancing lymph flow into the thoracic duct.

In addition to the 4 components of CDT (manual lymph drainage, skin care, compression therapy, and remedial exercise), additional treatments may be dictated by the occupational and physical therapists' findings during patient evaluation. Rehabilitation may focus on improving range of motion, strength, self-care skills, joint mobility, posture, adhesions, and pain management. Psychological and nutritional guidance for patients is supported through referral assistance.

Evidence of Efficacy

By way of introduction, all of the studies cited in this section for evidence of efficacy have been performed by highly acclaimed specialists in lymphedema management. The study descriptions, patient characteristics, treatment methods, and results allow the systematic evaluation of intervention strategies for the individual with lymphedema. Volume estimations by circumferential measurements have been shown to be highly correlated ($r = 0.93$ to 0.98) with water displacement. The types of studies are cohort. Statistical analyses for the studies include paired student t-test, descriptive, and measures of covariance.

CDT represents a multimodal intervention strategy recommended by several National Institutes of Health consensus panels and is currently the most efficacious treatment for both primary and secondary lymphedema.[39,77-79] In fact, it is recommended as the initial conservative treatment for lymphedema.[43,68,80-83] Treatment of lymphedema involves interstitial fluid mobilization and removal, and the reabsorption of stagnant proteins.[11,84] In addition, fibrosis reduction and limb recontouring may be needed to provide comprehensive and desired outcomes.

The Földis treat approximately 2500 patients with CDT each year.[85] Földi et al have conducted clinical studies in which CDT resulted in volume reductions in 95% of 399 patients; 50% reduction in 56% of patients; 25% to 49% in 31% of patients; 1% to 24% in 8% of patients; 89% sustained their results at 3 years.[3] Casley-Smith and Casley-Smith[41] reported over 60% reductions in 618 lymphedematous limbs. Boris et al[53,73] treated 119 patients with CDT. Reductions averaged 62% in 56 patients with one affected arm and 68% in 38 single-leg patients. After 36 months, follow-up reductions were 63% for the arm patients and 62% for the single-leg patients. The authors showed that compliance significantly influenced outcomes.[53,73] Szuba et al[86] prospectively analyzed 79 treated patients with moderate to severe lymphedema. Duration of treatment was 8±3 days. Mean short-term reductions in the upper extremities and the lower extremities were 44%±62% and 42%±40%, respectively. After 38±52 days, the reductions in the upper extremities and the lower extremities were sustained at 38%±56% and 41%±27%, respectively.[86] Ko et al[83] treated 299 patients over a duration of 15.7 days. Lymphedema reductions averaged 59.1% in the upper extremities and 67.7% in the lower extremities. Follow-up at 9 months demonstrated compliant patient reductions (86%) at 90% for upper and lower extremities. Noncompliant patients lost 33% of their reductions. Incidence of infections reduced per patient per year from 1.10 to 0.65.[83]

Since the first edition of *Complementary Therapies in Rehabilitation* was published in 1997, several issues have been raised by health care practitioners in the field of lymphedema management proposing the need for future investigations into practice methods. Rising health care costs, fiscal restraints, inadequate availability of trained personnel, and delayed and misdiagnosed lymphedema are impacting the comprehensive service utilization of CDT. The complex biology of lymphedema impacts the chronicity of the disease. Early intervention may have the ability to forestall, minimize, or even eliminate the consequences of lymphedema.[87] Suggestions for future research opportunities include early intervention strategies as a preventive approach for high-risk individuals; large, randomized controlled trials to investigate the effectiveness and efficiency of CDT interventions, in both the individual components and in combination; and studies on the effect of treatment on disease progression.

A study that reviewed 75 articles from 2009 to 2014 supported the use of CDT with the highest evidence for the best clinical practice.[88] It was also determined that additional interventions, including weight management, full-body exercise, information delivery, prevention awareness, and early intervention, can be effective in the treatment of lymphedema.

CASE EXAMPLE

Mrs. B. is a 58-year-old school teacher with a diagnosis of secondary lymphedema of the right dominant upper extremity. She had a radical mastectomy in 1995, followed by radiation therapy. During her hospital stay, she was briefly instructed in a home range-of-motion program. In 1997, Mrs. B. had a cellulitis infection in her right arm, which is when her swelling began. She was on antibiotics for 2 months and was then referred to the outpatient rehabilitation clinic. Her physician gave her medical clearance to participate in all components of the CDT program.

Findings on Initial Evaluation

The findings on initial evaluation include the following:

- Restricted range of motion in the glenohumeral joint following capsular pattern
- Postural imbalances
- Paresthesias in axilla along the lateral border of the right chest wall, in the right index finger, and in the thumb
- Reduced right upper-extremity strength, including grip and pinch

- Self-care restrictions with dressing, hygiene, cooking, home-maintenance tasks, and writing on a chalk board

- Pain in the right chest extending to the cap of the shoulder (4 to 6 out of 10)

- Stage II lymphedema with swelling throughout the limb and anterior chest wall, greatest along the lateral border of the forearm. Pitting and fibrosis in the lower arm, soft tissue texture in upper arm and in digits. Total edema volume of the right upper extremity was 38% higher than that of the left upper extremity (3798.2 cm^3 vs 2735.4 cm^3)

- Myofascial restrictions (anterior and lateral chest wall, right lateral trunk, anterior throat, and lateral cervical regions)

- Insurance plan and prescription dictate 12 visits within 30 days for lymphedema

Treatment Plan

Mrs. B. has typical rehabilitation issues regarding her musculoskeletal system and her lymphedema condition. As joint immobility of the shoulder negatively influences the lymphatic flow and function, it is important that this be addressed as soon as possible. Initially, Mrs. B. was treated daily for 12 visits with a major focus on CDT. The second diagnosis related to the shoulder was added once the lymphedema management was under way, allowing the authorization of 9 additional treatment sessions.

Program

The components of Mrs. B.'s program include the following:

- Mrs. B. received educational materials on the lymphatic system, limb precautions, written pictures, review of home exercises (passive range of motion, strengthening, deep breathing, aerobics), and community support groups.

- Rehabilitation intervention: joint mobilization, neuromuscular training, myofascial release and scar mobilization, postural training, neural gliding, and functional strengthening

- Self-care training/adaptations

- CDT

- Daily MLD followed by compression wrap with short-stretch bandages. Exercises were performed with bandages. Mrs. B. and her husband were trained in the bandaging process. Mrs. B. received her elastic glove and sleeve, which she wore during the day by week 4. Compression bandages were worn while sleeping and in the early morning during home exercises.

Discharge Status

Mrs. B. has full range of motion of the right shoulder, with reduced pain reported at 2 out of 10. Strength is functional for activities such as dressing, hygiene, cooking, and leisure interests. Chalkboard writing activities were adapted by using an overhead projector. Continued gains in strength are anticipated over the next several months. As myofascial restrictions were reduced significantly, alterations in posture were normalized and paresthesia reduced by 90%. Limb volume reductions were 48.5% after the first 12 visits and 68% after total completion of the rehabilitation program. Tissue texture is soft throughout with minimal fibrosis at the lateral border of the ulna. Mrs. B. has continued trying to reduce the fibrosis with her bandaging method and through a massage technique she has been shown. Numbness in the hand is no longer an issue as long as compression methods are utilized and swelling is controlled.

Mrs. B. was instructed to continue daily exercises, use daytime elastic garment wear, and sleep with bandages. Due to insurance restrictions, Mrs. B. has a follow-up visit with her physician, who would initiate additional treatment if there were any significant limb changes. Mrs. B. will need a prescription from her physician for a new glove and sleeve in 6 months.

Training in Complete Decongestive Therapy

Current programs vary in their comprehensiveness of treatment and, therefore, in their success in management of lymphedema. Effective lymph management is directly related to therapist training and experience, insurance availability, and patient compliance. General standardization of treatment and the education of professionals would facilitate the consistency of treatment outcomes required for research and efficacy, and would offer policymakers and insurance companies the needed information to favorably influence reimbursement. There is an urgent need to develop legislative advocacy groups to facilitate the care of individuals with lymphedema.

Licensure for certification in lymphedema management became available in spring 2001 through LANA, a nonprofit corporation composed of health care professionals developing standards of qualification for individuals who treat lymphedema. Once lymphedema therapists are certified, they can utilize the acronym CLT-LANA (Certified Lymphedema Therapist-Lymphedema Association of North America). This is an important step toward qualifying care standards. Information regarding professional training programs that offer the didactic and manual training (a component of the certification) is available through the National Lymphedema Network (NLN).[89] The NLN, a nonprofit organization, is dedicated to making information on the prevention and treatment of lymphedema available to the general public and the medical community.

Conclusion

Lymphedema is a chronic condition requiring lifelong consideration. The disease currently has many available treatment options that demonstrate efficacy for reducing edema volume, preventing the re-accumulation of fluid, and reducing the frequency of infections. Patients who participate in a CDT program with a qualified therapist have the opportunity to achieve greater functional usage of their limb(s), improved quality of life, and a sense of control in their disease management.

References

1. Merchant SJ, Chen SL. Prevention and management of lymphedema after breast cancer treatment. *Breast J.* 2015; 21(3):276-284.
2. Lymphology Association of North America. Mission statement. www.clt-lana.org/mission-statement.html. Published 2016. Accessed February 6, 2016.
3. Ward RC. *Foundations for Osteopathic Medicine.* 2nd edition. Philadelphia, PA: Lippincott Williams & Wilkins; 2003.
4. Oschman JL. *Energy Medicine: The Scientific Basis.* New York, NY: Churchill Livingstone; 2000.
5. Choi I, Lee S, Hong YK. The new era of the lymphatic system: no longer secondary to the blood vascular system. *Cold Spring Harb Perspect Med.* 2012;2(4):a006445.
6. Alitalo K. The lymphatic vasculature in disease. *Nat Med.* 2011;17(11):1371-1380.
7. Ali Khan A, Mudassir J, Mohtar N, Darwis Y. Advanced drug delivery to the lymphatic system: lipid-based nano-formulations. *Int J Nanomedicine.* 2013;8:2733-2744.
8. Margaris KN, Black RA. Modelling the lymphatic system: challenges and opportunities. *J R Soc Interface.* 2012;9(69):601-612.
9. Guyton AC, Hall JE. The microcirculation and the lymphatic system: capillary fluid exchange, interstitial fluid and lymph flow. In: *Textbook of Medical Physiology.* Philadelphia, PA: Saunders Elsevier; 1996: 183-197.
10. Wiig H, Swartz MA. Interstitial fluid and lymph formation and transport: physiological regulation and roles in inflammation and cancer. *Physiol Rev.* 2012;92(3):1005-1060.
11. Földi E, Földi M, Clodius L. The lymphedema chaos: a lancet. *Ann Plast Surg.* 1989;22(6):505-515.
12. Barnes JF. *Myofascial Release: The Search for Excellence: A Comprehensive Evaluatory and Treatment Approach.* Paoli, PA: MFR Seminars; 1990.
13. Wittlinger H, Wittlinger G. *Textbook of Dr Vodder's Manual Lymph Drainage. Vol 1. Basic Course.* 3rd rev. Heidelberg, Germany: Haug; 1982.
14. Casley-Smith JR, Casley-Smith JR. *Modern Treatment of Lymphedema.* 5th edition. Malvern, PA: Lymphedema Association of Australia; 1997.

15. Casley-Smith JR. The structure and functioning of the blood vessels, interstitial tissues, and lymphatics. In: Casley-Smith JR, Földi M, eds. *Lymphangiology.* New York, NY: New Schattauer; 1983: 27-143.
16. Weissleder H, Schuchhardt C. *Lymphedema: Diagnosis and Therapy.* 2nd ed. Bonn, Germany: Kagerer Kommunikation: 1997.
17. Guyton, AC. Immunity and allergy. In: Guyton AC, ed. *Textbook of Medical Physiology.* 4th ed. Philadelphia, PA: WB Saunders; 1971: 118-125.
18. Wang TY, Liu M, Portincasa P, Wang DQ. New insights into the molecular mechanism of intestinal fatty acid absorption. *Eur J Clin Invest.* 2013;43(11):1203-1223.
19. Glickman RM. Fat absorption and malabsorption. *Role Gastrointestinal Tract Nutrient Del.* 2013;3:145.
20. Ochałek K, Grądalski T. The use of manual lymph drainage in vascular diseases. *Acta Angiologica.* 2011;17(3):189-198.
21. Rusznyák I, Földi M, Szabó G, *Lymphatics and Lymph Circulation: Physiology and Pathology.* Philadelphia, PA: Elsevier; 2013.
22. Kiyonaga M, Mori H, Matsumoto S, Yamada Y, Sai M, Okada F. Thoracic duct and cisterna chyli: evaluation with multidetector row CT. *Br J Radiol.* 2012; 85(1016):1052-1058.
23. Gregoire V, Scalliet P, Ang KK. *Clinical Target Volumes in Conformal and Intensity Modulated Radiation Therapy: A Clinical Guide to Cancer Treatment.* Berlin, Germany: Springer Science & Business Media; 2004.
24. World Health Organization. *International Classification of Diseases.* Geneva, Switzerland: World Health Organization; 2010.
25. Petrek JA, Lerner R. Lymphedema. In: Harris JR, Lippman ME, eds. *Diseases of the Breast.* Philadelphia, PA: Lippincott Williams & Wilkins; 1996: 896-903
26. United States Department of Health and Human Services. *The Breast Cancer Digest: A Guide to Medical Care, Emotional Support, Educational Programs, and Resources.* 2nd ed. Bethesda, MD: Office of Cancer Communications, National Cancer Institute; 1984.
27. Lerner R. Chronic lymphedema. In: Chang JB, ed. *Textbook of Angiology.* New York, NY: Springer Link; 2000: 1227-1236.
28. Maunsell E, Brisson J, Deschênes L. Arm problems and psychological distress after surgery for breast cancer. *Can J Surg.* 1993;36(4):315-320.
29. Sneeuw KC, Aaronson NK, Yarnold JR, et al. Cosmetic and functional outcomes of breast conserving treatment for early stage breast cancer. 2. Relationship with psychosocial functioning. *Radiother Oncol.* 1992;25(3):160-166.
30. Segerström K, Bjerle P, Nyström A. Importance of time in assessing arm and hand function after treatment of breast cancer. *Scand J Plast Reconstr Surg Hand Surg.* 1991;25(3):241-244.
31. Passik SD, Newman ML, Brennan M, Tunkel R. Predictors of psychological distress, sexual dysfunction and physical functioning among women with upper extremity lymphedema related to breast cancer. *Psycho-Oncology.* 1995;4(4):255-263.
32. Velanovich V, Szymanski W. Quality of life of breast cancer patients with lymphedema. *Am J Surg.* 1999;177(3):184-187; discussion 188.
33. Tobin MB, Lacey HJ, Meyer L, Mortimer PS. The psychological morbidity of breast cancer-related arm swelling. Psychological morbidity of lymphoedema. *Cancer.* 1993;72(11):3248-3252.
34. Schlögel MJ, Brouillard P, Boon LM, Vikkula M. Genetic causes of lymphedema. In: Greene AK, Slavin SA, Borson H, eds. *Lymphedema: Presentation, Diagnosis, and Treatment.* New York, NY: Springer; 2015: 19-31.
35. Klose G, Norton S. *Course Manual for Manual Lymph Drainage (MLD), Complete Decongestive Therapy (CDT).* Red Bank, NJ: Red Klose Norton Training and Consulting; 2000.
36. Földi E, Földi M, Weissleder H. Conservative treatment of lymphoedema of the limbs. *Angiology.* 1985;36(3):171-180.
37. Piller NB. Pharmacological treatment of lymph stasis. In: Olszewski W, ed. *Lymph Stasis: Pathophysiology, Diagnosis and Treatment.* Boca Raton, FL: CRC Press; 1991: 501-529.
38. Clodius L. Secondary arm lymphedema. In: Clodius L, ed. *Lymphoedema.* Stuttgart, Germany: Georg Thieme; 1977:166-174.
39. Casley-Smith JR, Földi M, Ryan TJ, et al, Summary of the 10th International Congress of Lymphology working group discussions and recommendations, Adelaide, Australia, August 10-17, 1985. *Lymphology.* 1985;18:175-180.
40. Sitzia J, Stanton AW, Badger C. A review of outcome indicators in the treatment of chronic limb oedema. *Clin Rehabil.* 1997;11(3):181-191.
41. Casley-Smith JR, Casley-Smith JR. Treatment of lymphedema by complex physical therapy, with and without oral and topical benzopyrones: what should therapists and patients expect. *Lymphology.* 1996;29(2):76-82.
42. Casley-Smith JR. Measuring and representing peripheral oedema and its alterations. *Lymphology.* 1994;27(2):56-70.
43. Morgan RG, Casley-Smith JR, Mason MR, Casley-Smith JR. Complex physical therapy for the lymphoedematous arm. *J Hand Surg Br.* 1992;17(4):437-441.
44. Tan CW, Coutts F, Bulley C. Measurement of lower limb volume: agreement between the vertically oriented perometer and a tape measure method. *Physiotherapy.* 2013;99(3):247-251.
45. Ridner, SH. Pathophysiology of lymphedema. *Semin Oncol Nurs.* 2013;29(1):4-11.
46. Brennan MJ, DePompolo RW, Garden FH. Focused review: postmastectomy lymphedema. *Arch Phys Med Rehabil.* 1996;77(3 Suppl):S74-S80.

47. Mortimer PS, Bates DO, Brassington HD, Stanton AWB, Strachan DP, Levick JR. The prevalence of arm oedema following treatment for breast cancer. *QJM*. 1996;89:377-380.
48. Hafez HM, Wolfe JH. Basic data underlying clinical decision making: lymphedema. *Ann Vasc Surg*. 1996;10(1):88-95.
49. Fu MR. Lymphedema management. In: Paice JA, Ferrell BR. *Physical Aspects of Care: Nutritional, Dermatologic, Neurologic and Other Symptoms*. Oxford, United Kingdom: Oxford University Press; 2015.
50. A., VW. Die Elephantiasis, Deutsche Chirurgie. Stuttgart, Germany: Enke; 1892.
51. Kinmonth JB. Management of some abnormalities of the chylous return. *Proc R Soc Med*. 1972; 65(8):721-722.
52. Kubik ST, Manestar M. Some lymphological problems in anatomical view. Progress in lymphology. Proceeding of the VIIth International Congress of Lymphology, Florence 1979. Prague, Czech Republic: Avincenum Czcechoslovak Medical Press; 1981: 22-25.
53. Boris M, Weindorf S, Lasinksi S, Boris G. Lymphedema reduction by noninvasive complex lymphedema therapy. *Oncology (Williston Park)*. 1994;8(9):95-106; discussion 109-110.
54. Casley-Smith JR, Casley-Smith JR. Other physical therapy for lymphedema: pumps, heating, etc. In: Casley-Smith JR, Casley-Smith JR, eds. *Lymphedema*. Adelaide, Australia: Lymphedema Association of Australia; 1991: 155-159.
55. Leduc A, Leduc O. Physical treatment of oedema. *European Journal of Lymphology and Related Problems*. 1990;1:8-10.
56. Kurz, I. *Textbook of Dr. Vodder's Manual Lymph Drainage*. Stuttgart, Germany: Thieme; 1997.
57. Casley-Smith JR, Boris M, Weindorf S, Lasinski B. Treatment for lymphedema of the arm—the Casley-Smith method: a noninvasive method produces continued reduction. *Cancer*. 1998;83(12 Suppl American):2843-2860.
58. American Physical Therapy Association. Oklahoma 49th state to grant patients direct access to physical therapist treatment. www.apta.org/Media/Releases/Legislative/2014/5/29/. Published May 29, 2014. Accessed February 6, 2016.
59. Mortimer PS. Investigation and management of lymphoedema. *Vasc Med Rev*. 1990;1:1-20.
60. Barnes, JF. Pain relief for cancer patients. *PT and OT Today*. 1996;4:18-19.
61. Williams A. Manual lymphatic drainage: exploring the history and evidence base. *Br J Community Nurs*. 2010;15(4):S18-S24.
62. Thiadens SRJ. *Eighteen Steps to Prevention for the Upper Extremity/Lower Extremity*. San Francisco, CA: National Lymphedema Network; 1997.
63. Bergan JJ. Control of lower extremity lymphedema by semirigid support. *Natl Lymphed Net Newslett*. 1994;6:1-2.
64. Reid T. Reid sleeve for effective treatment for lymphedema. Abstract presented at: Lymphedema The Problem and the Challenge Second National Lymphedema Network Conference; September 1996; San Francisco, CA.
65. Woźniewski M. Value of intermittent pneumatic massage in the treatment of upper extremity lymphedema [article in Polish]. *Pol Tyg Lek*. 1991;46(30-31):550-552.
66. Mirolo BR, Bunce IH, Chapman M, et al. Psychosocial benefits of postmastectomy lymphedema therapy. *Cancer Nurs*. 1995;18(3):197-205.
67. Zelikowski A, Aviram R, Haddad M, Hadar H, Reiss R. The use of far distal arterial bypass for limb salvage. *J Cardiovasc Surg (Torino)*. 1986;27(1):38-41.
68. Bunce IH, Mirolo BR, Hennessy JM, Ward LC, Jones LC. Post-mastectomy lymphoedema treatment and measurement. *Med J Aust*. 1994;161(2):125-128.
69. Pappas CJ, O'Donnell TF Jr. Long-term results of compression treatment for lymphedema. *J Vasc Surg*. 1992;16(4):555-562; discussion 562-564.
70. Richmand DM, O'Donnell TF Jr, Zelikovski A. Sequential pneumatic compression for lymphedema. A controlled trial. *Arch Surg*. 1985;120(10):1116-1119.
71. Boris M, Weindorf S, Lasinski BB. The risk of genital edema after external pump compression for lower limb lymphedema. *Lymphology*. 1998;31(1):15-20.
72. Eliska O, Eliskova M. Are peripheral lymphatics damaged by high pressure manual massage? *Lymphology*. 1995;28(1):21-30.
73. Boris M, Weindorf S, Lasinkski S. Persistence of lymphedema reduction after noninvasive complex lymphedema therapy. *Oncology (Williston Park)*. 1997;11(1):99-109; discussion 110, 113.
74. Swedborg I. Effectiveness of combined methods of physiotherapy for post-mastectomy lymphoedema. *Scand J Rehabil Med*. 1980;12(2):77-85.
75. Miller LT. *Recovery in Motion: An Exercise Program to Assist in the Management of Upper Extremity Lymphedema*. Philadelphia, PA: LT Miller; 1992.
76. Miller LT. The enigma of exercise: participation in an exercise program after breast cancer surgery. *Natl Lymphed Net Newslett*. 1996;8:15-16.
77. International Society of Lymphology. The diagnosis and treatment of peripheral lymphedema: 2013 consensus document of the International Society of Lymphology. *Lymphology*. 2013;46(1):1-11.
78. Harris SR, Hugi MR, Olivotto IA, Levine M; The Steering Committee for Clinical Practice Guidelines for the Care and Treatment of Breast Cancer. Clinical practice guidelines for the care and treatment of breast cancer: 11. Lymphedema. *CMAJ*. 2001;164(2):191-199.
79. International Society of Lymphology. Consensus document of the International Society of Lymphology Executive Committee. The diagnosis and treatment of peripheral edema. *Lymphology*. 1995;28:113-117.

80. Rockson SG, Miller LT, Senie R, et al. American Cancer Society Lymphedema Workshop. Workgroup III: diagnosis and management of lymphedema. *Cancer.* 1998;83(12 Suppl American):2882-2885.

81. Kirshbaum M. The development, implementation and evaluation of guidelines for the management of breast cancer related lymphoedema. *Eur J Cancer Care (Engl).* 1996;5(4):246-251.

82. Asdonk J. Effectiveness, indications and contraindications of manual lymph drainage therapy in painful edema [article in German]. *Z Lymphol.* 1995;19(1):16-22.

83. Ko DS, Lerner R, Klose G, Cosimi AB. Effective treatment of lymphedema of the extremities. *Arch Surg.* 1998;133(4):452-458.

84. Janbon C, Ferrandez JC, Vinot JM, Serin D. A comparative lympho-scintigraphic evaluation of manual lymphatic drainage and pressotherapy in edema of the arm following treatment of a breast tumor [article in French]. *J Mal Vasc.* 1990;15(3):287-288.

85. Földi M. Treatment of lymphedema [Editorial]. *Lymphology.* 1994;27:1-5.

86. Szuba A, Cooke JP, Yousuf S, Rockson SG. Decongestive lymphatic therapy for patients with cancer-related or primary lymphedema. *Am J Med.* 2000;109(4):296-300.

87. Rockson SG. The lymphatic continuum continues. *Lymphat Res Biol.* 2006;4(1):1-2.

88. Fu MR, Deng J, Armer JM. Putting evidence into practice: cancer-related lymphedema. *Clin J Oncol Nurs.* 2014;18 Suppl:68-79.

89. National Lymphedema Network (NLN). *Resource Guide Training Programs.* www.lymphnet.org/patients/search-for-treatment/choosing-a-therapist. Accessed June 10, 2016.

BIBLIOGRAPHY

Brennan MJ, Miller LT. Overview of treatment options and review of the current role and use of compression garments, intermittent pumps, and exercise in the management of lymphedema. *Cancer.* 1998;83(12 Suppl American):2821-2827.

Földi E. Massage and damage to lymphatics. *Lymphology.* 1995;28(1):1-3.

Passik S, Newman M, Brennan M, Holland J. Psychiatric consultation for women undergoing rehabilitation for upper-extremity lymphedema following breast cancer treatment. *J Pain Symptom Manage.* 1993;8(4):226-233.

Schmid-Schönbein GW. Microlymphatics and lymph flow. *Physiol Rev.* 1990;70(4):987-1028.

Smith RO. Lymphatic contractility; a possible intrinsic mechanism of lymphatic vessels for the transport of lymph. *J Exp Med.* 1949;90(5):497-509.

ADDITIONAL RESOURCES

Lymphology Association of North America (LANA). Available at www.clt-lana.org.

Medical Advisory Committee, National Lymphedema Network. Choosing a lymphedema therapist. Available at www.lymphnet.org/patients/search-for-treatment/choosing-a-therapist.

National Certification for Lymphedema Therapists. Available at www.clt-lana.org/download-your-lana-certificate.html

National Lymphedema Network. Resource guide. Available at www. lymphnet.org.

The Ida Rolf Method of Structural Integration

Judith E. Deutsch, PT, PhD, FAPTA

Dr. Ida P. Rolf, who was trained as a biochemist, developed the Ida Rolf Method of Structural Integration (SI) in the late 1960s. She first described her theoretical framework and concepts supporting the method in an article published in *Confinia Psychiatrica*[1] followed by a book she authored titled *Rolfing: The Integration of Human Structures*.[2] Additional information about the approach can be gained from a book in which Rolf is interviewed titled *Ida Rolf Talks About Rolfing and Physical Reality*.[3] The method is based on her personal interest with the human body and its response to use and injury, and, especially, its relationship to gravity.

SI, or Rolfing, was classified as a manual body-based therapy by the National Center for Complementary and Alternative Medicine.[4] However, more recently it is listed as a mind-body practice by the National Center for Complementary and Integrative Health (formerly known as the Office of Alternative Medicine and the National Center for Complementary and Alternative Medicine). It is, like many of the mind-body therapies, an approach to the examination and intervention of the body that focuses on the relationship between structure and function. In this chapter, the main ideas in Rolfing are described and the evidence that exists to support the approach is reviewed.

BACKGROUND AND DESCRIPTION OF STRUCTURAL INTEGRATION

Based on her observations of the human body, Rolf organized her approach around 3 main principles: (1) the role of gravity in shaping posture and movement; (2) the importance of the myofascial system as the organ that connects and supports all structures; and (3) the belief that structure (tissues of the human body) can be changed.[5] These principles guide the examination and intervention, which can be described as a 10-session process of soft tissue mobilization and movement education.

Rolf believed that the body was shaped or organized by the effects of gravity and that the fascia was the central organ in this process. The examination process in Rolfing is to view the body using a 3-dimensional postural analysis referenced to a column of blocks. Each block represents a section of the body, with the pelvis being the central block. This allows for descriptions of the body segments in all 3 planes using terms such as *rotations* and *obliquities*. Because the fascial system supports posture, the examination also includes observing and describing the quality of tissues. For example, the

Davis CM.
Integrative Therapies in Rehabilitation: Evidence for Efficacy in Therapy, Prevention, and Wellness, Fourth Edition (pp 131-138).
© 2017 Taylor & Francis Group.

practitioner observes whether tissues appear tight or restricted in a particular area. Bony and soft tissue structures are also observed during movement. Specific movements are selected because they relate to the goals of a session. For example, the anterior chest is one of the main structures worked on during the first session, so the practitioner will observe the person's breathing. Thus, the identification of deviations in posture and tissue restrictions serves to locate dysfunction and to guide the practitioner's interventions.

The 10 sessions of SI are sometimes referred to as a *recipe*.[3] To some extent, this is an accurate description because there is a systematic approach to each examination and intervention. Each session has a specific purpose, and the practitioner focuses on a set of soft tissue structures and then provides movement cues. For example, during the second session, practitioners focus on lower extremity alignment and work primarily on the superficial soft tissue of the feet and legs, such as the retinaculum on the dorsum of the foot, perimalleolar structures (eg, peroneal tendons), gastrocnemius muscles, medial and lateral collateral ligaments, tibial crest, Achilles tendon to the calcaneus, and medial and lateral arches. Following this, the client is given movement awareness cues, such as to "walk vertical" and attend to the weight distribution of the feet. While the elements of the second session would be recognized by all Rolfing practitioners, the intent and rendering of the session vary depending on each client's needs.

The focus of each session and the depth of the soft tissue work are varied systematically. Sessions 1 through 6 alternate their emphasis on either the upper (odd numbered: 1, 3, and 5) or lower (even numbered: 2, 4, and 6) part of the body. Sessions 7 through 10 are focused on work directed toward large fascial planes that connect the upper and lower parts of the body. The depth of the work begins superficially during the first session as the practitioner works on the fascia of the sternocleidomastoid in the neck; he or she moves to the deepest structures during the fourth session, such as the insertion of the adductors on the pubic ramus. The manual soft tissue work is performed with the intention of freeing the structures of adhesions so that they move freely. The focus of each session, the main structures that are worked on, and the depth of the work are summarized in Table 10-1. A more detailed description of the first 6 sessions can be found in the *Guild News*[6,7] and of the entire series in the *Journal of Bodywork and Movement Therapies*.[8-10]

As previously mentioned, each session has a specific focus and certain structures are evaluated and worked on in each of the 10 sessions. A 3-dimensional assessment of posture is always performed. The central structure of the body is the pelvis, so a pelvic lift is performed during each session. The pelvic lift is performed with the client in the supine position with his or her knees flexed. One hand is placed on the patient's sacrum with the fingertips resting on the lumbosacral junction, while the second hand is placed on his or her epigastrium to stabilize the trunk. A cranial traction force is applied using the hand on the lumbosacral junction to rotate the pelvis posteriorly.[11] There is evidence that using this pelvic lift increases parasympathetic tone and is therefore associated with a relaxation response.[11,12]

Sessions are typically performed with 1 week of rest in between. This schedule allows the body to reorganize itself with respect to gravity. After the 10-session process is completed, individuals may be reevaluated if their symptoms persist. This is more likely to occur in those who return to the habitual movement patterns and postures that created their original myofascial imbalances. Additional lessons are offered that have a greater emphasis on movement reeducation or as tune-up sessions.[13]

EVIDENCE OF EFFICACY: VALIDATION AND OUTCOME STUDIES

The literature that describes and supports Rolfing is modest and varied. Early papers were mechanistic and will be presented first, followed by studies of clinical efficacy. The first articles about Rolfing were published in 1973 in the psychiatry literature. Rolf described the assumptions underlying Rolfing and made a connection between imbalances in the structural system with disease, both physical and psychological.[1] An accompanying paper attempted to validate the assumptions

TABLE 10-1
KEY ELEMENTS OF EACH STRUCTURAL INTEGRATION SESSION

SESSION	GOALS	DEPTH	KEY
1	• Establish a rapport with the patient • Increase movement with each breath of the thorax and ribs • "Horizontalize" the pelvis	Superficial	Rib cage and costal arch
2	• Restore the alignment between the calcaneus and the ischial tuberosities • Restore balanced movement between the hip, knee, and ankles • Direct attention to the relationship of the feet to the ground	Superficial	Periarticular ankle retinaculum, plantar fascia, and lateral arch
3	• Lengthen the lateral line • Increase the space between the pelvis and the 12th rib • Release the shoulder and pelvic girdles	Superficial	Quadratus lumborum, 12th rib
4	• Reduce excessive rotation of the lower limb • Align the pelvis in all planes • Align the foot with respect to the spine	Deep	Medial retinaculum of the ankle, attachments of the adductors and hamstrings to the pubic ramus
5	• Lengthen the anterior thorax • Align the clavicles in all planes • Facilitate movement of the arm with proper scapular alignment • Facilitate movements of hip flexion	Deep	Psoas, pectoralis minor, rectus abdominus, and diaphragm
6	• Vertically align the lower limb • Align the pelvis, sacrum, and spine	Deep	Hip rotators, sacrotuberous ligament, thorocolumbar fascia
7	• Align the head • Separate the fascia of the head and arms	Superficial to deep	Sternocleidomastoid, scalenes, masseter, occipital atlantic ligaments, deep cervical muscles, and cranial fascia *(continued)*

TABLE 10-1(CONTINUED) KEY ELEMENTS OF EACH STRUCTURAL INTEGRATION SESSION			
SESSION	**GOALS**	**DEPTH**	**KEY**
8 and 9	• Focus on either the upper or lower body • "Balance and relate the girdles" to the "dorsal lumbar hinge" • Relate the limbs to the spine	Varied	Mobility of fascial planes
10	• Integrate a functional whole • Maximize movement strategies and efficiency	Varied	Fascial planes across joints

Reprinted with permission from *Ortho Phys Ther Clin North Amer,* 9(3), Deutsch JE, Derr L, Judd P, Reuven B, Structural integration applied to patients with chronic pain. 1059-1061. ©2000 with permission from Elsevier.

of Rolfing by using electrophysiological and biochemical measures to quantify the effects of Rolfing on 15 healthy individuals.[14] Significant changes were found when comparing pre- and post-SI measures, suggesting that there was an effect observed with the use of Rolfing. Using cluster analysis, the authors identified 4 groups of responders that correlated well with a blinded review by an SI practitioner characterizing the outcome of the patients. The authors concluded that they had provided preliminary evidence for relating the outcomes of SI to their prototypical model of an "open, receptive, efficient sensory information processor."[14] They argued that there was a connection between the muscular system and the sensory system.

Another study was designed to examine energy in motor behavior using electromyography (EMG). Muscle activity was recorded using EMG on 13 individuals executing a variety of tasks before and after receiving 10 sessions of SI.[15] After receiving the 10 sessions of SI, subjects performed the same motor tasks with a shorter duration of muscle contraction and a greater force amplitude during the contraction. The authors interpreted this finding as evidence for subjects being able to overcome the resistances from inertia, gravity, and friction more rapidly, thus making their movements more efficient. Post-SI, subjects exhibited more sequential contraction and less co-contraction for all movements tested. This finding was interpreted as having the control of the movement accomplished by agonists by using either better recruitment of motor units or a change in frequency of motor unit firing. The authors also noted that this EMG pattern of firing was similar to the patterns identified of individuals who were in nonstressful situations, suggesting that SI may reduce stress. The authors reported another interesting finding: a decrease in neuromuscular excitation after SI for areas that were not related functionally to the motor task. The combined results of the specificity of muscle action with decreased overall motor activity post-SI can be interpreted as improved neuromuscular organization consistent with more efficient movement.[12] Finally, after SI, EMG patterns between static and rhythmic activities were performed with a clear distinction between isotonic and isometric contractions. The absence of random action potentials of EMG activity in between rhythmic activities is interpreted as a nonhyperactive neuromuscular system. The relationship between the observed EMG patterns of subjects post-SI and those who were not anxious was highlighted by the authors.[15]

Additional work testing the association between elements of Rolfing and the autonomic nervous system was reported by Cottingham et al[11,12] in 2 quasi-experimental design studies in which the effect of the pelvic lift (a standard part of an SI lesson) on autonomic nervous system function is reported. They found that participants significantly decreased their anterior pelvic tilt (measured by an inclinometer) and increased their vagal tone (measured with heart rate variability) after a pelvic lift. The results persisted for 24 hours. These findings support the assumption that there is relationship between posture and tone. Causality, however, remains to be tested.

In more recent work by Langevin and Sherman,[16] mechanical deformation of connective tissue, which is an integral component of SI therapy, was associated with nervous system changes, offering an additional mechanistic explanation for the effects of manual body-based therapies. Specifically, investigators proposed a pathophysiological model integrating connective tissue changes with nervous system mechanisms. In this model, the proponents link the connective tissue remodeling and resultant stiffness that occurs during a lower back injury with chronic pain, fear avoidance, and movement dysfunction. The model also proposes that this cycle may be reversed as a result of neuroplastic changes in the fascia by using mechanical deformation.[16] Their hypothesis that the stretching of nonspecific connective tissue or fascia can reduce inflammation, mechanical sensitivity, and gait was supported in a controlled study using a rodent model by Corey et al.[17] This type of research on the effects of mechanical stretch begins to elucidate the role of manual body-based approaches from the cellular level to activity.

Taken together, these validation or mechanistic studies aim to test the assumptions about the approach, such as the effect of soft tissue mobilization on increasing parasympathetic tone[11,12] and improved movement efficiency,[15,17] which may be explained at the cellular level. The model proposed by Langevin and Sherman[16] may guide future research focused on explaining the efficacy of manual body-based interventions that have physical, emotional, and psychological components.

Clinical studies supporting the use of SI were extensively reviewed by Jacobson[18] in 2011. Many papers contained in the review are not easy to access, as they are published in *Conference Proceedings*, which makes this article especially useful. Outcomes of clinical studies can be found in the pediatric, complementary therapy, and physical therapy literatures published as early as 1981 through 2014. The findings will be commented on based on patient population.

Studies of pediatric patients have focused on movement outcomes of those with cerebral palsy with mild to moderate disease presentation.[19-21] In a single group pre-test post-study, Perry and colleagues[19] reported changes in temporal spatial measures of gait before and after a 10-series session and at 3 and 6 months after treatment. After treatment, participants with mild deficits improved gait speed by increasing stride length and cadence, and those with mild deficits increased gait speed only.[19] Hansen et al[20] reported positive outcomes on the Gross Motor Function Measure and on parents' reports of improved mobility. In another article, Hansen and colleagues[21] discussed the cases of a child with spastic diplegia and another child with hemiplegia, both of whom experienced improved cadence at the end of treatment and continued to improve at 3 months, but then experienced drops in their improvement to close to baseline at 6 months.

Case studies on adults with neuromuscular conditions who have received the complete SI series have demonstrated improvements in balance, mobility, and well-being.[22,23] The cases included persons with a traumatic brain injury, multiple sclerosis, and amyotrophic lateral sclerosis (ALS). All reported favorable outcomes when using SI both at the impairment and functional levels. In the case of the patient with ALS, the author reported an association between reports of well-being and the measured increases in parasympathetic tone.[23]

Persons with musculoskeletal conditions, low back and cervical pain, chronic pain, and chronic fatigue syndrome have been evaluated using case reports[24] and retrospective chart reviews.[25-27] Interestingly, in the case report about a patient with low back pain, the authors attributed the patient's positive outcome to the movement reeducation component of the therapy and not the soft tissue work.[24] Persons with cervical spine dysfunction (n = 31) were assessed for neck motion and pain before and after a 10-series SI intervention.[25] Authors reported improvements in range and reductions in pain that were greater for older individuals. In another study, Deutsch et al[26] examined persons (n = 33) with chronic musculoskeletal pain in 2 or more sites (median pain duration, 37 months) whose charts were retrospectively reviewed after receiving, on average, 8 SI sessions from a group of physical therapists who were trained as SI practitioners. Significant improvements (with the percent of documented improvements in the chart) were reported in range of motion (ROM; 85%), pain (74%), function (75%), and patient reports of treatment effectiveness (79%).[26] Talty and colleagues[27] reported on 11 participants with chronic fatigue syndrome who received SI combined with a cardiovascular training program. The physical therapists who treated the participants reported that most (90%) of them achieved 2 or more functional goals, experienced improvements in their sleep, and presented with improved breathing and posture.[27] It appears that SI targets soft tissue, resulting in improvements in flexibility, pain reduction, and movement.

In sum, the literature supporting the efficacy of SI is modest and weak, with not a single controlled trial. Although most of the reported findings are positive, encouraging, and appear applicable to diverse patient populations, they are, at best, preliminary. The rate at which the evidence is accumulating is very slow, suggesting that this therapy has not been a target for funded research, which is surprising given that it is systematic and could be ensured for reliability. The barrier to research is likely the requirement of a 10-session process and the level of training required to properly train a practitioner. While it may not be the first line of therapy, persons with chronic conditions who have not responded to other therapies may consider a course of SI to address flexibility, posture, pain management, and function.

CASE EXAMPLE

A 71-year-old woman who had a right cerebrovascular accident (CVA) 3 months earlier was referred for SI to reduce musculoskeletal and neuromuscular impairments that were interfering with balance and gait. The patient had a history of 2 previous left CVAs 3 months and 1 year prior to presentation, for which she had received both in- and outpatient services. Her medical history was also remarkable for coronary bypass graft surgery 3 years prior and a history of coronary artery disease, arrhythmias, hypertension, and borderline diabetes mellitus. Her personal goal for this outpatient referral was to "walk taller and with more energy."

The patient presented with bilateral loss of ROM and weakness in all hip and ankle musculature on initial examination. She had residual right shoulder ROM loss from the previous strokes. Her sitting posture was flexed at the thoracic spine with a posterior pelvic tilt and her standing posture was flexed. Her vital capacity, measured an average of 3 trials with an incentive spirometer, was 950 cc. She ambulated at a speed of 0.45 m/second and exhibited shortness of breath. Her score on the Tinetti Balance Test was 14 out of 28. It was determined that she may benefit from a full course of SI. The therapist's rationale for selecting SI was based on the assumption that reversing some of the ROM losses and postural deficits may have a positive impact on breathing and may potentially improve the mechanics of walking.

She received 6 sessions of SI that were not concurrent with physical therapy. (She was unable to complete the 10 sessions because of inclement weather.) She tolerated the sessions well. Upon completion of the 6 sessions, the following improvements were noted: ROM increased for both lower extremities (improvements were greater in the right side than the left), in particular the hip extensors, abductors, and internal rotators. There were no remarkable changes noted in ROM of the right upper extremity or in her strength. Her posture was less flexed upon observation, her vital capacity increased by 500 to 1450 cc, and her Tinetti score increased by 2 points to 16 out of 28, which still put her in the high falls–risk category. Ambulation speed increased to 0.58 m/second, with a decrease in shortness of breath. The patient reported pain when reaching behind her back. She also reported feeling less shortness of breath when she walked and a "little stronger," but said that otherwise she felt unchanged.

Consistent with the therapist's prediction, the patient did make improvements with flexibility and posture and, in turn, experienced improvements in respiratory capacity and walking. The appearance of new pain symptoms is interesting and may be attributed to a change in posture and available range without the appropriate mechanics to support movement in a new ROM. Since the patient remained in the high falls–risk category based on her Tinetti score, she was recommended for outpatient physical therapy to address balance and to increase endurance during ambulation. The SI intervention in this instance served to lay the groundwork for additional rehabilitation services and was likely a complement to physical therapy.

ACKNOWLEDGMENTS

I wish to thank Patricia Judd, PT; Irene DeMasi, MA, PT; Barbara Reuven, PT; and Thomas Findley, MD, PhD, who have taught me much of what I know about SI.

REFERENCES

1. Rolf IP. Structural integration: a contribution to the understanding of stress. *Confin Psychiatr.* 1973;16(2):69-79.
2. Rolf IP. *Rolfing: The Integration of Human Structures.* New York, NY: Harper & Row; 1977.
3. Feitis R. *Ida Rolf Talks About Rolfing and Physical Reality.* New York, NY: Harper and Row; 1978.
4. National Center for Complementary and Integrative Health. What is complementary, alternative or integrative health? https://nccih.nih.gov/health/integrative-health#types. Published October 2008. Accessed February 7, 2016.
5. Oschman J. Connective tissue as an energetic and informational continuum. *Structural Integration.* 2003;31(3):5-15.
6. Urbanczik A. A tour of the first three sessions. *Guild News.* 1994;4:32-35.
7. Urbanczik A. A tour of the basic series: sessions 4, 5, and 6. *Guild News.* 1995;5:21-23.
8. Myers TW. Structural integration: developments in Ida Rolf's "recipe"—part 1. *J Bodyw Mov Ther.* 2004;8(2):131-142.
9. Myers TW. Structural integration: developments in Ida Rolf's "recipe"—part 2. *J Bodyw Mov Ther.* 2004;8(3):189-198.
10. Myers TW. Structural integration: developments in Ida Rolf's "recipe"—part 3. An alternative form. *J Bodyw Mov Ther.* 2004;8(4):249-264.
11. Cottingham JT, Porges SW, Lyon T. Effects of soft tissue mobilization (Rolfing pelvic lift) on parasympathetic tone in two age groups. *Phys Ther.* 1988;68(3):352-356.
12. Cottingham JT, Porges SW, Richmond K. Shifts in pelvic inclination angle and parasympathetic tone produced by Rolfing soft tissue manipulation. *Phys Ther.* 1988;68(9):1364-1370.
13. Kotzsch E. Restructure the body with Rolfing: deep massage that realigns the human form. *East West Natural Health.* 1993:35.
14. Silverman J, Rappaport M, Hopkins K, et al. Stress intensity control and the structural integration technique. *Confin Psychiatr.* 1973;16:201-219.
15. Hunt VV, Massey WW. Electromyographic evaluation of structural integration techniques. *Psychoenergetic Systems.* 1977;2:199-210.
16. Langevin HM, Sherman KJ. Pathophysiological model for chronic low back pain integrating connective tissue and nervous system mechanisms. *Med Hypotheses.* 2007;68(1):74-80.
17. Corey SM, Vizzard MA, Bouffard NA, Badger GJ, Langevin HM. Stretching of the back improves gait, mechanical sensitivity and connective tissue inflammation in a rodent model. *PLoS One.* 2012;7(1):e29831.
18. Jacobson E. Structural integration, an alternative method of manual therapy and sensorimotor education. *J Altern Complement Med.* 2011;17(10):891-899.
19. Perry J, Jones M, Thomas L. Functional evaluation of Rolfing in cerebral palsy. *Dev Med Child Neurol.* 1981;23(6):717-729.
20. Hansen AB, Price KS, Feldman HM. Myofascial structural integration: a promising complementary therapy for young children with spastic cerebral palsy. *J Evid Based Complementary Altern Med.* 2012;17(2):131-135.
21. Hansen AB, Price KS, Loi EC, et al. Gait changes following myofascial structural integration (Rolfing) observed in 2 children with cerebral palsy. *J Evid Based Complementary Altern Med.* 2014;19(4):297-300.
22. Deutsch JE, Judd P, DeMasi I. Structural integration applied to patients with a primary neurologic diagnosis: two case studies. *Neurology Report.* 1997;21(5):161-162.
23. Cottingham JT, Maitland J. Integrating manual and movement therapy with philosophical counseling for treatment of a patient with amyotrophic lateral sclerosis: a case study that explores the principles of holistic intervention. *Altern Ther Health Med.* 2000;6(2):128, 120-7.
24. Cottingham JT, Maitland J. A three paradigm treatment model using soft tissue mobilization and guided movement-awareness techniques for a patient with chronic low back pain: a case study. *J Orthop Sports Phys Ther.* 1997;26(3):155-167.

25. James H, Castaneda L, Miller ME, Findley T. Rolfing structural integration treatment of cervical spine dysfunction. *J Bodyw Mov Ther.* 2009;13(3):229-238.

26. Deutsch JE, Derr L, Judd P, Reuven B. Structural integration applied to patients with chronic pain. *Phys Ther Clin North Am.* 2000;9(3):411-427.

27. Talty C, DeMassi I, Deutsch JE. Structural integration applied to patients with chronic fatigue syndrome: a retrospective chart review. *J Orthop Sports Phys Ther.* 1998;27(1):83.

IV

Mind-Body Work

11

T'ai Chi
Choreography of Body and Mind

Jennifer M. Bottomley, PhD, MS, PT

If there is light in the soul. There will be beauty in the person. If there is beauty in the person. There will be harmony in the house. If there is harmony in the house. There will be order in the nation. If there is order in the nation. There will be peace in the world.

Chinese Proverb

T'ai Chi is an alternative therapeutic approach that can greatly enhance the practice of physical therapy. It is a form of exercise that recognizes the mind/body connection.[1,2] The movements are graceful, the tempo is slow, the benefits are great. It can positively augment physical therapy programs aimed at improving balance and posture, coordination and integration of movement, endurance, strength, flexibility, and relaxation.[1-13] T'ai Chi exercise has cardiovascular, neuromuscular, and psychological benefits[7-12,14-17] that are clinically observed. It is a form of exercise that allows the individual to assume an active role in obtaining maximal health and focusing on the prevention of disease, rather than the passive acceptance of illness as a consequence of life, aging, fate, or genetics. It is an exercise form that is particularly helpful in the elderly population because of its slow-controlled, nonimpact-type movement that displaces, thereby "exercises," the center of gravity. This exercise form incorporates all of the motions that often become restricted with inactivity and aging. It improves respiratory status, stresses trunk control, expands the base of support, improves rotation of the trunk and coordination of isolated extremity motions, and helps to facilitate awareness of movement and position.[3,5-8,10,18] Studies of elders participating in T'ai Chi programs have also indicated a significant improvement in self-reported well-being and quality-of-life measures.[14-18] Even in the frailest and most inactive elderly individuals, studies have shown that T'ai Chi is effective for improving functional status and enhancing health-related quality-of-life measures.[19-21] An additional benefit is the opportunity for social interaction, as most T'ai Chi is performed in group settings.

WHAT IS T'AI CHI?

T'ai Chi is an ancient physical art form, originally a martial art, where the defendant actually uses his or her attacker's own energy against him- or herself by drawing the attack, sidestepping the

Davis CM.
Integrative Therapies in Rehabilitation: Evidence for Efficacy in Therapy, Prevention, and Wellness, Fourth Edition (pp 141-160).
© 2017 Taylor & Francis Group.

attacker, and throwing the opponent off balance. There are numerous forms of T'ai Chi[22] involving as many as 108 postures and transitions of controlled movement, each style with slightly different philosophical foundations. Family surnames came to be associated with the different styles of T'ai Chi that have been passed on from generation to generation (eg, Wu style, Yang style, Ch'en style, Chuan style). Each style is distinctive, but all follow the classic T'ai Chi principles.

T'ai Chi is a way of life that has been practiced by the Chinese for thousands of years. It is a Taoist philosophical perspective that forms the foundation of an exercise regime developed to balance the mind and body. Unlike Western civilization, which separates the body from the mind and allows spiritual development only in terms of religions and mystical beliefs, T'ai Chi integrates the connections between the mind, body, and spirit in a quest for the highest form of harmony in life through the combination of exercise and meditation.[23-25] The Chinese conceived the human mind to be an unlimited dimension and focused on simplification of beliefs. They also viewed the human body as limitless in its physical capabilities. These beliefs were the keystones for the evolution of what we refer to as T'ai Chi Ch'uan today (see the historical background section in this chapter for a description of the evolution of T'ai Chi to T'ai Chi Ch'uan).[22]

Since ancient times, Taoist philosophy has been concerned with the question of how to reproduce and maintain the essential type of energy required to prolong life and enhance creativity of the individual. The answer can be found in the T'ai Chi methods of Taoist meditation, in which a combination of movement, breathing, and mental concentration is used to purify the essential life energies, distill out its pure Yang aspect, the vital energy (ch'i), and transmit it through the body/mind's 8 channels to every cell in the body. The regular practice of these methods has been shown to result in longevity, good health, vigor, mental alertness, and creativity far beyond what is experienced by most people.[1,26]

To obtain the full benefits of T'ai Chi, it is essential to understand the principles underlying its methods. Hence, it is the aim of this chapter to describe the methods of meditation and exercise and explain how they are based on the philosophy of Taoism.

Many Westerners feel uncomfortable with the "spiritual" component of T'ai Chi and of other Eastern practices.[23-25] However, the concentration required to accomplish the rhythmic and coordinated movement patterns and integrate these motions with respiration in T'ai Chi induces a level of concentration that edges on meditation.[1,2,11] Movement is vital to preventing disability and maintaining health and well-being. The capability of understanding the movements is an essential element in the successful practice of the T'ai Chi exercise form. T'ai Chi requires practice (preferably throughout the life cycle) and commitment.[11,12] Further, there would be a total lack of consistency and benefit from this exercise form if the mind/body connection was not made.

PHILOSOPHICAL BACKGROUND OF T'AI CHI

Behind every T'ai Chi movement is the philosophy of Yin and Yang. Traditional Chinese Medicine, the principle of Yin and Yang has been the basis of the Chinese understanding of health and sickness since ancient times.[1,2,26] Good health requires a balance between opposing forces within the body. Sickness results if one is too predominant. It is the aim of Eastern medical practices, including acupuncture, Qi gong, and herbal medicine, to discover the source of the imbalance and restore the forces to their proper proportions. In the Western world, exercise concentrates on outer movements and the development of the physical body. T'ai Chi develops both the mind and the body.[1,2] It embodies a philosophy that not only promotes health but can also be applied to every aspect of life. T'ai Chi emphasizes the development of the whole person, promoting personal growth in all areas.[26]

T'ai Chi means "the ultimate" energy. This ultimate power is ch'i. According to the legendary theory of Yin and Yang, ch'i exercises its power, creating a balance between the positive and negative energies of nature.[22] T'ai Chi's philosophical basis is directed toward improving and progressing toward the unlimited and immense interrelationship between the self and all other things in existence. T'ai Chi is guided by the theory of opposites: the Yin and the Yang, the negative and the positive. This is the original principle of Taoist thought.[27] According to the T'ai Chi theory, the human body's abilities are capable of being developed beyond their commonly conceived potential. Creativity has no boundaries, and the human mind should have no restrictions or barriers placed upon its capabilities.

The fundamental principle of Taoist philosophy—the joining together of opposites—is the basis for the practice of T'ai Chi. The Taoist philosophy that underlies T'ai Chi exercise and meditation is somewhat more complex in its application of the relationship between Yin and Yang within the body. It is not denied that a general balance is necessary to avoid illness; however, it is the aim of meditation to greatly increase the Yin and to reduce and diminish the Yang. One of the fundamental beliefs of Taoist philosophy is that the reason people become old and weak and eventually die is that they lack essential energy (ch'i) that sustains life.[22,26,28] Thus, the goal of exercise is to greatly reduce Yin and to increase and *enhance* Yang.[26,28] The combined practice of meditation and exercise balances these opposing energies.

One reaches the ultimate level of health and physical and mental well-being through exercise and meditative means of balancing the opposing powers and their natural motions. Yin, the negative (yielding) power, and Yang, the positive (action) power. The theory is that the interplay and balance between opposite yet complementary forces of equal strength promotes health. These two opposing manifestations have universal significance and apply to the phenomena of the cosmos and the operations of the human body. On the largest scale, heaven is *Yang* and the earth is *Yin*. Day is *Yang* and night is *Yin*. Bright and clear weather is *Yang* and dark and stormy weather is *Yin*. On the scale of living things, a man is *Yang* and a woman is *Yin*. Spirit is *Yang* and body is *Yin*. This opposition also applies to the different parts of the body and their functions. For instance, in the circulatory system, the arteries are *Yang* and the veins are *Yin*. Muscle contraction is *Yang* and relaxation is *Yin*. In breathing, exhalation is *Yang* and inhalation is *Yin*. In human activities, movement is *Yang* and rest is *Yin*.[29]

Hundreds of years ago, those who searched for a way to elevate the human body and spirit to their ultimate level developed the ingenious system known as T'ai Chi exercise. It has since proven to be the most advanced system of body exercise and mind conditioning ever to be created.[22,29] It makes intuitive sense from a clinical perspective to apply the idea of a natural harmony and a balancing of life forces to the integration of body and mind.

HISTORICAL BACKGROUND OF T'AI CHI

A systematic description of the relationships of Yin and Yang is found in the hexagrams of *I Ching: The Book of Changes*, the oldest and most important book of Chinese philosophy.[27] One of the pioneers of the philosophy of Taoism was Lao Tzu.[22] He emphasized that "the soft overcomes the hard." Later, this idea permeated the practice of T'ai Chi Ch'uan. After Lao Tzu, the second great master of Taoism was Chuang Tzu.[30] To the philosophy of soft over hard, he added the component of "breathing," not only as the process of the movement of air in and out of the lungs, but also the process involving the whole body, including the circulation of oxygen to the extremities through the blood. In other words, the flow of ch'i, or vital energy. T'ai Chi Ch'uan was not actually developed until centuries after Chuang Tzu, although there is clear evidence that he was practicing methods of exercise coordinated with breathing,[31] which is the basis of T'ai Chi exercise.

Approximately 1700 years ago (3rd century AD), the famous Chinese medical doctor Hua Tuo emphasized physical and mental exercise as a means of improving health.[29] He believed that human beings should exercise and imitate the movements of animals to recover physical/cognitive abilities that had been lost to "civilization." Hua Tuo organized a martial arts form called the Five Animal Games.[22] Since then, these exercises have become popular with Chinese individuals who wish to maximize their health through exercise.

Huang Ti, the so-called Yellow Emperor of 2700 BC, practiced a form of exercise called *Tao Yin* with the aim of increasing his life span.[22] *Tao* means "guide" and *Yin* is translated here as "leading." These terms give a hint of how the exercise works: the movement of the limbs guides the circulation of the blood so that the tissues throughout the body can be repaired and cleansed more efficiently. The movement also leads the breath in and out of the lungs to nourish and energize the body through inhalation and to rid the body of poisons through exhalation. Thus, movement is the foundation of a discipline that guides and leads the automatic bodily processes so that they will function efficiently.[26] The essential element of Tao Yin was the way in which the movements of the limbs were combined with breathing. Huang Ti's exercises were also known as T'u Na (t'u = exhale; na = inhale) exercises.[29] There is little doubt that Huang Ti's health practices, consisting of an alternation of movement and rest, and form of exercise involving breathing in and out were direct applications of the principle of Yin and Yang.

Alchemist Ko Hung (325 AD) developed a series of 18 forms of "health exercise" to complete the evolution. His system is only for health, not for self-defense.[28] He also combined exercise, breathing, and meditation.

These exercise forms were precursors of the methods of Taoist meditation and T'ai Chi Ch'uan. Unlike the movements of martial arts, which are generally strenuous and sometimes very quick, the movements developed in what we know as T'ai Chi Ch'uan today are done slowly, gently, and evenly from beginning to end, each posture unfolding with the same continuous rhythm. In this evolutionary way, the modified form of T'ai Chi became today's T'ai Chi Ch'uan, or the so-called *T'ai Chi exercise*. This is the T'ai Chi practiced publicly in China today.[22] It is the "T'ai Chi dance," also referred to as the "Chinese Ballet" by some Westerners.[6]

PRINCIPLES OF T'AI CHI CH'UAN

An important insight to be attained through an understanding of Taoist philosophy concerns the way in which the practice of exercise, such as T'ai Chi Ch'uan and meditation, should complement one another. The relationship between them manifests as a subtle interweaving of opposite tendencies. This relationship can be seen in the famous diagram known as the T'ai Chi T'u—Diagram of the Supreme Ultimate (Figure 11-1). The black portion of this diagram (called the *greater Yin*) represents rest and the white portion (called the *greater Yang*) represents movement. Within each figure there is a smaller circle of the opposite color. The black circle within the white figure is called the *lesser Yin* and the white circle within the black portion is called the *lesser Yang*. This inner component represents the way in which each of the opposing forces, *Yin* and *Yang*, contains its opposite and continuously originates from its opposite. T'ai Chi, essentially a form of movement, is *Yang*—the white portion of the T'ai Chi T'u; meditation, which involves quiet and rest, is *Yin*—the black segment. This distinction takes into account only the external aspects of these activities. To perform T'ai Chi Ch'uan exercise effectively requires inner peacefulness and quiet while executing outwardly visible movements. Conversely, the meditator uses breath and mental concentration to move the vital energy through the psychic channels while remaining externally at rest. Thus, the inner aspect of each of these practices is opposite to its outer aspect. In other words, just as the greater Yang contains the lesser Yin within it, the greater Yin embraces the lesser Yang. This diagram is a pictorial representation of how exercise and meditation grow out of one another as alternating practices. The movements of T'ai Chi Ch'uan tend to increase the Yang side of the Yin-Yang balance. When the Yang reaches a high point of energy and vitality, it generates the need to sit quietly, or meditate, which encourages a more peaceful condition and increases the Yin side of balance. And this is cyclic. When Yin reaches its peak, it generates a need to increase the Yang once again. Thus, it is through the alternate practice of these 2 opposite methods that one can obtain the beneficial effects of the T'ai Chi Ch'uan form of exercise/meditation.[26,28-31]

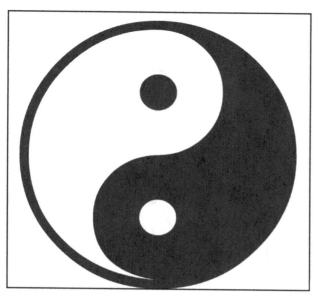

Figure 11-1. Yin and Yang. Diagram of the Supreme Ultimate: T'ai Chi T'u.

The traditional Chinese concept of the human body differs somewhat from the Western concept. Physiological foundations are based in descriptions of ch'i. As previously mentioned, the body is hypothetically composed of 8 energy (psychic) channels and has 12 meridians that run along the surface of the body. These channels and meridians form the basis of the highly sophisticated theories in acupuncture and acupressure.[24-26]

The 8 channels systematically include all parts of the trunk and extremities. The Tu Mo, or channel of control, runs along the spinal column from the coccyx through the base of the skull and over the crown to the head to the roof of the mouth. The Jen Mo, or channel of functions, goes through the center and front of the body from the genital organs to the base of the mouth. The Tai Mo, or belt channel, circles the waist from the navel to the small of the back. The Ch'ueng Mo, or thrusting channel, passes through the center of the body between Tu Mo and Jen Mo, extending from the genitals to the base of the heart. The Yang Yu Wei Mo, or positive arm channel, begins at the navel, passes through the chest, and goes down the posterior aspect of the arms to the middle fingers. The Yin Yu Wei Mo, or negative arm channel, extends along the inner aspect of the arms from the palms and ends in the chest. Likewise, there are positive and negative channels for both lower extremities. The Yang Chiao Mo is the positive channel that goes down the sides of the body, down the outer aspect of the lower extremity, and ending in the soles. The negative channel is called the Yin Chiao Mo, and it starts in the soles and extends upward on the inside of the legs through the center of the body to a point just below the eyebrows.[29] These energy channels are represented in Figure 11-2.

Twelve "psychic centers" of the human body are identified in Taoist thought.[22,27,29] In *I Ching: The Book of Changes,*[27] these 12 centers of the body, or 12 hexagrams, represent the 12 pathways in the body, the 12 months of the year, and the 12 times of the day (Table 11-1). According to Taoist thought, the circulation of energy through these 12 psychic centers reflects the cyclic pattern of the universe that brings about the alteration of light and darkness and the changing of the seasons.[29] Table 11-1 relates the 12 psychic centers to the 12 hexagrams that symbolize them, and indicates how the cycle reflects the times of the day and year and the center of the body that it represents.

According to Chinese astrologers, the Yang movement begins with the eleventh month, which is identified with fu. This Yang movement increases through the twelfth month up to the fourth month as represented by the increase in solid lines in the hexagrams. At the fifth month, the Yang movement begins to decrease until it reaches the tenth month, when Yin reaches complete dominance. The Yin movement is the opposite of the Yang.[26,27,29]

Figure 11-2. The 8 energy channels.

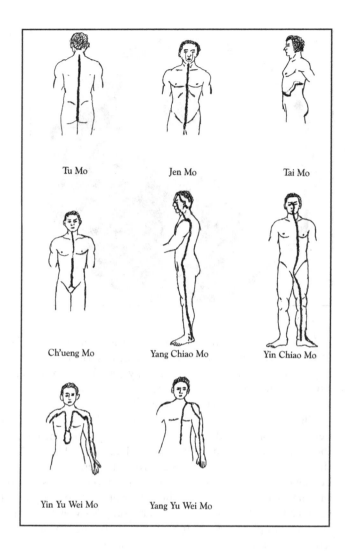

Tu Mo   Jen Mo   Tai Mo

Ch'ueng Mo   Yang Chiao Mo   Yin Chiao Mo

Yin Yu Wei Mo   Yang Yu Wei Mo

In addition to the psychic centers, there are 12 pathways of energy at the surface of the body called *meridians* (refer to Chapter 18). The 12 pathways take their names from the specific inner organs to which they correspond. The development of the T'ai Chi postures and movements are related to these meridians in the human body.[22,26,29] The transition from one posture to the next, combined with breathing, reflects the flow of energy through these meridians.

The importance of breathing techniques has long been stressed in Chinese medicine as a means of preventing illness, prolonging youth, and achieving longevity.[32] The rationale behind this is that the air we breathe contains many other essential elements besides oxygen, such as iron, copper, zinc, fluorite, quartz, zincite, and magnesium,[22,26,28,29,32,33] and that the combination of exercise and breathing provides an efficient and effective method of taking these precious elements in and getting rid of wastes and poisons. It is believed that the breathing techniques of abdominal or "inner" breathing facilitate the flow of energy throughout the body. Inhalation "stores" energy while exhalation "releases" energy.[33]

As previously mentioned, the classic methods of T'ai Chi combine movement with breathing. The movements are performed to assist and guide the circulation of vital energy (ch'i) through the 8 channels and 12 meridians. The mind consciously "lifts" the energy during inward breathing from the solar plexus region, which is considered the central energy source of the body.[22,28,29,33] During

TABLE 11-1						
WAXING AND WANING OF ENERGY REPRESENTED BY THE I CHING HEXAGRAMS						
NAME:	Fu	Lin	T'ai	Ta-Chung	Kuai	Ch'ien
MONTH:	11	12	1	2	3	4
CENTER:	Wei-Lu	Shun-Fu	Hsuan-Hsu	Chai-Chi	T'ao-Tao	Yu-Chen
	䷗	䷒	䷊	䷡	䷪	䷀
NAME:	Kou	Tou	P'i	Kuan	Po	K'un
MONTH:	5	6	7	8	9	10
CENTER:	Ni-Wan	Ming-T'ang	Tan-Chung	Chung-Huan	Shen-Chueh	Ch'i-Hai
	䷫	䷠	䷋	䷓	䷖	䷁

Along the **Tu Mo Centers:** *Wei-Lu*=tip of the spine; *Shun-Fu*=slightly below the middle of the spine; *Hsuan-Hsu*=middle of the spine; *Chai-Chi*=slightly above the middle of the spine; *T'ao-Tao*=below the neck; *Yu-Chen*=back of the head; *Ni-Wan*=top of the head; *Ming-T'ang*=between the eyebrows.

Along the **Jen Mo Centers:** *Tan-Chung*=in the chest; *Chung-Huan*=above the navel; *Shen-Chueh*=in the navel; *Ch'i-Hai*=about 3 inches above the navel.

exhalation concentrated directing of the energy is from the solar plexus region toward the lower abdomen.[22,26,28,29,33] It is through this conscious directing of the energy that each of the 8 channels is supplied with energy during the movement of T'ai Chi. It is hypothesized that in T'ai Chi exercise, the circulation of ch'i through the channels does not occur automatically as a result of the arm and leg movements combined with breathing. Rather, it is the mind's power of concentration that combines with the breathing to move the ch'i through the channels. The outer movements aid and guide the inner concentration. T'ai Chi is regarded as a method of "moving meditation."[28,29]

Both the movements of the limbs and the way they are coordinated with the breathing cycle constitute the T'ai Chi form of exercise. The movements are relatively simple, involving only the bending and unbending of the knees while the hands are lowered or raised. The movements are an effective way of directing the flow of energy through the channels. Several kinds of movement of the body and limbs during T'ai Chi exercise involve shifting the weight from one leg to another, rotating the body to the right or left, taking a step, moving forward or backward, and fine hand and foot movements, all put together and coordinated in more or less complicated combinations and sequences.

A T'AI CHI ROUTINE

The mastering of the T'ai Chi exercise form requires the guidance of a knowledgeable teacher. However, the following is offered as a recommended routine for the elderly. This progression is an example of movement through a sequence of 45 classic T'ai Chi postures, diagrammed with their Chinese names. Each movement should be practiced several times until it can be performed fluidly. It is recommended that transition through each posture be built upon so that the individual starts with the first 15 postures and gradually adds additional postures in the sequence until all 45 postures are perfected. Any exercise can be omitted if it presents difficulty for the individual. It is important to take note of the positions of the hands and feet and to keep the spine straight. For comfort, wearing loose-fitting clothing and slippers or aerobic sneakers is recommended. This author generally divides this exercise routine into 3 segments starting with double-stance exercises (Figure 11-3A), progressing to single-stance postures (Figure 11-3B), and cooling down with mostly double-stance, stretching-type postures (Figure 11-3C).

Each T'ai Chi exercise session should be preceded by stretching. It is essential to stretch before a T'ai Chi workout to prevent injury and prepare for the best possible practice. Flexibility allows one to concentrate on breathing, posit, pace, etc, rather than on the limits of motion in poorly stretched muscles. General flexibility improves the effectiveness and benefits of T'ai Chi exercises.

To start the exercise routine, assume an erect standing posture. Turn your right foot out 45 degrees and sink down slightly on your right leg. Shift all of your weight onto the right leg and extend your left leg, flexing your foot and crossing your hands in front of your chest (1. Salutation to the Buddha). Step back onto your left foot, turning it out, and move your hands to waist level as you shift your weight to the left leg (2. Grasp Bird's Tail). Swing your arms to the right and press forward, shifting some of your weight to the right leg (3. Grasp Bird's Tail). Pivot your left, shifting your weight to your right leg, bringing your left foot around and opening your arms (4. Single Whip). Step forward, leading with your right leg (5. White Crane Spreads Its Wings). Your right hand, elbow, knee, and toes should be in alignment. Slide your left foot forward and move your right arm parallel to the floor (6. White Crane Spreads Its Wings). Step back on your left foot as you raise your left hand and twist to the right (7. Brush, Knee, Twist, Step). Step back on your right foot (8. Parry, Punch); parry with your left arm and punch with your right. Rock back onto your right leg and bring your arms up (9. Closing). Pivot 90 degrees to the right, crossing your arms (10. Embracing Tiger). Slide forward, dropping your left hand to waist level and extending your right hand (11. Fist Under Elbow). Step back with your left foot and straighten your right leg and arm (12. Repulse Monkey). Pivot and step out, opening your arms (13. Diagonal Flying). Come forward, shifting your weight to your right leg, and extend your left arm (14. Raise Left Hand). Then pivot and step out with your left foot, moving your right hand up to your temple (15. Fan Through the Arms). Pivot right (16. Green Dragon Dropping Water). Step up, with knees bent, and push out with hands flexed (17. Step Up and Push). Pivot right, so that you face straight ahead, and extend your left leg out as your arms and torso rotate right (18. Cloud Hands). Rotate to the left as you bring your feet together (19. Cloud Hands). Rotate right and then left 4 times, ending in a single whip position (4. Single Whip). This ends the portion of exercise postures in which both feet are in contact with the ground. As this is mastered, progress to the single leg stance postures.

From the single whip position (4. Single Whip), rotate your torso right and kick your right leg straight out as you open your arms (20. Separation of Legs). Shift your weight to your right leg and kick with your left (21. Separation of Legs). Lower your left leg almost to the floor, turn your right foot out, and kick again with your left leg (22. Separation of Legs). Drop your left leg back, shift your weight onto it, and parry high and low with your arms (23. Wind Blowing Lotus). Pivot on your left foot and switch hand positions (24. Wind Blowing Lotus). Then pivot on your right foot, jump onto your left foot, and kick your right leg—without straining—toward your extended right arm (25. Double Jump Kick). Step back on your right leg, drop your arms, and shift backward onto your left foot (26. Step Back, Hands to the Side). Pivot in a full circle, coming around to stand on your left leg, and kick with your right (27. Kick With the Sole). Drop down on your left leg, keeping your right leg straight and your feet parallel; cover your right wrist with your left palm (28. Clap Opponent with Fist). Swing your right leg back and open your arms (29. Diagonal Single Whip). Step forward, moving your fists to your chest and hip (30. Parting of Wild Horse's Mane). This concludes the second segment of the exercise routine.

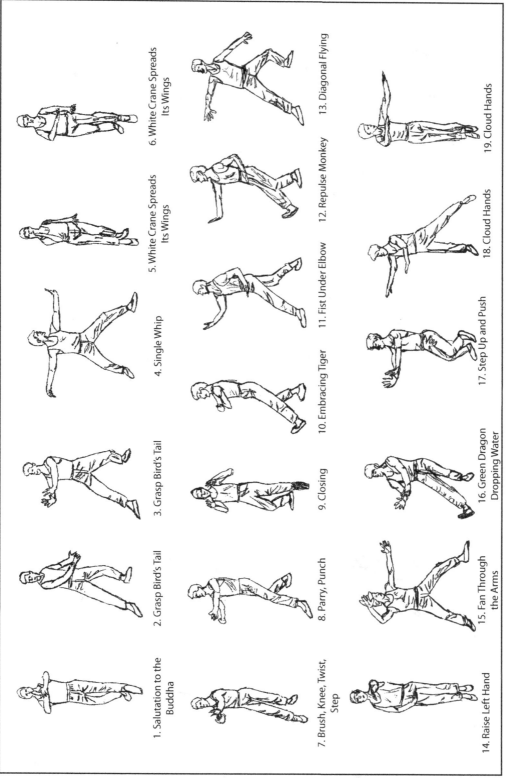

1. Salutation to the Buddha
2. Grasp Bird's Tail
3. Grasp Bird's Tail
4. Single Whip
5. White Crane Spreads Its Wings
6. White Crane Spreads Its Wings
7. Brush, Knee, Twist, Step
8. Parry, Punch
9. Closing
10. Embracing Tiger
11. Fist Under Elbow
12. Repulse Monkey
13. Diagonal Flying
14. Raise Left Hand
15. Fan Through the Arms
16. Green Dragon Dropping Water
17. Step Up and Push
18. Cloud Hands
19. Cloud Hands

Figure 11-3A. Double-stance postures.

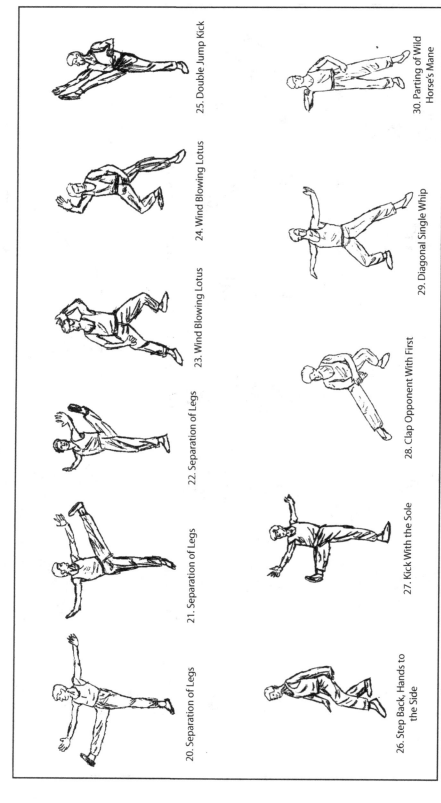

Figure 11-3B. Single-stance postures.

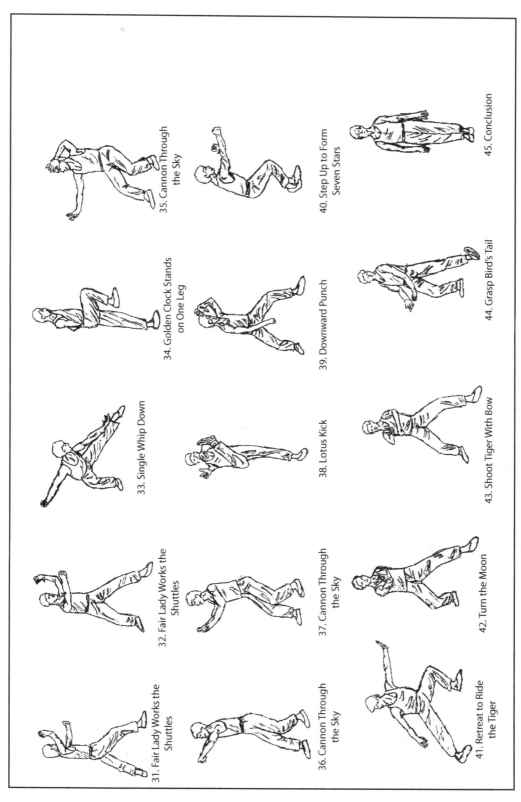

Figure 11-3C. Double-stance, stretching-type postures.

31. Fair Lady Works the Shuttles

32. Fair Lady Works the Shuttles

33. Single Whip Down

34. Golden Clock Stands on One Leg

35. Cannon Through the Sky

36. Cannon Through the Sky

37. Cannon Through the Sky

38. Lotus Kick

39. Downward Punch

40. Step Up to Form Seven Stars

41. Retreat to Ride the Tiger

42. Turn the Moon

43. Shoot Tiger With Bow

44. Grasp Bird's Tail

45. Conclusion

The third portion of this exercise routine starts with the Fair Lady Works the Shuttles (31 and 32) by turning to one side. Parry with one hand and punch with the other. Then pivot 90 degrees to your left and punch and parry again. Repeat the 90-degree pivot, along with the punch and parry, 2 more times, bringing you full circle. Finish with a single whip position (4. Single Whip). Shift your weight to your right leg and extend your torso and left arm toward your left foot (33. Single Whip Down). Swing around to face left; shift your weight onto your left leg and raise your right leg (34. Golden Cock Stands on One Leg). Extend your right leg straight out and step forward. Turn and block your temple with your left hand as you move your right arm and leg forward (35. Cannon Through the Sky). Step onto your right foot. Bring your arms out in loose fists, as though you were punching an opponent's ears (36. Cannon Through the Sky). Then repeat the stepping movement and punch both fists in an uppercut (37. Cannon Through the Sky). Step onto your left foot and kick your right leg high and slightly left, so that it moves across your extended palms (38. Lotus Kick). Step to bring your feet into a T-position and block up with your left hand. Pivot to face left, sink down on your left leg and punch and parry at chest level (39. Downward Punch). Slide forward foot back on the ball of your foot to the weight-bearing foot, squatting so knees are in line with the toes; flex arm on the weight-bearing side with fisted hand and extend opposite arm upward with a fisted hand. The seven stars are created by the head, 2 firsts, 2 knees, and 2 toes. Extend your right leg and arm back in a reverse lunge (41. Retreat to Ride the Tiger). Shift back onto your right leg and pivot to face forward, extending your right arm (42. Turn the Moon). Follow up with 2 short punches (43. Shoot Tiger With Bow). Form a mirror image of position 2, but with your forward foot flexed (44. Grasp Bird's Tail). Swing your hands up, crossing your palms at chest level, then lower your arms and turn so that you face forward in an erect posture (45. Conclusion).

Once this routine is mastered, it takes approximately 20 minutes to complete. Stretching exercises should be added to complete the T'ai Chi exercise routine.

MODIFYING A T'AI CHI EXERCISE ROUTINE FOR THE FRAIL ELDERLY

Although research has yet to be done on the modification of T'ai Chi exercises to accommodate increasingly frail patients, this author has had vast clinical experience in the modification of T'ai Chi routines. For instance, an individual who is unable to stand to do the T'ai Chi routine as recommended above can modify the exercise by sitting in a chair or on the edge of a mat and performing the upper trunk and extremity movements. These activities reflexively facilitate postural responses in the lower extremities, and ultimately result in the strengthening of the trunk and lower extremities. This therapist progresses the patient to less stable surfaces by placing a thick foam cushion or a SitFit cushion (Sissel Inc) on the chair or mat. A rocker board can also be used as a sitting surface to further facilitate balance responses and challenge the postural mechanisms.

As the patient gains agility and trunk strength, moving him or her onto a therapeutic ball, with the feet touching the ground, is a means of progressing toward the standing postures. Clinical experience lends credence to the fact that even the frailest patient can start T'ai Chi exercises in seated postures and progress to double-stance exercise routines.

T'AI CHI'S PREVENTIVE QUALITIES

More than 80% of all illnesses have been shown to have stress-related etiologies.[34] Medical and rehabilitation practices that seek only to "fix" the physical symptoms (body) without addressing the impact of emotional well-being on disease are missing the target. Although the origins of T'ai Chi exercise are based in ancient Eastern philosophy, it is a suitable form of exercise for tense Westerners. It has the advantage of regular exercise[1-18] combined with an emphasis on gracefulness and slowness of pace that Western society so conspicuously lacks. T'ai Chi can give those who live in a fast-paced environment a compensating factor in their lives.

From ancient Chinese medicine, it has long been recognized that there are mental and physical aspects of disease.[30-34] Traditionally, according to Eastern philosophies, the mental state of the individual was considered to be more important than the physical symptoms. Recently, a new basic science of Western medical research, called *psychoneuroimmunology*, has emerged.[1,2,11,12,34] This area of science is the study of the effect of emotions on disease. The new studies strongly indicate that virtually every illness, from a common cold to cancer and heart disease, can be influenced either positively or negatively by an individual's mental status. Today, Western health care professionals in both the physical and mental health fields are increasingly recognizing the role of the mind in the prevention and cure of illness. The health practitioner may encounter clients who do not seem to respond to traditional health care. Psychoneuroimmunology confronts these problems by employing the health traditions of other cultures and viewing the body and mind as a balanced whole.[1,2]

T'ai Chi is a specific technique for attaining peaceful mental states and therefore it can be extrapolated that it may help prevent or reverse disease processes. T'ai Chi integrates the body and mind through breathing and movement. The open and closed movements of T'ai Chi are coordinated with breathing. The benefits of this exercise form seem to be based in the fundamental combination of movements and breathing techniques in the basic T'ai Chi exercise routines. The entry level of the exercise has many similarities with medical treatments for respiratory illness (eg, deep breathing exercises, segmental expansion exercises) and with walking exercise, which is the most highly recommended aerobic exercise for patients with coronary artery disease.[4,6,9]

CURRENT RESEARCH ON THE EFFECTS OF T'AI CHI

Recent research that investigated the physiological effects of T'ai Chi exercise found that it has measurable effects on cardiorespiratory function, mental control, immune capacity, and falls prevention through the improvement in muscle strength, flexibility, and balance parameters.[35,36] Circulatory status has also been found to improve in elderly individuals participating in T'ai Chi exercise routines.[37]

Cardiorespiratory Function and T'ai Chi

In a study by Chan et al,[6] it was determined that elderly T'ai Chi exercisers showed a significant improvement in VO_2 uptake compared with an age-matched control group of sedentary elders. Chan and colleagues concluded that the data substantiated the practice of T'ai Chi as a means of delaying the decline in cardiorespiratory function commonly considered "normal" for aging individuals and complicated by conditions such as chronic obstructive pulmonary disease or other respiratory and cardiac conditions. In addition, T'ai Chi was shown to be a suitable aerobic exercise for older adults.[6] A subsequent study by Lu and Kuo[9] further substantiated that T'ai Chi exercise is aerobic exercise of moderate intensity. In the past, it was believed, although never studied, that T'ai Chi exercise forms did not have a significant cardiorespiratory component and therefore were deemed nonaerobic. It has been clearly demonstrated in these studies that, despite the slow, steady, smooth pace of T'ai Chi exercise routines, there is a significant positive effect on the cardiorespiratory system.[3,6,9]

The low, slow intensity of the T'ai Chi exercise form has long been a point of therapeutic contention. It is argued that this type of movement is not intense enough to produce cardiovascular and respiratory effects. Sato and coworkers[38] obtained vital sign measures, heart rate responses, VO_2 measurements, breath-by-breath measurement of cardiorespiratory function, and sequential determination of blood lactate levels during T'ai Chi routines. The same measures were collected on another exercise group that was performing incremental aerobic exercise of leg cycling. The results of comparing the 2 exercise groups clearly demonstrated that T'ai Chi is an exercise with moderate intensity (despite its appearance) and is aerobic in nature.[38] T'ai Chi exercise routines were found to be comparable to programs of moderate intensity aerobic exercise in reducing blood pressure in previously sedentary, hypertensive, elderly individuals in a study by Siddarth et al.[39]

Pan and colleagues[40] found that movements used to perform T'ai Chi require energy expenditure that is comparable with that for activities of daily living and for the low-level exercises that are currently recommended for persons with low exercise tolerance.

A program of T'ai Chi Chih, a modified T'ai Chi exercise, was piloted in a study composed of a small sample of individuals with heart failure.[41] Comparisons of pre- and post-measures of heart failure symptoms, general health, mental health, functional capacity, and energy perceptions support the potential of T'ai Chi Chih in managing heart failure symptoms and improving quality of life.[41] Lorenc and associates[42] studied the effects of T'ai Chi Ch'uan on patients following diagnosis with any pathologies that involved the respiratory status and demonstrated that this exercise form favorably enhances cardiorespiratory function and improves functional outcomes following implementation. Danusantoso and Heijnen[43] established that T'ai Chi Ch'uan has a positive impact on the outcomes in patients with hemophilia. Overall strength, flexibility, and functional measures improved in this population, and the number and severity of bleeding episodes decreased as a result of participation in T'ai Chi exercise routines.[43] Further, complementary therapies and healing practices have been found to reduce stress, anxiety, and lifestyle patterns known to contribute to cardiovascular disease.[44] In fact, T'ai Chi has been established as a primary component in cardiac rehabilitation programs.

Balance, Falls, and Postural Control and T'ai Chi

The potential value of T'ai Chi exercise in promoting postural control, improving balance, and preventing falls has also been substantiated by several researchers.[3,5,7,8,10,18] Liu and colleagues[3] found that T'ai Chi practitioners had significantly better postural control than the sedentary nonpractitioner. Kayama et al[5] found that treatments directed toward flexibility, balance, dynamic balance, and resistance, all components of T'ai Chi exercise, reduced the risk of falls in elderly adults, significantly improving balance ability when an older adult is challenged by dual tasks. Leung et al[7] demonstrated that short-term exposure to "altered sensory input or destabilizing platform movement" during a treatment session, in addition to home-based T'ai Chi exercises, elicited significant improvements in sway control and inhibited inappropriate motor responses. The outcome measure of functional balance improved more substantially in the exercise group that combined the treatment sessions with the home program of T'ai Chi. Wolf et al[8] compared a balance training group, in which balance was stressed on a static to moving platform using biofeedback, with a group of T'ai Chi Quan exercisers. A third group served as a control for exercise intervention. This article did not provide information on the results of the effects of the 2 different exercise approaches on balance and frailty measures, although it did provide a superb set of assessment tools for measuring balance. The authors spoke positively about the therapeutic value of exercise forms such as T'ai Chi in delaying or possibly preventing the onset of frailty. The benefits of T'ai Chi in fall prevention have also been supported by the findings of a study by Guan et al[10] that demonstrated improvements in single-stance postural sway in older women with T'ai Chi exercises. Wolf[13] in a summary of a series of investigations comparing computerized balance machines with T'ai Chi, ultimately found that T'ai Chi as an exercise form for older adults can have a substantially favorable effect in delaying the onset of fall events.

Taylor-Piliae et al[45] examined whether T'ai Chi practice could influence endurance and reduce the inconsistency of movement force and movement pattern output in older adults, a problem often associated with the increased incidence of falling. The findings suggest that T'ai Chi participants significantly reduce the variability of movement patterns and the inconsistency of muscle force reducing energy expenditure compared with participants in a traditional activity group after 8 weeks of practice. This study provides evidence that proposes that T'ai Chi practice may serve as a better real-world exercise for reducing endurance, movement, and muscle force variability in older adults.[45] Lan and associates[46] evaluated the effect of T'ai Chi Ch'uan on knee extensor strength and endurance in elderly individuals. As this muscle group weakness is directly associated with the increased risk of falling, the findings of this study are important. A significant improvement in muscular strength and endurance of knee extensors was observed following a 6-month program in T'ai Chi.[46]

The volume of research substantiating the use of T'ai Chi as a means of preventing falls has grown in the past few years. Regardless of the setting, evidence consistently supports the effectiveness of T'ai Chi exercise in improving balance and preventing falls.[18,47-53]

Neurological Conditions and T'ai Chi

Recently, research using T'ai Chi exercise as an exercise form has included neurological conditions of stroke, head trauma, and multiple sclerosis.[54,55] Rehabilitation after either stroke or severe head injury is a complex process that can be long and frustrating. New, more holistic methods for rehabilitation are constantly sought. The utilization of the slow, rhythmical movements in T'ai Chi have been found to significantly improve movement patterns and trunk stability, reduce tone, and improve balance in severely involved neurological patients.[54] Burschka and coworkers[55] reported that patients with multiple sclerosis who participated in T'ai Chi exercise showed consistent improvements in balance, coordination, and depression compared with patients who participated in traditional exercise programs. The results demonstrated an increase in walking speed and greater flexibility, especially in the hamstrings. Patients who participated in T'ai Chi exercise also experienced improvements in vitality, social functioning, mental health, and the ability to carry out physical and emotional roles. Traditional exercise showed a more significant impact on fatigue compared with T'ai Chi.[55] This suggests that integrating traditional exercise with T'ai Chi may have a greater impact on those with multiple sclerosis. T'ai Chi and other health promotion programs offer help toward achieving the goals of increasing access to a person's environment and services, maximizing independence, and improving quality of life for people with chronic disabling conditions.

T'ai Chi has also been found to be an efficient and feasible addition to a traditional rehabilitation program for stroke patients in the recovery phase.[56]

Musculoskeletal Conditions and T'ai Chi

Researchers have reported the beneficial effects of T'ai Chi in individuals with musculoskeletal problems. For instance, Wang et al[57] found that T'ai Chi may modulate complex factors and improve health outcomes in patients with chronic musculoskeletal problems. As a form of physical exercise, T'ai Chi enhances cardiovascular fitness, muscular strength, balance, and physical function. It also appears to reduce stress, anxiety, and depression. T'ai Chi can be safely recommended to patients with fibromyalgia, osteoarthritis, and rheumatoid arthritis.[57] Other researchers have reported that T'ai Chi was efficacious primarily as a complementary intervention for musculoskeletal disease and related disorders.[58] Their findings indicated that moderate T'ai Chi intervention can enhance all of these parameters and is a safe and effective means of managing pain and improving lower-extremity osteoarthritis.[58] These studies demonstrate that programs using alternative therapies, such as T'ai Chi and meditation, in combination with traditional medications appear to be beneficial in managing the complex stress and pain mechanisms, which share many central nervous system pathways, in patients with fibromyalgia, osteoarthritis, and rheumatoid arthritis. A long-term benefit was associated with quality-of-life measures. Patients with rheumatoid arthritis who practiced T'ai Chi showed positive results in functional measures, social involvement, and long-term outcomes.[58]

Strategies for the prevention and treatment of osteoporosis are directed at maximizing peak bone mass by optimizing physiologic intake of calcium and vitamin D and providing instruction in exercise that adds mechanical stress to bone.[59] Woo et al[59] determined that the combined stretching, strengthening, and balance components of exercise provided by T'ai Chi was the most effective in the prevention of bone loss and in decreasing falls. Prevention of bone loss is obviously preferable to any remedial measures, but, according to this study, T'ai Chi strategies provide a hopeful means of restoring deficient bone.[59,60]

One year of T'ai Chi training demonstrated the added musculoskeletal benefits of faster hamstring and gastrocnemius reflex reaction and improved knee joint position senses. These changes are not only associated with stronger and faster muscle contractions, but also improved dynamic standing and dynamic balance leading to significant balance improvements during exercise and sport activities and functional activities of daily living.[61] The influence of T'ai Chi training on reducing the risk of falling improved postural control by altering the center of pressure trajectory during gait initiation. T'ai Chi improved the mechanism by which forward momentum is generated and improved coordination during gait initiation, suggesting improvements in postural control.[62,63]

Cancer and T'ai Chi

T'ai Chi is among the many complementary and alternative therapies that have been studied for management of pain, treatment side effects, and functional losses associated with the treatment of cancer.[19,64,65] T'ai Chi has been found to be an exercise technique that relieves stress and enhances well-being in the patient with cancer. Researchers have reported T'ai Chi's effectiveness in decreasing pain and improving functional outcomes, even in the frailest of patients with a cancer diagnosis.[64,65]

Stress, Emotional, and Psychological Considerations and T'ai Chi

The stress reduction effects of T'ai Chi exercise, as measured by heart rate, blood pressure, urinary catecholamine, and salivary cortisol levels, were compared among groups of brisk walkers, meditators, and quiet readers.[11] In general, it was found that the stress-reduction effect of T'ai Chi characterized those physiological changes produced by moderate exercise. Heart rate, blood pressure, and urinary catecholamine changes for the T'ai Chi exercise group were similar to those changes occurring in the walking group. Additionally, it was reported that the T'ai Chi group expressed the enhancement of "vigor" and a reduction in anxiety states. In a study by Cheng et al,[12] unequivocal support is provided for the hypothesis that T'ai Chi exercise, which incorporates a cognitive strategy as part of the training program, is more effective than exercises lacking a structured cognitive component in promoting psychological benefits.

Self-rated health is a powerful and consistent predictor of self-care capability and health outcomes, including mobility, morbidity, and mortality.[14] Additionally, exercise is important for maintaining health and improving functioning in older adults.[66] T'ai Chi has been found to not only improve an elder's perception of health, but also to have a significant therapeutic value in improving overall quality-of-life measures.[14-17]

A very important component of quality-of-life measures is the measure of functional independence. Recent research has provided sound evidence that the practice of T'ai Chi leads to an improvement in functional and quality-of-life measures.[19-21] Li and associates[20,21] indicated that compared to a control group of inactive older adults, participants in the T'ai Chi group experienced significant improvements in all aspects of physical functioning over a 6-month intervention period. Overall, improvement occurred across all functional status measures from daily activities such as walking and lifting to moderate-vigorous activities such as running.[20,21] This strongly indicates that a self-paced and self-controlled activity such as T'ai Chi has the potential of being an effective, low-cost means of improving functional status in older persons.

As the above research indicates, there is clearly a positive effect on the sense of well-being of elders practicing T'ai Chi. A study by Blake and Hawley[66] added a new dimension to the study of T'ai Chi by exploring the reasons (eg, facilitators, barriers) that elders seemingly practice T'ai Chi on a more consistent basis than other exercise forms. The results showed that encouragement from others was the most important factor for elders to regularly practice T'ai Chi, whereas positive health outcomes were the reason they continued to practice it beyond group settings.[61,62] Interestingly, most of the initial non–T'ai Chi group participants felt that they were too weak to perform the T'ai Chi exercise. When this group was instructed in this exercise form following the comparative portion of the study, the significant and immediate improvements in health status and well-being measures prompted an even greater participation rate. This group was highly motivated and very enthusiastic about attending daily T'ai Chi sessions.[65] One of the reasons given by a member of this non–T'ai-Chi-turned-T'ai-Chi-group was, "T'ai Chi works better than regular exercise. It is not boring at all, in fact, it is rather enjoyable—like a dance."

A recent study looked at perceived health status in frail older adults who participated in 1 year of T'ai Chi exercise.[67] These findings suggest that older women who are becoming frail benefited from T'ai Chi, demonstrated by an improved perceived health status and a sense that they were able to do more functional activities, including ambulation. These findings have significant implications for the potential of near-frail elderly individuals remaining in the community or being admitted to skilled nursing facilities or requiring higher levels of assisted living environments. Practicing T'ai Chi offers the potential to enhance the physical and mental health of older adults.[68] A short-style T'ai Chi program found that older women practicing this form of exercise improved overall fitness levels, such as lower-extremity strength, balance, and flexibility, and demonstrated significantly faster brisk walking speeds and reduction of risk of falling in community-dwelling elders.[69]

CASE EXAMPLE: MANAGED CARE AND T'AI CHI

Mr. K. was an 84-year-old White male who was admitted to a nursing home in a markedly reconditioned state with diagnoses of coronary heart disease, tuberculosis, confusion, recent history of falls, depression, and malnutrition. The patient was referred to physical and occupational therapy for screening and recommendations. Screening by physical therapy resulted in an initial evaluation that revealed a significantly compromised cardiopulmonary response to any activity, flexed posturing in standing with occasional loss of balance during directional changes, ambulation with moderate assistance of one requiring verbal cueing, and a fluctuating cognitive status. Mr. K. was quite congested and occasionally expectorated blood, especially with exertion. He had remarkable shortness of breath at rest and significant rubor of all extremities with 1+ pulses distally. The patient was withdrawn, minimally verbal, and obviously quite depressed. Based on our assessment, his prognosis was deemed poor for functional recovery to his premorbid state and discharge was unlikely.

Mr. K. was placed on a fall-prevention program that included trunk extensor strengthening, extremity strengthening, and flexibility exercises. Deep breathing exercises were initiated and a reconditioning walking program using a 12-minute test protocol was started. Buerger-Allen exercises were initiated for his circulation and to promote postural changes and mobility. He was also referred to a nutritionist and nursing was consulted regarding his skin and circulatory status. Patient gains were marginal in both physical and occupational therapy over a 3-week period. Mr. K. continued to require minimal to moderate assistance during ambulation, had a poor physiological response to activity of any sort, remained short of breath at rest, and was still withdrawn, now being virtually nonverbal and severely depressed.

Due to the restrictions placed on duration of intervention in a managed care delivery system driven by critical pathways, aggressive "skilled" intervention could no longer be justified. The insurer agreed to a 4-week trial of T'ai Chi exercises to be done 5 days/week in a group setting. The patient was initially instructed in breathing techniques and standing postures utilizing a set of T'ai Chi movements that did not significantly displace his center of gravity. By the end of the first week, remarkable improvements were noted in Mr. K.'s respiratory status (ie, he was no longer short of breath at rest), and his standing posture was distinctively improved. It was noted that this elderly gentleman was much more alert and responsive to his surroundings and appeared to be less depressed. The T'ai Chi routine was expanded to encompass his increasing capabilities and weight shifting postures were started, although single-leg stance T'ai Chi activities were still omitted from his routine. By the end of the second week, this patient was ambulating to and from all activities with stand-by assistance and no verbal cueing. His extremity pulses had improved to 2+ with no extremity rubor. Mr. K. still experienced shortness of breath on exertion, but was no longer short of breath at rest and he was not expectorating blood. He was noted to be spontaneously telling stories and joking with the staff and other residents. He reported amiably "where" his energy was going from time to time and stated that he was "eating everything on my plate."

Mr. K. continued to progress in all areas of functional status. By the end of the third week, he was ambulating to all activities independently and safely. He was alert and obviously happy. We were able to start single-legged stance postures in his T'ai Chi routine. He was independently taking a shower, which pleased him to no end. He was quite fondly acknowledged by his fellow residents due to his sense of humor, optimism, and compassion for their concerns.

By the end of the fourth week, Mr. K. was happily discharged on a home program inclusive of T'ai Chi exercises. Since his discharge, he has enrolled in a T'ai Chi program at a local martial arts facility that he participates in for 2 hours, 3 times/week, and he comes back to the nursing home twice a week to assist as an instructor for our T'ai Chi classes.

Perhaps Mr. K.'s progress sounds too good to be true, but the reality of his improvement has been observed in many of our patients participating in the T'ai Chi classes. Beyond the physical aspects of this exercise form, the most notable improvement appears to be in the area of "outlook." Elderly individuals participating in the T'ai Chi classes express pure enjoyment in the slow, rhythmic movements and the group interaction. They report that they "feel stronger, more balanced" and that they feel as if they are "dancing not exercising." And, the insurers are overwhelmed with the functional successes that seem to be inherent in this mode of exercise. T'ai Chi is a low-cost, low-tech group activity.

CONCLUSION

The increasing body of research related to the use of T'ai Chi as a valuable therapeutic intervention substantiates our need as professionals, in a cost-containment arena, to evaluate the merits of this exercise form.[1-12] T'ai Chi is viewed as an "alternative" therapy and often perceived as "flaky"; however, it has clinically been observed and has now been scientifically shown to enhance function in our elderly patients. This author cautions, however, that while individual complementary modalities, such as T'ai Chi, hold considerable merit, it is critical that the philosophy underlying these therapies be understood and honored.

Recently, the use of T'ai Chi has been identified by the National Institutes of Health as one of a list of "alternative therapies" that will be targeted for research funding as a legitimate area for investigation. We should seize the opportunity to provide leadership in this emerging area in rehabilitative medicine. T'ai Chi, although a nontraditional approach to therapeutic intervention, merits further traditional scientific analysis to quantify its apparent therapeutic validity.

REFERENCES

1. Zhu W, Guan S, Yang Y. Clinical implications of tai chi interventions: a review. *Am J Lifestyle Med.* 2010;4(5):418-432.
2. Lan C, Lai JS, Chen SY. Tai Chi Chuan: an ancient wisdom on exercise and health promotion. *Sports Med.* 2002;32(4):217-224.
3. Liu J, Wang XQ, Zheng JJ, et al. Effects of Tai chi versus proprioception exercise program on neuromuscular function of the ankle in elderly people: a randomized controlled trial. *Evid Based Complement Alternat Med.* 2012;2012:265486.
4. Li JY, Zhang YF, Smith GX, et al. Quality of reporting of randomized clinical trials in Tai Chi interventions—a systematic review. *Evid Based Complement Alternat Med.* 2011;2011:3832425.
5. Kayama H, Okamoto K, Nishiguchi S, Yamada M, Kuroda T, Aoyama T. Effect of kinect-based exercise game on improving cognitive performance in community-dwelling elderly: case control study. *J Med Internet Res.* 2014;16(2):e61.
6. Chan AW, Lee A, Lee DT, et al. The sustaining effects of Tai chi Qigong on physiological health for COPD patients: a randomized controlled trial. *Complement Ther Med.* 2013;21(6):585-594.
7. Leung DP, Chan CK, Tsang HW, Tsang WW, Jones AY. Tai chi as an intervention to improve balance and reduce falls in older adults: a systematic and meta-analytical review. *Altern Ther Health Med.* 2011;17(1):40-48.

8. Wolf SL, Kutner NG, Green RC, McNeely E. The Atlanta FICSIT study: two exercise interventions to reduce frailty in elders. *J Am Geriatr Soc.* 1993;41(3):329-332.

9. Lu WA, Kuo CD. Three months of Tai Chi Chuan exercise can reduce serum triglyceride and endothelin-1 in the elderly. *Complement Ther Clin Prac.* 2013;19(4):204-208.

10. Guan H, Koceja DM. Effects of long-term tai chi practice on balance and H-reflex characteristics. *Am J Chin Med.* 2011;39(2):251-260.

11. Miller SM, Taylor-Piliae RE. Effects of Tai Chi on cognitive function in community-dwelling older adults: a review. *Geriatr Nurs.* 2014;35(1):9-19.

12. Cheng ST, Chow PK, Song YQ, et al. Mental and physical activities delay cognitive decline in older persons with dementia. *Am J Geriatr Psychiatry.* 2014;22(1):63-74.

13. Rand D, Miller WC, Yiu J, Eng JJ. Interventions for addressing low balance confidence in older adults: a systematic review and meta-analysis. *Age Ageing.* 2011;40(3):297-306.

14. Cheng ST, Chow PK, Song YQ, Yu EC, Lam JH. Can leisure activities slow dementia progression in nursing home residents? A cluster-randomized controlled trial. *Int Psychogeriatr.* 2014;26(4):637-643.

15. Chen KM, Snyder M, Krichbaum K. Clinical use of tai chi in elderly populations. *Geriatr Nurs.* 2001;22(4):198-200.

16. Woo J, Hong A, Lau E, Lynn H. A randomized controlled trial of Tai Chi and resistance exercises on bone health, muscle strength and balance in community-living elderly people. *Age Ageing.* 2007;36(3):262-268.

17. Mat S, Tan MP, Kamaruzzaman SB, Ng CT. Physical therapies for improving balance and reducing falls risk in osteoarthritis of the knee: a systematic review. *Age Ageing.* 2015;44(1):16-24.

18. Wang C, Schmid CH, Rones R, et al. A randomized trial of tai chi for fibromyalgia. *N Engl J Med.* 2010;363(8):743-754.

19. Galantino ML, Callens ML, Cardena GJ, Piela NL, Mao JJ. Tai chi for well-being of breast cancer survivors with aromatase inhibitor-associated arthralgias: a feasibility study. *Altern Ther Health Med.* 2013;19(6):38-44.

20. Zhuang J, Huang L, Wu Y, Zhang Y. The effectiveness of a combined exercise intervention on physical fitness factors related to falls in community-dwelling older adults. *Clin Interv Aging.* 2014;9:131-140.

21. Cheon SM, Chae BK, Sung HR, Lee GC, Kim JW. The efficacy of exercise programs for Parkinson's disease: Tai Chi versus combined exercise. *J Clin Neurol.* 2013;9(4):237-243.

22. Liao W. *T'ai Chi Classics: New Translations of Three Essential Texts of T'ai Chi Ch'uan With Commentary and Practical Instruction by Waysun Liao.* Boston, MA: Shambhala Publications; 1990.

23. Lynöe N. Ethical and professional aspects of the practice of alternative medicine. *Scand J Soc Med.* 1992;20(4):217-225.

24. Hoerster KD, Butler DA, Mayer JA, Finlayson T, Gallo LC. Use of conventional care and complementary/alternative medicine among US adults with arthritis. *Prev Med.* 2012;54(1):13-17.

25. Mak JC, Mak LY, Shen Q, Faux S. Perceptions and attitudes of rehabilitation medicine physicians on complementary and alternative medicine in Australia. *Intern Med J.* 2009;39(3):164-169.

26. Jou TH. *The Dao of Taijiquan: Way to Rejuvenation.* Warwick, NY: T'ai Chi Foundation; 1988.

27. Blofeld J (trans, ed). *I Ching: The Book of Changes.* New York, NY: E.P. Dutton & Co; 1965.

28. Liu D. *T'ai Chi Ch'uan and I Ching: A Choreography of Body and Soul.* New York, NY: Harper & Row Publishers; 1987.

29. Liu D. *T'ai Chi Ch'uan & Meditation.* New York, NY: Schocken Books; 1991.

30. Chu WK. *Tao & Longevity: Mind-Body Transformation.* New York, NY: Weiser Books; 1984:8-12.

31. Legge J. *The Texts of Taoism: The Tao Te Ching of Lao Tzu: The Writings of Chuang Tzu: The Sacred Books of China.* Part 1. New York, NY: Dover Publications; 1962:256-257.

32. Fung YL. *A History of Chinese Philosophy: The Period of Classical Learning.* Volume II. Princeton, NJ: Princeton University Press; 1953:436-444.

33. Sohn RC. *Tao and T'ai Chi Kung.* Rochester, VT: Destiny Books; 1989.

34. Palumbo MV, Wu G, Shaner-McRae H, Rambur B, McIntosh B. Tai Chi for older nurses: a workplace wellness pilot study. *Appl Nurs Res.* 2012;25(1):54-59.

35. Esch T, Duckstein J, Welke J, Braun V. Mind/body techniques for physiological and psychological stress reduction: stress management via Tai Chi training—a pilot study. *Med Sci Monit.* 2007;13(11):CR488-CR497.

36. Hong Y, Li JX, Robinson P. Balance control, flexibility, and cardiorespiratory fitness among older Tai Chi practitioners. *Br J Sports Med.* 2000;34(1):29-34.

37. Jahnke R, Larkey L, Rogers C, Etnier J, Lin F. A comprehensive review of health benefits of Qigong and Tai Chi. *Am J Health Promot.* 2010; 24(6):e1-e25.

38. Sato S, Makita S, Uchida R, Ishihara S, Masuda M. Effect of Tai Chi training on baroreflex sensitivity and heart rate variability in patients with coronary heart disease. *Int Heart J.* 2010;51(4):238-241.

39. Siddarth D, Siddarth P, Lavretsky H. An observational study of the health benefits of yoga or tai chi compared with aerobic exercise in community-dwelling middle-aged and older adults. *Am J Geriatr Psychiatry.* 2014;22(3):272-273.

40. Pan L, Yan JY, Guo YZ, Yan JN. Effects of Tai Chi training on exercise capacity and quality of life in patients with chronic heart failure: a meta-analysis. *Eur J Heart Fail.* 2013;15(3):316-323.

41. Wang J, Feng B, Yang X, et al. Tai chi for essential hypertension. *Evid Based Complement Alternat Med.* 2013; 2013:215254.

42. Lorenc AB, Wang Y, Madge SL, Hu X, Mian AM, Robinson N. Meditative movement for respiratory function: a systematic review. *Respir Care.* 2014;59(3):427-440.
43. Danusantoso H, Heijnen L. T'ai Chi Ch'uan for people with haemophilia. *Haemophilia.* 2001;7(4):437-439.
44. Kreitzer MJ, Snyder M. Healing the heart: integrating complementary therapies and healing practices into the care of cardiovascular patients. *Prog Cardiovasc Nurs.* 2002;17(2):73-80.
45. Taylor-Piliae RE, Silva E, Sheremeta SP. Tai Chi as an adjunct physical activity for adults aged 45 years and older enrolled in phase III cardiac rehabilitation. *Eur J Cardiovasc Nurs.* 2012;11(1):34-43.
46. Lan C, Lai JS, Chen SY, Wong MK. Tai Chi Chuan to improve muscular strength and endurance in elderly individuals: a pilot study. *Arch Phys Med Rehabil.* 2000;81(5):604-607.
47. Zeeuwe PE, Verhagen AP, Bierma-Zeinstra SM, van Rossum E, Faber MJ, Koes BW. The effect of Tai Chi Chuan in reducing falls among elderly people: design of a randomized clinical trial in the Netherlands [ISRCTN98840266]. *BMC Geriatr.* 2006;6:6.
48. Zhuang J, Haung L, Wu Y, Zhang Y. The effectiveness of a combined exercise intervention on physical fitness factors related to falls in community-dwelling older adults. *Clin Interv Aging.* 2014;9:131-140.
49. Choi JH, Moon JS, Song R. Effects of Sun-style Tai Chi exercise on physical fitness and fall prevention in fall-prone older adults. *J Adv Nurs.* 2005;51(2):150-157.
50. Tsang WW, Wong VS, Fu SN, Hui-Chan CW. Tai Chi improves standing balance control under reduced or conflicting sensory conditions. *Arch Phys Med Rehabil.* 2004;85(1):129-137.
51. Lin MR, Hwang HF, Wang Yw, Chang SH, Wolf SL. Community-based tai chi and its effect on injurious falls, balance, gait, and fear of falling in older people. *Phys Ther.* 2006;86(9):1189-1201.
52. Li F, Harmer P, Fisher KJ, et al. Tai Chi and fall reductions in older adults: a randomized controlled trial. *J Gerontol A Biol Sci Med Sci.* 2005;60(2):187-194.
53. Zhang JB, Ishikawa-Takata K, Yamazaki H, Morita T, Ohta T. The effects of Tai Chi Chuan on physiological function and fear of falling in the less robust elderly: an intervention study for preventing falls. *Arch Gerontol Geriatr.* 2006;42(2):107-116.
54. Purohit MP, Wells RE, Zafonte R, Davis RB, Yeh GY, Phillips RS. Neuropsychiatric symptoms and the use of mind-body therapies. *J Clin Psychiatry.* 2013;74(6):e520-526.
55. Burschka JM, Keune PM, Oy UH, Oschmann P, Kuhn P. Mindfulness-based interventions in multiple sclerosis: beneficial effects of Tai Chi on balance, coordination, fatigue and depression. *BMC Neurol.* 2014;14:165.
56. Zhang Y, Liu H, Zhou L, et al. Applying Tai Chi as a rehabilitation program for stroke patients in the recovery phase: study protocol for a randomized controlled trial. *Trials.* 2014; 15:484.
57. Wang C. Role of Tai Chi in the treatment of rheumatologic diseases. *Curr Rheumatol Rep.* 2012;14(6):598-603.
58. Waite-Jones JM, Hale CA, Lee HY. Psychosocial effects of Tai Chi exercise on people with rheumatoid arthritis. *J Clin Nurs.* 2013;22(21-22):3053-3061.
59. Woo J, Hong A, Lau E, Lynn H. A randomized controlled trial of Tai Chi and resistance exercise on bone health, muscle strength and balance in community-living elderly people. *Age Ageing.* 2007;36(3):262-268.
60. Chan K, Qin L, Lau M, et al. A randomized, prospective study of the effects of Tai Chi Chun exercise on bone mineral density in postmenopausal women. *Arch Phys Med Rehabil.* 2004;85(5):717-722.
61. Fong SM, Ng GY. The effects on sensorimotor performance and balance with Tai Chi training. *Arch Phys Med Rehabil.* 2006;87(1):82-87.
62. Hass CJ, Gregor RJ, Waddell DE, et al. The influence of Tai Chi training on the center of pressure trajectory during gait initiation in older adults. *Arch Phys Med Rehabil.* 2004;85:1593-1598.
63. Maciaszek J, Osinski W, Szeklicki R, Stemplewski R. Effect of Tai Chi on body balance: randomized controlled trial in men with osteopenia or osteoporosis. *Am J Chin Med.* 2007;35(1):1-9.
64. Campo RA, O'Connor K, Light KC, et al. Feasibility and acceptability of a Tai Chi Chih randomized controlled trial in senior female cancer survivors. *Integr Cancer Ther.* 2013;12(6):464-474.
65. Garland SN, Valentine D, Desai K, et al. Complementary and alternative medicine use and benefit finding among cancer patients. *J Altern Complement Med.* 2013;19(11):876-881.
66. Blake H, Hawley H. Effects of Tai Chi exercise on physical and psychological health of older people. *Curr Aging Sci.* 2012;5(1):19-27.
67. Greenspan AI, Wolf SL, Kelley ME, O'Grady M. Tai chi and perceived health status in older adults who are transitionally frail: a randomized controlled trial. *Phys Ther.* 2007;87(5):525-535.
68. Chen KM, Li CH, Lin JN, Chen WT, Lin HS, Wu HC. A feasible method to enhance and maintain the health of elderly living in long-term care facilities through long-term, simplified tai chi exercises. *J Nurs Res.* 2007;15(2):156-164.
69. Audette JF, Jin YS, Newcomer R, Stein L, Duncan G, Frontera WR. Tai chi versus brisk walking in elderly women. *Age Ageing.* 2006;35(4):388-393.

12

Biofeedback
Connecting the Body and Mind

Jennifer M. Bottomley, PhD, MS, PT

The suggestion that hemiplegia, migraine and tension headaches, asthma, hypertension, cardiac arrhythmias, visual acuity, torticollis spasms, pain, hyperkinesis, and functional and cognitive disorders of any of the body's systems may all be relieved by a single form of treatment sounds more like a 19th century pitch for snake oil than a true reflection of research. Yet, biofeedback has been investigated extensively and has promising clinical applications in an astounding number of conditions.[1-98]

The last 2 decades have seen an increasing convergence of body and mind therapies. These new therapies are often labeled as *psychosomatic or psychophysical medicine.*[1] As both names imply, these approaches to healing deal with the effect of the mind on the body. Tremendous strides have been made in the understanding of mental influences on body systems with the many mind-body integrative therapies that are currently being practiced. These connections range from the muscular to the immune system. This has led to the development of treatment procedures that incorporate this connection between mind and body. Biofeedback techniques for stress-related disorders and dysfunction and mental imaging using autogenic (a method of mind-over-body control based on a specific discipline for relaxing parts of the body by means of autosuggestion) feedback to enhance the responsiveness of the autonomic nervous system and/or the immune system response are 2 good examples of this process. Biofeedback is one of the earliest and most accepted methods employed by rehabilitation professions of integrating rather than separating the mind and body.[2]

Biofeedback, meaning "life-feedback," is a process of electronically utilizing information from the body to teach an individual to recognize what is going on inside of his or her own brain, nervous system, and muscles. Biofeedback refers to any technique that uses instrumentation to give a person immediate and continuing signals of bodily function changes that he or she is not usually conscious of, such as fluctuations in blood pressure, brainwave activity, or muscle tension. Theoretically and very often in practice, information input enables the individual to learn to control the involuntary function.[3,4]

Biofeedback acts as an output-input system whereby output is based in the motor unit and the input is via sensory pathways comprising proprioceptors, exteroceptors, and interoceptors.[1,3] Biofeedback provides a means of measuring a physiological response using an electronic device. It aids the sensory side of a feedback mechanism assisting a compensated sensation, such as with a cerebrovascular accident (CVA) or other brain injury, in responding appropriately (ie, motor unit training) by increasing conscious awareness of intact, but usually unfelt, sensation. Basically,

Davis CM.
*Integrative Therapies in Rehabilitation: Evidence for Efficacy in Therapy,
Prevention, and Wellness, Fourth Edition* (pp 161-180).
© 2017 Taylor & Francis Group.

biofeedback acts as a sixth sense by providing an artificial proprioception feedback. Via operant conditioning, a new association between a stimuli and a response is developed. The action that is taken by the learner is voluntary and under his or her own control. The response is instrumental in producing a reward or removing a negative stimulus, and this reinforcement shapes behavior and function with successive stages.

Biofeedback transfers the responsibility for final success to the patient. Often, individuals seek medical help, hoping to place the responsibility of "curing" their problems on the clinician, while the patients take an almost passive role in the treatment process. This is commonly known as an *external locus of control.*[5] The patient should understand that he or she has the ability, with assistance from the appropriate medical professionals, to help him- or herself. Biofeedback provides a modality to accomplish this.

PRINCIPLES OF BIOFEEDBACK

The prefix *myo* is derived from the Greek word for muscle. In combination with the Greek word *graphos*, meaning to write, and the additional prefix *electro*, the word becomes *electromyograph*, an instrument for recording the electrical activity of the muscles. Electromyographic (EMG) biofeedback is a modality for measuring and displaying muscle activity, and is used primarily where any modification of muscular behavior is indicated. With its use, an individual can learn to become more aware of his or her own muscle activity, thereby gaining more complete control of functional activity. EMG biofeedback also provides an ideal method for rehabilitation practitioners to record a patient's day-to-day progress.

The biofeedback device imparts objective information about the degree of activity occurring in a muscle through surface electrodes, in audio and/or visual form, in much the same way that an electrocardiogram (EKG) provides information about cardiac activity or an electroencephalogram (EEG) displays brainwave activity. In an EMG biofeedback system, the electrical signal originating in the muscle under study is amplified and then translated into sound and visual reading, which corresponds to increased and decreased muscle activity. EMG is the process of recording and interpreting the electrical activity of muscle. When a muscle contracts, it produces a characteristic spike (pulse) waveform that can be detected easily by placing an electrode on the skin over the muscle belly. For example, if you tightly grasp an object in your hand, the muscles in your arm will generate a specific electrical voltage, usually measured in millivolts (0.001 volt) or microvolts (0.000001 volt). As you squeeze the object tighter, the electrical voltage will increase as more motor units are recruited. As you relax your hand, the electrical voltage will decrease dramatically. EMG is, therefore, a direct physiological index of muscular activity and the state of relaxation.

The interior of a nerve cell is electrically negative with respect to the exterior during its resting phase. This negative potential, typically 50 to 100 millivolts, exists because of the "selective permeability" of the cell wall. On the outside of the cell membrane, Na+ ions are more concentrated; on the inside, K+ ions are more concentrated, along with Cl- and other large, negative ions. The semipermeable membrane acts as a barrier to the free interchange of these ions, bringing about a condition like that of a charged battery. The membrane is, therefore, polarized, giving rise to a potential gradient across the cell membrane. This phenomenon is known as the *resting potential of the cell.*[2,5]

When a nerve cell is stimulated, its normal resting potential disappears. The permeability of the cell wall changes, permitting Na+, K+, and Cl- ion migration through the wall. The Na+ ions move from the interstitial tissue fluid surrounding the nerve cell into the nerve fiber. Eventually, the Na+ ion concentration inside the nerve fiber exceeds that in the interstitial fluid. The K+ ions move from within the nerve fiber to the interstitial fluid. The Na+ and K+ ion movements cause a reverse potential to build up (ie, the interior of the cell becomes more positive than the exterior) because the inside of the cell has been flooded with Na+ ions. This reverse potential may reach a value of 30 to 50 millivolts. After a short time, the membrane regains its original permeability characteristics, and the normal ion distribution is reestablished via the sodium-potassium pump. This changing potential produced when the nerve cell "fires" and then regains its resting voltage is known as the *action potential*.[2,4,5]

When a nerve cell fires, it influences adjacent cells and causes them to fire. These cells, in turn, cause the nerve cells adjacent to them to fire. In this manner, the action potential spreads rapidly from cell to cell. This traveling action potential is known as an *impulse*. Impulses move along nerve fibers to stimulate the associated muscle fibers and move along the muscle fibers to cause contraction. An impulse can travel in both directions away from the point of stimulation, but it cannot reverse direction toward the starting point. Such reversal of direction is prevented because each nerve cell along the path of the impulse becomes momentarily refractory (ie, insensitive to stimulation for a short time after it has fired).[2,5]

The motor unit is a basic configuration of neuromuscular activity. It consists of a collection of muscle fibers controlled by a single nerve fiber. When the nerve provides the "triggering" electrical impulse, the muscle fibers contract practically simultaneously. A motor unit may have only a few muscle fibers or it may have thousands, and many motor units are needed to provide the mechanical force required to impart movement to the body.

The motor point is normally the most excitable point of a muscle and represents the area of the greatest concentration of nerve endings. It generally corresponds to the level at which the nerve enters the belly of the muscle.

The frequency spectrum is the range of frequencies present in a given electrical event, as measured in hertz. An example of such a frequency is the 60-cycle (hertz) waves given off from wall outlet voltage. The frequency spectrum of EMG signals covers the range of 20 to 5000 hertz.[5]

The raw, unprocessed EMG signal can be heard in a set of earphones or a speaker when amplified. These "muscle sounds" have been described as popping, crackling, hissing, freight train, airplane, and chugging sounds.[2] The raw EMG sound, however, is of little use as a feedback signal since the ear's ability to discern changes in signal amplitude is very limited. For this reason, the EMG signal is usually processed and converted to a variable frequency signal because the ear is much more sensitive to changes in tone.[5,6]

Both surface and needle electrodes have been used in EMG. Although the voltage from a single muscle fiber can be monitored by the use of a fine-tipped needle electrode, surface electrodes are commonly used for biofeedback in the rehabilitation setting. The voltage picked up by the surface electrodes is actually an average for the many muscle fibers below and near the electrodes. Although muscle action potentials as picked up by the electrodes could possibly be as high as 1000 microvolts, values between 100 and 500 microvolts are more representative.[1]

The principal advantage of needle electrodes is their high sensitivity to individual motor unit potentials, usually without interference from nearby muscles.[2] Therefore, they are usually used for diagnostic purposes. However, since physical therapists normally use EMG biofeedback for muscle reeducation and relaxation purposes, surface electrodes have a number of advantages. For example, they eliminate the necessity of keeping all materials sterile and can be used easily at home by the patient.

EMG biofeedback has been reported as being a successful procedure for assisting in the rehabilitation of patients with a wide variety of neuromuscular problems,[2,6,7] for providing muscle reeducation, and/or for providing muscle relaxation. It can be used for the following:

- Relaxation[1-8,61]
- Relief of migraine-headache pain[9-15]
- Relief of tension-headache pain[9-15]
- Treatment of temporomandibular joint (TMJ) disorders[16,17]
- Improvement of functional deficits in paraplegia and quadriplegia[18,19]
- Improvement of postural instability, proprioception, and reduction of falls[20-23]
- Treatment of vestibular disorders[24]

- Muscle reeducation and relaxation for children with cerebral palsy[25,26]
- CVA rehabilitation[27-33] for the following:
  - Foot drop and other gait problems
  - Posture and muscle tone improvement
  - Improved voluntary control of involved muscles
  - Muscle relaxation in associated reactions
  - Speech problems
- Gait training[34-36]
- Muscular training after nerve, muscle, ligament, or tendon injury, repair, or transfers[37-39,41,42,57]
  - Carpal tunnel syndrome
  - Hand dystonia
  - Rotator cuff and other shoulder pathologies
  - Lateral epicondylitis
  - Thoracic outlet syndrome
  - Patellofemoral pain
- Achilles tendon repairs
- Early joint mobilization after surgery[40,43,45]
  - Total joint replacements and other orthopedic surgeries
  - Reeducation of affected muscle following radical mastectomy
- Measurement of endurance with sustained activity[44-46]
- Functional training and reduction of myoclonus following brain injury[47-49]
- Control of urinary incontinence and other pelvic floor disorders and labor pain[50-54,58,60,87,89]
- Relaxation for intractable constipation symptoms and fecal incontinence[55-56,59,61-63]
- Respiratory control in asthma, emphysema, and chronic obstructive pulmonary disease[64-68,77]
- Modification of hypertension[69-71]
- Treatment of diabetes, vascular disease, and symptoms of intermittent claudication[72-75]
- Parasympathetic control of cardiac arrhythmias[77,78]
- Stress management[77-82]
- Treatment of affective disorders; depression, anxiety, addiction[83-98]
- Intervention for dysphagia and other swallowing disorders[83,84]
- Muscle reeducation following Bell's palsy[85,86]
- Pain management and reduction in chemotherapy-related symptoms in patients with cancer[88-92]
- Improvement of memory functioning[93]
- Wound healing[94]

TYPES OF BIOFEEDBACK INTERVENTIONS

Primarily, in the field of rehabilitation medicine, biofeedback techniques are used that focus on muscle reeducation or the voluntary inhibition (relaxation) of the muscle.[6,7] In these approaches, electrodes are placed directly over the belly of the target muscle. Success is measured by appropriate muscle activation or relaxation. Techniques that are aimed at autonomic nervous system control include placement of surface electrodes on the frontalis muscle and measurement of physiologic variables, such as heart rate, blood pressure, breathing pattern and rate, and galvanic skin response. Another approach for biofeedback intervention is the use of a digital temperature monitor for the measurement of physiologic response through body temperature.[8]

In addition to instrumentation for feedback purposes, treatment techniques often include guided imagery training or progressive muscle relaxation, which are forms of autogenic relaxation techniques.[5,7] Deep-breathing techniques have been shown to effectively regulate mental states[9,10] and are often employed in combination with the previously-mentioned biofeedback techniques to enhance a state of relaxation. Guided imagery is frequently used as an adjunct to biofeedback to facilitate a state of excitation for athletic training. Kaushik et al[11] observed significant tachypnea in participants during imagery of sprint running and, in most cases studied, EMG biofeedback substantially augmented the physiological responses.

The mechanisms by which cognitive processes influence states of bodily arousal are important for understanding the pathogenesis and maintenance of stress-related morbidity. Yang and associates[2] investigated cerebral activity related to cognitively driven modulation of sympathetic activity and found that biofeedback-assisted relaxation was associated with significant increases in left anterior cingulated, vermal, and globus pallidus activity.[2] These findings have potential implications for a mechanistic account of how therapeutic interventions, such as relaxation training in stress-related disorders, mediate their effects.

Muscle Reeducation

When using biofeedback for muscle reeducation, it is important to place the muscle that needs to be examined in the easiest position for the patient to elicit movement. For example, in testing the strength of the vastus medialis of the quadriceps muscle group, the patient might be positioned on his or her side, attempting to straighten his or her lower leg. Another useful position might be with the patient supine and his or her lower leg hanging off of the edge of the table. For other patients, this movement might best be accomplished from a sitting position. It is generally easier to elicit motor unit firing when a muscle is in a fully stretched condition and the patient is asked to move through a full range of motion. Visual observation by the patient of the motion to be performed can often be of great benefit.[1,4,6,8]

At the initial treatment session, it is important for the therapist to familiarize the patient with the operation of the biofeedback unit. Placing electrodes on a normal muscle or on the corresponding muscle of the uninvolved extremity when possible, and going through the full range of motion or tensing and relaxing the muscle, will help to prepare the patient to work with the affected muscle or muscle group. This approach will also give the patient practice in reading the meter and hearing the "muscle sounds."[5,6]

To aid the patient in eliciting motor responses, all forms of exercise, proprioceptive neuromuscular facilitation techniques, and body positioning may be employed. The objective is to discover any functional motor units in the muscle. If no active motor units are discovered at a particular therapy session, it does not necessarily mean that none are present. There may be only a few active motor units in a weakened muscle, as compared with thousands in a normal muscle. What we are searching for is *potential activity* of motor units in what appears to be a "paralyzed" muscle.[1,3,8]

When active motor unit responses are found, the next step is to bring the responses under voluntary control. After detecting responses in an involved muscle, one should not expect these responses to remain at the same high level of activity at future therapy sessions. A great degree of variability can be expected initially, especially in the neurologically compromised muscle. Over an extended period of treatment, a muscle given regular, continued exercise is likely to show a continuing increase in strength and a reduced tendency toward wide fluctuations in readings.[4]

Motivation of the patient is the key. If the therapist approaches the patient optimistically with the attitude that EMG biofeedback can be of significant benefit in the rehabilitation process, and continually emphasizes reachable goals with good exercise programs, then real progress can be achieved and objectively measured. As the return of functional components for a desired task occurs, and as the speed and accuracy of performance improve, biofeedback instrumentation may be gradually withdrawn.[1]

It is important to remember that it is extremely easy for a person who has obtained some functional use of a muscle group to later let those muscles regress to a decreased level of function. This generally happens when muscles are not exercised for a period of time. It must be stressed to the patient that the natural sensory feedback mechanism of the muscles that he or she is attempting to strengthen has been diminished, and that constant attention on a daily basis is required to increase muscle strength and function to an optimum level.

EMG biofeedback can also be used as a monitor for the evaluation of progress with home exercise programs in subsequent follow-up sessions. A home unit is often helpful, and most EMG biofeedback units manufactured today have memory capabilities of 30+ treatment sessions so that progress can be downloaded and compliance with the exercise program can be monitored. Since it is a natural tendency to decrease exercise as strength increases, patients should be reevaluated on a periodic basis, and the therapist should reinforce the necessity of continuing their exercise programs. It is important to remember that if a total program of objective measurement of muscle activity is undertaken, clear, concise records must be kept to facilitate reimbursement by third-party payers.[1,4,7,9]

Muscle Relaxation

The procedure for training a patient in muscle relaxation techniques is much the same as for muscle reeducation training. The difference lies in the fact that instead of teaching the patient to increase motor unit firing, we are trying to inhibit or decrease the level of firing created by the tension or tone in the muscle. Again, electrodes should be attached over an unaffected muscle for demonstration of how muscle tension can be lowered after an initial muscle contraction. Only when the patient has thoroughly understood the relationship between muscle contraction, relaxation, and the corresponding changes in auditory and visual displays should the electrodes be placed on the affected muscle.

The patient must understand that relaxing a muscle that has abnormal tone will not be as easy as relaxing a normal muscle, but that it can be done with practice and perseverance. Repeated orientation is necessary. The individual must understand that he or she controls the feedback and that the equipment does not control him or her. Among the best tools to assist a patient in decreasing muscle tension are deep-breathing techniques focusing in on the abdominal region, music, relaxation tapes, and progressive relaxation exercises, such as those designed by Jacobson.[3]

To assist patients who have difficulty decreasing muscle activity, the therapist should point out any strained posture, labored breathing, noted lack of focus, or anything else that is interfering with the ability to relax. Ideally, for training practice sessions, the patient should be in a quiet, dimly lit room, free from outside distractions, and positioned for maximum comfort. It is sometimes helpful to begin training or practice sessions by having the individual imagine pleasant scenes or experiences. This allows the patient to clear his or her mind of any of the "built-in" tensions of everyday life. Clinical training sessions generally last 30 minutes, 2 to 3 times/week. After the patient makes progress in decreasing the microvolts level in a structured situation, he or she should be encouraged to practice these relaxation techniques in the environment where the tension arises.

For those individuals with muscle contraction or tension headaches, the electrodes are often placed on the skin over the frontalis muscle approximately 2 inches apart and approximately 1 inch above the eyebrows. It should be explained to the individual that the electrodes are measuring the amount of muscle tension that he or she is producing, and that this tension is a reflection of the tension throughout his or her whole body.[9,10]

Some clinicians feel that the frontalis is not necessarily the best reflector of body tension for every patient, and this author agrees. Another effective lead placement is suggested using a global technique. With this technique, the electrodes are attached to the flexor surface of each forearm. This electrode placement allows one to monitor the tension of all of the muscles of the upper body, which comprise approximately 60% of the controlled muscles of the body.[4]

To develop a complete program of muscle reeducation or relaxation, it is important that the patient be instructed in the use of the EMG biofeedback unit at home. This approach allows the patient to monitor and maintain the optimum level that he or she has achieved in the clinical environment.

CLINICAL RESEARCH IN THE USE OF BIOFEEDBACK TECHNIQUES

Migraine and Tension Headache Pain

Behavioral therapies, such as biofeedback, are commonly used to treat migraine and tension headaches.[13-15] Controlling sympathetic activity is effective for controlling the pain in both disturbances.[13] Grazzi and Bussone[13] confirmed the clinical efficacy of EMG biofeedback treatment for tension and common migraine headaches. In this study, the basal stress indices (plasma catecholamines and cortisol) were significantly different in the experiment group compared with no change in the controls, and the study group experienced a substantial decrease in the frequency of headaches reported.

Functional activities of daily living are often restricted in the presence of tension headaches.[8-10] In a study by Evetovich et al,[8] EMG biofeedback was used to decrease upper trapezius activity related to tension headaches. These authors believed that headaches were caused by general tension and anxiety and affected the individual's ability to adequately attend to activities of daily living, including child care, homemaking, and vocational activities. The program combined deep-breathing exercises, progressive muscular relaxation exercises, resisted shoulder elevation exercises, EMG monitoring during upper-extremity tasks, and a home exercise/relaxation program. EMG biofeedback was successful in assisting to eliminate tension headaches, and the patients reported an increased ability to attend to activities of daily living.[8]

Other studies also strongly support the use of biofeedback-assisted relaxation techniques in the treatment of tension[12] and migraine[13,15] headaches.

Temporomandibular Disorders

Often, individuals with TMJ disorders experience a great deal of jaw pain and can develop tension headaches. Crider et al[16] reviewed and performed a meta-analysis of the available literature to determine the efficacy of biofeedback-based treatments in subjects with TMJ disorders. They determined that, although the effects of biofeedback interventions were limited in extent (ie, duration), the available data support the efficacy of EMG biofeedback treatment for TMJ disorders.

An interesting comparison of muscular relaxation effects of transcutaneous electrical neuromuscular stimulation and EMG biofeedback in patients with bruxism during the night was studied by Foster.[17] The author reported that tendencies of nocturnal bruxism decreased mean EMG levels in individuals after biofeedback treatment sessions. The results indicated that not only did individuals exhibit fewer bruxing episodes following treatment, but also that gains from biofeedback were maintained 6 months following the termination of treatment.[17] This research has significant implications for rehabilitation professionals involved in the management of patients with TMJ disorders.

Functional Deficits in Paraplegia and Quadriplegia

The efficacy of enhancing muscle function in patients with spinal cord injury when administered in conjunction with physical rehabilitation therapy has been substantiated.[18] Evidence from the study by Ersal and Sienko,[19] for example, indicated that patients with spinal cord injury in the study group using biofeedback and a conventional exercise program experienced more improvements than the control group, who used a conventional exercise program alone to regain muscle strength and function.

Postural Instability, Proprioception, and Falls

Postural instability, deficits in proprioception, and kinesthesia are associated with many neuromuscular pathologies and increase the potential of falling. Postural instability may be developmental, as in the case of the severely motorically impaired child with cerebral palsy or acquired later in life secondary to neural disease or trauma.[20,21] Beyond the pathological conditions creating postural instability, aging is also associated with trunk weakness, alterations in neuromuscular and musculoskeletal efficiency, and an increased incidence of falling.[22,23] In contrast to the use of biofeedback for neuromuscular reeducation of muscles that are over- or underactive, biofeedback for postural instability has been used to augment achievement of functional skills, such as head or trunk control or symmetry of standing balance.[21] EMG biofeedback instrumentation is effective in detecting muscle activity and in giving the patient objective information about the physiological functioning and movements not ordinarily perceived by the individual. In the case of postural instability, auditory and visual biofeedback signals provide the patient with information regarding head and trunk orientation and about symmetry of weight bearing through the lower extremities.[23,24]

The possibility of using learned physiological responses in control of progressive adolescent idiopathic scoliosis has also been investigated. A study by Domagalska-Szopa and Szopa[25] found that a long-lasting active spinal control could be achieved through the patient's own spinal muscles facilitated by auditory biofeedback. In another study, adolescent patients were able to decrease the use of, and, in some cases, eliminate the need for, bracing devices generally prescribed until skeletal maturity or cessation of curve progression.[26]

Cerebral Palsy

In addition to the physical problems inherent in cerebral palsy, speech problems can often create a frustrating communication deficit in these individuals. In a study by Yoo and associates,[26] electropalatography biofeedback was used to treat patients with severe speech production problems affecting articulation, phonation, and resonance. The authors found that this form of instrumented biofeedback provided a valuable form of visual feedback for patients and revealed and clarified aspects of oral movements for speech and nonspeech activity that had been difficult to capture via auditory perception.[25,26]

Vestibular Disorders

It is well known that diseases of the vestibular system can be compensated by increased spontaneous activity of other systems engaged in maintaining equilibrium (eg, proprioceptive and visual systems). A complex approach using multisensory stimulation is the optimal way to achieve vestibular compensation. Cakrt et al[24] studied the effect of vestibular rehabilitative therapy using biofeedback techniques in patients with vestibular disorders, such as Meniere's disease, neuritis vestibularis, and vertebrobasilar insufficiency. All of these subjects showed improvement in equilibrium by visual and proprioceptive biofeedback mechanisms, indicating a clear value and usefulness of biofeedback techniques in the treatment of vestibular disorders.[24]

Cerebrovascular Accident

Rehabilitation for individuals sustaining a CVA has been shown to be enhanced by employing EMG biofeedback for neuromuscular reeducation.[27] Shumway-Cook and colleagues[27] found that problems such as foot drop and other gait problems, posture and muscle tone, voluntary control of involved muscles, and muscle relaxation in associated reactions were all improved with the use of biofeedback as an adjunct to physical and occupational therapy. A recent study investigated whether visual biofeedback/force-plate training could enhance the effects of other physical therapy interventions on balance and mobility following stroke.[27] Post-intervention scores were higher among both the biofeedback and control groups on the balance measures. Research indicates no significant advantage to the use of visual biofeedback training combined with other physical therapy interventions. However, virtual reality training has been successfully used to rehabilitate functional balance and mobility.[27-30]

Hsu et al[31] performed a detailed study to determine the recovery of upper-extremity function following an acute stroke, comparing orthodox physical therapy interventions with therapy regimes enhanced by the use of EMG biofeedback to encourage motor learning with behavioral methods. Six months following strokes, it was found that study subjects had a statistically significant advantage in recovery of strength, range of motion, and speed of movement. This research demonstrated a small but significant effect on muscle function with EMG biofeedback compared with conventional physical therapy for improving upper-extremity function in patients following a stroke.

Gait Training

As discussed in relation to posture and balance, biofeedback techniques are often successfully employed to improve gait patterns. For example, residual limb recovery after surgery depends largely on close monitoring of the weight-bearing activities during the early postoperative stage. Del Din and co-workers[32] investigated the ability of individuals to increase weight bearing following biofeedback training and determined that weight bearing was well maintained and that partial weight bearing was more appropriately obtained with biofeedback. These findings could conceivably be employed in any condition where the amount of weight bearing during gait training was a consideration. The use of EMG biofeedback reduced the likelihood of tripping during gait and was found to consistently lead to a reduced fall risk and a more normal gait pattern among patients who had a stroke in a study by De Nunzio et al.[33]

Bisson and colleagues[34] examined the use of physical therapy in older adults involving muscle strengthening and gait training in which biofeedback was used for a portion of each therapy session. A subset of patients was also given an EMG biofeedback training device for neuromuscular reeducation outside of the clinic. It was found that the strength of gluteus medius contraction was improved through auditory input. If too little gluteus medius activity occurred on the affected side or the step was too short in duration, an audio cue alerted the individual so that he or she could correct the deficit. Subjects undergoing clinical therapy showed approximately a 50% reduction in tripping, whereas those participants who used the traditional methods showed almost normal gait after the 2-month treatment period.[34] Other studies have substantiated this improvement in lower-extremity weight bearing over time and better toe clearance through the use of biofeedback as a therapeutic modality.[35,36]

Muscular Reeducation/Relaxation Following Injury

The effects of biofeedback on carpal tunnel syndrome show promise in preventing this problem from reoccurring. In a study by Vedsted et al,[37] behavioral modification based on audible EMG biofeedback signals was used to discourage awkward hand postures and the exertion of excessive force with the fingers, which are suspected of causing carpal tunnel syndrome. They found a reduction in symptomatology and a learning affect related to proper ergonomic posturing, upper extremity positioning, and reduced key pressure during computer typing tasks.

Work-related upper-extremity disorders present a significant challenge to health care providers, employers, and insurers.[37] Verhagen and associates[39] described rehabilitation approaches for keyboard operators following radial tunnel compression and release of the extensor origin of the right elbow. An EMG biofeedback device was employed in this study to determine which work activities individuals should avoid or alter to reduce strain in the wrist musculature. It was found that reoccurrence of carpal tunnel symptoms was significantly reduced by reeducating workers through the use of biofeedback.[39]

Adding symmetry retraining to postoperative protocols following arthroplasty of the knee is clinically viable, safe, and may have the additional benefits of enhancing normal muscle contractions and normalizing range and strength. A return to independence was more rapidly obtained through the use of biofeedback.[40]

Rotator cuff and other shoulder pathologies are often accompanied by protective muscle guarding in the supraspinatus, infraspinatus, anterior and middle portions of the deltoid, and descending part of the trapezius. By using biofeedback surface electrodes, it has been found that subjects were able to reduce the EMG activity voluntarily in the trapezius.[40,41] This was not true for the other muscles investigated. When the trapezius activity was reduced there was a tendency toward an increase in EMG activity in the other shoulder muscle, particularly the infraspinatus. Jaggi and Lambert[42] suggest that the findings may be related to relaxation from an initial over-stabilization of the shoulder, or redistribution of load among synergists. It is suggested that the possibility of reducing trapezius activity may be of ergonomic significance.[42]

Voluntary posterior dislocation of the shoulder is a difficult condition to treat successfully. It has been shown that EMG biofeedback is a nonoperative treatment that has been successfully used to prevent recurrent dislocation.[42]

To determine the effects of EMG biofeedback in patients with patellofemoral pain syndrome, a recent study demonstrated that an effective treatment modality for improving quadriceps muscle strength after arthroscopic meniscectomy surgery is biofeedback.[43]

Measurement of Endurance

The effect of psychological strategies upon cardiorespiratory and muscular activity during aerobic exercise has been widely employed in sports therapy. Kranitz and Lehrer[44] demonstrated that all cardiovascular parameters (eg, heart rate, respiratory rate, depth of ventilation, blood pressure) could be consciously altered using biofeedback monitoring. Leisman et al[45] investigated the effects of fatigue and task repetition on the relationship between integrated electromyogram and force output of working muscles. This study showed that with fatigue, integrated EMG activity increased strongly and functional force output of the muscle remained stable or decreased. Fatigue results in a less efficient muscle process. Through training using biofeedback, the efficiency of muscle contraction could be improved with volitional control and the level of fatigue reduced.[45]

As it is difficult to produce conditions of aerobic training in bedrest or sedentary environments, the use of biofeedback to facilitate aerobic cardiac responses may assist in maintaining endurance under these circumstances. Applicability of biofeedback-induced endurance training with bedridden and otherwise immobilized individuals could hold great potential and should be evaluated in future research.

Brain Injury

Biofeedback has traditionally been used in the context of relaxation therapy along with stress management. Some recent studies have looked to extend the applicability of biofeedback by using it as a didactic tool for neuromotor rehabilitation. Guercio and colleagues[47] examined the effects of behavioral relaxation training and biofeedback on ataxic tremor of adults with acquired brain injury. Relaxation techniques were used as the foundation for biofeedback training. The results for specific skills (ie, use of a letter board for communication) when the participants were able to relax the appropriate musculature were positive. The research demonstrated that the individual was able to learn to significantly decrease the severity of tremor to accomplish a functional task. As a result, each participant became more proficient at communicating with a letter board. Collateral effects were increased attempts at communication and fewer episodes of anger.[47]

The mechanisms of feedback not controlled by our consciousness play an essential role in the functions of the central nervous system in the process of programming of activities, behavior, and control of these functions. In cases of deviations or errors of activities, imposed by brain injury and stroke, the possibility of their immediate correction exists.[48] Brain damage after trauma or caused by a tumor disturbs normal feedback mechanisms, producing varying symptom complexes. Nelson and Esty[49] found that EMG biofeedback was advantageous in providing afferent information to the brain-damaged patient and enhancing the return of motor function more substantially than conventional physical therapy interventions in patients with brain injury and post-traumatic stress symptoms.

Urinary Incontinence and Other Pelvic Floor Disorders

Stress incontinence is a debilitating condition affecting a large proportion of the female population. Pelvic floor exercising with the aid of EMG biofeedback is well established as an effective treatment regime.[50-56,58] Current EMG monitoring devices are effective, as they may also be employed in community-based home therapy.[53,54] Many of the units are compact, accurate, and suitable for the ambulatory monitoring of vaginal pressure.

Vonthein et al[59] found that both urinary and fecal incontinence was improved through the use of EMG biofeedback-assisted pelvic floor exercise. These authors clearly demonstrated that a pelvic floor rehabilitation program was an effective alternative to surgical intervention in reducing the frequency of urinary and fecal leakage. Numerous studies provide confirmation that both urinary and fecal incontinence can conservatively be managed through physical therapy interventions utilizing biofeedback-assisted pelvic floor muscle training.[50-63] Postoperative complications following radical prostatectomy usually include urinary incontinence.[60]

The effective use of biofeedback for gynecological problems, such as vulvar vestibulitis syndrome, marked by moderate to severe chronic introital dyspareunia and tenderness of the vulvar vestibule, has also been clearly demonstrated.[62] Women instructed in a home program employing biofeedback-assisted pelvic floor muscle rehabilitation exercises experienced an increase in pelvic floor muscle contraction strength, a decrease in resting tension levels of the pelvic floor muscle, a decrease in the muscle instability associated with this syndrome, and a remarkable decrease in pain.[52,53]

Recent systematic reviews on the conservative management of urinary incontinence in women have identified evidence for firm recommendations to include biofeedback in the conservative strategies for treating this condition.[58] A comparative study looking at the effectiveness of an intensive group physical therapy program with individual biofeedback training for female patients with stress incontinence showed improvement in both groups. Both the intensive therapy group and the biofeedback group resulted in a significantly reduced nocturnal urinary frequency and improved subjective outcome. Only group therapy resulted in reduced daytime urinary frequency. Biofeedback resulted in a better subjective outcome and higher contraction pressures of the pelvic floor muscle.[58]

Intractable Constipation and Fecal Incontinence

Some individuals have difficulty relaxing the striated muscles of the anal sphincters, sometimes referred to as *animus*. Fecal incontinence is often underreported by the older population. It is especially common in elderly persons residing in community or long-term care settings. Physiological changes, including sphincter muscle and sensory abnormalities in the anorectal region, contribute to this problem and respond effectively to biofeedback techniques.[59-63] Once fecal incontinence is identified, management is important. Treatment with biofeedback is feasible in many older adults.

Although immediate results are good to excellent in a great majority of patients who undergo biofeedback treatment for chronic constipation and fecal incontinence, it tends to lose its benefits over time.[61] Therefore, it is important that patients be reevaluated and that biofeedback intervention be performed on an ongoing basis. Although behavioral treatment (biofeedback) successfully treats the pelvic floor abnormalities in patients with idiopathic constipation, many patients also normalize their impaired bowel frequency. Patcharatrakul and Gonlachanvit[62] postulated that this response may be associated with altered cerebral outflow via extrinsic autonomic nerves to the gut. They found that a successful outcome after biofeedback treatment in irritable bowel syndrome is associated with improved activity of the direct cerebral innervation to the gut and improved gut transit. Treating dyssynergic defecation patients with irritable bowel syndrome by biofeedback therapy improved both constipation and symptoms.[62] Most programs implemented to treat fecal incontinence result in improvements. Biofeedback is a nonsurgical, less costly means of treatment that reportedly produces good results in fecally incontinent patients. Sensory retraining appears to be more relevant than strength training to the success of biofeedback.[63]

Asthma, Emphysema, and Chronic Obstructive Pulmonary Disease

The use of biofeedback techniques has also been shown to have an impact on respiratory resistance in conditions of asthma and other resistive lung problems.[64-68] Hypothesis for the positive impact of visual and auditory biofeedback effectiveness in these respiratory conditions is the activation of the parasympathetic nervous system providing more available oxygen and the influence of relaxation and deep-breathing techniques in calming the system, thereby reducing respiratory resistance.[64,66] Lehrer et al[64] provided substantial evidence supporting the learning effect facilitated by the use of feedback in control of respiratory pattern. This information indicates that EMG biofeedback could have a great deal of merit in the treatment of asthma and other stress-related breathing problems.

Laryngeal dyskinesia is a functional asthma-like disorder refractory to bronchodilator regimes. Age-related attenuation of biofeedback effects on cardiovascular variability does not diminish the usefulness of the method for treating asthma among older adults.[66]

Lehrer and associates[64] demonstrated that biofeedback techniques were effective as a nonpharmacological psychophysiological treatment for improving pulmonary function in asthmatic children. Biofeedback training in these children resulted in an increase in the amplitude of respiratory sinus arrhythmia with significant improvements in forced expiratory maneuvers from maximum vital capacity.[64] Likewise, Courtney et al[65] conducted a randomized controlled study examining the effects of biofeedback-assisted relaxation in individuals with asthma. Data were collected on asthma symptoms, pulmonary function, indicators of arousal, and cellular immune factors. Participants in the trained group evidenced a decrease in forehead muscle tension compared with participants in the control group, although the former showed no changes in peripheral skin temperature. Decreases in asthma severity, bronchodilator medication usage, and cardiovascular stress were observed among the experimental group. Pulmonary function testing revealed a significant difference between groups in forced expiratory volume (FEV) and forced vital capacity (FVC), with the biofeedback group having a higher ratio of FEV1/FVC at post-test compared with the controls. The cellular immune data showed no significant group differences in total white blood cell or lymphocyte counts, but decreases over time were observed. Further, researchers reported significant differences in the numbers of neutrophils and basophils in the trained group compared with the control group, which supports the concept of decreased inflammation.

These studies clearly support the use of biofeedback techniques in pulmonary diseases characterized by hyperresponsiveness of the airway, inflammation, and reversible obstruction. Respiratory tract infection, allergies, air pollution, and psychosocial factors impact the severity and frequency of asthma symptoms, and biofeedback has the potential of being a major component in the management of asthma.[64,67,68]

Modification of Hypertension

The central mechanisms and possibilities of biofeedback of the systemic arterial pressure have been investigated extensively.[69,70,71] Lin[70] studied a group of patients with essential hypertension for the effects of group relaxation training and thermal biofeedback on blood pressure and on other psychophysiologic measures: heart rate, frontalis muscle tension, finger temperature, depression, anxiety, plasma aldosterone, plasma renin activity, and plasma and urinary cortisol. A significant decline in blood pressure was observed in 49% of the experimental group. Of that group, 51% maintained a lower blood pressure at a 10-month follow-up examination, suggesting that relaxation training has beneficial effects for short-term and long-term adjunctive therapy of essential hypertension in selected individuals.

In a study to determine the effectiveness of biofeedback in the treatment of stages 1 and 2 essential hypertension, Yucha and associates[71] found that both biofeedback and active control treatments (ie, medications) resulted in a reduction in systolic and diastolic blood pressure. However, only biofeedback, with related cognitive and relaxation training, show a significantly greater reduction in both blood pressure measures. Researchers also reported a significant latent effect of biofeedback interventions, whereas active treatment approaches lost their effectiveness soon after cessation of the drug.[71]

Diabetes, Vascular Disease, and Intermittent Claudication

Saunders et al[72] examined the therapeutic effects of biofeedback-assisted autogenic training in a group of patients with diabetes and vascular disease who had symptoms of intermittent claudication. The individuals received thermal feedback from the hand for 5 sessions, then from the foot for 16 sessions, while hand and foot temperatures were monitored simultaneously. Within the session, foot temperatures rose specifically in response to foot temperature biofeedback, and starting foot temperature rose between sessions. Nicolai and coworkers[73] compared biofeedback with walking on intermittent claudication. Post-treatment blood pressure was reduced to a normal level following both interventions. Attacks of intermittent claudication were reduced to 0 after 12 sessions and walking distance increased by about 1 mile per day over the course of the treatment. Walking produced a more immediate improvement; however, the biofeedback group showed longer affects when the interventions were paused to determine latency. It would appear that thermal and auditory biofeedback, as well as autogenic training, are potentially promising therapies for persons with diabetes and peripheral vascular disease.[72,73]

McGinnis et al[74] investigated the effect of relaxation training/thermal biofeedback on blood circulation in the lower extremities of patients with diabetes. A within-subject experimental design was used. During phase 1, all subjects used a self-selected relaxation method and recorded toe temperatures daily. During phase 2, subjects were taught a biofeedback-assisted relaxation technique designed to elicit sensations of warmth in the lower extremities and increase circulation and temperature. Subjects relaxed at home with the use of a designated relaxation tape. Each phase of the study lasted 4 weeks. Mean temperature change scores between phases 1 and 2 were 8.73% (phase 1) and 31.88% (phase 2). The greater increase in phase 2 was attributed to the biofeedback-assisted relaxation technique. These authors concluded that patients with diabetes show significant increases in peripheral blood circulation with this technique. This noninvasive method could serve as an adjunct treatment for limited blood flow in some complications of diabetes, such as ulceration.

Of noted interest, stressful life events and negative mood have been associated with elevated blood glucose and poor self-care in individuals with diabetes. McGinnis et al[74] studied the outcome of biofeedback-assisted relaxation to determine its effect on mood state, specifically depression, anxiety, and means of dealing with daily hassles (ie, stress). Statistically significant correlations were found between high scores on stress, anxiety, and depression inventories and higher glucose levels. Biofeedback-assisted relaxation interventions resulted in an overall improvement in the psychological measures and a reduction in blood glucose levels without other adjunct therapies.[74] These findings hold great clinical significance in the management of persons with insulin-dependent diabetes.

Phantom pain is a frequent consequence of the amputation of an extremity and causes considerable discomfort and disruption of daily activities. Harden et al[75] demonstrated complete elimination of phantom limb pain after biofeedback techniques were employed.

Cardiac Arrhythmias

Respiratory sinus arrhythmia, the peak-to-peak variations in heart rate caused by respiration, can be used as a noninvasive measure of parasympathetic cardiac control. Vaschillo et al[76] demonstrated that individuals were able to modify their heart rates volitionally when instructed in relaxation techniques using EKG biofeedback monitoring. Additionally, resonant frequency heart rate variability biofeedback increased baroreflex gain and peak expiratory flow. Biofeedback readily produces large oscillations in heart rate, blood pressure, vascular tone, and pulse amplitude via paced breathing.

Stress Management

When we are truly relaxed, very definite and measurable changes take place in the body.[77,78] These changes distinguish relaxation from the opposite states of tension or arousal. Some of the most significant changes are triggered by the 2 branches of the autonomic nervous system. The sympathetic branch of the nervous system controls body temperature, digestion, heart rate, respiratory rate, blood flow and pressure, and muscular tension. The parasympathetic nervous system lowers oxygen consumption and carbon dioxide elimination, heart and respiratory rates, blood pressure, blood lactate, and blood cortisol levels.[77,78] These bodily changes are collectively referred to as the *relaxation response*.

Research also suggests that among the biochemical changes triggered by relaxation there is an increase in the body's manufacture of certain mood-altering neurotransmitters.[78] In particular, production of serotonin (the biochemical equivalent to Prozac [fluoxetine]) is increased. Serotonin is associated with feelings of calmness and contentment.

Lehrer et al[78] isolated the types of biofeedback techniques that worked most effectively in various conditions. Their study showed that instrumentation using biofeedback electrodes placed over the involved muscles was most effective in treating disorders with a predominant muscular component (eg, muscle strength and/or tone changes, tension headaches, carpal tunnel). Disorders in which autonomic dysfunction predominates (eg, hypertension, migraine headaches) are more effectively treated by techniques with a strong autonomic component, such as lead placement on the frontalis muscle, or digital temperature monitoring, and progressive relaxation techniques.

Affective Disorders

Biofeedback interventions have been proposed as a promising modality in the treatment of affective disorders.[79,80] Biofeedback was evaluated in relation to its effects on epilepsy and found to be an effective method of calming brain wave activity down and reducing the frequency and intensity of epileptic seizure.[79] It has been determined that brainwave activity can be altered using biofeedback techniques.[80,81] Moore[81] found that alpha, theta, and alpha-theta enhancements are effective treatments of the anxiety disorders. This research also demonstrated the alpha wave suppression is also effective, but less so. Perceived success in carrying out specific tasks seems to play a big role in clinical improvement and results in changes in alpha and theta rhythms.[81] Allen and colleagues demonstrated that individual differences in resting asymmetrical frontal brain activity can be used to predict subsequent emotional responses and is alterable utilizing biofeedback training.[82] Therefore, it is hypothesized that using biofeedback in the treatment of affective disorders can offer a nondrug approach to managing depression, anxiety, and other emotional disturbances. Trudeau[83] provides evidence that biofeedback is an effective treatment approach for addictive disorders. Employing brainwave biofeedback, addicts can alter their emotional response to external stimulus (the psychological components of addiction) and change their physiological need for the substance to which they are addicted.[83] The mind is clearly a powerful thing.

Dysphagia

EMG and biofeedback techniques are well established in the disciplines of physical medicine for the retraining of muscle groups to approximate functional performance in swallowing.[84,85] Dysphagia is a swallowing disorder frequently encountered in the rehabilitation of stroke and head injury patients. *Oral dysphagia* refers to abnormalities in the oral phase of the swallowing mechanism.[84,85] As this disorder is primarily based in muscle over- or underactivity, biofeedback devices rendering feedback of biomechanical parameters characterizing the oral phase of swallowing have been shown to be extremely effective in reestablishing swallowing patterns in neuromuscularly impaired individuals.[84] Leplow et al[28] demonstrated that the use of biofeedback was instrumental in the assessment of muscle activity in facial and oral musculature. These authors demonstrated that proprioception of neuromuscularly involved patients was enhanced, especially in muscles richly supplied with muscle spindles and afferent fibers (ie, masseter muscle, zygomatus major muscle).

Bell's Palsy

Neuromuscular rehabilitation can reduce the severity of chronic facial paralysis, but complete recovery is frequently impeded by synkinesis.[86,87] It has been determined that synkinesis could be minimized by preventing its possible reinforcement during rehabilitation by employing EMG biofeedback with the goal of eliciting smaller movements. Muscular reeducation in patients with Bell's palsy who have intact facial-motor innervation has clearly been found to be enhanced by the use of EMG biofeedback. Facial function typically improves with a more rapid recovery of symmetry and a decrease in synkinesis.[86,87]

Pain Management in Patients With Cancer

Pain is one of the most feared consequences of cancer. Control of pain from cancer has been shown to decrease discomfort and diminish the need for drugs that may induce other negative side effects.[88-90] Relaxation and related biofeedback techniques have been shown to be effective in the management of cancer pain.[89-91] Utilizing such interventions as progressive muscle relaxation, relaxation and systemic desensitization, hypnosis, and biofeedback and relaxation, researchers have determined that nonpharmaceutical interventions for pain management have a great deal of potential.[89-91] Tsai et al,[91] comparing many specific methods in the management of pain (including electrical nerve stimulation, acupuncture, sympathetic blockade, epidural and intrathecal blocks, and neurosurgical and psychological biofeedback techniques) showed that the noninvasive procedure of relaxation and biofeedback had the greatest overall effect on pain.

Chemotherapy protocols that induce severe protracted nausea and vomiting are stressful for patients with cancer, and the fear that may be associated with chemotherapy often outweighs other negative aspects of the cancer experience. Barragán Loayza and coworkers[88] showed that many of the associated side effects of chemotherapy could be managed through pharmacologic approaches and maintenance of hydration, in addition to reducing stress levels through emotional support and the use of behavioral relaxation techniques supported by EMG biofeedback. Recent research provides evidence that sensory-behavioral pretreatments can ameliorate radiation therapy-induced nausea and vomiting[92] and significantly diminish, and, in some cases, eliminate, pain in the patient with cancer.[93]

Immunology

The role of the mind in healing the body is a fascinating subject that is steadily gaining in importance even within traditional medical practice. Mentally influencing the immune system, for example, is an exciting new field given the name *psychoneuroimmunology* (literally the effect of the mind through the nervous system on the immune system). This topic has been extensively covered in Chapter 2 of this book and is only mentioned here as it relates to the utilization of biofeedback techniques.

The effect of biofeedback-assisted relaxation on cell-mediated immunity, cortisol, and white blood cell count was investigated by McGrady et al[94] under low-stress conditions. Interestingly, the group of subjects trained in biofeedback-assisted relaxation techniques showed increased blastogenesis and a decreased white blood cell count, indicating a clear effect on the immune system.

The results of immunological responses of patients with breast cancer to behavioral interventions is remarkable and promising. Jeong[95] reports the results of a study of immune system and psychological changes in patients with cancer provided with relaxation, guided imagery, and biofeedback training. Significant effects were found in natural killer cell activity, lymphocyte responsiveness, and the number of peripheral blood lymphocytes. This study clearly indicates that relaxation, guided imagery, and related biofeedback techniques have the potential for modifying the immune systems response in a positive manner.

Memory Functioning

Remediation of memory deficits through the application of biofeedback techniques has been found to be effective.[96] Cassetta[96] studied electrophysiological functioning involved in memory while applying biofeedback techniques (ie, the individual's ability to alter EEG wave patterns) and determined that memory could be improved in all subjects performing auditory memory tasks (prose passages and word lists). EEG biofeedback interventions were designed to increase the value of specific electrophysiological variables related to successful memory function. Memory improved in all the study participants as a result of the biofeedback interventions.[96]

Cognitive Function

Recent research shows that neurofeedback is an effective EEG biofeedback technique for training individuals with cognitive disorders via operant conditioning. It is of interest that biofeedback has been shown to have a positive effect on improving cognitive function in the elderly.[97]

Visual Acuity

Visual acuity has also been shown to be affected by biofeedback, which could have tremendous implications for many individuals as they age. Persons with visual acuity problems caused by different ocular disorders, including macular degeneration, myopic macular degeneration, and presbyopia, underwent visual rehabilitation with an instrument for biofeedback. Visual acuity was found to improve.[98]

CONCLUSION

As a literate civilization, we are now more than 5000 years old. Physical needs have always kept the mind well occupied. Technologies have granted us a comfortable control over our environment. Yet, these technologies are costly. It is clear that medical problems can be caused by or aggravated by the mental status of the individual. Understanding this, it is an intriguing paradox that Western medicine has created in its concentrated efforts on developing extensive drugs and elaborate surgical techniques to deal with physical and mental compensations. With the evolution of managed care, the trend needs now to seek less costly alternative of care. This involves reaching inward and developing technologies that will allow us some insight into our inner world. It is time to equal the balance and attempt to solve some of the physical manifestations of pathologies from within.

Biofeedback has shown a remarkably positive benefit on the functional and treatment outcomes of numerous conditions.[1,96] Biofeedback instrumentation has been a growing part of physical therapy practice for over 20 years,[94] and physical therapists have contributed to researching its efficacy in treating varying conditions. Sophisticated contemporary equipment does much more in quantifying biofeedback techniques' worth than was originally envisioned. The importance of relating quantified movement-based data to functional measures has influenced the level of appropriate reimbursement for physical therapy services utilizing biofeedback. Physical therapy, as an integral member of the medical community, needs to continue to investigate self-awareness and self-control as a probable rehabilitative tool in the treatment of a multitude of conditions.

REFERENCES

1. Giggins OM, Persson UM, Caulfield B. Biofeedback in rehabilitation. *J Neuroeng Rehabil.* 2013;10:60.
2. Yang J, Yamamoto T, Cho B, Seo Y, Keall PJ. The impact of audio-visual biofeedback on 4D PET images: results of a phantom study. *Med Phys.* 2012;39(2):1046-1057.
3. Jacobson E. *Progressive Relaxation.* Chicago, Illinois: University of Chicago Press; 1938.

4. Faith A, Chen Y, Rikakis T, Iasemidis L. Interactive rehabilitation and dynamical analysis of scalp EEG. *Conf Proc IEEE Eng Med Biol Soc.* 2011;2011:1387-1390.

5. Nelson LA. The role of biofeedback in stroke rehabilitation: past and future directions. *Top Stroke Rehabil.* 2007;14(4):59-66.

6. Prinsloo GE, Rauch HG, Derman WE. A brief review and clinical application of heart rate variability biofeedback in sports, exercise, and rehabilitation medicine. *Phys Sportsmed.* 2014;42(2):88-99.

7. Biondi M, Valentini M. Relaxation treatments and biofeedback for anxiety and somatic stress-related disorders [article in Italian]. *Riv Psichiatr.* 2014;49(5):217-226.

8. Evetovich TK, Conley DS, Todd JB, Rogers DC, Stone TL. Effect of mechanomyography as a biofeedback method to enhance muscle relaxation and performance. *J Strength Cond Res.* 2007;21(1):96-99.

9. Mullally WJ, Hall K, Goldstein R. Efficacy of biofeedback in the treatment of migraine and tension type headaches. *Pain Physician.* 2009;12(6):1005-1011.

10. Blume HK, Brockman LN, Breuner CC. Biofeedback therapy for pediatric headache: factors associated with response. *Headache.* 2012;52(9):1377-1386.

11. Kaushik R, Kaushik RM, Mahajan SK, Rajesh V. Biofeedback assisted diaphragmatic breathing and systematic relaxation versus propranolol in long term prophylaxis of migraine. *Complement Ther Med.* 2005;13(3):165-174.

12. Wang LN, Tao H, Zhao Y, Zhou YQ, Jiang SR. Optimal timing for initiation of biofeedback-assisted relaxation training in hospitalized coronary heart disease patients with sleep disturbances. *J Cardiovasc Nurs.* 2014;29(4):367-376.

13. Grazzi L, Andrasik F, D'Amico D, Usai S, Kass S, Bussone G. Disability in chronic migraine patients with medication overuse: Treatment effects at 1 year follow-up. *Headache.* 2004;44:678-683.

14. Singer AB, Buse DC, Seng EK. Behavioral treatments for migraine management: useful at each step of migraine care. *Curr Neurol Neurosci Rep.* 2015;15(4):14.

15. Scharff L, Marcus DA, Masek BJ. A controlled study of minimal-contact thermal biofeedback treatment in children with migraine. *J Pediatr Psychol.* 2002;27(2):109-119.

16. Crider A, Glaros AG, Gevirtz RN. Efficacy of biofeedback-based treatments for temporomandibular disorders. *Appl Psychophysiol Biofeedback.* 2005;30(4):333-345.

17. Foster PS. Use of the Calmset 3 biofeedback/relaxation system in the assessment and treatment of chronic nocturnal bruxism. *Appl Psychophysiol Biofeedback.* 2004;29(2):141-147.

18. Jensen MP, Sherlin LH, Fregni F, Gianas A, Howe JD, Hakimian S. Baseline brain activity predicts response to neuromodulatory pain treatment. *Pain Med.* 2014; 15(12):2055-2063.

19. Ersal T, Sienko KH. A mathematical model for incorporating biofeedback into human postural control. *J Neuroeng Rehabil.* 2013;10:14.

20. van Dijk H, Hermens HJ. Artificial feedback for remotely supervised training of motor skills. *J Telemed Telecare.* 2006;12(Suppl 1):50-52.

21. Allum JH, Carpenter MG. A speedy solution for balance and gait analysis: angular velocity measured at the centre of body mass. *Curr Opin Neurol.* 2005;18(1):15-21.

22. Zarzycka M, Rozek K, Zarzychi M. Alternative methods of conservative treatment of idiopathic scoliosis [article in English, Polish]. *Ortop Traumatol Rehabil.* 2009;11(5):396-412.

23. Horak F, King L, Mancini M. Role of body-worn movement monitor technology for balance and gait rehabilitation. *Phys Ther.* 2015;95(3):461-470.

24. Cakrt O, Vyhnalek M, Slaby K, et al. Balance rehabilitation therapy by tongue electrotactile biofeedback in patients with degenerative cerebellar disease. *NeuroRehabilitation.* 2012;31(4):429-434.

25. Domagalska-Szopa A, Szopa A. Gait pattern differences between children with mild scoliosis and children with unilateral cerebral palsy. *PLoS One.* 2014;9(8):e103095.

26. Yoo JW, Lee DR, Sim YJ, You JH, Kim CJ. Effects of innovative virtual reality game and EMG biofeedback on neuromotor control in cerebral palsy. *Biomed Mater Eng.* 2014;24(6):3613-3618.

27. Shumway-Cook A, Anson D, Haller S. Postural sway biofeedback: its effect on reestablishing stance stability in hemiplegic patients. *Arch Phys Med Rehabil.* 1988;69(6):395-400.

28. Leplow B, Schluter V, Ferstl R. A new procedure for assessment of proprioception. *Percept Mot Skills.* 1992;74(1):91-98.

29. Austermann Hula SN, Robin DA, Maas E, Ballard KJ, Schmidt RA. Effects of feedback frequency and timing on acquisition, retention, and transfer of speech skills in acquired apraxia of speech. *J Speech Lang Hear Res.* 2008;51(5):1088-1113.

30. Heller F, Beuret-Blanquart F, Weber J. Postural biofeedback and locomotion reeducation in stroke patients [article in French]. *Ann Readapt Med Phys.* 2005;48(4):187-195.

31. Hsu HY, Lin CF, Su FC, Kuo HT, Chiu HY, Kuo LC. Clinical application of computerized evaluation and re-education biofeedback prototype for sensorimotor control of the hand in stroke patients. *J Neuroeng Rehabil.* 2012;9:26.

32. Del Din S, Bertoldo A, Sawacha Z, et al. Assessment of biofeedback rehabilitation in post-stroke patients combining fMRI and gait analysis: a case study. *J Neuroeng Rehabil.* 2014;11:53.

33. De Nunzio A, Zucchella C, Spicciato F, et al. Biofeedback rehabilitation of posture and weightbearing distribution in stroke: a center of foot pressure analysis. *Funct Neurol.* 2014;29(2):127-134.
34. Bisson E, Contant B, Sveistrup H, Lajoie Y. Functional balance and dual-task reaction times in older adults are improved by virtual reality and biofeedback training. *Cyberpsychol Behav.* 2007;10(1):16-23.
35. Hustedt JW, Blizzard DJ, Baumgaetner MR, Leslie MP, Grauer JN. Lower-extremity weight-bearing compliance is maintained over time after biofeedback training. *Orthopedics.* 2012;35(11):e1644-e1648.
36. Tirosh O, Cambell A, Begg RK, Sparrow WA. Biofeedback training effects on minimum toe clearance variability during treadmill walking. *Ann Biomed Eng.* 2013;41(8):1661-1669.
37. Vedsted P, Sjøgaard K, Blangsted AK, Madeleine P, Sjøgaard G. Biofeedback effectiveness to reduce upper limb muscle activity during computer work is muscle specific and time pressure dependent. *J Electromyogr Kinesiol.* 2011;21(1):49-58.
38. Doğan-Aslan M, Nakipoğlu-Yüzer GF, Doğan A, Karabay I, Özgirgin N. The effect of electromyographic biofeedback treatment in improving upper extremity functioning of patients with hemiplegic stroke. *J Stroke Cerebrovasc Dis.* 2012;21(3):187-192.
39. Verhagen AP, Bierma-Zeinstra SM, Feleus A, et al. Ergonomic and physiotherapeutic interventions for treating upper extremity work related disorders in adults. *Cochrane Database Syst Rev.* 2004;(1):CD003471.
40. Zeni J Jr, Abujaber S, Flowers P, Pozzi F, Snyder-Mackler L. Biofeedback to promote movement symmetry after total knee arthroplasty: a feasibility study. *J Orthop Sports Phys Ther.* 2013;43(10):715-726.
41. Palmerud G, Kadefors R, Sporrong H, et al. Voluntary redistribution of muscle activity in human shoulder muscles. *Ergonomics.* 1995;38(4):806-815.
42. Jaggi A, Lambert S. Rehabilitation for shoulder instability. *Br J Sports Med.* 2010;44(5):333-340.
43. Akkaya N, Ardic F, Ozgen M, Akkaya S, Sahin F, Kilic A. Efficacy of electromyographic biofeedback and electrical stimulation following arthroscopic partial meniscectomy: a randomized controlled trial. *Clin Rehabil.* 2012;26(3):224-236.
44. Kranitz L, Lehrer P. Biofeedback applications in the treatment of cardiovascular diseases. *Cardiol Rev.* 2004;12(3):177-181.
45. Leisman G, Zenhausern R, Ferentz A, Tefera T, Zemcov A. Electromyographic effects of fatigue and task repetition on the validity of estimates of strong and weak muscles in applied kinesiological muscle-testing procedures. *Percept Mot Skills.* 1995;80(3 Pt 1):963-977.
46. Climov D, Lysy C, Berteau S, et al. Biofeedback on heart rate variability in cardiac rehabilitation: practical feasibility and psycho-physiological effects. *Acta Cardiol.* 2014;69(3):299-307.
47. Guercio JM, Ferguson KE, McMorrow MJ. Increasing functional communication through relaxation training and neuromuscular feedback. *Brain Inj.* 2001;15(12):1073-1082.
48. May G, Benson R, Balon R, Boutros N. Neurofeedback and traumatic brain injury: a literature review. *Ann Clin Psychiatry.* 2013;25(4):289-296.
49. Nelson DV, Esty ML. Neurotherapy of traumatic brain injury/posttraumatic stress symptoms in OEF/OIF veterans. *J Neuropsychiatry Clin Neurosci.* 2012;24(2):237-240.
50. Herderschee R, Hay-Smith EJ, Herbison GP, Roovers JP, Heineman JM. Feedback or biofeedback to augment pelvic floor muscle training for urinary incontinence in women. *Cochrane Database Syst Rev.* 2011;(7):CD009252.
51. Teunissen TA, de Jonge A, van Weel C, Lagro-Janssen AL. Treating urinary incontinence in the elderly—conservative therapies that work: a systematic review. *J Fam Pract.* 2004;53(1):25-30,32.
52. Newman DK. Pelvic floor muscle rehabilitation using biofeedback. *Urol Nurs.* 2014;34(4):193-202.
53. Pedraza R, Nieto J, Ibarra S, Haas EM. Pelvic muscle rehabilitation: a standardized protocol for pelvic floor dysfunction. *Adv Urol.* 2014;2014:487436.
54. Stern RM, Vitellaro K, Thomas M, Higgins SC, Koch KL. Electrogastrographic biofeedback: a technique for enhancing normal gastric activity. *Neurogastroenterol Motil.* 2004;16(6):753-757.
55. Bosshard W, Dreher R, Schnegg JF, Bula CJ. The treatment of chronic constipation in elderly people: an update. *Drugs Aging.* 2004;21(14):911-930.
56. Rayome RG, Johnson V, Gray M. Stress urinary incontinence after radical prostatectomy. *J Wound Ostomy Continence Nurs.* 1994;21(6):264-269.
57. Lepley AS, Gribble PA, Pietrosimone BG. Effects of electromyographic biofeedback on quadriceps strength: a systematic review. *J Strength Cond Res.* 2012;26(3):873-882.
58. Pages IH, Jahr S, Schaufele MK, Conradi E. Comparative analysis of biofeedback and physical therapy for treatment of urinary stress incontinence in women. *Am J Phys Med Rehabil.* 2001;80(7):494-502.
59. Vonthein R, Heimerl T, Schwandner T, Ziegler A. Electrical stimulation and biofeedback for the treatment of fecal incontinence: a systematic review. *Int J Colorectal Dis.* 2013;28(11):1567-1577.
60. Bartlett LM, Sloots K, Nowak M, Ho YH. Biofeedback therapy for faecal incontinence: a rural and regional perspective. *Rural Remote Health.* 2011;11(2):1630.
61. Ferrara A, De Jesus S, Gallagher JT, et al. Time-related decay of the benefits of biofeedback therapy. *Tech Coloproctol.* 2001;5(3):131-135.
62. Patcharatrakul T, Gonlachanvit S. Outcome of biofeedback therapy in dyssynergic defecation patients with and without irritable bowel syndrome. *J Clin Gastroenterol.* 2011;45(7):593-598.

63. Bartlett L, Sloots K, Nowak M, Ho YH. Biofeedback for fecal incontinence: a randomized study comparing exercise regimens. *Dis Colon Rectum*. 2011;54(7):846-856.
64. Lehrer PM, Vaschillo E, Vaschillo B, et al. Biofeedback treatment for asthma. *Chest*. 2004;126(2):352-361.
65. Courtney R, Cohen M, van Dixhoorn J. Relationship between dysfunctional breathing patterns and ability to achieve target heart rate variability with features of "coherence" during biofeedback. *Altern Ther Health Med*. 2011;17(3):38-44.
66. Lehrer P, Vaschillo E, Lu SE, et al. Heart rate variability biofeedback: effects of age on heart rate variability, baroreflex gain, and asthma. *Chest*. 2006;129(2):278-284.
67. Nishigaki Y, Mizuguchi H, Takeda E, et al. Development of new measurement system of thoracic excursion with biofeedback: reliability and validity. *J Neuroeng Rehabil*. 2013;10:45.
68. Jeter AM, Kim HC, Simon E, Ritz T, Meuret AE. Hypoventilation training for asthma: a case illustration. *Appl Psychophysiol Biofeedback*. 2012;37(1):63-72.
69. Wheat AL, Larkin KT. Biofeedback of heart rate variability and related physiology: a critical review. *Appl Psychophysiol Biofeedback*. 2010;35(3):229-242.
70. Lin G, Xiang Q, Fu X, et al. Heart rate variability biofeedback decreases blood pressure in prehypertensive subjects by improving autonomic function and baroreflex. *J Altern Complement Med*. 2012;18(2):143-152.
71. Yucha CB, Tsai PS, Calderon KS, Tian L. Biofeedback-assisted relaxation training for essential hypertension: who is most likely to benefit? *J Cardiovasc Nurs*. 2005;20(3):198-205.
72. Saunders JT, Cox DJ, Teates CD, Pohl SL. Thermal biofeedback in the treatment of intermittent claudication in diabetes: a case study. *Biofeedback Self Regul*. 1994;19(4):337-345.
73. Nicolai SP, Teijink JA, Prins MH; Exercise Therapy in Peripheral Arterial Disease Study Group. Multicenter randomized clinical trial of supervised exercise therapy with or without feedback versus walking advice for intermittent claudication. *J Vasc Surg*. 2010;52(2):348-355.
74. McGinnis RA, McGrady A, Cox SA, Grower-Dowling KA. Biofeedback-assisted relaxation in type 2 diabetes. *Diabetes Care*. 2005;28(9):2145-2149.
75. Harden RN, Houle TT, Green S, et al. Biofeedback in the treatment of phantom limb pain: a time-series analysis. *Appl Psychophysiol Biofeedback*. 2005;30(1):83-93.
76. Vaschillo EG, Vaschillo B, Lehrer PM. Characteristics of resonance in heart rate variability stimulated by biofeedback. *Appl Psychophysiol Biofeedback*. 2006;31(2):129-142.
77. Blumenstein B, Breslav I, Bar-Eli M, Tenenbaum G, Weinstein Y. Regulation of mental states and biofeedback techniques: effects on breathing pattern. *Biofeedback Self Regul*. 1995;20(2):169-183.
78. Lehrer PM, Carr P, Sargunaraj D, Woolfolk RL. Stress management techniques: are they all equivalent, or do they have specific effects? *Biofeedback Self Regul*. 1994;19(4):353-401.
79. Nagai Y, Matsuura M. Biofeedback treatment for epilepsy [article in Japanese]. *Brain Nerve*. 2011;63(4): 385-392.
80. Tschacher W, Junghan UM, Pfammatter M. Towards a taxonomy of common factors in psychotherapy-results of an expert survey. *Clin Psychol Psychother*. 2014;21(1):82-96.
81. Moore NC. A review of EEG biofeedback treatment of anxiety disorders. *Clin Electroencephalogr*. 2000;31(1):1-6.
82. O'Neill B, Findlay G. Single case methodology in neurobehavioral rehabilitation: preliminary findings on biofeedback in the treatment of challenging behaviour. *Neuropsychol Rehabil*. 2014;24(3-4):365-381.
83. Trudeau DL. The treatment of addictive disorders by brainwave biofeedback: a review and suggestions for future research. *Clin Electroencephalogr*. 2000;31(1):13-22.
84. Bogaardt HC, Grolman W, Fokkens WJ. The use of biofeedback in the treatment of chronic dysphagia in stroke patients. *Folia Phoniatr Logop*. 2009;61(4):200-205.
85. Thottam PJ, Silva RC, McLevy JD, Simons JP, Mehta DK. Use of fiberoptic endoscopic evaluation of swallowing (FEES) in the management of psychogenic dysphagia in children. *Int J Pediatr Otorhinolaryngol*. 2015;79(2):108-110.
86. Dalla Toffola E, Tinelli C, Lozza A, et al. Choosing the best rehabilitation treatment for Bell's palsy. *Eur J Phys Rehabil Med*. 2012;48(4):635-642.
87. Lee JM, Choi KH, Lim BW, Kim MW, Kim J. Half-mirror biofeedback exercise in combination with three botulinum toxin A injections long-lasting treatment of facial sequelae after facial paralysis. *J Plast Reconstr Aesthet Surg*. 2015;68(1):71-78.
88. Barragán Loayza IM, Sola I, Juando Prats C. Biofeedback for pain management during labour. *Cochrane Database Syst Rev*. 2011;(6):CD006168.
89. Shockey DP, Menzies V, Glick DF, Taylor AG, Boitnott A, Rovnyak V. Preprocedural distress in children with cancer: an intervention using biofeedback and relaxation. *J Pediatr Oncol Nurs*. 2013;30(3):129-138.
90. Kim T, Pollock S, Lee D, O'Brien R, Keall P. Audiovisual biofeedback improves diaphragm motion reproducibility in MRI. *Med Phys*. 2012;39(11):6921-6928.
91. Tsai PS, Chen PL, Lai YL, Lee MB, Lin CC. Effects of electromyography biofeedback-assisted relaxation on pain in patients with advanced cancer in a palliative care unit. *Cancer Nurs*. 2007; 30(5):347-353.
92. Biondi M, Valentini M. Relaxation treatments and biofeedback for anxiety and somatic stress-related disorders [article in Italian]. *Riv Psichiatr*. 2014;49(5):217-226.
93. Mertens AC, Sencer S, Myers CD, et al. Complementary and alternative therapy use in adult survivors of childhood cancer: a report from the Childhood Cancer Survivor Study. *Pediatr Blood Cancer*. 2008;50(1):90-97.

94. McGrady A, Conran P, Dickey D, et al. The effects of biofeedback-assisted relaxation on cell-mediated immunity, cortisol, and white blood cell count in healthy adult subjects. *J Behav Med.* 1992;15(4):343-354.

95. Jeong IS. Effect of progressive muscle relaxation using biofeedback on perceived stress, stress response, immune response and climacteric symptoms of middle-aged women [article in Korean]. *Taehan Kanho Hakhoe Chi.* 2014;34(2):213-224.

96. Cassetta RA. Biofeedback can improve patient outcome. *Am Nurse.* 1993;25(9):25.

97. Angelakis E, Stathopoulou S, Frymiare JL, et al. EEG neurofeedback: a brief overview and an example of peak alpha frequency training for cognitive enhancement in the elderly. *Clin Neuropsychol.* 2007;21(1):110-129.

98. Giorgi D, Contestabile MT, Pacella E, Barieli CB. An instrument for biofeedback applied to vision. *Appl Psychophysiol Biofeedback.* 2005;30(4):389-395.

13

Yoga Therapeutics
An Ancient Practice in a Twenty-First Century Setting

Matthew J. Taylor, PT, PhD, RYT

Yoga is the control of the fluctuations of the mind.

Yoga Sūtras of Patañjali 1.2; c. 150 CE

The current popularity of hatha yoga appropriately presents a dichotomy of its own. The term *hatha* is composed of 2 Sanskrit words: *ha*, which means sun, and *tha*, which means moon. The polarized nature of these 2 terms is a metaphor for the spectrum of reality that life presents to the human being. On one hand, the popularity has exposed many Westerners to this ancient psycho-spiritual practice who may never have had an opportunity to experience it. There are presently more yoga teachers in California than in all of India. Yoga is practiced in studios, corporate settings, sports facilities, and major hospitals. The physical performance bias of our culture obviously suggests a direct application in physical rehabilitation as well. The opposite pole in the spectrum is that, while yoga is incorporated within the framework of our physically based, consumptive culture, it is now used to sell everything from pharmaceuticals to brokerage services. Yesterday's step aerobics instructor can now be certified in 2 days as a yoga teacher.

While the popularity and commercialization might appear to jeopardize the heart of yoga, the quantum impact of the transformative nature of the practice is bound to remain after the market frenzy recedes. The true power of yoga lies not in slick, lithe, and limber glossy images, but within the classic definition above. Feuerstein's[1] review of the term *yoga* further reveals that, technically, yoga refers to that enormous body of precepts, attitudes, techniques, and spiritual values that have been developed in India for more than 5000 years. In other words, the physical postures and motor performance outcomes that characterize so much of yoga within our culture is actually a by-product of what is more accurately described as a technology for the evolution of the mind or consciousness. The essence of yoga is the experiential bridge it provides to the mind-body science. The emerging awareness by Western science of the mind-body connection is actually a rediscovery of what has been the basis of the practice of yoga for thousands of years. A brief overview and history of yoga will set the stage for further discussion and the potential application of yoga within the rehabilitation professions.

Davis CM.
Integrative Therapies in Rehabilitation: Evidence for Efficacy in Therapy, Prevention, and Wellness, Fourth Edition (pp 181-202).
© 2017 Taylor & Francis Group.

TABLE 13-1
PATANJALI'S EIGHT-FOLD PATH

PATH	DESCRIPTION
Yama	Moral precepts: nonharming, truthfulness, nonstealing, chastity, greedlessness
Niyama	Qualities to nourish: purity, contentment, austerity (exercise), self-study, devotion
Asana	Postures/movements: a calm, firm, steady stance in relation to life
Pranayama	Breathing exercises: the ability to channel and direct breath and life energy
Pratyahara	Decreased reactivity to sensation: focusing on senses inward, nonreactivity to stimuli
Dharana	Concentration
Dhyana	Meditation
Samadhi	Ecstatic union, flow, "in the zone," spiritual support/connection

OVERVIEW

The elements of yoga that directly address health concerns are known as *yoga therapeutics* and have been developed through the millennia. The Ayurvedic medical system of India and yoga therapeutics share many commonalties in their development to include a rich, allegorical language (ie, earth, ether, chakra, prana) that is employed to this day. While these terms may sound foreign to many Western-trained medical professionals, closer examination reveals some striking similarities with modern terminology in their descriptions of disease and health.

The term *yoga* is derived from the Sanskrit verb *yuj*, meaning to yoke or unite, as in uniting the body, mind, and spirit. This union is achieved through various methods and technologies that include the familiar postures. A complete classic yoga practice (Table 13-1) has 8 components that equate to moral restraints, personal behavioral observances, postures, regulation of breath, drawing the senses inward, concentration, and meditation.

Over time, this complete yoga practice results in increased strength, balance, stamina, flexibility, and relaxation.[2-5] These outcomes can be achieved without the stereotypes that yoga requires bizarre body positions and occult religious practices. Simple body movements (*asanas*) performed with mindfulness and attention achieve the outcomes without pain or extremes of range of motion (ROM). Yoga, as a life science philosophy, also makes no statement about any specific religious practice or spiritual belief; it can be used to support all major faith traditions. The comprehensive approach of yoga (see Table 13-1) can be likened to the widely embraced, present-day self-development theories that extol the virtues of the marketing theme "Body-Mind-Spirit."

YOGA THERAPY HEALTH MODEL

Yoga therapy is a broad philosophical model of health based on the human experience; as such, it is a powerful tool in linking the historical "parts" paradigm to a biopsychosocial or integral model of human movement. This model was developed in an Eastern culture that used concrete images (eg, bodies, sheaths) to describe what was understood to be an interwoven, indivisible whole—or, in Western terminology, an *integrative model*. The yoga model of health includes all dimensions of the patient's human experience and traces back c. 3000 to 4000 years to the Taittiriya Upanishad,

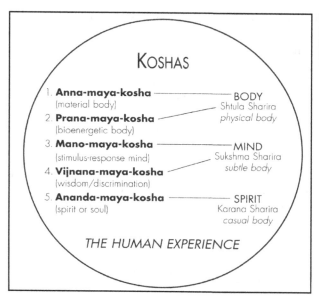

Figure 13-1. The Kosha and Sharira model. (Adapted with permission from Taylor MJ. What is health and illness? In: Taylor MJ, ed. *Integrating Yoga Therapy Into Rehabilitation.* Embug, IL: Galena; 1999:15.)

TABLE 13-2 CLINICAL TRANSLATIONS OF THE KOSHAS		
SANSKRIT	**COMMON NAME**	**DESCRIPTION**
Anna-maya-kosha	Food sheath	Composed of the physical solid aspect of the person (ie, cells, organs, bones, joints)
Prana-maya-kosha	Life force sheath	The bioelectric forces and breath are a portion of the prana; similar to Chi or Qi concepts in Chinese medicine
Mano-maya-kosha	Thought/primitive mind sheath	Includes emotions, reactive thinking reflexes, or subcortical function; is largely shared with the rest of the animal kingdom
Vijnana-maya-kosha	Wisdom/higher mind sheath	Includes the higher cortical functions of reflection, intuition, planning, and creativity; not as developed in animals
Ananda-maya-kosha	Bliss sheath	Sometimes equated to the soul or spirit of the patient

which hints at the Vedanta doctrine of the sheaths or koshas.[1] The koshas are illustrated in Figure 13-1, denoting 5 layers or envelopes of reality within the realm of the patient's experience. It demonstrates how, centuries later, these sheaths were organized into 3 shariras (bodies) summarized as the body, mind, and spirit, or "physical, subtle, and causal bodies" in yogic terminology.[6] The modern-day clinical translations of the koshas are listed in Table 13-2.

These bodies, beginning with the physical level, by definition are each progressively more subtle to perceive. Physical therapy training and practice focus primarily on the first 2 levels, but addresses all 5. Koshas may be better understood by the example of a patient with multiple sclerosis having an acute exacerbation of increased spasticity (first kosha), creating a bioenergetic hypertonicity (second kosha), triggering the pain cycle, functional self-consciousness, and varied emotional reactions (third kosha), making creativity, focus, and compassion challenging (fourth kosha), while generally sapping spirit, sense of support, and enthusiasm (fifth kosha). Clinically, this can also manifest as the opposite experience where the therapist senses that a physical impairment's etiology is the result of one or more other koshas, such as fear, depression, or inappropriate stress/energy management.[7]

The yogic model describes health as balance and awareness within a free-flowing systemic interaction between all 5 of the allegorically porous, "thin" sheaths. Theoretically, imbalance or absence of awareness at any of the 5 levels results in dysfunction or disease, manifesting either directly or indirectly in one or more of the koshas. The biopsychosocial view also maintains that no rehabilitation condition exists, impacts, or results as a consequence of a single kosha level and, thus, thorough care must include consideration at each level.[6] A metatarsal fracture would appear to be a purely physical condition. If the fracture resulted from an angry kick into a wall, the holistic view would state that the condition was not healed or "whole" until the individual worked at other kosha levels to determine the source and reaction to the anger, and developed appropriate strategies for the future. The right mix of higher kosha imbalances may trigger the sympathetic condition of a chronic regional pain syndrome, which presently defies reductionist explanation.

How Do Yoga Therapists Use the Model?

Yoga therapists (YTs) are trained to identify barriers to optimal function, to create strategies or environments for enhanced proprioception and function, and to retest outcomes. Their practice includes the assessment of structure and faulty motor sequencing/recruitment, and the prescription of remedial solutions. YTs also understand closed-chain kinematics, anatomical detail, motor sequencing, and the use of supports and manual facilitation techniques in managing their patients. On the surface, these roles share much in common with those of traditional rehabilitation therapists. It is the frame of reference of this yogic health model that differentiates the 2 practices.

YTs recognize that health conditions create stress for the patient, are exacerbated by stress, or that stress is a significant antecedent factor.[8] The yogic model defines *stress* as separation, or the sympathetic response, brought on by an imbalance or lack of integrity between koshas or within a particular kosha. The YT considers positive outcomes, or health, to occur as balance or homeostasis is achieved through a parasympathetic response and an integration of all 5 koshas. Herbert Benson, Physician and Founder of the Benson-Henry Institute for Mind Body Medicine at Massachusetts General Hospital, coined "remembered wellness,"[8] that includes accessing earlier motor strategies and the placebo effect, are additional outcomes present in this model that is focused on health optimization vs the crisis- or pathology-based system of conventional medicine.

Consider a YT working with a patient with hemiplegia post-cerebrovascular accident (CVA). A CVA presents by definition as a physical (first kosha) disruption of circulation. However, in addition to the physical impairment, if the stroke was preceded by an episode or pattern of rage, anger, or depression, the holistic view would say that the condition was not healed or "whole" until the individual worked at other kosha levels to determine the source and reaction to the emotion and developed appropriate strategies for the future. As such, the therapist would select interventions for both the current conditions and prophylactically, since the subtler imbalances would also be addressed.

Clinically, the YT's assessment of the patient is composed of various stress or kosha-imbalanced factors, and the treatment goals generally include measurable relaxation response. The YT assesses first and second kosha imbalances, such as spasticity, low tone, guarding, decreased ROM and strength, splinting, thoracic/chest breathing, poor balance, and hypertension. The assessment also encompasses the remaining higher kosha presentations, such as anger, depression, lethargy, anxiety, and fear. The goals, or intentions in the yoga vernacular, are to create an environment in which the student becomes aware of the present imbalances, is offered options for responding to those imbalances, and then experiences changes toward balance or health. Those changes might present as decreased spasticity, balanced affect, full diaphragmatic breath, enhanced postural balance, decreased impairment, increased functional mobility, and a sense of efficacy.

The YT also directly addresses the fact that, in addition to the host of functional challenges that patients face, many also often face a review of their life in the presence of the disease, disability, and, in some circumstances, end-of-life concerns. They may ask such questions as, Who am I? Did or do I make a difference? What is next? Can I handle it? What will become of me? All are very "spirit-oriented" (fifth kosha) questions that impact the role of the YT and the movement system of the lower koshas. This reflection of spiritual searching by the patient demands a complementary approach in assisting the patient to identify, understand, and achieve his or her goals. The broad depth of yoga addresses these concerns: changing the roles and level of function, shifts between independence and dependence, fears and anxieties, end-of-life concerns and questions, and a strong support of faith or spiritual tradition. Yoga therapeutics supports this stage of rehabilitation by offering expanded tools beyond the mechanical (first and second kosha) movement of exercise.

The YT then selects from the 8 paths (see Table 13-1), techniques, and methodologies that have been observed to create an environment for reconciling the imbalances of the koshas. The attractive simplicity of yoga therapeutics to the rehabilitation professional is that all of the koshas can be accessed through the therapeutic rehabilitation skills of positioning, movement, and breathing without having to directly address the more esoteric paths of yoga.

STRESS/RELAXATION RESPONSE MODEL

Benson first coined the term *relaxation response* in the early 1970s while studying transcendental meditators.[8] He documented the ability of the meditator to consciously elicit the relaxation response. The relaxation response's physiological mechanism is not fully understood. The relaxation response elicited by yoga has been associated with the psychophysiological responses that inhibit pituitary-adrenal activity by significantly decreasing cortisol blood levels during and somewhat after practice.[9,10] Further, a decrease in blood pressure readings and anxiety scores has been demonstrated in several studies, one of which included children and adolescents.[11-16] Harte et al[17] studied the effects of running and meditation on beta-endorphin, corticotropin-releasing hormone (CRH) and cortisol in plasma, and mood. They found similar changes in mood and increased CRH immunoreactivity, indicating that CRH release could be achieved with meditation without the physical exercise of running. Women practicing yoga produced improvements in scales of life satisfaction, mood, and coping with stress, while producing decreased scores in excitability and aggressiveness.[18]

Clinically, the rehabilitation therapist's systems assessment is composed of various stress-related factors, and the treatment goals generally include measurable relaxation phenomena, achieved by traditional therapy treatments, as listed in Table 13-3. The previously mentioned studies suggest the potential benefit of yoga in reducing the stress response, and Hannibal and Bishop's perspective piece on pain and stress[19] provides an excellent current reference list. A deeper examination of the physiology of yoga breath regulation and postures (asana) will stimulate critical evaluation of the forthcoming literature review.

TOOLS OF PRANAYAMA AND ASANA

One of the first physiologic responses produced under stress is an increase in respiration rate and a decrease in tidal volume, accompanied by a shift from a diaphragmatic pattern to upper chest breathing. Miller[20] provides a thorough summary of the psychophysiological effects of both breathing patterns. There are more than 100 different combinations of yoga breath regulation patterns. These are used in yoga as energy management tools to affect either the high-energy, anxious response to stress or the opposite, low-energy, withdrawn, depressed pattern.[6] Raju et al[21] demonstrated that subjects who practiced pranayama could achieve higher work rates with reduced oxygen consumption per unit of work and without increased blood lactate, as well as significantly lower resting blood lactate levels. The full practice of pranayama is a complex one, requiring careful instruction by an experienced YT. For the purposes of this introduction, the focus will be on the

TABLE 13-3	
THERAPEUTIC ASSESSMENT AND TREATMENT GOALS	
STRESS ASSESSMENT	**TREATMENT GOAL/RELAXATION/RESPONSE**
Increased muscle tone	Normalized tone
Cardiovascular stress	Cardiovascular ease
Anxiety/panic	Calm/relaxed
Elevated blood pressure	Normalized blood pressure
Fear/pessimism	Confidence/optimism
Dependent/passive	Independent/active
Distracted	Focused
Angry	Tolerant
Depressed	Balanced affect
Guarded, splinting	Fluid, graceful
Off balance	Balanced
Low energy	High energy
Thoracic/chest breathing	Diaphragmatic breathing
Adapted from Taylor MJ. *Integrating Yoga Therapy Into Rehabilitation.* Galena, IL: Embug; 1999:24.	

establishment of breath awareness and facilitating a full diaphragmatic breath, well within the competence and ethical realm of the rehabilitation professional. The yoga health model maintains that by having the patient direct the thinking mind (third kosha) to sensing and moving with the breath, there is little opportunity for that thinking mind to worry, despair, or become distracted. The focus of the mind on the sensation of breath and movement reduces stress, or the sympathetic response, which the model postulates allows the autonomic nervous system to move toward homeostasis with an inherent facilitation of sensorimotor integration (SMI). Instructing patients in diaphragmatic breathing with the intention of eliciting the treatment goals (see Table 13-3) is supported by research and is a simple, cost-effective form of yoga therapy.

Asanas, or postures, are the other yoga therapeutic tools that share much in common with the rehabilitation counterpart, therapeutic exercise. There are literally thousands of asanas to choose from to create an environment of mindfulness and kosha awareness. One definition of asana is that of a postural pattern created by deviating the head and trunk from the center of gravity and having the pattern maintained purposefully for a length of time, then released in a smooth and effortless manner.[22] This postural pattern is initiated slowly and with attention to internal sensation and maintaining a full diaphragmatic breath. These patterns are prescribed and ideally performed using a minimum amount of voluntary effort and a minimum expenditure of energy for its maintenance and adjustment. True asana is classically described as having the qualities of stability (sthira), ease (sukha), and effortlessness or minimized effort (prayatna shaithilya).[1,23] An asana is not, however, a braced or artificially sustained "posture" or a "pose." An experimental electromyogram (EMG) study revealed that, in an asana performed isometrically, there is a 30% increase in heart rate over the initial resting rate compared with only a 6% increase over resting rate when practiced the yoga way (ie, effortlessly and with full awareness).[24]

Another helpful description of asana is that the final stage of an asana (the "picture" in the book) is achieved through a natural sequence of mini-stages challenging the patient from midline stability to distal control, restoring stability and motor sequencing to address both primary and secondary impairments. The YT considers that each mini-stage may create a potential temporary disequilibrium by deviating the position of the center of gravity relative to midline or the base of support. Progressing the asana slowly, through all key components of functional movement along a continuum moving from the core, proximal to distal, then toward the full postural pattern with symmetry along the midline to ensure that each mini-stage is mastered through integration of the koshas.

From the yoga therapeutic perspective, asana is also an attitude that is psychophysiological in nature in which state of mind or mindfulness is of the utmost importance, hence linking the physical position with the higher koshas. Every asana has the potential to have an effect on each of the five koshas. The YT utilizes this understanding to facilitate system balance based on the assessed imbalances. Since yoga is an experiential philosophy, the author directs his students and patients, "Do not believe what is written; experience it." Try the following: sit in a slumped, forward head sitting posture for 10 breaths and sense the joy and enthusiasm of the asana. Now contrast that with upright, heart open, and arms spread wide overhead, face soft for 10 breaths. Feel the attitudinal difference? Every asana contains some of those subtle experiences and the physiological responses that are discussed in the following section.

The YT's neurophysiological rationale of yoga therapeutics has been documented by Taylor and Majmundar.[22] Briefly, the rationale is that performance in the human movement system is impacted by not only structure and physiology, but also by emotional, psychological, and spiritual conditions. The increased perception of proprioceptive information, awareness of thoughts and emotions, decreased cortical activity, and the development of nonreactivity to physical sensation result in the attainment of positive functional outcomes. Classically, the functional goal of the yogi was the elimination of postural sway, and from this practice it is believed comes the objective measures of increased flexibility, strength, and balance/postural stability.

To bridge the language of the 2 traditions, consider this yogic interpretation of the following Western motor concepts. Such an appreciation also resolves the dilemma of how one might document and record yoga therapeutic interventions. The above-stated postural efficiency depends on well-integrated and counteracting postural reflexes. There must be highly coordinated actions between numerous muscles and joints, and an adequate foundation of muscle tone. All the while, proprioceptors, exteroceptors, and visceroceptors convey moment-to-moment information of head and body position in space to the lower brain structures of the midbrain, cerebellum, basal ganglia, and reticular activating system (pons and medulla).[25] This maintenance of a postural pattern and the equilibrium of the body during movement or stability in the asana is performed subcortically as an autonomic nervous system function. Muscles, ligaments, and joints are stretched statically in a passive response to gravity during the mini-stage, or maintenance phase, of asana. There is minimum muscular contraction and minimal voluntary effort as the decreased cortical activity and inward focus allows for the integration of the tonic system responsible for postural control and stability. There should be minimal energy expenditure to avoid cortical stimulation and subcortical compensatory motor patterns. Muscle tone is regulated as the feedback from the various muscle spindle fibers (types Ia and II) as the Golgi tendon organs are allowed to integrate both peripherally and subcortically in a balanced or homeostatic autonomic nervous system.[26] The general rehabilitation goal of posture is stability and equilibrium of the body mass for safe interaction with the environment.

Asanas are often practiced as pairs, known as *counterposes*.[27] Biomechanically, this creates balance by soft tissue lengthening, hyaline cartilage compression and distraction, and reversing intervertebral disc pressures and dural stretch. These counterforces are also delivered to the internal organs, composed of smooth muscle, or the glands of the endocrine system. The patient experiences the more subtle effects of the higher koshas through this counterbalance, bringing about a balance in emotions and the subsequent biochemical signatures of that balance. This mechanical stimulation, coupled with the relaxation response, is cited as one potential source of many of the nonmusculoskeletal benefits of yoga.[28]

Weaving the principles of yoga with neurophysiological terminology not only facilitates communication within the medical community, but also creates an internal subjective reconciliation for the therapist between the hemispheric dichotomies of linear and circular understanding. For a thorough review of the physiology of mindful movement, the reader is referred to Jennifer Bottomley's coverage of the topic in Chapter 11. The tools of asana and pranayama precede meditation, or, in medical parlance, *psychosensorimotor integration*. For a review of the neurophysiology of meditation, the reader is referred to King and Brownstone's review.[29]

LITERATURE REVIEW

In addition to thousands of years of "clinical trials," there is an increasing amount of objective, outcomes-based research on yoga as it applies directly to rehabilitation. While there is the design problem of creating a sham yoga intervention because any movement done mindfully and with focus on the breath is technically yoga, the number of yoga therapy studies is increasing geometrically. There is now a MEDLINE-indexed, peer-reviewed *International Journal of Yoga Therapy* and over 400 studies on mindfulness-based stress reduction.

The psychophysiological literature on yoga documents some of the effects of practice to include improved ideal body weight, body density, cardiovascular endurance, and anaerobic power over a 1-year period of time.[30,31] The effect of long-term combined yoga practice has demonstrated a significant decrease in basal metabolic rate in healthy adults as a proposed result of reduced arousal.[32] A study of a group of 287 college students confirmed other research studies reporting the positive effect of yoga on the vital capacity of the lungs.[33] A short-term study of 6 weeks confirmed increased aerobic power, but demonstrated decreased anaerobic power.[24] Contrary to the Western aerobic prescription of sustained moderate exercise for increasing energy metabolism, yoga has been demonstrated to create an increased thermic effect that persisted greater than 90 minutes after practice.[30] In the elderly, yoga has been shown to decrease resting heart rate, increase VO_2 max, and increase parasympathetic baroreflex sensitivity.[11] A study of women found that yoga increased their maximum work output and decreased their oxygen consumption per unit of work.[34] A 6-month trial with seniors resulted in improved sense of well-being, energy, timed one-legged standing, and forward flexibility.[35] Yoga also induces a state of blood hypocoagulability with decreased fibrinogen; increased fibrinolytic activity, hemoglobin, and hematocrit; and prolonged activated partial thromboplastin and platelet aggregation time.[36] Could this suggest that preventive medical management of patients at risk for thrombosis and emboli benefit from these effects of yoga?

Finally, appropriate since it is the final asana of every yoga class, the relaxation pose of Shavasana, or corpse pose, has been demonstrated to significantly facilitate recovery from induced physiological stress compared with 2 other postures (resting in chair and resting supine posture).[37]

ORTHOPEDICS

A summary review of yoga application in orthopedics is available in the aforementioned article by Taylor and Majmundar.[22] Yoga as rehabilitative intervention gained national attention with the study on yoga for carpal tunnel syndrome by Garfinkel et al.[38] Utilizing a single-blind, randomized controlled trial, the subjects received 11 yoga postures and a relaxation twice weekly for 8 weeks. Controls wore a wrist splint to supplement their treatment. The yoga group experienced significant changes in improved grip strength (from 162 to 187 mm Hg; $P = .009$) and pain reduction (decreased from 5.0 to 2.9 mm Hg; $P = .02$), with no significant changes experienced by the control group. Further, more individuals in the yoga group demonstrated improvements in Phalen sign than in the control group (12 subjects vs 2 subjects, respectively; $P = .008$). The yoga group tended to improve, but without significant differences, in sleep disturbance, Tinel's sign, and median nerve motor and sensory conduction time. As a preliminary study, the sample size and generalizability were limited.

A study on yoga as treatment for osteoarthritis of the hands, also led by Garfinkel,[39] demonstrated significantly decreased pain during activity, tenderness, and increased finger ROM. Emphasis was placed on attention to respiration and upper-body alignment. There were favorable, although not statistically significant, differences in the treatment group's hand pain at rest and hand function. It was also noted that there were no reported exacerbations while performing the asana. In both of Garfinkel's studies,[38,39] a majority of the postures chosen either maintained the local tissue in a functional midrange position or in end-range without substantial overpressure for soft tissue deformation. There is considerable focus on proximal kinesthetic chain biomechanics, with special emphasis on core alignment and opening the chest. The yogic interpretation would describe both conditions as energetic imbalances and point to balancing the metaphoric heart and the musculoskeletal alignment. There are now chapters in 2 major hand/upper-quarter textbooks dedicated to the use of yoga therapeutics in rehabilitation.[39,40]

Iyengar yoga for the reduction of symptoms of osteoarthritis of the knee was examined in a pilot study with a very small sample. Seven participants utilized a 90-minute Iyengar yoga practice once weekly for 8 weeks.[40] After the 8-week intervention, participants reported a significant reduction in pain, physical impairments, and negative emotions associated with their condition. Of note by the authors, 6 of the 7 participants were obese, and they suggested that the study findings demonstrate the feasibility of using yoga as an intervention for individuals with obesity.

A designed yoga program on age-related changes in gait in a healthy senior population included 19 healthy adults (aged 62 to 83 years), all new to yoga, who participated in an 8-week Iyengar yoga program (2 90-minute yoga classes/week). The program was specifically structured for seniors and was designed to improve lower-body strength and flexibility.[40] Participants were also asked to complete at least 20 minutes of home practice on alternate days. The study examined pre- and post-intervention changes in peak hip extension, average anterior pelvic tilt, and stride length at comfortable walking speed. Peak hip extension and stride length significantly increased, and there was a marginally significant trend toward reduced average pelvic tilt. Participants who completed the home yoga practices were more likely to show this improvement. Both the frequency and duration of yoga home practice predicted changes in hip extension and average pelvic tilt, leading the authors to conclude that home practice is an important part of yoga interventions.

Energetically, yoga also describes right nostril breathing as stimulating and left nostril breathing as relaxing. The pranayama technique of alternate nostril breathing is a powerful balancing technique to produce homeostasis.[19] In a 1997 study involving children aged 11 to 18 years, grip strength increased by 4.1% to 6.5% after participating in single-nostril or alternate-nostril breath regulation (pranayama) without lateralization to one hand or the other over a 10-day period.[41] There were no changes in the other 2 groups in which participants maintained breath awareness or practiced mudras (hand positions that direct prana).

The yogic goal of drawing the senses inward to enhance focus and concentration, referred to as *dharana*, points to many interesting sport- and function-specific tasks requiring optimal performance levels. Yoga meditation combined with balance board training produced an enhanced balance index comprised of balance time and error for 5-minute duration trials.[42] The comparison group utilized amphetamine, which resulted in deterioration of task performance. There may also be an application in the patient with concomitant mental or neurological trouble attending to a task, or lack of dharana.

How does yoga compare with traditional therapeutic exercise intervention, and what can the technique achieve in the presence of acute spasm? In "normals," yoga has been demonstrated to produce a 58% decrease in EMG muscle activity below basal rate for men and women.[43] One descriptive study of asana-based exercises for low back pain offers a series of test protocols and assignment of asanas based on the results.[41] More than 70% of the participants reported significant improvement. However, there are a number of major design flaws and some anatomical inaccuracies in the figures presented. For instance, there was a nonstatistical report of correlation between compliance and those who reported no improvement. Adding the simple variables of attention to and synchronization of movement with breath to the plethora of hamstring flexibility studies may yield new information.

Although not described as a yoga intervention, the release of the anterior pelvis prior to forward bends or straight leg raises is common yogic practice. Clark et al[44] demonstrated increased passive unilateral straight-leg raise with ipsilateral anterior thigh soft tissue stretch. Both the study authors and Sahrmann in a commentary were unable to explain the results based on strict biomechanics (first kosha). The yoga explanation points to the second and third kosha issues of security, fear, and anger, with those biomechanical areas said to be the psychoneuroimmunology storehouses of that emotional energy. Opening those areas biomechanically is thought to allow for balance and integration of that energy, manifested as enhanced hip flexion or forward bending. Do these emotions exist in patients with acute or chronic low back pain? In the yoga model, there is almost always some emotional stored energy, even in "normals," providing an Eastern interpretation of a documented Western orthopedic outcome.

BACK PAIN

Yoga therapy for back pain gained national coverage with the publication of Sherman et al's study[45] comparing viniyoga-style yoga, physical therapy–led exercise, and a self-care book for chronic low back pain. The subjects included 101 adults (66% women; mean age, 44 years) with chronic low back pain, the majority of whom had experienced pain for more than 1 year, and had experienced pain for more than 45 of the past 90 days prior to entering the study. After 12 weeks, patients in the yoga group had better back-related function than patients in the exercise or education groups. Reports of pain were similar in all 3 groups. At 26 weeks, patients in the yoga group reported better back-related function and less pain. The authors concluded that over 3 to 6 months, yoga appeared to be more effective than traditional exercise or an educational book for improving function and pain in patients with chronic low back pain.

Galantino et al[46] observed trends in improvement of balance, flexibility, decreased disability, and depression in their modified hatha yoga pilot study. Another study by Williams and colleagues[47] examined the effect of Iyengar yoga in people who had been experiencing back pain for an average of 11.2 years. Participants in the 16-week yoga group reported on a variety of outcomes at baseline, the end of the 16-week intervention, and 3-month follow-up. The yoga practice was associated with significant reductions in pain intensity, functional disability, and the use of pain medication at both the 16-week point and the 3-month follow-up. Researchers from the Duke University Medical Center examined the benefits of a traditional Buddhist loving-kindness meditation for chronic low back pain in a 2005 study.[48] Participants were randomly assigned to either the loving-kindness intervention or to standard care. The authors assessed patients' pain, anger, and psychological distress before and after the intervention. The loving-kindness group showed significant improvements in pain and psychological distress, but the standard care group did not. In addition, the more an individual practiced loving-kindness meditation on a specific day, the less pain he or she experienced that day and the less anger he or she experienced the following day. These are interesting results, bearing in mind that this analysis included only meditation and no exercise or asana.

In a joint clinical practice guideline from the American College of Physicians and the American Pain Society, yoga was included in their recommendations for people with low back pain.[49] Further, three meta-analyses of yoga and back pain/function were published in 2012 to 2013.[50-52]

POST-STROKE HEMIPARESIS

A preliminary investigation of a yoga-based exercise program for people with chronic post-stroke hemiparesis lent support for improvement in impairments and mobility in this patient population.[53] The primary outcome measures for the four subjects were the Berg Balance Scale and the Timed

Movement Battery. The 8-week intervention consisted of twice-weekly, 1.5-hour yoga sessions in the subjects' homes. The authors concluded that further investigation is warranted to examine the effects of yoga in this population. A small pilot study reported improvements in fine motor control and aphasia in individuals using yoga.[54] A larger study by Schmid et al[55] found promising results using modified postures in twice-weekly, 1-hour classes for 8 weeks. Participants improved by 17% and 34% their Berg Balance and Fullerton Advanced Balance Scales, respectively. There was also measureable gain in confidence in their balance, and the investigators found wide acceptance from the participants. The data analysis examined gains in functional strength, flexibility, and endurance as a result of the yoga, and researchers reported significant improvements in all areas. Further, there was an unexpected improvement in gait with limb speed and increased stride length.[55]

SLEEP

The effects of yoga postures, self-regulated breathing, and yoga relaxation techniques on sleep in a geriatric population were compared with the effects of Ayurveda and a wait-list control in a 2005 study.[56] After 6 months, the yoga group (n = 40) experienced a statistically significant decrease in time to fall asleep and an increase in total number of hours slept (average increase, 60 minutes) and in the feeling of being rested in the morning. In addition to improving the participants' quality of life, being able to decrease their dependence on pharmaceuticals and the number of times up at night may lower the risks for fall in this population.

MOOD

Given that depression and anxiety are key factors in treating pain, the ways in which yoga might impact both is of interest to physical therapists. Significant reductions were shown for depression, anger, anxiety, neurotic symptoms, and low-frequency heart rate variability in the 17 completers of a study by Shapiro et al.[57] Eleven of the completers achieved remission levels post-intervention. Participants who remitted differed from the nonremitters at intake on several traits and on physiological measures indicative of a greater capacity for emotional regulation. Moods improved from before to after the yoga classes, leading to the conclusion that yoga appears to be a promising intervention for depression, is cost effective, and is easy to implement.

In a study on yoga and fibromyalgia, the yoga group showed significant improvements in depression compared with the control group.[58] This randomized controlled trial examined the effects of yoga on depressive symptoms in 91 women with fibromyalgia who were randomly assigned to treatment (n = 51) or a waiting list control group (n = 40). Somatic and cognitive symptoms of depression were assessed using the Beck Depression Inventory, which was administered at baseline, immediately post-program, and at follow-up 2 months after the conclusion of the intervention.

There are many more studies beyond the scope of this chapter, but therapists working with patients with mood disorders should note that in 2010 the *American Family Physicians* recommended yoga therapy as indicated along with cognitive behavioral therapy and pharmaceutical support for the treatment of anxiety and depression.[59] This strong endorsement points to many possibilities for rehabilitation professions that also use movement and breathing within their scope of practice for offering biopsychosocial interventions.

PAIN MANAGEMENT

The effects of chemical dependence and affective disorders, particularly depression, on pain management is well documented.[60,61] The perception and management of pain is closely linked to the mind-body connection. Yoga has been demonstrated to decrease somatic complaints in normal women.[18] Shavasana (lying supine) proved to be an effective technique for alleviating depression and significantly increasing positive change in a 1993 study.[62]

Kabat-Zinn[63] reported large and significant reductions in mood disturbance and psychiatric disorders (third and fourth koshas) using simple asana and meditation. He also found that they produced a more than 33% decrease in pain in 65% of the chronic pain subjects and a more than 50% relief on the pain index in 505 patients.[63] Kabat-Zinn's *Full Catastrophe Living: Using the Wisdom of Your Body and Mind to Face Stress, Pain, and Illness*[64] provides a thorough description of the methodology of breath and movement.

What is the mood change that one experiences following therapeutic exercise compared with the mood change following asana, and could it impact compliance to home programs? Berger and Owen[65] reported that men performing yoga experienced significantly decreased tension, anger, and fatigue compared with those who swam. They also noted that greater mood changes correlated positively with compliance to the exercise.

There is one meta-analysis available on pain and yoga detailing the literature and, despite some limitations, it demonstrates evidence that yoga may be useful for several pain-associated disorders.[66] Moreover, there are hints that even short-term interventions might be effective. The analysis concluded that additional large-scale studies have to identify which patients may benefit from the respective interventions.

BALANCE AND FALL PREVENTION

A preliminary study was completed by Majmundar et al on yoga for postural control and fall prevention in the elderly (Matra Majmundar, OTR, personal communication, August 2001). Citing falling as a major risk factor in the aging population, they compared a control group with a group that performed yoga asanas and breathing over a 12-week period. Utilizing a Wearable Accelerometric Motion Analysis System developed at the Department of Veterans Affairs Health Care System Rehabilitation Research and Development Center in Palo Alto, CA, researchers were able to gather 3-dimensional upper-body acceleration data through a variety of standard balance tests, measured pre- and post-experiment. They found decreased postural sway in tandem (toe-to-heel) standing with eyes closed in the yoga-trained group. Participants in the yoga group also reported subjective functional improvements, including relief of arthritis pain, enhanced stair climbing, increased ease in rising from and sitting down on the floor, and decreased frequency of urination through the night. Further, the previously mentioned study from Schmid et al[55] includes a quality literature review for yoga and balance.

RESPIRATORY CONDITIONS

It is well documented that yoga has a positive impact on the pulmonary and autonomic function of patients with asthma.[4,5,67-74] Tandon[71] found that yoga, when compared with standard physical therapy treatment for chronic obstructive pulmonary disease, produced symptomatic improvement and significantly increased the mean maximum work by 60.55 kpm, whereas no change occurred with physical therapy. The use of various hand mudras, bhandas, kriyas, pranayama patterns, and sustained restorative postures that mobilize the thoracic spine and chest wall have been valuable yoga therapeutic tools for the author. These easy-to-perform techniques are performed by the patient as a home program and are very comfortable.

END-OF-LIFE SUPPORT

Yoga therapeutics as a psychospiritual practice lends itself well to supporting patients and their families at the end of life and literally through transition to death. Taylor[75,76] has published 2 practice-oriented articles that can easily be adapted by rehabilitation professionals in end-of-life care.

CASE EXAMPLE

The following intervention illustrates the clinical nuances of a yoga therapeutic approach to therapy for a chronic orthopedic diagnosis of mechanical low back pain.

History

A 38-year-old man with a 10-year history of progressively severe episodes of central low back pain with acute debilitating lateral shifts was seen weekly for 8 60-minute visits—1 initial evaluation with 7 1-week follow-up visits. He had received many physical therapy interventions over the years to include spinal mobilization, craniosacral/myofascial release, and many of the approaches from existing schools of spine management. He reported a high level of compliance to therapeutic exercises, as well as utilizing various postural supports, such as rolls, wedges, and ergonomically designed seating. His primary reports were intolerance to sitting for longer than 30 minutes and an inability to garden vigorously without resulting in 3- to 4-day acute exacerbations. His activity level included running 30 minutes, 5 days/week with quality shoes, post-exercise stretching, and twice-weekly strength training with good form and moderate resistance. Secondary reports included an inability to comfortably play with his children on the floor, a fear of participating in nonlinear sports, and chronic stiffness across the entire lumbosacral region (fourth, third, and first koshas). He related 2 different 1-week episodes that required complete bed rest. He took over-the-counter nonsteroidal anti-inflammatory drugs at prescription dosages as needed. He had a comprehensive knowledge base of postural care, ergonomics, and adaptive positioning because of a background in physical rehabilitation and fitness. He verbalized concern over continued symptom progression leading to a need for surgical intervention and/or chronic pain (third kosha). Socioeconomically, he had a busy social life but few close friends (fourth kosha). He had no acute financial concerns, but had a constant focus on the performance and balances of his financial accounts (first kosha). When questioned about past experience with yoga or breathing exercises, he related that he had no prior instruction in either, but that he had been to several Feldenkrais workshops on back pain.

Examination

Static examination of posture revealed minimal forward head posture, well-developed musculature, and normal spinal curves; foot posture was symmetrical with slight pronation bilaterally but with a well-maintained longitudinal arch, and he reported greater weight bearing along the medial heels. There was no postural shift, and his hips and shoulders were level. Functionally, he moved freely and without pain. Forward bending in standing was limited to mid-tibia with flattened lumbar spine; back bending was smooth and within normal limits. The patient's hamstrings were tight, with left at 45 degrees in 90/90 supine and right at 50 degrees. His hips had 25 degrees of internal rotation left and 35 degrees right; hip extension was 5 degrees bilaterally. He was nontender to palpation and no active trigger points were identified. His gait was within normal limits but with very little anterior/posterior scapular or pelvic movement. In standing, he exhibited no discernible movement associated with breath (second kosha). His respiration was shallow, originating in the chest, and at a rate of 17 breaths per minute. There was no observable spinal, shoulder, or abdominal movement associated with the breath. He was observed to maintain the left hand in a closed position relative to his open right hand (third kosha). During conversation, he was observed to lean forward, appearing to almost strain himself to hear or comprehend (first 3 koshas). When questioned, he related maintaining his tongue firmly against his lower teeth. Running gait was forward leaning, with short strides and a flat, immobile spine with bracing across the shoulders. On attempted long sitting forward bend, the patient's knees were bent with shaking quadriceps, collapsed across the chest, little breath, and excessive upper cervical extension.

Assessment

The focus of the assessment was on the patient's trunk stiffness, secondary impairments of lower-quarter dysfunction, and inefficient gait (first kosha), and was primarily directed at the his restricted breath pattern (second kosha). A yoga therapeutic approach balances physical (first kosha) interventions by including asanas that not only address that level, but also the more subtle koshas to include restricted breath pattern (second kosha), concerns/fears of surgery/chronic pain (third kosha), and the bracing or fearful attitude suggested by the noted apprehensive postural patterns (fourth and fifth koshas).

Interventions

To that end, over the 8 visits, he was instructed in both a diaphragmatic and a full 3-part yoga breath, prone, and supine. Recruitment early on was inconsistent, ratcheted, and frequently out of sequence with upper chest accessory activity and regular queuing required to release the tongue, hand, and hips. He verbalized frustration at his inability to overcome the clumsiness and awkwardness of many of the standing and seated poses, necessitating constant reminders to ease up, engage the full breath, and utilize props or supports for comfort. He was reassured that this was an almost universal initial experience. Maintaining core awareness and the relaxation response through the diaphragmatic breath, he was then instructed in a supine back-of-the-leg stretch with a strap. Emphasis was placed on waiting for the breath (fifth kosha) and initiating all movement as a radiation or wave from the belly. The next progression was a standing-supported lunge with chairs and blocks. Mountain and Warrior II followed, with emphasis on symmetric and complete foot contact broadening the breath from pelvic floor to throat. Again, he verbalized frustration at sequencing, but his sequencing improved steadily with hand and verbal cues. He was cautioned against excessive upper-cervical extension and chin thrust on standing-forward bends. To address the lack of pelvic mobility (first and second koshas), he was instructed in a supported pigeon pose to open both hip rotators and flexors. The right side was well tolerated, but he noted a deep ache within the posterior hip on the left side along with a strong sense of anger/fear when reclining forward over the left knee for more than 20 seconds. He cooperated, but stated dislike for legs up the wall as a restorative pose. He was unable to articulate why he did not enjoy the pose. During final relaxation, he reported difficulty maintaining attention, with distracting thoughts either rehearsing or remembering numerous other parts of the day, causing him to have difficulty maintaining concentration. Modifying guided imageries to a more active, physically based reference helped, as did instruction in a pranayama technique of alternate nostril breathing, as both tend to provide a grounding task for the mind, making reflective ideation more difficult to pursue. The patient was instructed to attempt a gradual increase in endurance by extending the number of breaths he maintained in each posture, but without shaking or other signs of striving. He was given written instructions each time a new asana was assigned and was told to perform the exercises daily. Weekly follow-up eventually led to a 40-minute session 5 to 7 days per week, including a 10-minute final relaxation.

Outcomes

Subjective

At 8 weeks, the patient noted an increased awareness of how "small," or restricted, his breath had been most of the time (second kosha) and a strong correlation of the breath to the sensation of stiffness in his back. He noted that the breath was both comforting and relaxing (third through fifth koshas). He had experienced no acute pain or postural shifts during the treatment period. His compliance had been high, with at least 5 times per week. He related significant improvement in sitting tolerance to where a recent 5-hour drive had been symptom free (first kosha). Morning stiffness and post-sitting stiffness were rare, and when they did occur, they were less than 25% of the previous level. He noted increased awareness of physical tension (tongue, hand, and back) corresponding with perception of emotions, such as frustration, anger, and fear (third and fifth koshas). His running gait felt more efficient (first kosha), but he also noted the insight as to how in the past he ran to get away from stress or to experience the post-exercise relaxation. Lately, he had become more aware of running when he wanted to move, rather than running "away from or because of something else" going on in his life. He incorporated the breath work at night, especially early morning when sleep was difficult, and found it both comforting and restorative (third and fifth koshas). He reported being able to comfortably play board games on the floor and wrestle with his children without discomfort or fear.

Objective

Static examination of posture was unchanged but he related full-foot weight-bearing contact. Forward bending in standing was to mid-ankle with reversed lumbar curve. Hamstrings were left at 65 degrees in 90/90 supine and 70 degrees right. Hips measured 40 degrees internal rotation left and 45 degrees right. Hip extension was 10 degrees bilaterally. His gait was within normal limits with both anterior/posterior scapular and pelvic movement. In standing, he had discernible movement associated with breath (second kosha) through the abdomen, flanks, shoulders, and chest. There was no observable spinal, shoulder, or abdominal movement associated with the breath. He demonstrated a fluid, full 3-part sequenced breath at 9 breaths per minute (47% decrease in rate). He was observed to maintain an open hand position (third kosha). During conversation, he sat comfortably erect, but with a casual ease, not gripping forward in a leaning posture, and he had a softer facial expression (first 3 koshas). On questioning, he related still catching himself maintaining his tongue firmly against his lower teeth, but that presently his tongue had been resting in the floor of his mouth. Running gait was an erect, natural stride length and a suppler spine with natural swing across the shoulders. On attempted long-sitting forward bend, the knees were bent slightly but with no shaking, sustaining a neutral spine with open chest, full breath, and neutral upper-cervical spine.

Disposition

He was directed to continue with the series while gradually increasing the number of breaths, not to skip the final relaxation, and to monitor his physical comfort in relation to emotional stressors. He was discharged to his home program and planned to continue active participation in the local yoga class.

PRACTICAL APPLICATIONS OF YOGA

How can yoga therapeutics be incorporated in a rehabilitation practice? Table 13-4 describes the rationale behind incorporating certain yoga therapy techniques into a practice; these methods are practical, seamless, and conservative in application. Utilizing yoga techniques has the ethical considerations of knowing one's limits, receiving appropriate training for competency dependent on the skill level of the technique, and marketing in such a manner as to preserve the integrity of yoga therapeutics. Networking with a local YT will create business opportunities and lead to professional development for each party. Because yoga therapy is provided literally across the entire lifespan, from prenatal to end-of-life care, there are a wide variety of program development possibilities through such a relationship. Yoga therapy can be shared through the use of props, straps, bolsters, and restorative yoga (supported postures that are maintained for extended lengths of time).[77,78] Yoga therapy is very accessible for all levels of movement capacity.

The primary principles in Table 13-4 involve bringing the patient's focus and attention internally. This focus requires the patient to be attentive to the feedback that he or she is experiencing from all of the koshas, and within his or her capacity to communicate or manage this feedback responsibly in the moment. The only prerequisite for participating in yoga therapeutics is to be breathing, so please

TABLE 13-4
PRACTICAL THERAPEUTIC YOGA APPLICATIONS

THERAPEUTIC TECHNIQUE	RATIONALE
Breath assessment instruction (pranayama)	Optimize the autonomic nervous system through the relaxation response
Verbal cues (asana)	More imagery for proximal-distal sequencing and greater recall
Guided imagery/restorative yoga (meditation and samadhi)	Capture Benson's "remembered wellness" for motor patterns
Pre-/post-body scan (asana)	Embody proprioceptive baseline and intervention effects
Activities of daily living (ADLs) instruction (asana)	Create conscious movement awareness
Journaling (niyamas—self-study)	Explore, analyze, and deal with psychoemotional-stress issues
Clinic environment (niyamas—purity)	Facilitate a mindful, introspective, and stress-reduced environment
Home programs (asana)	Create movement sequences that are whole body, core initiated for subtle awareness and increased compliance
Group therapy (yamas and niyamas)	Economical, socially, and emotionally rewarding to address chronic needs
Therapeutic exercise (asana)	Synchronized with breath, whole body, core initiated

consider how you may already be utilizing, or how you may begin to utilize, these yoga techniques with all of your patients.

Professional Qualifications for Yoga Instruction

The rehabilitation professions are the branches of medicine that specialize in the functional human movement system and related pathologies. As a profession, they seek new related knowledge and create clinical application with outcome-based research. These professions' licensing processes and knowledge base of anatomy, kinesiology, and physiology (to include respiration) justify academic, legal, and ethical use of the yoga techniques of postures with breath awareness. In the United States, there presently are no standards or legal restrictions as to who may instruct yoga or practice yoga therapy.

How to decide if and when a rehabilitation professional is "qualified" to use yoga therapeutic techniques is not clearly defined. Deciding to use yoga therapeutically is almost always a gray, rather than a black or white, standard. The question of who is qualified to teach yoga is no exception. Points of reflection and consideration are as follows:

- Yoga is far more than just asanas and breath regulation. See the emerging individual and school standards being set by the International Association of Yoga Therapists (www.iayt.org).
- Limiting the instruction to just postures and breath misses an opportunity to address the deeper health model issues of the spirit being the causal body, and as such, those issues might not be supported in a traditional clinical setting with those limitations.

- Because yoga instructors share an expertise in movement and balance, are they practicing physical therapy?

- What could be gained from a collaborative effort?

There are no easy answers to these points, but if held in awareness by practitioners, a rich potential exists for better serving patients and clients. The author's experience is that physical and occupational therapists possess academic knowledge and scientific rigor that is sometimes lacking in the yoga community. The yoga community's intimate kinesthetic awareness and skills, coupled with being able to address higher kosha issues through breath and movement, could facilitate rehabilitation outcomes.[77,78] What follows is intended to initiate that bridge building (yoking or yoga) between the 2 paradigms.

Bridges

Just as there are barriers or obstacles at all kosha levels in assisting a patient to achieve rehabilitation goals, so too do barriers exist for us when we expand professional paradigms. The largest barrier in the author's experience is the misconception about the word *yoga*, which may necessitate using descriptors such as *movement therapy, mindful exercise, stretch and relax, integrative medicine,* and *mind-body science* as more acceptable terminology. Yoga defined as a spiritual vehicle or life science philosophy can often be misunderstood as being a religion or in conflict with an individual's religious beliefs. Originating from the Hindu tradition, it makes no direct claims about a specific deity or dogma and can be adapted to conform to all of the world's major religions.[26]

Documentation is another barrier addressed earlier in the asana section. Initially, documentation appears daunting, such as envisioning a code for pranayama. In the allegorical language, the YT may prescribe bhujangasana (cobra) with hands-on correction for release of the particular chakra determined to be out of balance. Generically, describing the intervention in traditional therapeutic jargon solves the charting, coding, and outcomes dilemma. The yogic principles are used independently or in conjunction with standard therapeutic tools. The previous example becomes performing prone press-ups with posterior-anterior glides while verbally directing attention to synchronizing movement with the breath, which can be coded as directed therapeutic exercise, neuromotor re-education, manual therapy, or some combination of codes dependent on time and emphasis. The outcomes might be documented as increased ROM for task-specific ADLs, increased sitting tolerance, among others, without any yoga-type language.

Breath Assessment and Instruction

The breath is a mirror of the individual's autonomic nervous system, a key source of postural control, and a tool for direct modulation. It is a tool to maintain internal focus by the patient with such techniques as incorporating all movement in synchrony with the breath (ie, opening the front of the body with inhale and closing the front of the body with exhale through the sagittal plane), or by counting breaths rather than repetitions, necessitating the patient to maintain internal and present focus. Diaphragmatic breathing is a cost-effective, simple form of yoga therapy. Remember that the patient will model or entrain with the therapist's breathing pattern, so your breathing pattern needs to be integrated too!

Verbal Cues and Language

Monitoring the patient's vocabulary is a "safe," conservative method of addressing the higher, subtler aspects of the patient. Word selection is a window into the patient's relationship with his or her body, illness, and overall health responsibility. Does the patient claim ownership of his or her body and current complaint? Does he or she speak in the first or second person? Who is responsible for him or her getting better? Remember to also change your verbal cues to correlate with the way the mind works by using more visual imagery and active language vs Western measurable instruction (eg, soften vs relax, telescope vs reach, lengthen/inflate vs stabilize). These cue changes augment proximal to distal sequencing more fluidly than linear, component directions.

Guided Imagery/Restorative Yoga

Use techniques of visualization, music, and guided imagery/relaxation (bhavana or yoga nidra), particularly during passive modalities. Provide enough time for SMI to occur during and after interventions rather than "rushing the patient out the door." Anatomical, regional, or diagnosis-specific audiotapes can reinforce extero-/interoception and kinesthetic awareness. A portable audio player and an audio file make this an easy intervention that can be recorded directly on a smartphone. Emphasize the skill of relaxation vs the patient's typical distraction/recreation scheme as a means of allowing the body to move into a full relaxation response and its consequent SMI. Judith Lasater, PhD, PT, authored a book, *Relax and Renew: Restful Yoga for Stressful Times*,[79] which is a rich introduction to this skill.

Pre-/Post-Intervention Body Scans

Insist that the patient form a pre-intervention baseline of internal awareness or exteroception, followed by a post-intervention comparison, allowing SMI to reach a cognitive level of appreciation and discrimination. Five minutes sensing the breath in and out is as complicated and expensive as this gets! An axiom of yoga of unknown origin is, "They can't heal what they don't feel." In rehab-speak, "Afferent-efferent-afferent" becomes the mantra to repeat.

Activities of Daily Living Instruction

Given what we now know about the number of repetitions for motor learning and neuroplastic change, how does the therapist create mindfulness in movements throughout the day? The key is to create increased emphasis on self-awareness during ADLs. This might include asking the patient to note the direction of the breath (inhalation/exhalation) through activities, the sensations involved at various aspects of the body during an activity, or the altering of movements based on a focus of various areas of the body (eg "Sense the sensation in your shoulder and how it changes if you breathe in or out as you reach," "...as you press down more firmly with the big toe").

Journaling

The use of a personal journal (self-study or svadhyaya) to include reflections on the patient's impairment and all other experiences can be an excellent tool for broadening the patient's awareness of more subtle issues and also expanding the therapist's understanding of the patient's situation. Whether this journal is kept privately or shared with the therapist is up to the patient's discretion. The act of journaling, if encouraged, can become a powerful tool for the patient to develop a deeper mind-body connection and sense of responsibility for his or her own health.

Passive Modalities/Clinic Environment

The holistic approach can be as simple as turning off the TV or radio; utilizing art, music, and color tastefully; providing positive waiting room material; and creating a quiet, warm environment. From the waiting room to departure, attention to breath can be tactfully encouraged. During passive modalities, breath awareness and listening to guided imagery relaxation tapes rather than reading an outdated news magazine can deepen the relaxation response. Anatomical, body region–specific tapes can reinforce proprioceptive and kinesthetic awareness. Kabat-Zinn[63] and others, using mindfulness meditation and asanas, demonstrated an uncoupling of the sensory dimension of the pain experience from the affective/evaluative alarm reaction so often found in patients experiencing pain. This type of mindful movement provides a powerful interruption of the pain-spasm cycle at a higher kosha level.

Home Programs

Asanas tend to be, by definition, whole-body exercise and, as such, generally do not require as many different forms. They can also be sequenced in a pleasant, functional flowing manner of progression called *vinyasas* rather than linear, calisthenic-type sections. There is some evidence that exercise that improves mood is positively correlated with compliance.[55] While not yet studied, fewer more relaxing and flowing movements may enhance patient compliance.

Therapeutic Exercise

Many of the therapeutic exercises traditionally prescribed resemble asanas in form. McKenzie exercises in physical therapy look very much like crocodile (prone-lying), sphinx (prone-on-elbows), cobra (press-ups), and initiation of the triangle (lateral glides).[3] The focus on the breath, movement synchronized with breath, decreased perceived exertion, and therapeutic intention differentiate asanas from therapeutic exercise. Therapeutic progression is similar within the parameters of intensity and gravity modification. Counting by breaths for duration rather than repetitions facilitates attention. Disruption of a smooth, full breath signals the need for a modification of intensity.

Asanas are identified with creating certain effects on all of the kosha levels. Similar biomechanical stretches may have very different "attitudes" or "emotional responses." The verbal and tactile cues utilized in yoga make use of the mind's ability to think in image, motion, and color by being more colorful and image-oriented to enhance kinesthetic learning ("drift" vs "reach"; "soften and release" rather than "relax"). Yoga asanas have been integrated into other movement therapies because of their effectiveness and complement to SMI. There is aquatic yoga, yogassage (soft tissue work in sustained asana), and Eleanor Criswell's somatic yoga,[80] which blends the work of Moshé Feldenkrais and yoga.

Group Rehabilitation

The group setting of yoga has produced numerous improvements in a wide range of health conditions. Chronic spinal pain, post-stroke, fibromyalgia, multiple sclerosis, osteoarthritis, and joint replacement are just a few of the group classes being offered. While this contradicts our detailed, patient-specific evaluation and treatment prescription, it should compel us to inquire what this phenomenon is and how it can be utilized. Ornish[81] contends that group support may be the single most important factor in his studies. Would delivering therapy to a group of similar diagnostic codes be cost effective in making services more affordable to those who are dependent on discretionary funds, yet maintain revenue rates for the rehabilitation yoga instructor? As direct access and increased financial responsibility fall to the individual, this may be a valuable model for delivery of services.

Professional Networking

Establishing a working relationship with the yoga community offers many personal, professional, and business opportunities. The therapist who develops a personal yoga practice enjoys the health benefits, increased kinesthetic awareness, and expanded teaching tools of technique and vocabulary. As experts in movement science, this ongoing, mindful motor practice enhances both entry-level and continuing education for professionals while providing a psychomotor learning base of clinical mastery not available from conceptual academic study.

There can also be bottom-line enhancements to practice management by offering workshops in the rehabilitation and yoga communities on common topics, such as back pain or women's health, off-hour space utilization, the introduction of cash-based programming, and increased market traffic. Referrals that ensue between the professions will increase as familiarity with each other's capabilities expands. Cooperative program development in ergonomics, stress management, pain management, osteoporosis, and numerous other shared clientele areas can lead to additional revenue streams in niche markets via seminar presentations, books, and instructional audio and video resources that include yoga and rehabilitation. As the field of biopsychosocial science expands and delineates how the body, mind, and emotions interact to impact movement, the rehabilitation professional who understands how asanas express all of the koshas will be well positioned to incorporate the emerging science. Rather than turf wars and a scarcity mentality, this world view of integral perspective embraces collaboration and partnering with yoga therapy professionals.[77,78]

CONCLUSION

The profession of yoga therapy is a broad and ancient practice that continues to evolve while gaining acceptance in the West. Sufficient evidence exists to warrant further scientific investigation of yoga therapeutic properties as they apply to human performance. Five thousand years of field testing held under the rigors of Western science promises to bring additional knowledge to this healing science. The knowledge held within this experiential science will expand our vision of integrative medicine and serve as an invaluable rediscovery of these biopsychosocial practices for the 21st century integral rehabilitation professional.

ACKNOWLEDGMENTS

Special thanks to Mary Lou Galantino, PT, MS, PhD, who phoned in 1998 and convinced me that I could write an article on yoga therapy in physical therapy. Thanks also to our editor, Carol Davis, DPT, EdD, MS, FAPTA, who later insisted that I could contribute an entire chapter in a textbook. Their trust has introduced many colleagues to a fuller biopsychosocial practice. Finally, thanks to Neil Pearson, PT, MSc, BA-BPHE, for his help with the references.

REFERENCES

1. Feuerstein G. *The Yoga Tradition*. Prescott, AZ: Hohm Press; 1998.
2. Horak FB. Clinical measurement of postural control in adults. *Phys Ther*. 1987;67:1881-1885.
3. Iyengar BKS. *The Tree of Yoga*. Boston, MA: Shambhala; 1989.
4. Jain SC, Rai L, Valecha A, Jha UK, Bhatnagar SO, Ram K. Effect of yoga training on exercise tolerance in adolescents with childhood asthma. *J Asthma*. 1991;28(6):437-442.
5. Jain SC, Uppal A, Bhatnagar SO, Talukdar BA. Study of response pattern of non-insulin dependent diabetics to yoga therapy. *Diabetes Res Clin Prac*. 1993;19(1):69-74.
6. LePage J. *Integrative Yoga Therapy Training Manual*. Aptos, CA: Printsmith; 1994.
7. Taylor MJ. Yoga therapeutics in neurologic physical therapy: application to a patient with Parkinson's disease. *Neurology Report*. 2001;25:56.
8. Benson H, Stark M. *Timeless Healing: The Power and Biology of Belief*. New York, NY: Fireside; 1997.
9. Blackwell B, Bloomfield S, Gartside P. Transcendental meditation in hypertension. Individual response patterns. *Lancet*. 1976;1(7953):223-226.
10. Jevning R, Wilson AF, Davidson JM. Adrenocortical activity during meditation. *Horm Behav*. 1978;10(1):54-60.
11. Bowman AJ, Clayton RH, Murray A, Reed JW, Subhan MM, Ford GA. Effects of aerobic exercise training and yoga on the baroreflex in healthy elderly persons. *Eur J Clin Invest*. 1997;27(5):443-449.
12. Platania-Solazzo A, Field TM, Blank J, et al. Relaxation therapy reduces anxiety in child and adolescent psychiatric patients. *Acta Paedopsychiatr*. 1992;55(2):115-120.
13. Sahasi G, Mohan D, Kacker C. Effectiveness of yogic techniques in the management of anxiety. *J Pers*. 1989;5(1):51-55.
14. Miller JJ, Fletcher K, Kabat-Zinn J. Three-year follow-up and clinical implications of a mindfulness meditation-based stress reduction intervention in the treatment of anxiety disorders. *Gen Hosp Psychiatry*. 1995;17(3):192-200.
15. Murugesan R, Govindarajulu N, Bera TK. Effect of selected yogic practices on the management of hypertension. *Indian J Physiol Pharmacol*. 2000;44(2):207-210.
16. Grossman E, Grossman A, Schein MH, Zimlichman R, Gavish B. Breathing control lowers blood pressure. *J Hum Hypertens*. 2001;15(4):263-269.
17. Harte JL, Eifert GH, Smith R. The effects of running and meditation on beta-endorphin, corticotropin-releasing hormone and cortisol in plasma, and on mood. *Biol Psychol*. 1995;40(3):251-265.
18. Schell FJ, Allolio B, Schonecke OW. Physiological and psychological effects of hatha-yoga exercise in healthy women. *Int J Psychosom*. 1994;41(1-4):46-52.
19. Hannibal KE, Bishop MD. Chronic stress, cortisol dysfunction, and pain: a psychoneuroendocrine ratioanale for stress management in pain rehabilitation. *Phys Ther*. 2014;94(12):1816-1825.
20. Miller R. The psychophysiology of respiration: Eastern and Western perspectives. *Journal of the International Association of Yoga Therapists*. 1991;2(1):8-23.
21. Raju PS, Madhavi S, Prasad KV, et al. Comparison of effects of yoga & physical exercise in athletes. *Indian J Med Res*. 1994;100:81-86.

22. Taylor MJ, Majmundar M. Incorporating yoga therapeutics into orthopedic physical therapy. *Ortho Phys Ther Clinics N Amer.* 2000;9(3):341-360.
23. Iyengar BKS. *Light on Yoga.* New York, NY: Shocken; 1976.
24. Balasubramanian B, Pansare MS. Effect of yoga on aerobic and anaerobic power of muscles. *Indian J Physiol Pharmacol.* 1991;35(4):281-282.
25. Allum B, Hulliger M. Afferent control of posture and locomotion. In: Allum JHJ, Hulliger M, eds. *Progress in Brain Research.* New York, NY: Elsevier; 1989: 75-86.
26. Werner JK. *Neuroscience: A Clinical Perspective.* Philadelphia, PA: WB Saunders; 1980.
27. Desikachar TKV. *The Heart of Yoga.* Rochester, NY: Inner Traditions; 1995.
28. Monro R, Nagarathna R, Nagendra HR. *Yoga for Common Ailments.* New York, NY: Simon & Schuster; 1990.
29. King R, Brownstone A. Neurophysiology of yoga meditation. *International Journal of Yoga Therapy.* 1999;9:9-17.
30. Agte V, Chiplonkter S. Thermic responses to vegetarian meals and yogic exercise. *Ann Nutr Metab.* 1992;36:3.
31. Malathi A, Damodaran A, Iyar N, Patel L. Effect of yogic training on body composition and physical fitness. *The Journal of the Indian Association of Physiotherapists.* 1999;1:19-23.
32. Chaya MS, Kurpad AV, Nagendra HR, Nagarathna R. The effect of long term combined yoga practice on the basal metabolic rate of healthy adults. *BMC Complement Altern Med.* 2006;6:28.
33. Birkel DA, Edgren L. Hatha yoga: improved vital capacity of college students. *Altern Ther Health Med.* 2000;6(6):55-63.
34. Raju PS, Prasad KV, Venkata RY, Murthy KJ, Reddy MV. Influence of intensive yoga training on physiological changes in 6 adult women: a case report. *J Altern Complement Med.* 1997;3(3):291-295.
35. Oken BS, Zajdel D, Kishiyama S, et al. Randomized, controlled, six-month trial of yoga in healthy seniors: effects on cognition and quality of life. *Altern Ther Health Med.* 2006;12(1):40-47.
36. Chohan IS, Nayar HS, Thomas P. Influence of yoga on blood coagulation. *Thromb Haemost.* 1984;51(2):196-197.
37. Bera TK, Gore MM, Oak JP. Recovery from stress in two different postures and in Shavasana—a yogic relaxation posture. *Indian J Physiol Pharmacol.* 1998;42(4):473-478.
38. Garfinkel MS, Singhal A, Katz WA. Yoga-based intervention for carpal tunnel syndrome. *JAMA.* 1998;280(18):1601-1603.
39. Garfinkel MS, Schumacher HR, Husain A. Evaluation of a yoga based regimen for treatment of osteoarthritis of the hands. *J Rheumatol.* 1994;21:12.
40. Kolasinski SL, Garfinkel M, Tsai AG, et al. Iyengar yoga for treating symptoms of osteoarthritis of the knees: a pilot study. *J Altern Complement Med.* 2005;11:689-693.
41. Raghuraj P. Pranayama increases grip strength without lateralized effects. *Indian J Physiol Pharmacol.* 1997;41(2):129-133.
42. Dhume RR, Dhume RA. A comparative study of the driving effects of dextroamphetamine and yogic meditation on muscle control for the performance of balance on balance board. *Indian J Physiol Pharmacol.* 1991;35(3):191-194.
43. DiBenedetto M, Innes KE, Taylor AG, et al. Effect of a gentle Iyengar yoga program on gait in the elderly: an exploratory study. *Arch Phys Med Rehabil.* 2005;86(4):1830-1837.
44. Clark S, Christiansen A, Hellman DF, Hugunin JW, Hurst KM. Effects of ipsilateral anterior thigh soft tissue stretching on passive unilateral straight-leg raise. *JOSPT.* 1999;29(1):4-11.
45. Sherman KJ, Cherkin DC, Erro J, Miglioretti DL, Deyo RA. Comparing yoga, exercise, and a self-care book for chronic low back pain: a randomized, controlled trial. *Ann Intern Med.* 2005;143:849-856.
46. Galantino ML, Bzdewka TM, Eissler-Russo JL, et al. The impact of modified hatha yoga on chronic low back pain: a pilot study. *Altern Ther.* 2004;10(2):56-59.
47. Williams KA, Petronis J, Smith D, et al. Effect of Iyengar yoga therapy for chronic low back pain. *Pain.* 2005;115(1-2):107-117.
48. Carson JW, Keefe FJ, Lynch TR, et al. Loving-kindness meditation for chronic low back pain: results from a pilot trial. *J Holist Nursing.* 2005;23(3):287-304.
49. Chou R, Qaseem A, Snow V, et al. Diagnosis and treatment of low back pain: a joint clinical practice guideline from the American College of Physicians and the American Pain Society. *Ann Intern Med.* 2007;147(7):478-491.
50. Cramer H, Lauche R, Haller H, Dobos G. Systematic review and meta-analysis of yoga for low back pain. *Clin J Pain.* 2013;29(5):450-460.
51. Holtzman S, Beggs RT. Yoga for chronic low back pain: a meta-analysis of randomized controlled trials. *Pain Res Manag.* 2013;18(5):267-272.
52. Ward L, Stebbings S, Cherkin D, Baxter GD. Yoga for functional ability, pain and psychosocial outcomes in musculoskeletal conditions: a systematic review and meta-analysis. *Musculoskeletal Care.* 2013;11(4):203-217.
53. Bastille JV, Gill-Body KM. A yoga-based exercise program for people with chronic poststroke hemiparesis. *Phys Ther.* 2004;84(1):33-48.
54. Lynton H, Kligler B, Shiflett S. Yoga in stroke rehabilitation: a systematic review and results of a pilot study. *Top Stroke Rehabil.* 2007;14(4):1-8.
55. Schmid AA, Van Puymbroeck M, Altenburger PA, et al. Poststroke balance improves with yoga: a pilot study. *Stroke.* 2012;43(9):2402-2407.

56. Manjunath NK, Telles S. Influence of yoga and ayurveda on self-rated sleep in a geriatric population. *Indian J Med Res*. 2005;121(5):683-690.

57. Shapiro D, Cook IA, Davydov DM, et al. Yoga as a complementary treatment of depression: effects of traits and moods on treatment outcome. E-cam Feb, 2007.

58. Sephton SE, Salmon P, Weissbecker I, et al. Mindfulness meditation alleviates depressive symptoms in women with fibromyalgia: results of a randomized clinical trial. *Arthritis Rheum*. 2007;57(1):77-85.

59. Saeed SA, Antonacci DJ, Bloch R. Exercise, yoga, and meditation for anxiety and depression. *Am Fam Physician*. 2010;81(8):987.

60. Nespor K. Psychosomatics of back pain and the use of yoga. *Int J Psychosom*. 1989;36(1-4):72-78.

61. Nespor K. Pain management and yoga. *Int J Psychosom*. 1991;38(1-4):76-81.

62. Khumar SS, Kaur P, Kaur S. Effectiveness of Shavasana on depression among university students. *Indian J Clin Psychol*. 1993;20(2):82-87.

63. Kabat-Zinn J. An outpatient program in behavioral medicine for chronic pain patients based on the practice of mindfulness meditation: theoretical considerations and preliminary results. *Gen Hosp Psychiatry*. 1982;4(1):33.

64. Kabat-Zinn J. *Full Catastrophe Living*. New York, NY: Delta; 1990.

65. Berger BG, Owen DR. Mood alteration with yoga and swimming: aerobic exercise may not be necessary. *Percept Mot Skills*. 1992;75(3 Pt 2):1331-1343.

66. Bussing A, Osterman T, Ludtke R, Michalsen A. Effects of yoga interventions on pain and pain-associated disability: a meta-analysis. *J Pain*. 2012;13(1):1-9.

67. Nagarathna R, Nagendra HR. Yoga for bronchial asthma: a controlled study. *Brit Med J Clin Res Ed*. 1985;291(6502):1077-1079.

68. Nagendra HR, Nagarathna R. An integrated approach of yoga therapy for bronchial asthma: a 3-54-month prospective study. *J Asthma*. 1986;23(3):123-137.

69. Vijayalakshmi S, Satyanarayana M, Krishna-Rao PV, Prakash V. Combined effect of yoga and psychotherapy on management of asthma: a preliminary study. *J Indian Psychol*. 1988;7(2):32-39.

70. Wilson AF, Honsberger R, Chiu JT, Novey HS. Transcendental meditation and asthma. *Respiration*. 1975;32(1):74-80.

71. Tandon MK. Adjunct treatment with yoga in chronic severe airways obstruction. *Thorax*. 1978;33(4):514-517.

72. Sabina AB, Williams AL, Wall HK, Bansal S, Chupp G, Katz DL. Yoga intervention for adults with mild-to-moderate asthma: a pilot study. *Ann Allergy Asthma Immunol*. 2005;94(5):543-548.

73. Vedanthan PK, Kesavalu LN, Murthy KC, et al. Clinical study of yoga techniques in university students with asthma: a controlled study. *Allergy Asthma Proc*. 1998;19(1):3-9.

74. Sodhi C, Singh S, Dandona PK. A study of the effect of yoga training on pulmonary functions in patients with bronchial asthma. *Indian J Physiol Pharmacol*. 2009;53(2):169-174.

75. Taylor JC, Taylor MJ. Yoga therapeutics: preparation and support for end of life. *Top Geriatr Rehabil*. 2011;27(2):142-150.

76. Taylor JC. End of life yoga therapy: exploring life and death. *Int J Yoga Therap*. 2008;18:97-103.

77. Taylor M. Opportunities with the complementary and alternative medicine world. *Impact*. 2010:40-41.

78. Wojciechowski M. Integrative Medicine: New Opportunities for PTs. *PTinMotion*, 2014;July:22-27.

79. Lasater J. *Relax and Renew: Restful Yoga for Stressful Times*. Berkeley, CA: Rodmell Press; 2011.

80. Criswell E. *How Yoga Works: An Introduction to Somatic Yoga*. Phoenix, AZ: Freeperson Press; 1989.

81. Ornish D. *Love & Survival*. New York, NY: HarperCollins; 1997.

14

Feldenkrais Method in Rehabilitation
Using Functional Integration and Awareness Through Movement to Explore New Movements and Solve Clinical Problems

James Stephens, PT, PhD, GCFP and Teresa M. Miller, PT, PhD, GCFP

The authors have been impressed by the effectiveness that the use of the Feldenkrais Method has demonstrated in their clinical practice. Not only does the process usually allow the practitioner and client (also referred to as *student* throughout this chapter) to find an effective solution to the problems at hand, but it often subsequently empowers students to more effectively solve problems in pursuit of their own health and function. Support is beginning to appear in the literature for use of the Feldenkrais Method as a way to improve health and function.

The goal of this chapter is to introduce the conceptual and practical processes of the Feldenkrais Method. In this chapter, the authors will briefly introduce the man responsible for developing the method, Moshé Feldenkrais, by presenting a picture of his creative processes and thinking over time. A description of the different aspects of working with a client using Functional Integration (FI) and Awareness Through Movement (ATM) will be presented, which will include information on some of the related assessment and intervention processes and case studies for each approach. Current research on the method will also be reviewed and discussed. Finally, a list of resources for people who are interested in pursuing further learning on their own is included at the end of the chapter.

BACKGROUND

Moshé Feldenkrais' Life and Work

From a base in physics, the work of Feldenkrais expanded into many other areas, including Gestalt psychology, progressive relaxation,[1] bioenergetics,[2] sensory awareness,[3] the hypnosis of

Davis CM.
Integrative Therapies in Rehabilitation: Evidence for Efficacy in Therapy, Prevention, and Wellness, Fourth Edition (pp 203-225).
© 2017 Taylor & Francis Group.

Milton Erickson,[4] an ecological perspective on mind[5] and human perception,[6] and the physiological studies of Sherrington, Magnus, Pavlov, Fulton, and Schilder.[7]

Born in Russia in 1904, Feldenkrais grew up in an educated, middle class family. He was the grandson of a revered Jewish rabbi. At the age of 14, he trekked to Palestine. There he worked doing manual construction, surveying and tutoring children who had difficulty learning.[8,9] During this time in Palestine, under the British mandate, there were attacks made against the new Jewish settlers. Feldenkrais developed a form of hand-to-hand combat that was used by the settlers for self-defense, described in the book *Ju-Jitsu and Self-Defense*,[9] which he published in Paris in 1929.

Feldenkrais went to Paris in the late 1920s to continue his education at the University of Paris, where he studied mechanical and electrical engineering and later read for his doctorate in physics. While in Paris, he also studied the writings of Sigmund Freud and Emile Coué. In 1930 he published *Autosuggestion*, a Hebrew translation with commentary of Coué's work.[9] In 1934, Feldenkrais met Jigorō Kanō, the Japanese originator of Judo, who was doing demonstrations in Paris. Feldenkrais trained with Kanō and became one of the first Europeans to receive a black belt in Judo; he founded the Judo Club of France in 1936.[9] While playing soccer with a French club, he tore the meniscus of his left knee. He observed that there were times when he was able to move normally and other times when he would become incapacitated by the pain in his knee while he seemed to be doing the same activities. He took this as a challenge to improve himself, and, over time, he learned to walk and move without pain.[7] This was his initial experience in using awareness to improve function.

During World War II, Feldenkrais fled to England and was assigned to the British Admiralty unit on antisubmarine warfare. He found a group of people interested in studying Judo with him. These classes provided the opportunity for him to experiment with his own ideas that formed the beginning of his thinking on ATM.[8] In addition, he wrote and published several volumes on Judo during this time.[10,11] His study of Judo provided the practical experience of the biomechanics of movement engaging the whole body, which was foundational to his thinking. After World War II, Feldenkrais continued his study of psychology, anatomy, and neurophysiology in London. He became familiar with the work of Frederick Matthias Alexander (who developed a system for changing postural habits through awareness and exercise), Elsa Gindler (who was teaching the importance of sensory awareness), George Gurdjieff (who believed that most humans lived in a perpetual state of "walking sleep" and taught that personal development was a lifelong process of improving self-awareness of the body and the spirit), and Nikolai Bernstein in the Soviet Union (who was developing his now well-known ideas of a dynamic systems description of human movement and action). In London, Feldenkrais also worked with D.G. Morgan, a psychiatrist who believed that the history of a person's experience was locked in the body and could be released by neuromuscular work. This wide-ranging study by Feldenkrais culminated in his publication of *Body and Mature Behavior: A Study of Anxiety, Sex, Gravitation and Learning* in 1949,[12] which was the first comprehensive expression of the philosophy, science, and experience underlying his method of working.

In 1951, Feldenkrais returned to Israel to become head of armed forces research. He continued the development of his psychophysical methods by teaching small group classes during his spare time on weekends and evenings. In 1968, Feldenkrais began his first training program with 14 students in Tel Aviv.[13] This training lasted for 3 years. Later, some of these students traveled with him to the first American training in San Francisco from 1975 to 1977. Sixty people were trained at that program. After the San Francisco training, the Feldenkrais Guild of North America was established under his guidance to support graduates of the training program and to plan and conduct future training programs. In July 1984, on the first day of the author's (JS) training program in Toronto, Ontario, Canada, Feldenkrais died. The Toronto training program and subsequent training programs have been conducted by senior practitioners under the auspices of the Feldenkrais Guild. There are now many chapters of the Feldenkrais Guild and ongoing training programs throughout the world (see Additional Resources).

Philosophical and Theoretical Basis

The initial exposition of Feldenkrais' thinking is set out in *Body and Mature Behavior: A Study of Anxiety, Sex, Gravitation and Learning.*[12] The subtitle suggests the breadth of issues addressed, such as integration, habits, maturity, and learning.

Integration of Body, Mind, and Environment

Feldenkrais believed that the mind, body, and environment were indivisible.[14] He perceived functioning of higher levels of the nervous system as being extremely sensitive to what happens in the body and that the functioning of the body and mind could not be separated from each other or from the experiences of that individual. Feldenkrais also envisioned human nature as being dynamic or changeable, and he believed that the human frame and human behavior are influenced by inherited features and by personal experience. He saw human nature as being flexible, adjustable, and temporary, and he thought that "there is no such thing as a personality without an environment and no behavior without interaction between them."[14]

Habits, Individuality, and Support for Learning

Supporting individuality based on inheritance and personal experience is one of the major features of the Feldenkrais work.

> The manner of projecting the idea of action, the way of motivating and enacting our motivation, the way of rearranging the different body segments, and the way of leaving them after an act is performed, remain our own. They can be detected in our way of doing, our way of thinking, walking, sitting, gripping or letting go, speaking or having sex.[14]

The philosophy of the Feldenkrais Method includes supporting the individual in his or her current way of functioning and providing other choices for the individual that are just as good or even better, and that can be chosen spontaneously by the nervous system. As Feldenkrais wrote:[14]

> [F]aulty action, unnecessary tension, caricature, and holding of the body are not bad in themselves. When we adopted them, they met with our entire wholehearted approval, and with the approval of those who, not knowing any better, appraised our efforts and helped to make us what we are. To destroy these bad habits of use of self without providing better substitutes is not only difficult but foolish.

The patterns of action that were learned provided some useful purpose in our lives or they would not have been chosen as options.

Attempting to "correct" faulty postures, movements, or functions may create anxiety and increase the level of tension within the system. Presenting additional options that are nonjudgmental provides an environment for learning that is safe and allows the individual to explore what works better as opposed to a self-imposed environment that promotes external criticism.

There is no perfect or ideal way of functioning and therefore practitioners do not impose prescribed or correct ways of functioning. Rather, practitioners work to enhance the learning of alternatives that may be more efficient. According to the following passage from Feldenkrais[14]:

> [T]he way we make use of ourselves is the best we can muster with the means at our command at that moment, later we may become aware of other alternatives, but at the moment of action we could not do otherwise. Therefore our use is always the proper one as far as concerns our ability to adjust it at the moment of action. If, we say we stoop badly in walking, it is not because we can do otherwise; but nonetheless, we do make an improper use of the body. Our use of self is as good as our means at the moment permit. To be of any practical use, the mode of doing must not be ideal but expedient—one that can be normally used in our present-day society...The main object is to form an attitude and a new set of responses that permit an even and poised application of oneself to the business of living.

Patterns of movement that become habitual are reinforced by "abstract mental associations, by vegetative states of the body, by muscular and attitudinal patterns, all formed, in a most personal manner, in the course of one's personal history…Providing new options for function is accomplished through bringing awareness to current patterns which include complete perceptions, memory and sensations of action,"[14] whether conscious or unconscious. New patterns of movement can be formed by regrouping the existing patterns and by modifying our responses to intrinsic and extrinsic stimuli through thinking, imagining, inventing, and essentially learning new behaviors.

Enhancing Maturity of Function for a Potent Self

Feldenkrais was interested in developing a method that would assist people to function at a higher level of maturity. In this state of maturity, a person would bring to bear on present circumstance only those past experiences that were appropriate and necessary.[12] This image was embodied for him by the Judo concept of *shizentai*, balanced upright stance. This stance had the following 2 components: (1) posture from which a person could initiate movement in any direction with the same ease, without preliminary adjustments; and (2) performance of movements with the minimal amount of effort and maximum efficiency. Such a person would have the capacity to recover well from any kind of challenge or trauma. Basic to this ideal was a well-developed kinesthetic sense necessary for learning. Feldenkrais saw maturity as the state in which the capacity to learn had reached its highest level of development and a "potent self" as one in which the individual was prepared to act dynamically on a moment-to-moment basis, depending on the demands of the internal and/or external environment.[14]

Learning

Learning is defined as an organic process in which the mental and physical aspects are fully integrated.[14] It proceeds at its own pace; it is completely individualized and guided by the perception of an action feeling easier to do. It occurs most readily in short, focused intervals of attention and when the learner is in a good mood. The outcome of this process is the development of self-knowledge, the awareness of how we perform an action. "Learning is the acquisition of the skill to inhibit parasitic action (components of the action which are unrelated to the intention of the action resulting from some secondary intention) and the ability to direct clear motivations as a result of self knowledge,"[14] Feldenkrais wrote. When initially learning a new skill, many components of movement are performed that interfere with the overall intention of the action. One by one, the parasitic movements are eliminated, leaving only the essential, differentiated action. This learning is different from training, practice, or exercise. It involves the discovery of new ways to do functional activities by broadening the current repertoire of behavior. Children develop this capacity naturally. For example, a 3-year-old child will delight in demonstrating the many different ways that he or she is able to come down the stairs, such as sliding on his or her stomach head first, sliding on his or her stomach feet first, creeping backward, creeping forward, bumping on his or her butt while sitting, walking holding the rail, jumping 2 or 3 steps holding the rail, rolling, and, finally, walking without holding the rail. Learning to come down the stairs can be an exciting process.

Each person learns to satisfy his or her basic needs in his or her own individual way. For an infant, who is dependent on adults for fulfillment of many of those needs, much of the learning process is interpersonal. The infant can therefore develop what Feldenkrais called *cross-motivation*, in which gaining the approval of adults is more important than exploring and learning the task in an individualized way. Successful interpersonal learning occurs when adults support the exploration and satisfaction of needs in a positive and playful way while maintaining safety. However, adults may impose arbitrary and erroneous ideas of caution, prudence, and decent and indecent behavior on the child, and impose punishment or withdraw approval when the child does not perform to their expectations.[14]

Well-meaning adults may interfere with the process of organic learning, limiting the development of skills for performing an activity in multiple ways and constraining control over the subtleties of environmental interaction. Imagine you, as a parent, have anxiety that your child will get hurt coming down the stairs any way other than the conventional way of walking, and you withdraw approval from the child and even punish alternate ways of descending the stairs. Feldenkrais believed that anxiety related to fear of falling could be produced in a child. He also believed that anxiety would be produced when our options were removed and we had no alternative ways of acting.[12] Imagine that you are faced with failing in your professional training and have no other idea of what you might do with your life! Or imagine the difference between walking on a 6-inch-wide beam that rests on the ground compared with a 6-inch-wide beam that is raised 20 feet in the air, where stepping off is not an option.

Feldenkrais clearly conceived of the process of learning as producing new connections, pathways, and associations in the central nervous system. All of the different patterns of innervation involved in the control of voluntary movement develop as the control of action is being learned. So, the control of movement is integrated into "the vast background of vegetative and reflexive activity of the nervous system."[12] The imposition of anxiety, compulsion, or cross-motivation on this process of learning created what Feldenkrais referred to as *faulty learning*. The child learns to produce the behavior that is expected, the posture that is approved, or the expression that is acceptable, and does not learn to test behavior primarily against present reality. The continual learning process that might go on throughout life in a mature person could come to a standstill. How many 60- or 70-year-old adults can still come down the stairs 9 different ways? In the adult, habitual patterns formed over the years have molded the body to produce, for example, flat feet, stiff shoulders, a neck that will not turn, or a painful low back. The problem may not be with the feet, back, or neck. It may be with the stereotypical, parasitic neuromuscular patterns that have formed in which excessive effort is used, and the person has lost the ability to adapt to new situations by learning.[12]

Later in his career, Feldenkrais recognized that physical injury and malfunction of the nervous system interacted significantly with the process of neuromuscular habit formation. If the nervous system does not work properly in any of its motor, sensory, or integrative/cognitive components, it becomes difficult or impossible to produce the normal functional control patterns used in everyday life. A musculoskeletal injury, a stroke, or the development of multiple sclerosis may create pain or alter the anatomy, therefore interfering with normal function. Or a person who has rigid and maladaptive neuromuscular habit patterns will be more likely to be injured in an automobile accident and less likely to adapt and recover after the accident than a person who can learn and adapt quickly.[7] The challenge in these cases is to establish a process for learning new options for optimal ways of functioning based upon current structural, cognitive, emotional, sensory, and motor constraints.

What would it take for a 70-year-old individual to have a movement repertoire that included the 9 ways of coming down the stairs mentioned earlier? Or to return the arm and hand of a concert flutist, damaged by a bullet, to its previous world-class level of function? Or for a child born with cerebral palsy to learn to walk? Feldenkrais believed that the key to these transformations was the education or reeducation of the kinesthetic sense and the process of resetting function to new patterns that can self-adjust as demands on the individual change.

APPROACHES TO THE CLIENT

The Feldenkrais Method is practiced in 2 forms: FI and ATM.

Functional Integration

An FI lesson is a one-on-one, hands-on approach to learning that occurs in a safe, supportive, and nonjudgmental environment. The practitioner uses passive movement and resistance to passive movement through the skeleton to explore the student's current state of functioning in the world. Lessons are aimed at increasing the student's awareness of how he or she moves, discovering alternative ways of functioning in the world beyond what is already familiar, and increasing fluidity, ease, and efficiency of movement.[15]

Environment and Orientation to the World

Students are guided to become more familiar with their current organization of body segments in relation to other segments and to the support surface. The way that the student most often organizes his or her body segments at rest and during functional activities is a reflection of his or her orientation to the world and preparedness to move in different directions at a particular moment in time. There are generally commonalities in how an individual organizes while in different positions and while performing varying tasks. For example, an individual may demonstrate a forward head position while sitting, standing, lying, and performing all functional activities. The beginning of an FI lesson is generally performed with the student's body in a fully supported position, such as sitting or lying, so that his or her system is responding to a neutral, quiet environment in which learning can be optimized. Rollers, pillows, and bolsters may be used to support the student in his or her current organization, filling in spaces between the student and the surface to facilitate a sense of support.[15]

Communication Through "Passive Touch"

A minimal amount of verbal instruction is provided during an FI lesson. The practitioner uses gentle, "passive" movement to stimulate the student's self-awareness and a sense of curiosity about movement processes. Movement is not passive in the sense of the participant being inactive. It is movement that is introduced by the practitioner to ask questions about the student's nervous system, such as which direction is easiest, how does it translate to other body segments, what happens when the direction is varied, and how does it compare on different sides of the body? The practitioner's hands are not used to push or manipulate, although there is intent to convey how that person typically functions by drawing attention to motions that are easy and to how movement translates to other body segments. Alternatives to easy movements are explored by varying motions around those who are already easy.[15]

The quality of touch used in FI differs from other forms of manual guidance[16,17] or haptic guidance,[18,19] in which the practitioner or a machine provides passive movement with a prescriptive or corrective intent to augment learning. During an FI lesson, the practitioner has no preconceived notions of how the person should move. The passive guidance of an FI lesson is used to enhance the discovery of body awareness and to provide both intrinsic and extrinsic feedback to the student about movement affordances and limitations, functional relationships between body segments, and functioning of the whole.[15] The practitioner explores what movements are possible without neural resistance and what makes sense for that person based on inherent constraints and affordances to movements, alignment of bony segments in relationship to the support surface, and greater efficiency for movement during functional activities.

When the student's body is relaxed and moved passively, there is a chain reaction of movement throughout the skeleton that is similar to the observed phenomenon of knocking over a set of dominos. If no muscles were present to constrain or influence passive movement through the skeleton, movement would travel through the skeleton unimpeded. Attempts to correct someone's familiar habit patterns can stimulate fear and the subconscious tension of muscles. It is important to establish trust with the client. For example, if a practitioner were to try and realign an individual's standing alignment to an arbitrary posture, the person may feel unbalanced and fearful, resulting in the freezing or locking of adjacent body segments in an attempt to prevent falling. The imposed alignment may not be a good option for that person and is dependent upon many factors, including morphology, center of mass, increased excitation in the nervous system, and past experiences.[20] Passive touch is therefore used to augment what is already working for the student and helps the nervous system to spontaneously shift to other ways of functioning that may serve the student better.

In a hands-on FI lesson, the practitioner's ability to move freely and easily with the student can affect the student's ability to learn. The lesson is similar to ballroom dancing, in which 2 people move symbiotically, becoming one with each other by being in a place of physical, psychological, and emotional receptivity to the other person's movements. During an FI lesson, the practitioner's position relative to the student, the support surface, and the practitioner's own habit patterns play a role in the ability of the student and practitioner to become completely receptive and engaged in the exploration of movement at any moment in time. Practitioners spend a great deal of time during their formal training learning to organize themselves so that their own interactions in the world will be less likely to limit those of the students with whom they work.

Reducing Effort

Feldenkrais believed that use of effort and willpower to complete movements and maintain postures would tend to limit freedom of movement and thereby reduce choices for action.[7] FI lessons generally begin with "passive" movement by the practitioner to minimize the use of effort by the student. Effortful movements tend to reinforce embedded habit patterns and may limit access to movements that are new or unfamiliar. Movements are explored initially in small ranges and at slow speeds to reduce unnecessary effort. As the lesson progresses, the movements may become faster, larger, and more playful as the range of free, unguarded movement increases.

Learning to reduce muscular effort is also encouraged by passively supporting the student's body segments using rolls, pillows, bolsters, and/or the practitioner's hands to match and/or augment habit patterns. Matching and/or augmenting familiar, easy patterns set the stage for a safe, nonthreatening context for learning. This is analogous to the exploratory behavior of a toddler who runs back and forth between the safety of a parent and the curiosity of a new toy or person in the room. When the parent is not present, the child stops playing and becomes anxious. The presence of the parent provides a sense of security from which the child can explore. Likewise, matching rather than correcting or insisting upon change in posture or a movement pattern sets the stage for safe exploration and integration of alternative ways of using one's body.

Active Movements to Consolidate Learning

As an FI lesson progresses, the student may be asked to move some parts of his or her body actively while the practitioner moves other segments passively. Passive movements may also be followed by purely active movements on the part of the student. Current research shows that passive movements help with initial skill acquisition; however, active movements are generally better for retention of learning.[21] Novel movements and movement combinations are used to draw attention to the process of movement. The client may also be asked to imagine the movement using motor and/or visual imagery.[22] Movements are practiced in varied positions against gravity, in different contexts, and during functional activities to generalize the learning to other situations. Each repetition of a movement takes on a slightly different pathway within the habit or attractor pattern, which expands upon the student's options for easy movement. Repetition of movement is used not for the sake of practice but to familiarize the person with how he or she is moving and to bring attention and awareness to a particular function. Frequent, brief rest periods are provided to give the person time to process and integrate movement comparisons into memory. There are no exercises to practice following a lesson, although the student may be asked to explore and compare similar movements during the following week to reinforce concepts learned during a lesson.

Working With Specific Issues

When pain is present, the practitioner generally begins working at a distant area of the body to minimize the student's anxiety and muscle tension. For example, if the student has a painful shoulder or neck, the practitioner may choose to start the lesson at the person's feet and build upon the ease of movement there. Small, indirect movements may occur simultaneously at other segments as anxiety and co-contraction of muscles decrease. In a situation involving a person with a neurological injury, such as a stroke, the practitioner often works with the less-affected side of the body first, especially when sensory deficits limit the student's ability to feel what is happening on the more affected side. This process is less confrontational to the student and evokes less anxiety by focusing on movements that he or she is able to perceive easily and that he or she is successful in using for function. The practitioner uses passive movements to help the student actively compare what is happening on one side of the body with the other side and/or one body segment moving on another.

Examination, Evaluation, and Reassessment

The practitioner begins an FI session by observing the student's movements upon entering the room, analyzing aspects of functioning, such as affective state, alignment of body segments, base of support, coordination of movement, breathing patterns, and relative movement between different body segments. The student is queried about what he or she would like to improve about his or her functioning during the lesson.

The practitioner observes the student's initial postural configuration at rest (alignment of body segments relative to other segments, to gravity, and to the support surface [in sitting, standing, and/or lying]). Arrangement and folds of the student's clothing and body contours can provide additional information about the way the individual organizes him- or herself in relationship to the world.

Following the initial postural assessment, the practitioner may ask the student to actively move as part of a functional activity, such as reaching, bending forward, or turning. The practitioner makes notes of aspects of the movement, including eye gaze and tracking; facial expression; and the initiation, smoothness, speed, direction and excursion of movement. The practitioner observes how movement translates from one body segment to the next, and if there are restrictions to the flow of movement between segments.[15]

Passive movement is assessed using a very gentle, supportive contact of the practitioner's hands with the student's skeleton. The practitioner then assesses for the student's ease and willingness to be moved passively in various directions from the student's initial postural configuration. The practitioner makes a mental note of directions in which movement are easy or less easy, the quality of the movement and how that movement translates to other body segments, and through the skeleton as a whole. The practitioner feels for the first inkling of muscular resistance to passive movement, while observing for dampening of the chain reaction through the skeleton. Constraints to the flow of movement between body segments are noted and brought to the student's attention, as are areas of the body that are used as pivots around which functional movements occur easily.

Lesson Design and Focus

Information from the student's history and the practitioner's observations of the student's active and passive movements are considered and compared in relationship to the student's initial reports and requests.[15] The practitioner gathers this information and uses it to decide on a lesson for the student that will augment his or her current level of functioning. FI lessons are generally based on documented ATM lessons designed by Feldenkrais; they are modified by the practitioner on a moment-to-moment basis throughout the course of a lesson.[15] Ongoing judgments for how to proceed with the lesson are made based on what makes the most sense for that individual at that moment and not on preconceived notions of what is "normal" or "correct." The practitioner takes into account the student's reports and requests, knowledge of the student's background, knowledge, and experience when designing a lesson for the student.

Themes of a lesson include the following: (1) enhancing the student's orientation within the environment; (2) enhancing fluidity, ease, and efficiency of movement; and (3) enhancing the sense of differentiation or integration of body segments to the whole.[15]

Orientating the student to the environment includes working on postural control by enhancing the student's sense of weight shift; awareness of orientation of the eyes at rest and during functional activities; sense of support of the skeleton in relationship to gravity; and the support surface, self-image, and body image.[15]

Lessons focused on enhancing fluidity, efficiency, and ease of movement may include comparisons of effort, resistance and/or constraint to movement, segments of the body from which the student initiates movement most often, and changes in the tonus of the muscles. As the lesson proceeds, the practitioner engages the student's interest through the exploration of active and/or passive movement options, speed, direction, magnitude, and quality of movement.[15]

Practitioners also structure lessons to enhance the student's perception of how movement translates between body segments and through the whole skeleton during functional and passive movement activities. Lessons of this nature include enhancing the student's perception of the differentiation of movement of body segments from the whole and/or integrating movement of specific body segments to movements of the whole.

When the practitioner observes and/or palpates restrictions to movement through the skeleton from a particular vantage point, he or she may choose to change the point of contact of his or her hand(s) with the student's body segment, change the angle or direction of movement, or switch to a different body segment to affect the flow of movement through the skeleton.

Case Example 1

A woman in her early 50s with cerebral palsy requested Feldenkrais lessons to improve the smoothness and safety of her walking. She also wanted to be able to stand on one foot. Her movement assessment showed that she had difficulty uncoupling the joints of her lower extremities while sitting, standing, lying down, and on her hands and knees. Her lessons focused on supporting her initial configuration. When lying on her back, her pelvis was rotated to the right, both of her left lower extremities were rolled toward the right, and there was little, if any, movement at her hip joints. As part of the lesson, her pelvis and lower extremities were rolled further toward the right and were briefly compared with movement to the left. Her left lower extremity had greater availability of movement than the right, so movement on that leg was explored first. Rolling her leg to the right automatically brought the pelvis to the right so the pelvic motion was augmented and then differentiated from the leg. The practitioner also worked on gently pushing from the sole of the foot through the leg to initiate movement of the leg in the socket of the hip. As the practitioner did this subtle movement, she varied the amount of roll of the leg slightly each time so that the client could begin to feel the movement of the leg in the joint. In amazement, the client said, "I didn't know I had a joint there." She asked to see an anatomy book to confirm that there was supposed to be a joint at her hip where she had never felt one. During that lesson, the practitioner was also able to bring the client's knee up toward her body by rolling her leg further out and bending the knee. They then explored movement at the hip joint within the tiny zone of comfort that was available with the hip and knee bent. When the client's muscles would grab, the practitioner would wait for the contraction to let up before exploring another slight variation to the movement. The stiffness that had been so evident in her legs changed significantly. At the end of that lesson, they practiced lifting one leg in standing while holding onto the back of a chair. The client was able to march in place by raising her feet several inches off the floor without having to lean backward. She had learned to disassociate, or uncouple, her leg from her pelvis for the first time in her life.

Case Example 2

Often, the changes in postural configuration and functional abilities that occur are not linearly related to the lesson. For example, the author had a client in her 90s who came for lessons to improve the way she was walking. She arrived for her first lesson with a walker and had a great deal of difficulty climbing steps. She was very hunched over and she complained of weakness and stiffness in her knees. When lying down, she was unable to fully straighten her hips or knees and she needed 2 pillows under her head to accommodate her forward head position and rounded shoulders. Her FI lesson brought her further into her initial configuration of flexion of the trunk and lower extremities. By building upon her willingness to move into flexion and listening to her system for directions of ease versus resistance, eventually she was able to lie on her back while curled in a ball and holding her knees. In this position, the practitioner could roll her side to side. Briefly, toward the end of the session with the woman still lying on her back, the practitioner helped her to explore pushing with one foot or the other into the table with bent knees. When she stood up, her posture was much more erect, and she reported that her legs felt stronger and less stiff. Several days later, the practitioner received a phone call from the student. She reported that she had taken a bath by herself for the first time in 1 year and that she had no problems getting out of the tub. The changes in function were nonlinear in the sense that the practitioner never worked on teaching her how to get in or out of the tub and never worked directly on improving her erect standing or walking.

Case Example 3

In addition to identifying ways in which the initial configuration could be achieved more completely, the practitioner also helps to identify pathways of connections between body segments that are more consistent with the bony skeleton and with function. Take, for example, the case of a 74-year-old woman with a history of several falls and pain in her right groin and knee that had been present for years who came for FI lessons. She had received physical therapy and acupuncture treatments with some short-term relief. Movement assessment revealed that she was organized, with her pelvis rotated to the right and her upper body rotated to the left when sitting, standing, and lying down. In addition, her right shoulder was rolled forward and her right upper arm was held firmly at her side when lying down. When pressing down through her first rib to assess movement through her skeleton from the base of her neck toward her feet, her right side moved down easily while her left side did not. The body segment components of this configuration were augmented first. Then right and left side-bending of the trunk were compared. The right side bent easily in a direction of slight extension; however, when guiding the movement from the neck down, the motion traveled down to only the middle of the rib cage before moving off to the left. There was no connection to the feet. This was compared with the left side, which did not side bend. The opposing configuration between the pelvis and the lower ribs was augmented and held for her to take over the work of habitual muscle contraction. Providing support into her initial configuration allowed her to relax and let her pelvis and lower ribs move more easily together to the left. Movement through the skeleton from the right side of the neck became more clear in the direction of the left pelvis and left leg, but was still moving off to the left in the mid-rib area. As side bend of the trunk at different levels was again compared, side bend to the left became easier and movement down through the neck to the left foot was more consistent. From there, the lesson progressed to reversals of rolling to the left and onto the back, to sitting, and, eventually, to standing. Reaching toward the left with the right arm while in sitting and in standing positions was compared with reaching toward the right with the left arm while in the same positions. The client reported almost total relief of pain for several days and being able to perform heavy house cleaning, which she was previously unable to do, following the lesson.

Awareness Through Movement

ATM is a verbally directed movement process that can be performed with one person or in group settings. In fact, Feldenkrais held public workshops with as many as 300 participants. An ATM lesson can be held in person by a practitioner; presented on audiotape, CD, or DVD; or downloaded from the Internet in MP3 or other file format. Hundreds of ATM lessons are commercially available (see openATM.org from the list of Additional Resources at the end of the chapter as an example). Many practitioners record lessons for client to take home to work with. When many people participate in a lesson at the same time, different people respond in very individualized ways using action pieces from the lesson, as they are able, for mini-lessons at a level that they can manage.[23]

An ATM lesson is a structured movement exploration that makes use of common movement forms to explore how the individual organizes his or her control of movement. For the practitioner, it is like taking the client on a leisurely stroll along the edge of a canyon while feeling safe and in control, appreciating the view and knowing that there may be something different just over the edge. A lesson is commonly performed with the client lying supine, lying prone, sitting, or standing, and involves small turns, bends, or weight shifts. The goal is for the student to be able to perceive excessive effort, make the least amount of effort needed, and inhibit unnecessary efforts and movements while remaining in complete control of the movement process. The client may be manually or verbally cued during this process to facilitate recognition of what is happening. The guiding therapeutic idea for the practitioner physical therapist is to engage the client in a movement that will integrate involved areas of the body using the whole body, which have functional value for the client. Arriving at the functional movement may be the result of a longer process that addresses smaller component limitations along the way.

Slow, small, simple movements are done at first to reduce effort and optimize awareness. The Weber-Fechner principle in sensory physiology shows us that excessive effort interferes with our ability to perceive small changes.[24] A lesson might begin with a very small movement involving external rotation of the hip with flexion of the knee while the student is in the supine position. This movement would be repeated in slightly different ways 10 to 20 times. During this process, awareness would be directed to changes in other areas of the body related to this movement. There may be rotation of the spine so that the opposite hip lifts from the floor, a change in the pattern of breathing, a stiffening of the opposite leg or foot, or pressing into the floor with the opposite leg. When this simple movement is optimally performed using the whole body, the opposite leg will be fully relaxed and the spine will be able to turn as weight is transferred laterally with the core of the body controlling the movement. (One part of the body not doing anything, such as the leg resting during movement of another part of the body, can be an optimal part of a movement pattern depending on the intention of the movement. One of the recurrent themes in ATM lessons is for the client to learn to use the power of the core muscles to control movement effectively.) Other parts of the body would then be free to move in other directions; turning or nodding of the head, for example, should be easy. If a person is holding his or her leg or foot stiffly, holding his or her breath, or not experiencing a weight shift through the skeleton during movement, then he or she is making unnecessary, excessive muscular efforts to perform that movement. The effort spent on this habit interferes with the perception of action, the control of movement, and the integration of effort into subsequent continuing movement.

These kinds of observations are the bases of the assessment performed in conjunction with ATM. As practitioners, we look for how a person organizes his or her weight through the skeleton in relation to the base of support. Is the use of the skeleton efficient? How much effort does the person make to hold a position or to transition from a position? Are all of the body segments organized to participate optimally in the intention of the movement, or is one leg possibly anchoring with a different intention, thus making the movement less efficient and potentially dangerous? Is the timing of control of one body segment contributing optimally to the movement of other body segments? Is momentum being used and controlled effectively? The more a person is able to reduce effort and discriminate small changes, the more finely he or she can control any action.

ATM lessons commonly make use of novelty. Lessons can be structured in such a way that the outcome of the movement (eg, rolling over, standing up) is not obvious during the process. This use of novelty allows the client to develop better awareness of the details of the unfolding movement in progress without reverting back to habitual movement patterns. (We all know how to roll over, in the way that we roll over.) In this way, new patterns of motor control can be developed.

Case Example

A 41-year-old clinical psychologist and professional singer with a 20-year history of recurring headaches and chronic pain in her upper back, lower back, and neck was referred after sustaining an injury from trying to open a heavy door. The effort of opening the door had caused a spasm of pain in her right lower back, from which upper-back and neck stiffness developed over the next day without resolution. Her diagnoses included right sacroiliac joint dysfunction, pelvic hypermobility, cervical and thoracic facet joint malalignment, and mild (less than 20 degrees) scoliosis with apices at C5, T6, and L2. Lifting or carrying even very light objects also set off her back pain, often incapacitating her for weeks. Because of this type of onset, she had severely limited her activities, leading to further loss of function and loss of independence in many daily activities.

She had previously been treated in a variety of ways, including bed rest, heavy medication for pain, myofascial release, traditional strengthening and range of motion, and Pilates technique, all with limited success. Initial observations of her movement showed that she was unable to organize abdominal muscles well in supine transfers, depending more than usual on upper-extremity assistance during these transfers, and unable to lift her head off of the floor while in the supine position.

She was also fearful of making a lot of movement because of the frequent disastrous consequences she had experienced. Her demonstration of the precipitating event during the initial assessment clearly showed that she was unfamiliar with the process of stabilizing one's body from the floor up and transferring power from the legs through the abdominal core and into the upper extremities to exert force on the door.

She had a general problem with effective motor control, not simply a problem of weakness. The intervention lessons were designed around how she could learn to use her abdominal core again in a coordinated and powerful way. The ATM process outlined in the following bulleted list was a part of her treatment plan. It unfolded slowly over the course of 8 once-weekly sessions. As she developed mastery of these movement problems, she ceased having headaches, had much less tension in her upper back and neck, and experienced reduced low back pain. She was able to bend, reach, lift, and carry light objects with much more ease. She could lift her head up from the supine position and get up from the floor without any thought of difficulty. The process of learning abdominal control was organic, embedded in a variety of functional movement patterns.

Awareness Through Movement Lessons

Each of the following bullets is a movement sequence that was explored in many repetitions and variations in the order presented, with her responses marked in italics.

- From a long-sit position leaning back on the hands, slowly bend the legs and posteriorly tilt the pelvis until the feet come off of the floor. *Initially, she had difficulty with pain in her low back, upper back, and neck that eased as she found a way to take weight more symmetrically through her ischial bones and to bring her head forward, closer to her base of support.*

- While sitting with the legs flexed, the feet in the air, and the hands on the knees, slowly rock in different directions. A process of progressive approximation should be used to develop this movement sequence. For example, begin with lifting one foot off of the floor while shifting weight slightly toward the right ischium. Then lift both feet slightly off of the floor while shifting weight to the right. Repeat similar movements to the left side. With both feet in the air, move one knee in small circles, then move the other knee in small circles. *Initially, she was able to move very little without losing her balance. Her range and control of motion increased considerably as she discovered how she could laterally flex and rotate her spine to bring her head closer over her base of support.*

- While maintaining sitting balance with the hands on the knees and the feet in the air, slowly move and twist the legs side to side and turn the head in the same and opposite directions. *She developed skill in these movements as she discovered how to let her weight go further out to the side on her pelvis and turn her legs in a different direction at the same time.*

- From sitting with the hands on the knees, slowly roll backward with a rounded back so as to roll the back to the floor with the pelvis coming up into the air and the weight shifting onto the shoulders, then roll back up to sitting. *Initially, she was very afraid to do this; in fact, her back slapped flat against the floor during her first attempt. Slowly, she learned to curl her spine so that she could feel each vertebra as it met the floor. When she reached this stage of control, she was able to roll her back down onto the floor and roll back up with minimal effort and use of momentum. At this point, she was able to stabilize her core and control its rotation effectively as she opened a heavy door in her home, which she had been unable to do previously.*

- Roll down to the floor and then back up as she had learned per the previous bullet, coming all the way to standing. *Coming back up, it was suggested that she try flexing one leg, rolling up onto the flexed leg, placing her same-side hand onto the floor beside her, letting her momentum and a small push with the supporting hand and leg carry her up to standing. She had trouble with the placement of her hand and foot on the floor in optimal positions to support her into standing. Many positions were tried before she found that if she let her body weight come forward far enough over her hand and feet the natural extension of these limbs brought her to standing. An important*

point in her learning was realizing how to integrate the timing of the different parts of the move-
ment with having the movement be continuous without stopping anywhere until she was standing.
This last piece of the sequence allowed her to experience the integration of forceful movement from
her feet to her hand controlled and stabilized through her core.

A natural question might be: Why go to all of this apparent trouble over 8 weeks instead of just teaching her to brace herself with her legs when opening the door? The answer is simple enough. While going through this process of motor learning, she developed a whole new awareness of her body and how to control its movement. The process itself changed her brain, her perceptual/motor processing. The likelihood that this was the case is explained in the neuroplasticity portion of the following Evidence of Efficacy: Review of the Research section. She accessed other benefits from this process including the ability to reach objects from high and low shelves and to carry them easily; and a return to playing the piano and jogging, which she had not done in years. None of these things was practiced directly. She knew how to do them already, but now in a slightly different way.

EVIDENCE OF EFFICACY: REVIEW OF THE RESEARCH

In 1949, Feldenkrais wrote the following[12]:

> The human brain is such as to make…acquisition of new responses a normal activity… This great ability to form individual nervous paths makes it possible for faulty patterns to be learned. The faulty behavior will appear in the executive motor mechanisms, which will seem inherent to the person and unalterable. It will remain largely so unless the nervous paths producing the undesirable pattern of motility are undone and reshuffled into a better configuration.

Patterns of behavior are learned and etched into the brain. ATM and FI were the tools used to work with movement and action to "reshuffle to a better configuration."[12] Recently, researchers were able to draw a direct link between the tools of ATM and FI and the principles and processes of motor learning.[25]

There has been a growing body of neuroscience literature over the past 30 years that is expanding our understanding of brain plasticity and is linking it to motor learning in just the way that Feldenkrais imagined. This research is building a picture of modulation of excitation and inhibition playing an important role in changes in synaptic efficiency. These interactions are the basis for changes in behavior, enhancement of skill, and recovery from nervous system injury.[26-37] The idea of the rewiring synaptic connections and their pathways in the central nervous system as the basis for recovery of function is now widely accepted.[38,39] Nair et al[39] have used functional magnetic resonance imaging to demonstrate improved activation of the involved motor cortex paralleled by improved hand function following a Feldenkrais intervention in a patient 9 months after stroke. The basal ganglia is an area of the brain that is central to adaptive motor control processes and learning.[32] It has been suggested that the process of motor learning itself may be impaired in the basal ganglia in some cases and that some forms of dystonia may be exacerbated by intensive motor learning experiences.[40,41] This very process has been described as happening during a Feldenkrais training, which both provides evidence for the Feldenkrais Method as a motor learning modality and suggests caution about its use in this particular instance.[42] Feldenkrais developed a perceptual motor process that he imagined would produce plasticity in the brain. The question that we want to address here is, "Does this method produce significant and appropriate functional change and recovery?"

Much of the published work on the Feldenkrais Method is in the form of single or multiple case studies. These reports contain detailed information about interventions that have been highly successful in producing functional gains. Examples of this type of literature include reports of improved functional mobility in a group of people with spinal cord injury[43] and with a set of individual cases,[44] the reduction of stuttering in 3 people using FI,[50] dramatic functional improvements in

2 women with traumatic brain injury,[46] the resolution of back pain,[47,48] the reduction of pain and improved mobility in 4 women with rheumatoid arthritis,[49] improved mobility and well-being in 4 women with multiple sclerosis,[24] improved balance and mobility in a woman with multiple sclerosis,[50] improved flexibility and mobility in a woman with hereditary spastic paraparesis,[51] and improved function in patients with Parkinson's disease.[52] Stephens[53] has reported outcomes from clinical practice that demonstrate, out of a total of nearly 200 clients and approximately 90 different International Classification of Diseases-9 diagnostic codes, a greater than 80% rate of clients achieving 100% of initial goals and a greater than 90% rate of clients achieving at least 75% of initial goals. The number of visits per episode of care fell well within the guidelines suggested by the *Guide to Physical Therapist Practice*.[54]

Ives and Shelly[55] reviewed the research published through 1996 and noted that, in many cases, well-controlled research designs were not used or there were other flaws in the experimental procedures. However, they concluded that further research was warranted due to the "sheer number of positive reports that fit within a sound theoretical framework."[55] More recently, a number of studies incorporating more-effective methods, larger groups, and random assignment control groups have been conducted. Four general areas of clinical outcomes will be presented in the following sections: (1) pain management, (2) motor control, (3) mobility and postural control, and (4) psychological and quality-of-life effects.

Pain Management

Boudreau et al[56] have proposed that motor learning strategies and plasticity may play an important role in treatment strategies for musculoskeletal pain disorders. Pain is perhaps the most common complaint that brings people to a Feldenkrais practitioner.[53] This has been studied in a variety of ways. Fibromyalgia is an increasingly common diagnosis. A study of 5 women with fibromyalgia using ATM twice weekly for 2 months revealed a significant decrease in pain and improved posture, gait, sleep, and body awareness.[57] In an attempt to replicate this work, Stephens et al,[58] using a repeated measures design with 16 people with fibromyalgia, observed changes in pain and mobility variables. However, these were overshadowed by the high variability of repeated baseline measures. In another study of the fibromyalgia population, initial improvements found during the 15-week intervention were not maintained at the 6-month follow-up.[59] Again, methodological problems were cited in this study. Treatment of fibromyalgia using body awareness therapy, closely related to Feldenkrais Method, has also been studied, with positive effects on pain and movement quality.[60]

Edwards and colleagues[61] present the Feldenkrais Method as a philosophically different approach to the treatment of pain based on the approach of relearning skilled movement rather than focusing on pain management. This approach makes use of the growing idea that pain experience is largely cognitive.[62] Bearman and Shafarman[63] found large decreases in pain perception, improvements in functional status, reduction in use of pain medication, and a 40% reduction in the cost of medical care during a 1-year follow-up period for a group of 7 patients with chronic pain following an 8-week intensive Feldenkrais Method intervention. Working with 34 patients with chronic pain in a retrospective study, Phipps et al[64] showed that the Feldenkrais Method helped to reduce pain and improve function and that learned ATM methods were still used independently by patients 2 years post-discharge. In a study of 97 automobile workers in Sweden, Lundblad and colleagues[65] found significant decreases in reports of neck and shoulder pain and in disability during leisure activity in individuals in the Feldenkrais intervention group compared with those randomly assigned to physical therapy and no intervention control groups. In another large trial, the Feldenkrais Method was found to be an effective intervention for neck and scapular pain in a randomized control study of 61 visually impaired people.[66]

DeRosa and Porterfield[67] included the Feldenkrais Method among a number of intervention methods that would most successfully address the motor control elements underlying much of the presenting back pain seen in physical therapy clinics. Since this work, it has been widely recognized that active exercise is a more-effective intervention for back pain than other, more passive approaches. Maher[68] has recommended that the Feldenkrais Method not be considered as an intervention for low back pain based on the idea that there is little high-quality evidence supporting its efficacy. The same conclusion was reached with regard to mechanical neck pain in another study.[69] Both of these papers conclude that the lack of supporting evidence from large clinical trials is a reason to not use the Feldenkrais Method.

In other pain-related work, Rogers[70] has provided evidence that people who have used Feldenkrais ATM and other body awareness therapies have a greater awareness of the mechanisms of injury occurring during piano practice and therefore a better opportunity to develop preventative strategies. More recently, the Feldenkrais Method was used to significantly decrease the severity and frequency of tension and pain in 130 high school musicians.[71] O'Connor and Webb[72] have reported that the Feldenkrais Method can be used effectively as part of palliative care for people who are in chronic pain.

The Feldenkrais Method is based, in part, on the concept that awareness of body and movement are the basis for change in behavior and physiology. However, this has not yet been directly tested. Mehling et al[73] have developed an interesting tool to assess changes in awareness. This differentiates between interoceptive and other types of body awareness. Positive findings using this tool will make a stronger connection between the physical process of movement and the changes observed following movement. In summary, the Feldenkrais Method, which appears to have great potential as an intervention for pain, needs to be better supported by more large, randomized controlled trials.

Motor Control

In the area of motor control, 3 types of problems have been explored: (1) changes in the activity of a muscle group during a standard task, (2) changes in postural control related to breathing, and (3) changes in postural control related to standing balance and mobility. In a study involving 21 subjects, researchers found that an ATM lesson exploring cervical flexion led to a decrease in abdominal electromyogram activity and a perception of the standardized supine flexion task being easier.[74] A second group was used to control for the possible effects of imagery and suggestion used during the ATM process, suggesting that the changes noted were a result of the exploratory movements alone. In another study involving 30 subjects, the authors reported an increase in supine neck flexion range of motion and a decrease in perceived effort in this movement compared with a control group.[75]

Several groups have been interested in studying effects on hamstring length.[76-79] The initial studies of hamstring function by James et al[76] and Hopper et al[77] reported no change in hamstring length following a single ATM lesson designed to lengthen hamstrings compared with relaxation and normal-activity control groups. These studies looked at the effects of ATM following a single lesson. Stephens et al[78] studied the effects of a set of hamstring lengthening ATM lessons used over a period of 3 weeks. There was a significant increase in hamstring length observed in the ATM group compared with a normal-activity control group. The magnitude of length change seen in this study was equivalent to changes noted in the literature for muscle lengthening in various ways but without stretching, suggesting that a period of time longer than a single lesson may be required for adequate learning in most people. Researchers also observed that very short ATM sessions over the same time period had the same effect. Chowdhury[79] corroborated this result using a stretching control group.

Saraswati[80] showed changes in breathing patterns involving increased movement of the abdomen, postural changes involving increased use of erector spinae muscles, and increased peak flow rates in individuals who received a series of ATM lessons compared with a matched group of young, healthy controls. The use of ATM to improve breathing, mobility, and postural control has also been reported in a case study of a man with Parkinson's disease.[81]

Mobility and Postural Control

Improvement in balance and mobility was an early interest and observation of Feldenkrais research. Now, with increasing emphasis in the safety and well-being of the elderly, this is gaining in significance and is better supported by research. For example, in a study with 59 well, elderly women who were randomly divided into 3 groups, Hall et al[82] reported improvements in activities of daily living scores, Timed Up and Go scores, Berg Balance Scale scores, and 3 of 8 scales on the 36-Item Short Form Survey following a 10-week series of ATM lessons. In another study, Seegert and Shapiro[83] have also reported changes in static standing control in healthy, young subjects. Further, several studies[24,84-86] have shown improvements in functional mobility using Timed Up and Go and other measures. These studies have been conducted with well elderly people,[84,85] people with multiple sclerosis,[24,86] and people who suffer from cerebrovascular accidents (CVAs).[87]

These initial investigations have been followed recently by larger controlled studies with community-dwelling adults (mean age, 75 years), showing clinically significant improvements in gait speed, Timed up and Go scores, and Falls Efficacy scale scores[88]; and in gait speed, Four Step Square Test scores, and Activities-Specific Balance Confidence scale scores.[25] Ullmann et al[89] found similar results working with a similar population. These results are also supported by other more-recent studies, all using widely accepted outcome measures[90] and relatively large, controlled sample sizes.[91-93] Each study used between 15 to 20 total group ATM classes over a period of 5 to 10 weeks. All these results build a strong case for a significant role for ATM in improving the community functioning of healthy older adults.

Several studies suggest a possible mechanism for these improvements in balance and mobility. DellaGrotte and colleagues[94] have shown reorganization of global postural measures, including skeletal alignment and muscular control, using a process of intervention developed from the Feldenkrais Method called *Core Integration*. This approach uses both individual hands-on (FI) and group instruction (ATM) learning processes. Working with a more-cognitive aspect of postural control, Ullmann and Williams[95] looked at dual-task performance using a GAITRite Walkway system. They observed improvements in balance and gait under single-task conditions and positive changes ($P = .067$) in mobility under dual-task conditions.

In an initial study of 4 women with multiple sclerosis, Stephens et al[24] documented improvements in transfers and a subjective report of generally improved control of balance and movement. In a follow-up study with a group of 12 people with multiple sclerosis, Stephens et al[86] found significant improvements in balance performance and balance confidence in persons who participated in a set of ATM classes compared with individuals in a group meeting for educational purposes only, using a randomized control group design. Batson and Deutsch[87] have provided similar evidence of improved balance and mobility in a pilot study of stroke patients.

Psychological and Quality of Life Effects

As noted earlier, Feldenkrais' thinking was driven by theory from psychology and physiology. An overriding interest was to find a method of improving the level of maturity with which people function in their lives.[12] Frank[96] has discussed the role of proprioception, what he refers to as "awareness through movement," in the development and regulation of self-perception throughout life. He came to the conclusion, which was in agreement with Feldenkrais, that a cohesive experience of the body is at the core of individual health and maturity. This suggests that changes in psychological variables, such as body image, self-efficacy, anxiety, and life satisfaction, should be studied.

In a qualitative study of 10 people who had prolonged experience of FI, Steisel[97] reported improvements in body awareness, motivation, self-esteem, and decreases in anxiety. In a study using clay figure analysis, Deig[98] described expansion in the detail and form of body image after a series of ATM lessons. This work was extended by Elgelid,[99] who found improvements in body image resulting from a series of ATM lessons using the Jourard-Secord Cathexis Scale. Hutchinson[100] also used this scale and reported improvements in body image in a group of women who were overweight. The best-designed study in this area involved a matched, control group study of 30 patients with eating disorders by Laumer et al,[101] who used standardized psychological testing to measure outcomes. They concluded that a 9-hour course of ATM improved the level of acceptance of the body and self, decreased feelings of helplessness and dependence, increased self-confidence, and facilitated a general process of maturation of the whole personality in the experimental group. All of these studies lend support to the idea that one of the fundamental impacts of the Feldenkrais Method is on body image and awareness.

In 1977, Gutman et al[102] conducted the first research involving Feldenkrais Method in a well elderly population. Subjects were divided into 3 matched groups: ATM, standard exercise, and a no-exercise control. The interventions lasted over a period of 6 weeks. Although they were unable to show additional benefits of Feldenkrais sessions in functional or physiological measures compared with exercise and no exercise control groups because of measurement and design flaws, they did find a trend toward improvement in overall perception of health status in the Feldenkrais group. Also studying a well elderly population, Stephens et al[85] reported significant improvements in the vitality and mental health subscales of the SF-36 following a 2-day ATM workshop. This area of work has been extended by Malmgren-Olsson et al[103,104] in a group of 78 patients with a variety of musculoskeletal disorders, showing that Feldenkrais Method intervention was effective in reducing psychological distress and pain and in improving negative self-image. Lowe et al[105] suggested that the same effect may occur in people who are engaged in a process of rehabilitation acutely after myocardial infarction.

More extensive study of the effects of the Feldenkrais Method on anxiety has been done by Kolt and McConville[106] and Kerr et al.[107] Both studies found significant reduction of state anxiety across a single lesson and a continuing decrease in anxiety across the 10 weeks of the study. This conclusion was further supported by Netz and Lidor,[108] who compared the effects on state anxiety, depressive mood, and subjective well-being and found ATM, swimming, and yoga all more effective than aerobic dance or a computer class control groups in improving outcome measures in these areas.

Psychological and quality-of-life outcomes have also been studied with patients in neurological rehabilitation. In the first study in this area in people with multiple sclerosis, Bost et al[109] demonstrated an improvement in well-being in a controlled study of 50 subjects over 30 days. In a small, multiple case study involving 4 women, Stephens et al[24] reported large increases in well-being using the Index of Wellbeing. In a follow-up study in which balance was also demonstrated to be improved, Stephens et al[110] found that changes in perceived deficits and social support correlated with reduced fatigue impact in people with multiple sclerosis. And, in a randomly assigned, crossover design, Johnson et al[111] found a significant decrease in perceived stress and anxiety following Feldenkrais sessions in a group of 20 people with multiple sclerosis.

Research has begun in this area with the post-CVA population. Connors et al[112] described a patient with hemi-inattention who showed significant improvement on the Behavioral Inattention Test after a 4-week intervention with the Feldenkrais Method, acutely following a right frontal hemorrhage. This improvement was not accompanied by motor improvement at this early stage of rehabilitation. Finally, in a recent study that is in preparation for publication, Batson[113] has found improvement in the ability to image movement, using the Movement Imagery Quotient, in a group of people who had a CVA more than 1 year earlier. The most exciting aspect of this finding was the strong positive correlation found between improvement in motor imagery and improvement in balance and mobility measures. Recently, a group of 30 people with Parkinson's disease participated in a controlled study and demonstrated a significant improvement in quality of life and a decrease in depression compared with the controls over a period of 25 weeks.[114]

Research has begun to target 2 other areas: people with spinal cord injury and people with dementia. Bost[44] has reported a number of case studies of people with spinal cord injury with video documentation, showing improvements in mobility, sensing of the body, and body image. Study of the Feldenkrais Method has also begun with people with dementia. An individual case study has documented a 92-year-old man becoming more alert, improving his comfort in public situations, and communicating better.[115] This work is being expanded by a group of researchers in San Francisco who have used the Feldenkrais Method as an integrated piece of a somatic exercise intervention.[116] Their initial qualitative findings describe improvements in body image and physical function, reduction of anxiety, and improvement in social awareness and relationships. Quantitative assessments showed no significant physical changes but clinically meaningful improvements in physical performance, cognitive function, and quality of life, as well as caregiver quality of life and caregiver burden.[117] Lista and Sorrentino[118] and Mahncke et al[119] have provided a cellular level rationale, related to cellular mechanisms of learning, for reasons why a process method of learning like the Feldenkrais Method and physical exercise might be useful when facilitating improvement in states of dementia. In these fresh research areas, there is clearly a lot of work to be done to establish efficacy, but there is also reason to suggest positive clinical implications.

CONCLUSION

The Feldenkrais Method begins with a great respect for the individuality and dignity of the client and proceeds with gentle exploratory processes, actively and passively, to engage the client in a process of change. It has application to people with a wide range of disabilities, from very low to very high functional levels. The research supports efficacy in a variety of areas. Clearly, more research is needed to establish the range of useful application and to understand the processes by which this approach is effective.

ACKNOWLEDGMENTS

We would like to thank all of the students and patients with whom we have worked over the years for challenging our creativity and allowing us to challenge theirs.

REFERENCES

1. Jacobson E. *Progressive Relaxation*. Chicago, IL: University of Chicago Press; 1938.
2. Lowen A. *Bioenergetics*. New York, NY: Coward, McCann and Geoghegan, Inc; 1975.
3. Brooks CVW. *Sensory Awareness: The Rediscovery of Experiencing*. Great Neck, NY: Felix Morrow Publishing; 1974.
4. Erickson M. *Hypnotic Realities*. New York, NY: Irvington; 1976.
5. Bateson G. *Mind and Nature*. New York, NY: EP Dutton; 1979.
6. Gibson JJ. *The Senses Considered as a Perceptual System*. Boston, MA: Houghton Mifflin; 1966.
7. Feldenkrais M. *The Elusive Obvious*. Cupertino, CA: Meta Publications; 1981.
8. Newell G. Moshe Feldenkrais: a biographical sketch of his early years. *Somatics*. 1992;7:33-38.
9. Hanna T. Moshe Feldenkrais: the silent heritage. *Somatics*. 1984;5(1):8-15.
10. Feldenkrais M. *Higher Judo*. Volume 3. London, United Kingdom: Frederick Warne; 1942.
11. Feldenkrais M. *Judo*. London, United Kingdom: Frederick Warne; 1942.
12. Feldenkrais M. *Body and Mature Behavior: A Study of Anxiety, Sex, Gravitation and Learning*. New York, NY: International Universities Press; 1949.
13. Talmi A. First encounters with Feldenkrais. *Somatics*. 1980;3(1):18-25.
14. Feldenkrais M. *The Potent Self. A Guide to Spontaneity*. San Francisco, CA: Harper & Row; 1985.
15. Miller TM. Decision making processes of physical therapists and Feldenkrais practitioners. PhD dissertation. Temple University, Philadelphia, PA, May 2007.
16. Talvitie U. Socio-affective characteristics and properties of extrinsic feedback in physiotherapy. *Physiother Res Int*. 2000;5(3):173-188.
17. Lennon S, Ashburn A. The Bobath concept in stroke rehabilitation: a focus group study of the experienced physiotherapists' perspective. *Disabil Rehabil*. 2000;22(15):665-674.
18. Liu J, Cramer SC, Reinkensmeyer DJ. Learning to perform a new movement with robotic assistance: comparison of haptic guidance and visual demonstration. *J Neuroeng Rehabil*. 2006;3:20.
19. Marchal-Crespo L, Schneider J, Jaeger L, Riener R. Learning a locomotor task: with or without errors? *J Neuroeng Rehabil*. 2014;11:25.
20. Latash ML, Anson JG. What are "normal movements" in atypical populations? *Behav Brain Sci*. 1996;19(1):55-106.
21. Beets IA, Mace M', Meesen RL, Cuypers K, Levin O, Swinnen SP. Active versus passive training of a complex bimanual task: is prescriptive proprioceptive information sufficient for inducing motor learning? *PLoS One*. 2012;7(5):e37687.
22. Sirigu A, Duhamel JR. Motor and visual imagery as two complementary but neurally dissociable mental processes. *J Cogn Neurosci*. 2001;13(7):910-919.
23. Scott Kelso JA. *Dynamic Patterns: The Self-Organization of Brain and Behavior*. Cambridge, MA: MIT Press; 1997.

24. Stephens JL, Call S, Evans K, Glass M, Gould C, Lowe J. Responses to ten Feldenkrais awareness through movement lessons by four women with multiple sclerosis: improved quality of life. *Physical Therapy Case Reports.* 1999;2(2):58-69.

25. Connors KA, Galea MP, Said CM. Feldenkrais Method® balance classes improve balance in older adults: a controlled trial. *Evid Based Complement Alternat Med.* 2011;873672:1-9.

26. Manto M, Oulad ben Taib N, Luft AR. Modulation of excitability as an early change leading to structural adaptation in the motor cortex. *J Neurosci Res.* 2006;83(2):177-180.

27. Delgado-García JM, Gruart A. Building new motor responses: eyelid conditioning revisited. *Trends Neurosci.* 2006;29(6):330-338.

28. Thompson AK, Wolpaw JR. The simplest motor skill: mechanisms and applications of reflex operant conditioning. *Exerc Sport Sci Rev.* 2014;42(2):82-90.

29. Ziemann U, Siebner HR. Modifying motor learning through gating and homeostatic metaplasticity. *Brain Stimul.* 2008;1(1):60-66.

30. Ween JE. Functional imaging of stroke recovery: an ecological review from a neural network perspective with an emphasis on motor systems. *J Neuroimaging.* 2008;18(3):227-236.

31. Di Filippo M, Picconi B, Tantucci M, et al. Short-term and long-term plasticity at corticostriatal synapses: implications for learning and memory. *Behav Brain Res.* 2009;199(1):108-118.

32. Doyon J, Bellec P, Amsel R, et al. Contributions of the basal ganglia and functionally related brain structures to motor learning. *Behav Brain Res.* 2009;199(1):61-75.

33. Wittenberg GF. Experience, cortical remapping, and recovery in brain disease. *Neurobiol Dis.* 2010;37(2):252-258.

34. Francis JT, Song W. Neuroplasticity of the sensorimotor cortex during learning. *Neural Plast.* 2011;2011:310737.

35. Dayan E, Cohen LG. Neuroplasticity subserving motor skill learning. *Neuron.* 2011;72(3):443-454.

36. Beste C, Dinse HR. Learning without training. *Curr Biol.* 2013;23(11):R489-R499.

37. Lee KJ, Rhyu IJ, Pak DT. Synapses need coordination to learn motor skills. *Rev Neurosci.* 2014;25(2):223-230.

38. Kantak SS, Stinear JW, Buch ER, Cohen LG. Rewiring the brain: potential role of the premotor cortex in motor control, learning, and recovery of function following brain injury. *Neurorehabil Neural Repair.* 2012;26(3):282-292.

39. Nair DG, Fuchs A, Burkart S, Steinberg FL, Kelso JAS. Assessing recovery in middle cerebral artery stroke using fMRI. *Brain Inj.* 2005;19(13):1165-1176.

40. Quartarone A, Hallett M. Emerging concepts in the physiological basis of dystonia. *Mov Disord.* 2013;28(7):958-967.

41. Peterson DA, Sejnowski TJ, Poizner H. Convergent evidence for abnormal striatal synaptic plasticity in dystonia. *Neurobiol Dis.* 2010;37(3):558-573.

42. Burrell L. My journey with dystonia and the Feldenkrais Method®: beginning a discussion on contraindications for aspects of our practice. *Feldenkrais Journal.* 2015;28:7-19.

43. Ginsburg C. The Shake-A-Leg Body Awareness Training Program: dealing with spinal injury and recovery in a new setting. *Somatics.* 1986;Spring/Summer:31-42.

44. Bost H. Developing a new self-image with the help of the Feldenkrais Method. www.helgabost.de/seite29.html. February 23, 2012. Accessed February 12, 2016.

45. Gilman M, Yaruss JS. Stuttering and relaxation: applications for somatic education in stuttering treatment. *J Fluency Disord.* 2000;25(1):59-76.

46. Ofir R. A heuristic investigation of the process of motor learning using Feldenkrais Method® in physical rehabilitation of two young women with traumatic brain injury [unpublished doctoral dissertation]. New York, NY: Union Institute; 1993.

47. Lake B. Acute back pain: treatment by the application of Feldenkrais principles. *Aust Fam Physician.* 1985;14(11):53-77.

48. Panarello-Black D. PT's own back pain leads her to start Feldenkrais training. *PT Bulletin.* 1992;8:9-10.

49. Narula M, Jackson O, Kulig K. The effects of six-week Feldenkrais Method® on selected functional parameters in a subject with rheumatoid arthritis [abstract]. *Phys Ther.* 1992;72(Suppl):S86.

50. Stephens J. Feldenkrais Method: a case study of the application of Feldenkrais Method for a person with balance problems related to multiple sclerosis, evidence and practice. In: Deutsch J, Anderson E, eds. *Complementary Therapies for Physical Therapists: From Art to Practice.* Atlanta, GA: Elsevier; 2008: 273-286.

51. Stephens J. Feldenkrais Method of somatic education. In: Umphred D, ed. *Neurological Rehabilitation.* 5th ed. Philadelphia, PA: Mosby; 2007: 1141-1145.

52. Johnson M, Wendell LL. Some effects of the Feldenkrais Method® on Parkinson's symptoms and function. Paper presented at: Annual Conference of the Feldenkrais Guild of North America; October, 2001. San Francisco, CA.

53. Stephens J. Feldenkrais Method®: background, research and orthopedic case studies. *Orthopedic Physical Therapy Clinics of North America.* 2000;9(3):375-394.

54. American Physical Therapy Association. Guide to Physical Therapist Practice. 2nd ed. *Physical Therapy.* 2001;81(1):9-746.

55. Ives JC, Shelley GA. The Feldenkrais Method® in rehabilitation: a review. *Work.* 1998;11(1):75-90.

56. Boudreau SA, Farina D, Falla D. The role of motor learning and neuroplasticity in designing rehabilitation approaches for musculoskeletal pain disorders. *Man Ther.* 2010;15(5):410-414.

57. Dean JR, Yuen SA, Barrows SA. Effects of a Feldenkrais ATM sequence on fibromyalgia patients. Poster session presented at: Annual Conference of the Feldenkrais Guild of North America; August 1997. Tamiment, PA.

58. Stephens JL, Herrera S, Lawless R, Masaitis C, Woodling P. Evaluating the results of using Awareness Through Movement with people with fibromyalgia: comments on research design and measurement. Paper presented at: Annual Conference of the Feldenkrais Guild of North America; August 1997. Tamimet, PA.

59. Kendall SA, Ekselius L, Gerdle B, Soren B, Bengtsson A. Feldenkrais intervention in fibromyalgia patients: a pilot study. *J Musculoskelet Pain.* 2001;9(4):25-35.

60. Gard G. Body awareness therapy for patients with fibromyalgia and chronic pain. *Disabil Rehabil.* 2005;27(12):725-728.

61. Edwards I, Jones M, Hillier S. The interpretation of experience and its relationship to body movement: a clinical reasoning perspective. *Man Ther.* 2006;11:2-10.

62. Lotze M, Moseley GL. Theoretical considerations for chronic pain rehabilitation. *Phys Ther.* 2015;95(9):1316-1320.

63. Bearman D, Shafarman S. Feldenkrais Method® in the treatment of chronic pain: a study of efficacy and cost effectiveness. *Amer J Pain Manage.* 1999;9(1):22-27.

64. Phipps A, Lopez R, Powell R, Lundy-Ekman L, Maebori D. A functional outcome study on the use of movement re-education in chronic pain management [unpublished master's thesis]. Forest Grove, OR; Pacific University, School of Physical Therapy; 1997.

65. Lundblad I, Elert J, Gerdle B. Randomized controlled trial of physiotherapy and Feldenkrais interventions in female workers with neck-shoulder complaints. *J Occup Rehabil.* 1999;9(3):179-194.

66. Lundqvist L, Zetterlund C, Richter HO. Effects of Feldenkrais Method® on chronic neck/scapular pain in people with visual impairment: a randomized controlled trial with one-year follow-up. *Arch Phys Med Rehabil.* 2014;95:1656-1661.

67. DeRosa C, Porterfield J. A physical therapy model for the treatment of low back pain. *Phys Ther.* 1992;72(4):261-269.

68. Maher CG. Effective physical treatment for chronic low back pain. *Orthop Clin North Am.* 2004;35(1):57-64.

69. Kay TM, Gross A, Goldsmith C, Santaguida PL, Hoving J, Bronfort G. Exercises for mechanical neck disorders. *Cochrane Database Syst Rev.* 2007;3:CD004250.

70. Rogers SM. Survey of piano instructors: awareness and intervention of predisposing factors to piano-related injuries. Doctoral Dissertation, Columbia University Teachers College, 1999.

71. Rardin MA. The effects of an injury prevention intervention on playing-related pain, tension, and attitudes in the high school string orchestra classroom. Dissertation, Doctor of Musical Arts. University of Southern California—Los Angeles. 2007.

72. O'Connor M, Webb R. Learning to rest when in pain. *European Journal of Palliative Care.* 2002;9(2):68-71.

73. Mehling WE, Daubenmier J, Price CJ, Acree M, Bartmess E, Stewart AL. Self-reported interoceptive awareness in primary care patients with past or current low back pain. *J Pain Res.* 2013;6:403-418.

74. Brown E, Kegerris S. Electromyographic activity of trunk musculature during a Feldenkrais awareness through movement lesson. *Isokinet Exerc Sci.* 1991;1(4):216-221.

75. Ruth S, Kegerreis S. Facilitating cervical flexion using a Feldenkrais Method®: Awareness Through Movement. *J Sports Phys Ther.* 1992;16(1):25-29.

76. James ML, Kolt GS, Hopper C, McConville JC, Bate P. The effects of a Feldenkrais program and relaxation procedures on hamstring length. *Aust J Physiother.* 1998;44:49-54.

77. Hopper C, Kolt GS, McConville JC. The effects of Feldenkrais Awareness Through Movement on hamstring length, flexibility and perceived exertion. *J Bodyw Mov Ther.* 1999;3(4):238-247.

78. Stephens J, Davidson JA, DeRosa JT, Kriz ME, Saltzman NA. Lengthening the hamstring muscles without stretching using "awareness through movement." *Phys Ther.* 2006;86(12):1641-1650.

79. Chowdhury S. Static stretching versus awareness through movement in improving hamstring flexibility. Masters dissertation submitted to the Rajiv Gandhi University of Health Sciences, Bangalore, India, May 2011.

80. Saraswati S. Investigation of human postural muscles and respiratory movements. [unpublished master's thesis]. University of New South Wales; Australia; 1989.

81. Shenkman M, Donovan J, Tsubota J, Kluss M, Stebbins P, Butler R. Management of individuals with Parkinson's disease: rationale and case studies. *Phys Ther.* 1989;69:944-955.

82. Hall SE, Criddle A, Ring A, Bladen C, Tapper J, Yin R. Study of the effects of various forms of exercise on balance in older women [unpublished manuscript]. Healthway Starter Grant, File #7672, Department of Rehabilitation, Sir Charles Gairdner Hospital, Nedlands, Western Australia; 1999.

83. Seegert EM, Shapiro R. Effects of alternative exercise on posture. *Clinical Kinesiology.* 1999;53(2):41-47.

84. Bennett JL, Brown BJ, Finney SA, Sarantakis CP. Effects of a Feldenkrais based mobility program on function of a healthy elderly sample. Poster session presented at: Combined Sections Meeting of the American Physical Therapy Association; February 1998; Boston, MA.

85. Stephens JL, Pendergast C, Roller BA, Weiskittel RS. Learning to improve mobility and quality of life in a well elderly population: the benefits of Awareness Through Movement. *IFF Feldenkrais Research Journal.* 2005;2:17.

86. Stephens J, DuShuttle D, Hatcher C, Shmunes J, Slaninka C. Use of Awareness Through Movement improves balance and balance confidence in people with multiple sclerosis: a randomized controlled study. *Neurology Report.* 2001;25(2):39-49.

87. Batson G, Deutsch JE. Effects of Feldenkrais awareness through movement on balance in adults with chronic neurological deficits following stroke: a preliminary study. *Complement Health Pract Rev.* 2005;10(3):203-210.
88. Vrantsidis F, Hill KD, Moore K, Webb R, Hunt S, Dowson L. Getting grounded gracefully: effectiveness and acceptability of Feldenkrais in improving balance. *J Aging Phys Act.* 2009;17(1):57-76.
89. Ullmann G, Williams HG, Hussey J, Durstine JL, McClenaghan BA. Effects of Feldenkrais exercises on balance, mobility, balance confidence, and gait performance in community-dwelling adults age 65 and older. *J Altern Complement Med.* 2010;16(1):97-105.
90. Connors KA, Pile C, Nichols ME. Does the Feldenkrais Method® make a difference? An investigation into the use of outcome measurement tools for evaluating changes in students. *J Bodyw Mov Ther.* 2011;15(4):446-452.
91. Hillier S, Porter L, Jackson K, Petkov J. The effects of Feldenkrais classes on the health and function of an ageing Australian sample: a pilot study. *Open Rehabil J.* 2010;3:62-66.
92. Webb R, Cofré Lizama LE, Galea MP. Moving with ease: Feldenkrais Method® classes for people with osteoarthritis. *Evid Based Complement Alternat Med.* 2013;2013:479142.
93. Cook SB, LaRoche DP, Swartz EE, Hammond PR, King MA. A novel sensorimotor movement and walking intervention to improve balance and gait in women. *Complement Ther Clin Pract.* 2014;20(4):311-316.
94. DellaGrotte J, Ridi R, Landi M, Stephens J. Postural improvement using core integration to lengthen myofascia. *J Bodyw Mov Ther.* 2008;12(3):231-245.
95. Ullmann G, Williams HG. Effect of Feldenkrais exercises on dual task postural control in older adults. *Clin Interv Aging.* 2014;9:1039-1042.
96. Frank R. Body awareness: the development of self-perception. Dissertation Abstracts International: Section B: The Sciences and Engineering. Vol 58(6-B), Dec 1997, pp. 3315. Dissertation Abstract: 1997-95024-173.
97. Steisel SG. The student's experience of the psychological elements in functional integration. Dissertation Abstracts International, Massachusetts School of Professional Psychology. University Microfilms;1993; Ann Arbor, MI.
98. Deig D. Self image in relationship to Feldenkrais Awareness Through Movement classes [unpublished master's thesis]. Indianapolis, IN; University of Indianapolis, Krannert Graduate School of Physical Therapy; 1994.
99. Elgelid HS. Feldenkrais and body image [unpublished master's thesis]. Conway, AR; University of Central Arkansas; 1999.
100. Hutchinson MG. *Transforming Body Image. Learning to Love the Body You Have.* Freedom, CA: The Crossing Press; 1985.
101. Laumer U, Bauer M, Fichter M, Milz H. Therapeutic effects of Feldenkrais Method® "Awareness Through Movement" in patients with eating disorders. *Psychother Psychosom Med Psychol.* 1997;47(5):170-180.
102. Gutman G, Herbert C, Brown S. Feldenkrais vs conventional exercise for the elderly. *J Gerontol.* 1977;32(5):562-572.
103. Malmgren-Olsson E, Armelius B, Armelius K. A comparative outcome study of body awareness therapy (BAT), Feldenkrais, and conventional physiotherapy for patients with non-specific musculoskeletal disorders: changes in psychological symptoms, pain and self image. *Physiother Theory Pract.* 2001;17(2):77-95.
104. Malmgren-Olsson EB, Branholm IB. A comparison between three physiotherapy approaches with regard to health-related factors in patients with non-specific musculoskeletal disorders. *Disabil Rehabil.* 2002;24(6):308-317.
105. Lowe B, Breining K, Wilke S, Wellmann R, Zipfel S, Eich W. Quantitative and qualitative effects of Feldenkrais, progressive muscle relaxation, and standard medical treatment in patients after acute myocardial infarction. *Psychother Res.* 2002;12(2):179-191.
106. Kolt GS, McConville JC. The effects of a Feldenkrais Awareness Through Movement program on state anxiety. *J Bodyw MovTher.* 2000;4(3):216-220.
107. Kerr GA, Kotynia F, Kolt GS. Feldenkrais Awareness Through Movement and state anxiety. *J Bodyw Mov Ther.* 2002;6(2):102-107.
108. Netz Y, Lidor R. Mood alterations in mindful versus aerobic exercise modes. *J Psychol.* 2003;137(5):405-419.
109. Bost H, Burges S, Russell R, Ruttinger H, Schlafke U. Feldstudie zur wiiksamkeit der Feldenkrais-Methode bei MS-betroffenen. Deutsche Multiple Sklerose Gesellschaft. Saarbrucken, Germany; 1994. Unpublished manuscript.
110. Stephens J, Cates P, Jentes E, et al. Awareness improves quality of life in people with multiple sclerosis. *J Neurologic Phys Ther.* 2003;27(4):170.
111. Johnson SK, Frederick J, Kaufman M, Mountjoy B. A controlled investigation of bodywork in multiple sclerosis. *J Altern Complement Med.* 1999;5(3):237-243.
112. Connors K, Grenough P. Redevelopment of sense of self following stroke, using the Feldenkrais Method®. Poster abstract presented at: Movement and Development of Sense of Self Symposium, Annual Conference of Feldenkrais Guild of North America; August 2004. Seattle, WA.
113. Batson G. The effect of group delivery of Feldenkrais Awareness Through Movement on balance, functional mobility and quality of life in adults post-stroke. PhD Dissertation, Rocky Mountain University, Provo, UT, 2006.
114. Teixeira-Machado L, Araujo FM, Cunha FA, Menezes M, Menezes T, DeSantana JM. Feldenkrais Method®-based exercise improves quality of life in individuals with Parkinson's disease: a controlled, randomized clinical trial. *Alternative Therapies.* 2015;21(1):8-14.
115. Ann J. Individuals with dementia learn new habits and are empowered through the Feldenkrais method. *Alzheimers Care Q.* 2006;7(4):278-286.

116. Wu E, Barnes DE, Ackerman SL, Lee J, Chesney M, Mehling WE. Preventing Loss of Independence through Exercise (PLIÉ): qualitative analysis of a clinical trial in older adults with dementia. *Aging Ment Health.* 2015;19(4):353-362.

117. Barnes DE, Mehling W, Wu E, et al. Preventing Loss of Independence through Exercise (PLIÉ): a pilot clinical trial in older adults with dementia. *PLoS One.* 2015;10(2):e0113367.

118. Lista I, Sorrentino G. Biological mechanisms of physical activity in preventing cognitive decline. *Cell Mol Neurobiol.* 2010;30(4):493-503.

119. Mahncke HW, Bronstone A, Merzenich MM. Brain plasticity and functional losses in the aged: scientific bases for a novel intervention. *Prog Brain Res.* 2006;157:81-109.

BIBLIOGRAPHY

Florence SL, Boydston LA, Hackett TA, et al. Sensory enrichment after peripheral nerve injury restores cortical, but not thalamic, receptive field organization. *Eur J Neurosci.* 2001;13(9):1755-1766.

Friel KM, Heddings AA, Nudo RJ. Effects of postlesion experience on behavioral recovery and neurophysiologic reorganization after cortical injury in primates. *Neurorehabil Neural Repair.* 2000;14(3):187-198.

Kaas JH. Plasticity of sensory and motor maps in adult mammals. *Annu Rev Neurosci.* 1991;14:137-167.

Kandel ER, Schwartz JH, Jessell TM. *The Principles of Neural Science.* 4th ed. Norwalk, CT: Appleton and Lange; 2000.

Kolb B, Gibb R, Gorny G. Cortical plasticity and the development of behavior after early frontal cortical injury. *Dev Neuropsychol.* 2000;18(3):423-444.

Liepert J, Uhde I, Graf S, et al. Motor cortex plasticity during forced-use therapy in stroke patients: a preliminary study. *J Neurol.* 2001;248(4):315-321.

Nudo RJ, Friel KM. Cortical plasticity after stroke: implications for rehabilitation. *Rev Neurol (Paris).* 1999;155(9):713-717.

Nudo RJ, Milliken GW, Jenkins WM, Merzenich MM. Use-dependent alterations of movement representations in primary motor cortex of adult squirrel monkeys. *J Neurosci.* 1996;16(2):785-807.

ADDITIONAL RESOURCES

- Feldenkrais Guild of North America (FGNA)

  3611 SW Hood Avenue, Suite 100

  Portland, OR 97201

  Phone: 800-775-2118

  Fax: 503-221-6616

  Email: guild@feldenkrais.com

  Website: www.feldenkrais.com/fgna

Feldenkrais established the FGNA in 1977 as the professional organization of practitioners and teachers of the Feldenkrais Method. FGNA provides training, certification, and continuing education for practitioners; protection of the quality of the Feldenkrais work; and support for research. It is also a source of information about the Feldenkrais Method for the public. The Guild publishes *The Feldenkrais Journal* quarterly, which contains case stories, practitioner reflections, historical information, and artwork. It also publishes *In Touch*, a quarterly newsletter about practice issues and FGNA business. The role of the FGNA has been to establish professional standards for training and practice, to support the continued learning and growth of practitioners, to authorize and conduct training programs, to deal with ethical issues, and to support research.

- Feldenkrais Institute of New York (FINY)

  134 W 26th St

  New York, NY 10001

  Phone: (212) 727-1014

  Website: www.feldenkraisinstitute.com

FINY is a resource center in New York City that presents ATM classes and workshops, hosts training programs, has a store for educational materials, and provides a space for practitioners to conduct private FI lessons.

- Feldenkrais Resources

  3680 6th Avenue

  San Diego, CA 92103

  Phone: 800-765-1907 or 619-220-8776 (For the Berkeley Location (FRTI), please call 877-765-1907)

  Fax: 619-330-4993

  Website: www.feldenkraisresources.com

Feldenkrais Resources is a practitioner-owned and run organization that is a resource for audiotape, videotape, and print instructional information and practice support materials. It is also responsible for making available documentary materials about the life and work of Feldenkrais.

- International Feldenkrais Federation (IFF)

  Website: www.feldenkrais-method.org

The IFF is a virtual academy that publishes a regular newsletter and journal and maintains an information bureau. The mission of the IFF is to raise the level of competence of practitioners worldwide through continuous learning. To this end, it maintains a website that allows access to a video collection of work by Feldenkrais and more than 400 ATM lessons, sponsor conferences, training programs, and research promotion.

- OpenATM.org

  Free online resources for ATM lessons

- YouTube videos of the Feldenkrais Method from the Feldenkrais Institute and David Zemach-Bersin.

15

Pilates Rehabilitation

Brent Anderson, PhD, PT, OCS, PMA-CPT

As a child, German-born Joseph H. Pilates (Figure 15-1) suffered from a multitude of illnesses resulting in muscular weakness. Determined to overcome his frailties, he dedicated his life to becoming physically stronger. He studied yoga, martial arts, Zen meditation, and Greek and Roman exercises. He worked with medical professionals, including physicians and his wife Clara, a nurse. His experiences led to the development of his unique method of physical and mental conditioning, which he brought to the United States in 1923. In the 1930s and 1940s, popular dance artists and choreographers, such as Martha Graham, George Balanchine, and Jerome Robbins, embraced Pilates' exercise method. As elite performers, these dancers often suffered from injuries resulting in long recovery periods and an inability to reach peak performance. Unique at the time, Pilates' method allowed and encouraged movement early in the rehabilitation process by providing needed assistance. It was found that reintroducing movement with nondestructive forces early in the rehabilitation process hastened the patient's healing. As a result, it was not long before the dance community at large adopted his work.

More than 60 years later, these techniques began to gain popularity in the rehabilitation setting. In the 1990s, for instance, many rehabilitation practitioners were using the method in multiple fields of rehabilitation, including general orthopedic, geriatric, chronic pain, and neurological rehabilitation, among others. Within the rehabilitation setting, most Pilates exercises are performed on several types of apparatuses (Figures 15-2 to 15-5). The apparatus work evolved from Pilates' original mat work, which proved difficult as a result of the effect of gravity on the body (Figure 15-6). On the apparatus, springs and gravity are used to assist an injured individual to successfully complete movements that otherwise would be restricted for multiple reasons, aiding in a safe recovery (see Figure 15-3). Ultimately, by altering the spring tension or increasing the challenge of gravity, an individual may be progressed toward achieving functional movement. The use of the Pilates principles with the variations of the traditional repertoire to meet the needs of patients is often referred to in the Pilates community as *Pilates evolved*. The Pilates environment consists of equipment used by Pilates practitioners, including reformers, Cadillac or trapeze tables, chairs, ladder barrels, and mats.

Today, despite an increased number of health care practitioners using Pilates principles for rehabilitation, there is still a lack of supportive literature examining the efficacy associated with Pilates-evolved techniques. Current scientific theories in motor learning and biomechanics are examined to help explain the principles of this old method of movement reeducation.

Davis CM.
Integrative Therapies in Rehabilitation: Evidence for Efficacy in Therapy, Prevention, and Wellness, Fourth Edition(pp 227-238).
© 2017 Taylor & Francis Group.

Figure 15-1. Joseph H. Pilates. (Reprinted with permission from Polestar Education LLC.)

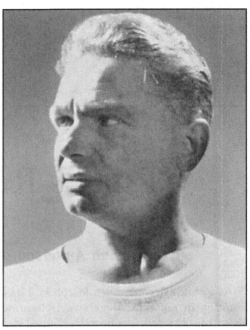

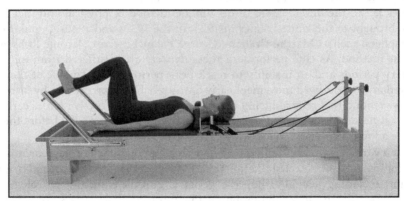

Figure 15-2. Footwork on a clinical reformer (Body Balance Inc). (Reprinted with permission from Polestar Education LLC.)

PILATES PRINCIPLES

Pilates originally developed 8 basic principles to guide his exercises, known as *contrology*. They consisted of concentration, control, precision and coordination, isolation and integration, centering, flowing movement, breathing, and routine.[1] However, Pilates was not a prolific writer and, unfortunately, much of what is known about Pilates principles has been passed down verbally from generation to generation. This has left much of his original work open to varying interpretations.

There are many avenues for Pilates certification around the world. Various Pilates education and treatment groups are known throughout the United States and advertised widely.

The founders of Polestar Pilates Education (a Pilates education company specializing in rehabilitation founded in 1992) studied with many of the first-generation Pilates enthusiasts and teachers. Although their repertoires were quite different from one another, they shared common principles. The therapists of Polestar took the opportunity to investigate the Pilates principles vs the original

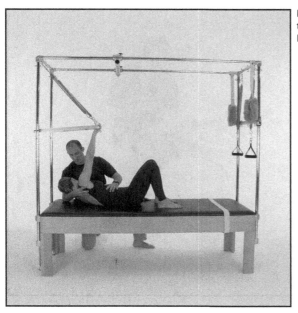

Figure 15-3. Neuromobilization with Tower Bar on the Cadillac. (Reprinted with permission from Polestar Education LLC.)

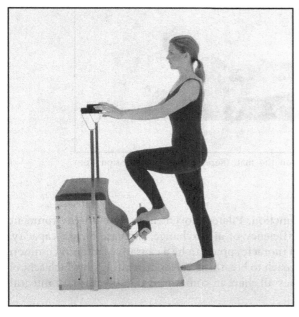

Figure 15-4. Single leg press on Combo-Chair (Body Balance Inc). (Reprinted with permission from Polestar Education LLC.)

repertoire of Pilates and came up with the following 6 principles, supported with scientific foundations, to better explain the applications of Pilates for rehabilitation: (1) breathing; (2) axial elongation/core control (centering); (3) spine articulation (isolation and integration); (4) efficient organization of head, neck, and shoulder girdle (flowing, efficient movement); (5) alignment and posture (centering, precision, and coordinating); and (6) movement integration (concentration, integration, flowing, and routine)[2] (Table 15-1).

Principle 1: Breathing

Breath, one of the key elements of Pilates training, is thought to be a facilitator for stabilization and mobilization of the spine and extremities. Faulty breath patterns are often associated with

Figure 15-5. Limited thoracic spine extension over the Ladder Barrel (Body Balance Inc). (Reprinted with permission from Polestar Education LLC.)

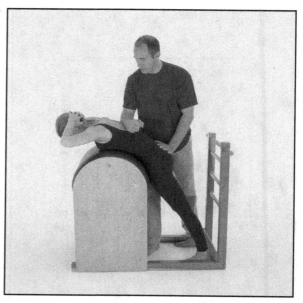

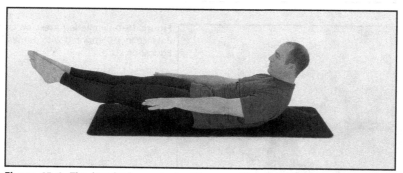

Figure 15-6. The hundred exercise on the mat. (Reprinted with permission from Polestar Education LLC.)

common reports of pain and movement dysfunction. Pilates movements create an environment whereby breath is facilitated to increase the efficiency of air exchange, increase breath capacity, and facilitate thoracic postural changes. A rigid thoracic spine can be a causative factor in common cervical and lumbar pathology. The Pilates approach to breathing varies depending on which school of Pilates you graduated from, but one thing they all share in common is that breath is an integral part of each and every exercise.

Principle 2: Axial Elongation/Core Control (Centering)

The principle of stabilization and axial elongation greatly relies on the research from Queensland, Australia. Such studies demonstrate that the transverse abdominus, multifidus, diaphragm, and abdominal oblique muscles are key organization muscles of movement in healthy individuals and are often lacking in individuals with chronic low back pain.[3-5] The principle of elongation has generated the greatest interest in Pilates rehabilitation. Stabilization is not always the best descriptor of what Pilates can do for an individual. Motor control studies and theories of trunk organization and stabilization teach us that subthreshold contraction of global stabilization muscles provide safe movement throughout one's daily activities.[6] Sahrmann[7] relates control of the trunk to a balance of stiffness between muscles to provide efficient control of dynamic posture.

TABLE 15-1
CLINICAL APPLICATIONS OF THE PILATES PRINCIPLES
BREATHING
Breath can facilitate spine stability, spine articulation, core control, and efficiency of movement, and movement can facilitate breath.
AXIAL ELONGATION/CORE CONTROL (CENTERING)
Axial elongation should be present in every Pilates exercise, providing the optimal space, stiffness, and orientation of joints and supporting tissues to move throughout the day without the risk of injury.
SPINE ARTICULATION (ISOLATION AND INTEGRATION)
Knowing the properties of the spine and the groupings of the vertebrae (cervical, thoracic, and lumbar) allows for accurate imagery, verbal cueing, and tactile cueing to optimize movement.
EFFICIENT ORGANIZATION OF THE HEAD, NECK, AND SHOULDER GIRDLE (FLOWING, EFFICIENT MOVEMENT)
Providing the efficient expenditure of energy while moving will help to maintain an optimal alignment of the head, neck, and shoulders on the trunk; this organization provides for safety, aesthetics, and energy conservation.
ALIGNMENT AND POSTURE (CENTERING, PRECISION, AND COORDINATING)
Proper alignment and organization of the upper and lower extremities as they pertain to the trunk allows for safe, efficient movement of the body; alignment often removes damaging stressors that prevent spontaneous healing.
MOVEMENT AND INTEGRATION (CONCENTRATION, INTEGRATION, FLOWING, AND ROUTINE)
Movement integration not only consists of musculoskeletal movement integration but also the integration of mind and body; maximizing the mental involvement with the exercise creates an almost meditative state for the patient, enhancing body awareness and exploring new movement opportunities without pain. When the mind, body, and spirit are thought to be one, if one moves the body, one moves all systems.

The principle of axial elongation is thought to organize the spine in its optimal orientation for efficient movement, thus avoiding working or resting at the end of range, which can place undue stresses on the inert and contractile structures of the trunk and extremities. This organization of spine and extremities also provides optimal potential for performance of sport and leisure activities. With an ever-growing population interested in feeling good and being able to perform daily activities and recreate without the risk of injury, axial elongation is a high priority and could account for many of the anecdotal spontaneous resolutions of low back pain that come with Pilates. Clinically, forces seem to be better distributed throughout the spine when a patient has the ability to reorganize his or her strategy of spine movement, spine stabilization, and movement of the extremities in conjunction with the spine, and these are less likely to introduce harmful effects to the soft tissues surrounding the spine. It also appears that those who are diagnosed with spine pathology, even as grievous as disc pathologies, can often minimize the provoking forces at the site of the lesion, thus minimizing the pain response and accelerating healing. Pilates exercises have an innate way of facilitating trunk

Figure 15-7. 90/90 on the Cadillac. (Reprinted with permission from Polestar Education LLC.)

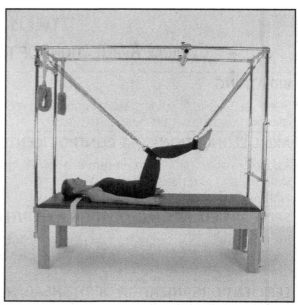

organization at a subconscious level, allowing the individual to explore and assimilate more efficient control of his or her trunk. These clinical observations warrant scientific investigation.

Pilates also provides an environment in which the difficulty of the exercise can be modified, thus facilitating successful execution of a desired movement outcome. The following 4 basic tools referred to by Polestar Education in the Pilates environment are familiar to neurological rehabilitation: (1) modify the base of support; (2) decrease the center of gravity; (3) shorten the length of the levers; and (4) vary the assistance (spring tension). One of the basic exercises, 90/90, uses the springs for assistance. The tables allow the practitioner to lower the center of gravity and increase the base of support, and the exercise can be modified by changing the length of the levers (Figure 15-7). This formula allows the therapist to facilitate motor changes of the trunk quickly, while giving ownership of the newly acquired movement to the patient or client.

Principle 3: Spine Articulation (Isolation and Integration)

The distribution of segmental movement through the spine is a topic that researchers are anxious to measure. Does distributing the motion between spinal segments significantly reduce stressful forces from causing micro- and macrotraumas to the hypermobile segment? Currently, there are no instruments that can measure this accurately. A study carried out at Mount Saint Mary's University's physical therapy program in Emmittsburg, Maryland, used the Metrecom Skeletal Analysis System to measure the phenomena of motion distribution following Pilates exercises. Pilot studies showed that following one session of Pilates, healthy subjects had a significant increase in overall forward bending, an increase in motion of less-mobile segments, and a decrease in motion of the previously measured hypermobile segments.[8] With limited research regarding this topic, it still can be hypothesized that by increasing the motor awareness of spinal motion in all directions, one can extrapolate that distribution of movement is equivalent to a distribution of sheer force to the spine.

Principle 4: Efficient Organization of Head, Neck, and Shoulder Girdle (Flowing, Efficient Movement)

This principle focuses on the patient's ability to align the head, neck, and shoulder girdle. Efficiency of movement can be observed by the tone and posture of the head, face, neck, and shoulder girdle in relationship to the thoracic spine and trunk. Many restrictions and unnecessary

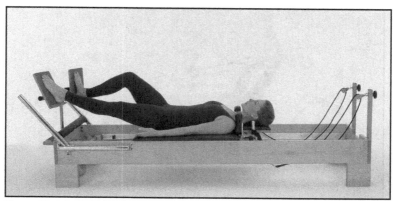

Figure 15-8. Footwork with proprioceptive T-bar on Clinical Reformer. (Reprinted with permission from Polestar Education LLC.)

stresses can occur in this area. The benefits of this principle are increased range of motion, energy conservation, and minimized risk of lesions. Lesions usually occur at the end of a range of motion. Increasing the available range of motion and improving the coordination of the scapulothoracic joints will decrease the likelihood of experiencing destructive forces to the shoulder and neck joints.

Principle 5: Alignment and Posture (Centering, Precision, and Coordinating)

Proper alignment and posture are foundational to efficient, coordinated movement. Postural organization can significantly decrease energy expenditure in daily activities. For example, if an individual allows his or her femurs to medially rotate while decelerating in gait, it will lead to a number of potential lesions, such as patellofemoral pain, foot and ankle tendonitis, and hip and pelvic pathologies. Faulty alignment in the extremities and spine can be the source of decreased range of motion, early muscle group fatigue, abnormal stresses on inert structures, and faulty movement patterns that can potentially become harmful to the individual.

Pilates pays attention to static alignment and posture but places greater emphasis on dynamic alignment and posture. With a device on the Clinical Reformer (Balanced Body; one of the basic pieces of apparatus used by Joseph Pilates and modified for rehabilitation) known as the rotating T-bar, a therapist can measure weight-bearing asymmetries while squatting. By using the closed-chain foot bar, one can assess asymmetries between hip rotators as they apply to alignment through a squatting range of motion (Figure 15-8). These diagnostic and treatment applications in the Pilates environment allow rehabilitation practitioners to better assess and treat alignment-related impairments not only in the lower extremity but also in the upper extremity and trunk.

Principle 6: Movement Integration (Concentration, Integration, Flowing, and Routine)

According to many Pilates rehabilitation specialists, this most important principle of rehabilitation could represent the unexplainable changes often experienced in the Pilates environment. The advanced mastery of movement requiring a connectedness between mind and body is thought by many Pilates rehabilitation practitioners to be one of the primary reasons for its success. Emphasizing holistic mind and body integration sometimes uncovers emotional causes for movement disorders.

One anecdotal account of a therapist with a patient suffering from chronic low back pain for 5 years could be a good example of this principle. The patient's magnetic resonance imaging, computed tomography scan, among other tests, were negative. She was referred to the therapist for an evaluation and Pilates intervention. After introducing the first few Pilates exercises, the hamstring

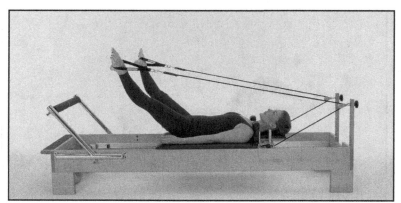

Figure 15-9. Leg circles on Clinical Reformer. (Reprinted with permission from Polestar Education LLC.)

arcs in particular (an exercise that supports the legs in straps while the patient lies supine; the legs were moved in circular motions; Figure 15-9), the patient began to cry and express emotional releases. After being escorted to a private room, she proceeded to confide an experience in her childhood involving sexual molestation by a family member. She had never shared this with anyone before, not even with her husband of 25 years. Within weeks, her symptoms significantly decreased and she was referred to the proper intervention.

According to experienced clinicians, this type of behavior is seen or expressed quite often. However, we usually do not talk about it because it does not fit within our current practice act. If movement integration is allowed to be expanded beyond just the musculoskeletal and allowed to incorporate the mind, emotions, subconscious, spirit, and physical body (including the digestive, circulatory, respiratory, and reproductive systems), this represents holistic movement integration of the entire person. Movement approaches that incorporate the movement of the whole person, such as Pilates, T'ai Chi, yoga, the Feldenkrais Method, and Gyrotonic Expansion System, are going to continue to receive greater attention due to the increasing incidence of anecdotal improvements. The rehabilitation sciences will do well to look for ways of measuring outcomes as they pertain to movement of the whole person. Examples of possible movement-related research efforts might include self-efficacy studies pertaining to one's perception of self and one's ability to move, depression scales as they pertain to one's perception of the ability or inability to move, and communication of disability through movement patterns.

An example of how perception influences motivation in movement was revealed in a man with a diagnosis of mechanical low back pain. He worked with the city street cleaning division, and was looking forward to a long leave from work due to his back injury. His pain was local, and was aggravated with forward bending, twisting, and prolonged sitting. During his second visit, the physical therapist initiated Pilates exercises to teach him to minimize the unnecessary guarding and begin to increase awareness of his center and trunk control. During this session, the patient observed an elite dancer next to him doing an advanced move on the trapeze table. He made the comment, "I could never do that." He was told that he could, in fact, do that exercise (hanging spine extension on the trapeze table; Figure 15-10). On his next visit, the Pilates environment was manipulated such that he was able to perform the exercise safely and without any discomfort whatsoever. As he sat on the edge of the table following his successful execution of what appeared to be an advanced exercise, he stated, "I can't believe I just did that exercise." The therapist waited a minute and then said to the patient, "That exercise is much harder than anything you would be required to do at work." There was silence and one could tell that the patient was reorganizing his neural network. What he thought was going to be a 6-month vacation now was reduced to 2 weeks. His previous motivation of the back

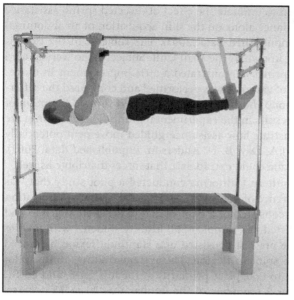

Figure 15-10. Hanging series on Cadillac. (Reprinted with permission from Polestar Education LLC.)

injury was in conflict with his successful execution of an advanced movement on his third visit. He experienced a paradigm shift in his perception of what his mechanical low back pain meant to him.

In another example, a 76-year-old retired radiologist with a diagnosis of lumbar stenosis and Parkinson-like tremors was unable to walk more than 100 yards without bilateral calf and lateral leg pain. He was taking medication for the tremor, pain, and inflammation. His previous activity included running, which he hadn't been able to do for more than 1 year. Objectively, his posture was very kyphotic with a significant forward head, with eye gaze on the feet. His gait was a slow shuffle and he often experienced a loss of balance. Active range of motion of his spine was limited to negative 15 degrees of extension, and he had no hip extension.

He did a once-weekly Pilates session for approximately 1 year, accompanied by a walking program. The focus of his program was to facilitate his upright posture, axial elongation of the lumbar and thoracic spine, and to increase his ability to walk 1 to 3 miles per day. The Pilates environment (basic equipment and principles of Pilates) provided him with the ability to use assistance from the springs and varying orientations to gravity to learn how to safely walk upright in spite of his spinal stenosis, increase his hip and thoracic extension, and bring his eye gaze into a parallel orientation to the floor while standing. Examples of two exercises used to help with balance, disassociation, and trunk extension are shown in Figures 15-4 and 15-5.

This patient now walks 1 to 3 miles/day with minimal reports of lower leg pain. His medications have been reduced, and although he continues to battle the tremors, he has noted a significant decrease in loss of balance and near falls.

EVIDENCE OF EFFICACY

Since the fist edition of this chapter was released, there have been several papers published pertaining to Pilates and health,[9-11] Pilates and aging,[12] and continued work on Pilates for low back care.[13-17] This number continues to grow as the interest in and the awareness of the use of Pilates for rehabilitation and health practices grow. There are still a number of studies analyzing low back pain management, motor learning with spring-assisted movement training, and imagery facilitation that are awaiting publication.

One study awaiting publication was designed to evaluate the effect of directed spring assistance and verbal guidance compared with verbal guidance alone on the skill acquisition of an abdominal curl-up (B. Carr, J.A. Day, B. D. Anderson, unpublished data, 2003). The subjects in the experimental group used a piece of Pilates equipment known as the Wall Unit. Subjects who were guided through movement with assistance from the springs demonstrated a 50% improvement in movement amplitude after intervention. An analysis of variance was performed and compared the differences between the control and experimental groups both pre- and post-test; it showed retention of benefit even higher than the original post-test results in the experimental group. These findings are important to the profession in that they demonstrate how assistance-guided movement potentially can affect the strategy of movement (B. Carr, J.A. Day, B. D. Anderson, unpublished data, 2003). If movement distributes throughout the spine, one could extrapolate that forces distribute as well.

In 1996, Mount Saint Mary's College in Southern California conducted a pilot study that was presented at the California State Chapter Conference of the American Physical Therapy Association as a poster presentation.[8] The research design consisted of a control and experimental group and pre- and post-test measures. The subjects consisted of a sample of all healthy students with no history of performing Pilates-based exercises. The pre-test consisted of a standing flexion measured with a device to assess segmental motion of the spine in flexion. The average findings in this pilot study identified the strategy of forward flexion to take place primarily at the hip, L4-5, and L5-S1. The average angle of displacement in the lower 2 segments of the lumbar was 20 to 25 degrees. The angles significantly decreased from L4 upward, with the majority of the thoracic spine at 0 to 2 degrees maximum. The experimental group then proceeded with a 45-minute session of Pilates on the Clinical Reformer. Following the session, they returned to take their post-test. The control group took the pre-test with similar results to those of the experimental group. They then rested for 45 minutes and returned to take the post-test; the results were similar to the pre-test. The interesting findings of the experimental post-group were as follows: overall flexion increased; segmental motion increased by as much as 25% in the thoracic and upper lumbar segments; and at the levels L4-5 and L5-S1, there was a significant reduction in the angle of flexion by more than 50%, approximately 10 to 15 degrees per segment—this was the most important finding. This pilot study could not be continued due to malfunction of the measurement instrument and the withdrawal of the company's ability to validate its findings.[8] However, the findings in the pilot study definitely laid the groundwork for further investigation regarding motor learning in the Pilates environment, which might explain how changing the strategy of movement can alleviate harmful forces that often continue the perturbation of lesions.

In January 2000, an article was published that discussed a case study using Pilates and the Gyrotonic Expansion System (Balanced Body Inc) with favorable results (D. M. Duschatko, unpublished data, 2000). Further, the most recent publications pertaining to low back care have shown a significant decrease in low back disability using the Oswestry Low Back Pain Questionnaire, the Roland-Morris Low Back Pain and Disability Questionnaire, and the 36-Item Short Form Survey scale.[13,15,17] A dissertation from the University of Miami demonstrated a significant improvement in back extension strength and the SF-36 vitality measure when compared with massage alone.[16] It is interesting that, of all measures in the SF-36, vitality demonstrated the strongest correlation with the Pilates intervention. It could be that this positive movement experience without pain provides hope for a vital life. A study by Rydeard et al[13] showed that Pilates-based approach was more efficacious than usual care in a population with chronic, unresolved low back pain. This growing trend in the research continues to support Pilates as a legitimate intervention for physical therapy and health-related professions.

Two publications looked at the effects of Pilates training on flexibility and body composition.[9,10] One showed a significant decrease in body fat composition and the other did not. The difference between the 2 studies probably was due to the frequency of intervention and the duration. Jago et al[10] instructed female high school students to take a Pilates class 5 days/week for 4 weeks. Segal et al[9] were not able to substantiate a significant decrease in body fat composition, but participants only participated in 1 class/week for 2 months, which is a significant decrease in actual contact hours compared to Jago et al's study. What Segal and colleagues did show was a significant increase in flexibility. Anderson's dissertation[16] also showed a trend of positive change in all of the physical measures for strength, flexibility, and coordination.

The Pilates Method Alliance (a nonprofit organization) and a few of its members, including Polestar Pilates, continue to promote evidence-based research to substantiate the Pilates approach as a viable and valid intervention for rehabilitation and fitness. Polestar is currently conducting a number of studies and is supporting students from universities who are interested in conducting Pilates-based research.

CONCLUSION

In addition to the principles described in this chapter, one of the greatest advantages that Pilates has to offer is its flexible environment to meet the specific needs of the client. By manipulating gravity, base of support, length of levers, and center of gravity, the practitioner is much more capable of facilitating the patient's successful movement with less effort, less fatigue, and greater movement awareness retention. Pilates has been a tool for successful intervention with a large variety of patients of all ages with ranging diagnoses, from neurological to rheumatological, pediatric to orthopedic, and women's health to performance enhancement. Two basic assumptions we make in Pilates rehabilitation are that movement exists within each person and that the ability to heal lies within each individual. Ongoing studies will add to our understanding of the mechanisms of action that support these assumptions.

REFERENCES

1. Pilates JH, Miller WJ. Result of contrology. In: Pilates JH, ed. *Return to Life Through Contrology*. New York, NY: JJ Augustin; 1945: 18-32.
2. Anderson BD. *Polestar Education Instruction Manual: Polestar Approach to Movement Principles*. Self-published education manual. 2001.
3. Richardson C, Jull G, Hodges P, et al. Local muscle dysfunction in low back pain. In: *Therapeutic Exercise for Spinal Segmental Stabilization in Low Back Pain*. London: Churchill Livingstone; 1999: 11-61.
4. Richardson C, Jull G, Toppenberg R, Comerford M. Techniques for active lumbar stabilization for spinal protection: a pilot study. *Aust J Physiother*. 1992;38(2):105-112.
5. Richardson C, Jull G, Hodges P, et al. Overview of the principles of clinical management of the deep muscle system for segmental stabilization. In: *Therapeutic Exercise for Spinal Segmental Stabilization in Low Back Pain*. London, United Kingdom: Churchill Livingstone; 1999: 93-102.
6. Porterfield JA. Dynamic stabilization of the trunk. *J Orthop Sports Phys Ther*. 1985;6:271.
7. Sahrmann S. Diagnosis and treatment of muscle imbalances and musculoskeletal pain syndromes. Workshop Manual. Self-published education manual. 1996.
8. Daack M, Huntingdon J, Isaacson AF, Anderson B. The effects of Pilates based exercises on hypomobility of the spine in a healthy population. Poster presentation at: California American Physical Therapy Association Conference; January 1996.
9. Segal NA, Hein J, Basford JR. The effects of Pilates training on flexibility and body composition: an observational study. *Arch Phys Med Rehabil*. 2004;85:1977-1981.
10. Jago R, Jonker ML, Missaghian M, Baranowski T. Effect of 4 weeks of Pilates on the body composition of young girls. *Prev Med*. 2006;42(3):177-180.
11. Hutchinson MR, Tremain L, Christiansen J, Beitzel J. Improving leaping ability in elite rhythmic gymnasts. *Med Sci Sports Exerc*. 1998;30(10):1543-1547.
12. Smith K, Smith E. Integrating Pilates–based core strengthening into older adult fitness programs: implications for practice. *Top Geriatr Rehabil*. 2005;21(1):57-67.
13. Rydeard R, Leger A, Smith D. Pilates-based therapeutic exercise: effect on subjects with nonspecific chronic low back pain and functional disability: a randomized controlled trial. *J Orthop Sports Phys Ther*. 2006;36(7):472-484.
14. Graves BS, Quinn JV, O'Kroy JA, Torok DJ. Influence of Pilates-based mat exercises on chronic coger back pain. *Med Sci Sports Exerc*. 2005;37(5 Supplement):S27.
15. Blum CL. Chiropractic and pilates therapy for the treatment of adult scoliosis. *J Manipulative Physiol Ther*. 2002;25(4):E3.

16. Anderson BD. Randomized clinical trial comparing active versus passive approaches to the treatment of recurrent and chronic low back pain. Dissertation, University of Miami, Department of Physical Therapy; 2005.

17. Cowan T, Lackner J, Anderson BD, Polina J, Morigerato G, Hopkins L. A pilot study of Pilates exercise for rehabilitation of sub acute low back patients. 2003 pending submission for publication.

ADDITIONAL RESOURCES

Pilates continues to grow at a rapid pace and, thus, there is an ongoing need for Pilates practitioners in rehabilitation and in fitness. If one is interested in learning more about becoming a Pilates rehabilitation practitioner, contact the following groups:

- Pilates Method Alliance

  1666 Kennedy Causeway, Suite 402

  North Bay Village, FL 33141

  Phone: (866) 573-4945

  Fax: (305) 573-4461

  Email: info@pilatesmethodalliance.org

  Website: www.pilatesmethodalliance.org Offers a more-extensive list of Pilates-certified therapists around the world.

- Polestar Physical Therapy and Pilates Center

  7171 SW 62nd Avenue, 3rd Floor

  Miami, FL 33143

  Phone: (305) 740-6001

  Fax: (305) 740-6998

  Website: www.polestarmiami.com

- Polestar Pilates Education

  7300 North Kendall Drive, Suite 550

  Miami, FL 33156

  Phone: (305) 666-0037

  Website: www.polestarpilates.com

V

Energy Work

Reiki
A Biofield Therapy

Sangeeta Singg, PhD, ACN

Although the notion that people with mental or physical disorders can be healed by someone's touch is contemporary in the Western world, such practice has been in existence in the world since ancient times. With the advent of the Internet, it has become impossible for the Western medical establishment to prevent the invasion of ancient knowledge and practice of alternative medicine from looming as a new movement of healing with the help of so-called *New Age modalities*. It is ironic that the alternative healing modalities are being assigned to the New Age movement (some say a misnomer), which burgeoned in the West in the 1960s, whereas most alternative modalities are ancient. Modalities such as hands-on healing, T'ai Chi, hatha yoga, Ayurveda, prayer, acupuncture, Qi gong, shiatsu, herbal remedies, and so on were the common practices in the ancient civilizations. All of these systems view injury, dysfunction, and disease as manifestations of weak, unbalanced, or blocked vital energy. Energy in such a state is optimized with the help of alternative modalities, which lead to facilitated health and wellness.

For the most part, what caused the gap between ancient belief and modern medical practice is the rigorous adherence to the scientific method by the modern medical community and the rejection of ancient healing methods. Allopathic medicine is based on scientific inquiry, whereas alternative medicine is based on tradition and belief. The most important criterion for any drug or treatment to meet before the United States Food and Drug Administration will allow it to reach the American consumer is that it is able to withstand a double-blind controlled trial. Because many energy-based alternative modalities lack the stringent testing with double-blind controlled trials, they have been shunned as viable methods of treatment. In spite of the lack of controlled research, however, alternative healing methods are seeping into the treatment regimen of many patients either by their own undertaking or as a part of professional intervention. Although many alternative modalities require involved training and internship, one modality called *Reiki* requires very little training and is the second most-accessible modality (the first being prayer).

Reiki (pronounced Ray-key) is a Japanese word, with *Rei* meaning universal or omnipresent and *Ki* meaning life force or energy. It is an all-knowing and all-encompassing universal life force that animates all living things.[1-4] It is the same as *ch'i* in Chinese, *prana* in Sanskrit, *mana* in Polynesian, *pneuma* in Greek, and *ruah* (breath of life) in Hebrew and in the Old Testament.[1,5]

There are as many words for the *universal life force* as there are the belief systems and languages. The author was interested in Reiki as a researcher and a psychologist for many years even though she did not know it by its Japanese name. As a result, she obtained training at all levels, from first degree

Davis CM.
Integrative Therapies in Rehabilitation: Evidence for Efficacy in Therapy, Prevention, and Wellness, Fourth Edition (pp 241-257).
© 2017 Taylor & Francis Group.

to master level, and subsequently conducted and published a controlled Reiki study with graduate student Linda Dressen.[5,6]

Reiki practice has become quite well known all over the world. The Internet is replete with information on Reiki. There are several national and international Reiki organizations, and many Internet websites, books, and anecdotal articles in magazines and professional journals. The National Center for Complementary and Integrative Health (formerly known as both the Office of Alternative Medicine and the National Center for Complementary and Alternative Medicine) has classified Reiki as energy medicine and a biofield therapy.[7] However, there are very few controlled studies in the scientific literature supporting the efficacy of Reiki healing. This chapter attempts to reconcile much anecdotal and limited empirical information, some of which is conflicting. Because the Reiki tradition is proudly referred to as "a rich oral tradition" by practitioners, most of the theoretical and historical information about Reiki lacks written verification. Much of the information presented in this regard was obtained from interviewing several practitioners and reading a large number of informal (and a few formal) sources. Contradictory information from many of these sources is confusing. Thus, this chapter presents a coherent and widely accepted version of the Reiki story. Because of the vast amount of public domain information available on the Internet and via other sources, citing of all such sources is neither possible nor fair. As a result, only formal sources are cited here. Also, because of discrepancies among many sources, only information that appeared to be accepted by a majority of practitioners is presented.

WHAT IS REIKI?

Reiki is a healing system that channels the universal life force through the practitioner's hands. The fundamental supposition of Reiki is that all living things are animated with the same infinite, monolithic, vital energy, and the source of this vital energy is spiritual. It is considered a holistic approach to health and well-being. The activation of Reiki is believed to promote energy balancing, healing, and a state of well-being in all living things. Therefore, Reiki may be called a form of *energy medicine.*[8] As such, it is practiced not only by professionals, but also by laypersons to heal themselves and others in a variety of settings. The medical community is beginning to recognize the inevitable arrival of energy medicine in treatment. Gerber[9] has aptly stated, "Within certain subspecialties of conventional medicine…The permutation from conventional drug and surgical therapy to electromagnetic healing represents the beginnings of a revolution in consciousness for the medical profession."

As a noninvasive modality, Reiki is believed to flow via the hands of a practitioner to a willing recipient. The practitioner serves as a conduit for the flow of this universal life force without using his or her own personal energy. This energy can be transmitted either by touching the recipient or intending its transmission from any distance. This universal life force is believed to be an intelligent energy that reaches the part of the body that needs it.[1,4,8] The practitioner does not need to know the ailment or diagnosis before administering a healing treatment. Although some alternatively think that Reiki can be channeled to a specific place or problem in the body, most practitioners believe that this energy cannot be controlled or regulated in any way, and the energy will not work if one tries to direct it. This nondirective approach to healing is the major difference between Reiki and other hands-on healing methods.

Another difference from other manual therapies lies in the training procedure of the Reiki practitioner. Anyone can learn Reiki. However, unlike other hands-on healing methods, Reiki is not taught. Instead, it is transferred from the Reiki master to the student during the induction process called *attunement.*[5,7,8] Becoming attuned is a way of allowing oneself to open up to channel the universal life force. Once a person opens up to channel this energy, it is believed that he or she never loses it. However, a few believe that Reiki will "weaken and fade away when it is not exercised."[2] Also, some claim that you do not need to be attuned to practice Reiki, because the ability to tap into the universal life force is inborn in all of us. The author agrees with this contention. There are many ways to tap into this energy. While some are more tedious than the others, Reiki is considered one of the easiest and quickest ways to achieve this goal.

Intentionality is a crucial factor for the success of all natural healing modalities. Intentionality was the theme of 2 1999 issues of *Bridges*,[10,11] the quarterly magazine of the International Society for the Study of Subtle Energies and Energy Medicine (ISSSEEM). *Intentionality* is described as the process of focusing attention of thought or concentration in a specific way so as to bring about a healing or balance by way of energy flow. Reiki practitioners are specifically taught to be cognizant of the recipient's voluntary intent to receive healing. Sending Reiki to an unwilling and unbelieving recipient is considered unethical. However, the situation is different when the recipients are children, animals, or seriously ill persons who cannot express their will in relation to receiving Reiki. It is believed that these recipients lack barriers and are, therefore, very responsive to this life force.[4] If they do not want it, they will let the practitioner know by moving away from the practitioner's hands or simply by not accepting it.

EXPERIENCE OF RECEIVING REIKI TREATMENT

The experience of Reiki differs from recipient to recipient. Some commonly reported sensations are warmth, tingling, coolness, and subsequent general relaxation. Also, some individuals feel a positive change in symptoms right away, while others report feeling a positive change after a longer period of time. Reiki treatments are reported to produce no negative side effects. Respecting individual freedom is an important tenant of Reiki. The belief is that Reiki cannot be used against an individual's will or in a negative way. It can only be used with a willing recipient for the best possible outcome or the highest good because the intelligent life force knows what is best for the person.[1,2,4,8]

Because Reiki can be used along with allopathic treatment, patients in the hospital or under conventional medical care are very good candidates to benefit from Reiki. Reiki as a complementary modality can accelerate the healing process and reduce negative side effects of medicines and other procedures. It permeates all aspects of self, from physical health to emotional well-being and spiritual awareness. Thus, it is believed to work simultaneously at the physical, mental, and spiritual levels. Because the universal life force is channeled through the practitioner, it benefits the practitioner as well.[1,2,4,8] As such, it is a double blessing; it blesses those who receive it and those who give it.

HISTORICAL ACCOUNT

Different authors have presented different versions of the Reiki story.[1-6,8,12] All agree that Hawayo Takata (1900-1980), who lived in Hawaii, introduced Reiki to the West around 1937. While visiting her family in Japan in 1935, she became very ill and was admitted to a hospital to undergo an operation. In the operating room before the surgery, she strongly felt that there was another way to get better. Upon her inquiring, she was directed to a clinic run by Dr. Chujiro Hayashi (1880-1940), who learned Reiki from Dr. Mikao Usui (1865-1926), the founder of the Usui System of Reiki. In 1925, Hayashi, a retired Naval officer, became impressed with Usui's commitment and dedication and joined him in his cause of helping people with Reiki. Following the Usui tradition, he established the first Reiki clinic after Usui's death in 1926. This is where Takata was treated. After her recovery, she received Reiki training from Hayashi and returned to Hawaii in 1937. A few weeks later and just before World War II, Hayashi came to Hawaii and further trained Takata to teach Reiki to others. In February 1938, she was named a Reiki master. It is believed that Hayashi trained approximately 17 masters. Takata returned to Japan per Hayashi's request, and Hayashi passed the Reiki torch to her as his successor. Soon after this, he died in 1940.[1-6,8,12]

Takata practiced Reiki in Hawaii and later moved to California. She continued using and teaching Reiki until her death in 1980. She trained 22 Reiki masters, including her granddaughter, Phyllis Furumoto, to carry out the Reiki tradition.[1-4] After her death, 2 leaders emerged, creating

2 different branches of the Usui system of Reiki. Furumoto founded The Reiki Alliance in 1981. In 1982, another student of Takata, Dr. Barbara Weber Ray, founded the American International Reiki Association, Inc.[1,2] Currently, there are several organizations and versions of Reiki claiming their authenticity. They can be located on the Internet.

Origins of Reiki

How did the originator, Usui, learn Reiki? The legend is that Usui, a Christian minister, was heading a Christian boys' school in Kyoto, Japan. Some believe that he was a Buddhist monk. Yet, others say that he was neither a Christian minister nor a Buddhist monk, but was simply a spiritual healer.[1-7,12] He may have been both because many Buddhist spiritualists are not bound by strict religious beliefs or boundaries. While working at the boys' school, he became interested in researching the miracles performed by Jesus. To learn the healing methods that Jesus might have used, he traveled to the United States, but did not find the information he sought in Christian schools. He was then directed to study Buddhist writings seeking knowledge of what Buddha had taught about healing.

There are conflicting statements about Usui's visit to America. Some say that he never came to America, while others contend that he received his doctorate in theology from the University of Chicago. In any event, many practitioners in old Eastern societies in the late 1800s were labeled as doctors without a medical degree if they learned the medical practice while assisting a doctor, many opening up an independent practice of their own after several years of training under a medical doctor.

In Japan, Usui searched for an answer in many temples and finally found Sanskrit writings in the form of Sutras, which explained how the healing was done. However, although he had found the information that explained the mechanisms of healing, he did not feel empowered to heal others. He then turned to another ancient Indian method of achieving enlightenment, one Buddha had used. He performed tapasya (penance) by fasting and meditating on Mount Koriyama, some 17 miles from Kyoto. At the end of the 21st day, he was enlightened with the knowledge of healing.

Usui used this knowledge to give healing to many people in Japan. He believed that to free humanity from illness and suffering, this healing method should be made available to the public. Therefore, he trained 18 or 19 Reiki masters before his death. Although most of the formal and informal information about Reiki practice pertains to healing others, the most important aspect of Reiki is self-healing. He also gave the following 5 spiritual precepts to his students to practice in daily life—for today only: do not anger, do not worry, be humble, be honest in your work, and be compassionate to yourself and others.[1-7,12]

It has been said that Usui rediscovered Reiki in the late 1800s; however, the author disagrees. *Rediscovery* denotes that some lost thing has been found again. Reiki is an ontological reality that always existed regardless of our knowledge of it. It was in existence before Usui and before Buddha. What might be a more accurate statement is that Usui practiced Reiki based on an ancient Buddhist practice, which was introduced to the Western world in late 1930s by Takata. However, after Takata's death in 1980, Reiki practice became more structured and formalized than the original oral intuitive method. The goal, however, remains the same as Usui envisioned it: personal and global healing.

Some believe that both Usui and Hayashi did not leave any written instructions about Reiki, yet there are others who claim that they both had written some sort of manual. During her training sessions, Takata maintained the oral tradition and did not allow her students to take notes. However, this changed after her death.[1-7,12] At present, it appears that there are as many manuals as there are Reiki masters, and several Reiki masters claim to have unique Reiki systems with different names; however, they all claim their lineage to Usui.

Because Reiki is not associated with any religion, both the practitioner and the recipient do not have to accept any religious beliefs as prerequisites to Reiki healing.[1-6,8,12] Although it comes from an ancient Tibetan Buddhist practice, it is not connected to Buddhism as such. It surpasses professional, cultural, and religious boundaries. Reiki practitioners include a variety of professionals and laypersons from many religions and cultures. For example, the International Association of Reiki

Professionals (IARP)[13] claims a global membership of Reiki practitioners and master teachers from 50 countries. There are several directories available on the Internet that list Reiki practitioners. *The Reiki Page,*[14] for instance, lists practitioners and masters from all over the world. Of course, not all persons attuned to be Reiki practitioners are included in these directories.

REIKI TRAINING

Reiki training is provided by Reiki masters at 3 to 4 levels presented in 3 to 10 stages, depending on the master's training and association. However, traditionally, Reiki training was divided into 3 levels: *Shoden* (first teachings), *Okuden* (inner teachings), and *Shinpiden* (mystery teachings). They are now called *first* (beginner's level), *second* (advanced level), and *third* (Reiki master level) degrees, respectively.[4] Usui, Hayashi, and Takata have been considered the Grand Masters among Reiki practitioners; however, Takata did not appoint a successor. In fact, some have tried to claim this title.[1-4] Since Takata's death, several modifications of the traditional Reiki system have come into existence. Proponents of different variations have altered the classification and training system according to their preferences.

Although the training methods may differ slightly, the ultimate goal at every level is a series of *attunements. Attunement* is a form of initiation that prepares one's body for channeling the universal life force. Attunement is believed to prime one to receive the flow of energy and empower to be able to channel this energy from the top of one's head through the palms. These cannot be explained in the text, however, because secrecy is maintained and disclosed only during master degree. Completion of the training is not heralded by any formal examination, because the major component of the training is the experience of attunement.

Keeping in line with Takata's tradition, the beginner's level, or first-degree training, begins with masters relating the Reiki story and sharing of anecdotal cases. The use of the word *master* is equivalent to teacher/mentor in the Western world. In the East, the title master, or guru, is bestowed on those who have achieved the highest levels of knowledge and enlightenment in a certain area and who are capable of imparting knowledge and mentoring others in that area. Some masters may also provide the information on research supporting the efficacy of Reiki. Students are then given attunements. They are also given a manual that shows different hand positions, which they then practice on themselves or others in class. Considerable time is spent on supervised practice. The number or sequence of laying hands on a recipient's body may differ from master to master, with the number of hand positions ranging from 5 to 15, depending on the master.

The advanced level, or second-degree training, is available to all of those who have completed the first degree. In second-degree training, additional attunements are given and a series of special symbols are revealed. This allows for a deeper Reiki experience involving work on a mental/emotional level and added ability to send Reiki to a distant source. It is also called *distant* or *absentee healing*.

The master level, or third-degree training, is for those who are experienced Reiki practitioners both at the first- and second-degree levels. Some divide this level into third degree and master's level, depending on a student's preparation and interest. During their attunement, participants learn a final symbol for attuning others and experiencing Reiki at the deepest level possible. This training empowers the participants to become Reiki masters who are capable of providing all 3 levels of Reiki training to others.

Each Reiki training workshop may last from a half day to several days. Certificates of completion are provided at the end of each workshop for each level of Reiki training. Many masters have developed their own manuals in an attempt to personalize their training, and students receive these manuals during their training.

REIKI TREATMENT

The process of attunement allows one to channel Reiki immediately. Practitioners usually place their palms (some specify to cup them) in a sequential pattern on or just above the body of a recipient who is fully clothed. The hand positions are designed to cover the head, front, back, and feet, providing Reiki to the body's major organs and endocrine and lymphatic systems. The complete process may take from 60 to 90 minutes.[1-6,8] However, the time spent in a Reiki session can vary from situation to situation and place to place. Sometimes, the Reiki touch may last for only a few moments.[6] Such flexibility has made Reiki very useful for those professionals who have a very limited amount of time for each patient and a large number of patients to care for. That is a major reason why Reiki is popular with nurses and why Reiki training is acceptable as part of their continuing education.[15] Sometimes the recipients may not wish to be touched or they may be in such condition that their skin cannot be touched (eg, burn victims). Reiki can be administered by holding hands 3 to 4 inches over the recipient's body, functioning as a distant healing.[1,8]

EVIDENCE OF EFFICACY FOR REIKI PRACTICE

Although the literature is full of anecdotes from Reiki practitioners and clients claiming healing at all levels, only a handful of scientific studies are found in support of such claims. Because these studies examine different physical and emotional problems using different research instruments, the results are difficult to compare. Also, most of the studies have small samples and methodological flaws due to the nature of the subject matter.[5] Five articles published between 2007 and 2014 conducted systematic reviews of clinical trials using Reiki as the treatment modality.[7,16-19] All 5 articles used online search, specific criteria for inclusion, and were comparative reviews of the Reiki studies. Because of the heterogeneity of the studies, their conclusions were guarded. However, in my review of the reviews, I found 2 articles to be too limiting in their scope because they eliminated animal studies and focused either only on randomized clinical trials[17] or on studies with test/control groups.[18] I believe that this robs the readers of some important information presented in the eliminated studies. Both of these reviews were inconclusive about the effectiveness of Reiki. The other 3 reviews discussed in this section provide a well-organized and complete knowledge of Reiki research to date.[7,16,19]

From December 2008 to June 2009, a team of researchers through the Center for Reiki Research (CRS) conducted a rigorous review of all United States studies published in the peer-reviewed journals.[7] If a study met the specified selection criteria, it entered the Touchstone Process for review by 2 independent doctoral-level researchers before being included in a final group of evidence-based studies. Initially, the team identified 7 qualitative and 19 quantitative peer-reviewed Reiki articles. The Touchstone Process consists of experts who conduct an ongoing critique of all Reiki research published in peer-reviewed journals. The team includes 7 researchers with doctoral degrees and 5 experienced nurses. All article summaries and the summary of the Touchstone Process evaluation are posted on the CRS website.[20]

This is by far the most comprehensive, objective, and systematic review I have found in the area of Reiki research.[7] The CRS website provides other useful information about Reiki as well. Of the 26 peer-reviewed articles selected by the Touchstone Process, only 13 articles[5,24,37-47] were assessed to have "robust research designs and well-established outcome parameters."[9] These articles were assessed as "very good" or "excellent" by at least one reviewer from the Touchstone Process team and were not considered "weak" by any reviewer. Our study was included in their list of 13 finalists and will be presented later in this chapter. The main conclusion of the Touchstone Process team was that 83% of these "top range" studies showed "moderate to strong evidence in support of Reiki as a therapeutic modality in conditions relating to pain, stress, anxiety and mood."[20]

Another noteworthy conclusion of the CRS Touchstone Project team was that the 2 carefully controlled studies on rats[21,26] yielded the "strongest demonstrable biological effect."[20] These studies showed that the Reiki significantly reduced stress compared with sham Reiki. The team further recognized the advantage of animal studies over the human studies because most extraneous variables can be controlled in the laboratory setting and they eliminate the placebo effect.[7,20] In the first experiment, Baldwin and Schwartz[21] divided 16 male Sprague Dawley rats into 4 groups housed in four separate, but similar, rooms. The rats in 3 of the 4 groups were subjected to 15 minutes of 90 dB white noise for 3 weeks and rats in the fourth room were the quiet control group. Because loud noise stress can damage the mesenteric microvasculature, causing leakage of plasma into the surrounding tissue, the rat groups were varied in 4 conditions to determine whether Reiki as a healing energy can reduce microvascular leakage. The 4 groups were no noise group, noise group, noise and sham Reiki group, and noise and Reiki group. The noise and Reiki group received a daily 15-minute Reiki treatment prior to the noise. The experiment was performed 3 times, and Reiki significantly reduced the average number and area of microvascular leaks compared with the other noise groups each time. However, authors questioned whether the effects were caused by Reiki itself or the relaxing effect of the Reiki practitioner and recommended using distant Reiki in the future experiments.

In a later experiment, Baldwin et al[26] used 3 male Sprague Dawley rats implanted with radio-telemetric transducers to monitor the heart rate and blood pressure. They were subjected to 90 dB white noise for 30 minutes a day for 8 days. During the last 5 days, 2 Reiki practitioners provided 15 minutes of Reiki before and 15 minutes after the noise. The experiment was repeated with the sham Reiki on the same animals. Mean heart rates and blood pressure were recorded before, during, and after Reiki treatment and during the noise. Results showed that Reiki as opposed to sham Reiki significantly reduced heart rate compared to the baseline. However, neither Reiki nor sham Reiki significantly affected blood pressure. It was concluded that Reiki was effective in modulating heart rate in rats as it has been found to be a stress reducer in humans.

The second major review was conducted by Thrane and Cohen,[19] who mainly examined the effect of Reiki for pain and anxiety in randomized clinical trials. Studies that used randomization, a control group, and were published in 2000 or later in peer-reviewed journals examining pain or anxiety were included in the review. Of the 12 relevant articles, only 7 met the inclusion criteria. Of the 7 studies, 4 used cancer patients, 1 included post-surgical patients, and 2 used older adults. The heterogeneity of participants and interventions made it difficult to make any generalizations, even though most of the 7 studies yielded statistically significant results, either for pain, anxiety, or both. Cohen's d was used to calculate effect sizes. This procedure allows the comparison of studies in a standardized way. The effect sizes ranged from $d=0.24$ (small) for decrease in anxiety in women undergoing breast biopsy to $d=2.08$ (large) for decreased pain in older adults. Based on the Cohen's d statistical results, the authors concluded that there is evidence to suggest that Reiki therapy may be effective for pain and anxiety. They offered suggestions for future research to use larger sample sizes, randomized groups, and standardized treatment protocols.[19]

Vitale[16] conducted an integrative review of 16 Reiki studies published from 1980 to 2006. She reported 8 studies showing effectiveness of Reiki therapy for stress reduction and depression,[33] anxiety reduction,[5,30,36] and pain reduction.[5,31,34,35] Upon completion of her review, Vitale questioned "…whether the randomized controlled trial design considered the 'criterion standard' in medical research is the optimal methodology for capturing the efficacy of energy work."[16] Even though the randomized controlled trial is the gold standard in medical research, some researchers are questioning its feasibility in relation to biofield therapies, such as Reiki.

Also, it is difficult to demonstrate whether sham Reiki used as a placebo is truly inert or whether it introduces another confounding variable.[29,35] Human touch is healing in itself, and then there is another uncontrollable variable of intentionality, which has not been addressed in the 5 major reviews.[7,16-19] The phenomenological findings of some studies suggest that the effects of biofield work, such as Reiki, may be better understood with help of qualitative research methods.[35] Several researchers have voiced their concern about using the linear research methods to study biofield therapies.[29,37,38] Perhaps they have a point. An experimental design may not be optimal for studying an individualized healing therapy, such as Reiki, which is used in a natural setting.[33] One major weakness of all of the studies evaluated by the Touchstone Process team was small sample size due to the exploratory nature of the studies and a lack of funding. The team has posted on the CRS website some research guidelines including Essential Components of Good Study Design for future Reiki research, and the team will also provide consultation service to those seeking help in designing their studies.[20]

Considering the current state of Reiki research, the following 3 conclusions by the Touchstone Process offer acceptable answers[20]:

1. Due to the subtle and complex nature of Reiki practice, the measures used in research to date may not be sensitive enough for capturing individualized experiences of Reiki recipients.

2. There are no reported negative effects of Reiki.

3. There is "enough scientific evidence to support the ability of Reiki to reduce anxiety and pain, induce relaxation, improve fatigue and depressive symptoms, and strengthen overall wellbeing."[20]

PERSONAL RESEARCH EXPERIENCE WITH REIKI

Hailing from India, I grew up knowing about many alternative healing modalities, such as yoga, Ayurvedic medicine, homeopathy, healing through touch and prayer, and herbal remedies, among others. Consequently, when I first learned about Reiki at the 1997 Annual Conference of the ISSSEEM, I was not surprised. I assumed that Reiki was similar to some healing practices that have been in existence for centuries in India. If you have ever seen the pictures of Hindu gods and goddesses, you would have noticed that they have their right hands up facing you, with energy bursting out of them. This energy represents the divine energy that heals and blesses. Also in India, when younger persons touch the feet of elders as a form of greeting, the elders place their palms on the younger persons' heads and shoulders, giving them *ashirwad*, which means blessings.

At any rate, having earned 3 graduate degrees in America and being involved in research for over 2 decades, I learned to put my subjective feelings about what constitutes effective healing practice aside and profess only that which was verified via scientific method. But my exposure to Reiki at the ISSSEEM awakened the memories of my experiences with the alternative healing methods of India. Also, I met doctors, bioengineers, nurses, psychologists, professional counselors, social workers, and laypersons at the ISSSEEM meeting who practiced Reiki and other forms of alternative and complementary therapies. Inspired by their testimonies, I sought the training and earned my first degree in Reiki on July 20, 1997.

I was very excited about being initiated into this art of healing, and I could not wait to share my experiences with my psychology students. In addition to telling them all about this hands-on healing modality, I shared my frustrations about the lack of scientific evidence demonstrating the efficacy of Reiki practice. I had decided to conduct research in this area to satisfy my own curiosity. One day after an undergraduate counseling psychology class, my previously mentioned student, Linda Dressen, stopped me and said, "I was looking for a mentor, and I think I have found her." She then shared with me her enthusiasm about Reiki and commented that she was a Reiki master. I shared my research ideas and hypotheses with Linda and asked her if she would like to get involved in the project. She agreed immediately and enrolled in an independent research class with me. Later, she participated in a Reiki study that I designed and directed in which 5 Reiki masters and 4 laypersons helped to collect data from chronically ill patients in the West Texas area. The impressive results prompted me to submit the study for presentation at the Ninth Annual Conference of the ISSSEEM in Boulder, Colorado. Our paper was one of the 4 technical papers accepted from over 110 submissions worldwide for the 1999 ISSSEEM conference.[6] Our study was published in *Subtle Energies & Energy Medicine*.[5] Following is a summary of the study.

This was the first experimental study that compared Reiki with progressive muscle relaxation, control, and placebo conditions to examine the efficacy of Reiki for emotional, personality, and spiritual changes in chronically ill patients.[5] Sex and type of treatment were the independent variables of the study. Treatment groups were the Reiki (R) group, progressive muscle relaxation (PMR) group, wait-list control (C) group, and placebo (P) group. The dependent variables included present pain intensity; total pain rating index-R (PRI-R); PRI-R: sensory quality of pain; PRI-R: affective quality of pain; PRI-R: evaluative quality of pain, depression, state anxiety, trait anxiety, self-esteem, locus of control, realistic sense of personal control, and belief in God's (higher power) assistance. These variables were measured by the following instruments: General Information Questionnaire, Social Readjustment Rating Scale, McGill Pain Questionnaire, Beck Depression Inventory-II, State-Trait Anxiety Inventory, Rotter Internal-External Locus of Control Scale, Rosenberg Self-Esteem Scale, and Belief in Personal Control Scale.[5]

The study included 48 men and 72 women (N = 120) who were chronically ill with headaches (45%), heart disease (10%), cancer (8%), arthritis (7%), peptic ulcer (6%), asthma (7%), hypertension (12%), or HIV infection (5%). They were predominantly White (92%) with average age of 41.34 years (standard deviation = 11.32). These participants had no prior experience with Reiki, PMR, or any type of hands-on healing therapy, and they all experienced some type of pain. These volunteers were randomly assigned to 1 of the 4 treatment groups, resulting in 8 (treatment x sex) subgroups (ns = 30). All participants received 10 twice-weekly 30-minute sessions. The R group received Reiki sessions and the PMR group received sessions involving PMR and deep breathing exercises. Participants in the C group read any material of their choice for 10 twice-weekly 30-minute sessions and did not receive Reiki treatment. The P group received false (sham) Reiki treatments by 4 lay assistants who did not receive Reiki attunement, but learned the hand positions used on R group participants. The R group participants were contacted after 3 months for follow-up testing to assess the change in dependent measures from post-test to follow-up.[5]

The results using the 4 x 2 factorial analysis of variance (ANOVA) and Omega Squared (ω^2) for pre-test/post-test change for all dependent variables are presented in Table 16-1. Although the ANOVA results for 10 independent variables were significant, only 3 main effects and 4 main effects showed medium and large effect sizes, respectively. Large treatment effects (ω^2 of 0.15 or larger is considered large treatment effect 0.24) were found on present pain intensity, depression, and state and trait anxiety. Medium treatment effects were noted on PRI-R: evaluative, locus of control, and unrealistic sense of control; while treatment effects were small on PRI-R: sensory, self-esteem, and faith in God. Significant interaction effects of treatment x sex were found only on depression and faith in God. The Tukey/Kramer procedure was used for all post hoc pairwise comparisons. The direction of significant Tukey/Kramer procedure results are documented in Table 16-2.

The post-test and follow-up comparison results of the R group showed significant reduction in sensory and affective qualities of pain along with the overall pain measure. All other comparisons did not yield significant results.

This was the first study of Reiki that randomly assigned men and women experiencing similar levels of life-event stress to experimental conditions and compared Reiki with PMR therapy, no therapy, and false Reiki. One of the major contributions of this study was to demonstrate how a placebo group can be used in Reiki studies. This strength was also recognized by the Touchstone Process team.[7,20] To my knowledge, no study prior to this study used a placebo group (false Reiki). After our study, several studies designed experiments and quasiexperiments that included a placebo or sham Reiki group.

Cooperation from patients and their health care providers was an important factor for the success of this study. Also, the patients were highly motivated to participate, perhaps due to their need to experience reduction in chronic pain resulting from their medical conditions. Some limitations of the study were that the sample was self-selected and some uncontrolled variables might have influenced the results; for example, "seriousness of the illness, multiple experimenters, multiple sites, religiosity, and social support available to the patient."[5] However, the random assignment of

TABLE 16-1

MAIN EFFECTS OF TREATMENT AND ONLY SIGNIFICANT TREATMENT X SEX ANOVA AND OMEGA SQUARED RESULTS USING PRE-TEST/POST-TEST CHANGE SCORES FOR TWELVE DEPENDENT VARIABLES

DEPENDENT VARIABLE	F	P	Ω^2
Global pain intensity	9.67	0.0001	0.18[a]
Pain Rating Index-R: Sensory	2.87	0.03	0.05
Pain Rating Index-R: Affective	0.17	0.91	ns
Pain Rating Index-R: Evaluative	5.43	0.001	0.13
Pain Rating Index-R: Total scale	2.24	0.09	ns
Depression	23.57	0.0001	0.34[a]
Depression x sex	2.98	0.03	0.03
State anxiety	18.56	0.0001	0.28[a]
Trait anxiety	17.29	0.0001	0.29[a]
Self-esteem	3.29	0.02	0.05
Locus of control	5.18	0.002	0.10
Unrealistic sense of control	3.79	0.01	0.07
Faith in God	2.80	0.04	0.04
Faith in God x sex	2.68	0.05	0.02

[a]Large effect size.

the participants and other controls used in the study provided some safeguards. The 6 major conclusions of the study are as follows[5]:

1. Reiki is an effective modality for reducing pain, depression, and state anxiety. Of those receiving Reiki, men tend to show greater reduction in depression than women after receiving Reiki.

2. Reiki is effective in enhancing desirable changes in personality. Persons tend to show decreased trait anxiety, self-esteem enhancement, and greater sense of internal locus of control. Further, their belief in their personal control tends to become more realistic.

3. Reiki enhances one's faith that God is a powerful agent whose help can be enlisted. Women tend to experience this enhancement in faith more than men.

4. Attunement is necessary for the practice of Reiki. A false Reiki practice would not be effective in enhancing desirable changes in pain, affective states, personality traits, and spirituality.

5. The gains made by Reiki tend to persist over longer periods of time. After a 3-month period, significant reduction tends to occur in sensory and affective qualities of pain and the Total Pain Rating Index.

6. Chronically ill patients experiencing high stress and pain would be receptive to Reiki practice.

TABLE 16-2	
ILLUSTRATION OF THE TUKEY/KRAMER PROCEDURE RESULTS FOR POST HOC PAIRWISE COMPARISONS	

VARIABLE	TUKEY/KRAMER PROCEDURE RESULTS PATTERN
Present pain intensity (A)	Group R > PMR) C) P
Pain Rating Index-R: Sensory (A)	Group R > PMR) P
Pain Rating Index-R: Evaluative (A)	Group R > PMR) C) P
Depression (A)	Group R > PMR) C) P
A x B	R ♂ > R ♀
State anxiety	Group R > PMR) C) P
Trait anxiety	Group R > PMR) C) P
Self-esteem	Group R > PMR) C) P
Locus of control	Group R > PMR) C) P
Unrealistic personal control	Group R > PMR) C
Faith in God (A)	Group R > PMR) C
A x B	R ♀ > PMR ♀) C ♀ ♂) P ♀
	P ♂ > PMR ♂ ♀) C ♂ ♀) P ♀

Key: A = Treatment; A x B = Treatment x sex interaction; R = Reiki group; PMR = progressive muscle relaxation group; C = control group; P = placebo group; > = significantly greater change;) = no significant difference in change; ♂ = men; ♀ = women

CURRENT APPLICATIONS AND FUTURE DIRECTIONS

Reiki is currently being used by many doctors and nurses in the United States as an adjunct to conventional medical practice. The major application of Reiki is in the areas of stress reduction and pain management in chronically ill patients.[4,8,15] Other areas in which Reiki is being used are physical healing, emotional healing, attitudinal changes, and facilitation of the dying process.[1,8,15,39,40] Some are using it as a psychotherapy tool. Barnett and Chambers[8] state, "Reiki accelerates the process of psychotherapy by eliciting additional insights regarding the client's situation as well as by allowing the emotional residue to gently release from the body's cells. The result is a sense of well-being and empowerment."

Because of medical and psychological applications, Reiki training has become acceptable as part of continuing education for many types of health professionals. For example, in 2015, I presented a 2-hour seminar on using Reiki for stress and pain management for continuing education at the Psychological Association of Greater West Texas (PAGWT).[41] The continuing education seminars are approved by PAGWT for the psychologists to use for renewal of their licenses in the state of Texas.

In last few years, Reiki practice has also entered the hospital setting. In 1997, all but one physician at the Columbia/HCA Portsmouth Regional Hospital in Portsmouth, New Hampshire, agreed to allow an option to receive a 15-minute Reiki treatment for preregistered surgery patients.[42] Sawyer[43] and Wing and Wolf[44] also took Reiki practice into the Dartmouth-Hitchcock Medical Center in Lebanon, New Hampshire, and the Department of Oncology at the Women and Infants Hospital in Province, Rhode Island, respectively. Their articles provide information that can be helpful to professionals in making similar attempts.

Rand[45] has an online article on the CRS website that discusses the efforts of several doctors, nurses, and Reiki practitioners who succeeded in having hospitals include Reiki as an adjunct therapy among their patient services.

Rand states that since the mid-1990s, Reiki has been used in hospital operating rooms and is now offered as a regular part of patient services in 15% of United States hospitals. A detailed description of 64 Reiki hospital programs is posted on the CRS website. Some of the hospitals are the Columbia Presbyterian Medical Center in New York, New York; the Tucson Medical Center in Tuscon, Arizona; the Manhattan Eye, Ear and Throat Hospital in New York, New York; the Memorial Sloane Kettering Hospital in New York, New York; the Marin General Hospital in Greenbrae, California; the California Pacific Medical Center in San Francisco, California; the University of Michigan Hospital in Ann Arbor, Michigan; and the Foote Hospital in Jackson, Michigan. Many benefits have been reported as a result of using Reiki as an adjunct therapy in hospitals, such as reduction in pain, reduction in anxiety, faster recovery, lessened blood loss during surgery, fewer side effects of chemo-therapy, and less use of medications.[1,4,8,15,39,40]

ETHICS AND INSURANCE

The IARP has been trying to regulate the practice of Reiki by creating a membership registration, a code of ethics, and a liability insurance program. The IARP has 2 slightly differing versions of the code of ethics, one for practitioners and another for master teachers. Of the 10 principles, principle 2 is the only one that differs in wording from the practitioner's version to the teacher's version. Therefore, the 2 wordings of principle 2 are presented in Table 16-3, along with the common wordings of the other 9 principles.[46]

A professional liability insurance program is also available through the IARP,[13] which covers Reiki practitioners and teachers in the United States and Canada. The insurance policy protects against malpractice suits resulting from services provided by these individuals. Besides providing the protection and support for its members, this program is believed to be useful because hospitals and other health care settings often require Reiki practitioners to have liability insurance to practice in these settings.

GUIDELINES FOR FUTURE RESEARCH

All research on Reiki to date is exploratory and preliminary because most findings have not been replicated under controlled conditions and lack extended follow-ups. However, findings of all types of studies serve as guidelines for future research. Science builds itself on all types of empirical studies, ranging from observational studies to rigorously controlled studies.

Nield-Anderson and Ameling[47] discuss several methodological and philosophical reasons for difficulty in conducting scientific research on the efficacy of Reiki. Although I agree with their general contention that it is difficult to conduct Reiki studies using traditional scientific method, I do not think that it is an impossible task. For example, they say, "This healing method cannot be masked, per se, so that double-blind studies involving random assignment of subjects to standard-ized treatment protocols and control groups are not possible."[47] Several Reiki studies[5,17-19,48] have shown that random assignment of participants, standardized treatment protocols, and placebo and control groups are possible. Another difficulty noted by Nield-Anderson and Ameling[47] is that randomization and group assignment render participants without choice in treatment, which may be a threat to a practitioner-client relationship. This problem can be handled by using a crossover experimental design and a wait-list control group, as done in several studies.[5,17-19,48] Yet, another problem with Reiki studies mentioned in the article by Nield-Anderson and Ameling[47] is that the studies of Reiki efficacy "deal almost exclusively with well populations." There are several studies that used patient samples.[5,17,39]

TABLE 16-3

INTERNATIONAL ASSOCIATION OF REIKI PROFESSIONALS CODE OF ETHICS FOR REIKI PRACTITIONERS AND REIKI MASTER TEACHERS

THE REGISTERED REIKI PRACTITIONER (RP)/REGISTERED REIKI MASTER PRACTITIONER AND TEACHER (RMT) AGREES TO:

1. Abide by a vow of confidentiality. Any information that is discussed within the context of a Reiki session is confidential between the client and practitioner.

2. Provide a safe and comfortable area for sessions or classes and work to provide an empowering and supportive environment for clients and students.

3. Always treat clients and students with the utmost respect and honor.

4. Have a pure and clear intention to offer your services for the highest healing good of the client and highest potential of the student.

5. Provide a brief oral or written description of what happens during a session and what to expect before a client's initial session. Provide a clear written description of subjects to be taught during each level of Reiki prior to class and list what the student will be able to do after taking the class.

6. Be respectful of all others' Reiki views and paths.

7. Educate clients/students on the value of Reiki and explain that sessions do not guarantee a cure, nor are they a substitute for qualified medical or professional care. Reiki is one part of an integrative healing or wellness program.

8. Suggest a consultation or referral for clients to qualified licensed professionals (medical doctor, licensed therapist, etc) when appropriate.

9. Never diagnose or prescribe. Never suggest that the client/student change prescribed treatment or interfere with the treatment of a licensed health care provider.

10. Be sensitive to the boundary needs of individual clients and students.

11. Never ask clients to disrobe (unless in the context of a licensed massage therapy session at the client's option). Do not touch the genital area or breasts. Practice hands-off healing of these areas if treatment is needed.

12. Be working to create harmony and friendly cooperation between Reiki Practitioners/ Master Teachers in the community and represent the IARP in a most professional manner.

13. Act as a beacon in your community by doing the best job possible.

14. Work to empower your students to heal themselves and to encourage and assist them in the development of their work with Reiki or their Reiki practices.

15. Be actively working on your own healing so as to embody and fully express the essence of Reiki in everything that you do.

Reproduced with permission from International Association of Reiki Professionals.

While some researchers are making efforts to investigate the efficacy of Reiki, there are still many research questions demanding answers. For example, do we need multiple hand positions? If it is to be believed that Reiki is a self-directing and intelligent force that goes where it is needed, why not use only one hand position? Research needs to be designed comparing the single hand position, such as shoulders, to multiple hand positions.

Another question arises. Do practitioners need to pay attention during the session or can they be talking, watching television, etc? It is believed that no focus or attention is required by the practitioner during the Reiki session. All one needs is to place the hands on another, and the Reiki will go where it is needed. Future studies should examine this axiom, for example, by comparing a group receiving Reiki while watching television to a group receiving Reiki in a quiet, private setting without any distractions for the practitioner and the recipient. This condition could be further varied by testing a session that is distracting for the practitioner (eg, use of headphones) but not for the recipient, and vice versa. Several other unanswered questions regarding Reiki are as follows:

- How long do Reiki sessions need to be?
- Do longer sessions produce better results than shorter sessions?
- How long should each hand position be held?
- Which hand positions are better for which disorders?
- Is the relaxed position in which the recipient is lying down better than a sitting or standing position?
- Could the attunements be removed if a person wished to have this done?

Reiki has a long way to go to be fully integrated into practice of medical professionals, because these unanswered questions might lead to their reluctance. Our scientific world rests on results of controlled studies, and that is what is needed to further the standing of Reiki in the medical field.

CASE EXAMPLE

A professional White woman, Mary (pseudonym), was 61 years old when she had her neck surgery for C4/5 disc herniation. Because of partial hearing loss and multiple allergies, Mary could not tolerate opioids, aminoglycosides, and several other ototoxic medications. Her neurosurgeon worked within her limitations and used only general anesthesia and intravenous antibiotics approved by her otolaryngologist. After the surgery, Mary was sent home the same day around 5:30 PM with instructions to take extra-strength acetaminophen if she experienced pain. After the effect of anesthesia wore off, Mary began experiencing severe pain and she took extra-strength acetaminophen as instructed, which made her sick to her stomach. Throwing up caused more even more pain, and she did not feel any relief from the medicine. She had a rigid cervical collar to limit neck mobility, and she sat on a recliner because she could not put her head down in the bed. It was 11:00 PM and she was still sitting in her recliner trying to cope with the pain. Out of desperation, her husband called me and asked if I could do anything for her. I came to their home and found Mary moaning and groaning with pain. I gently held her hand and stroked her forehead to calm her down. I asked her to relax her neck and shoulders muscles. I asked her if I could pray for her and she said, "Please." I said a prayer and both Mary and her husband said, "Amen." I asked her to rate her pain on a scale from 0 (no pain) to 10 (excruciating pain). She rated her pain to be 10 and said that it was the worst pain she ever had. I told her about the Reiki protocol and I gave her a 90-minute session the first night and 60-minute sessions for 3 more days, followed by 60-minute sessions every other day for 1 week and twice a week for 2 more weeks.

Because of the surgery and the cervical collar, during the first 4 sessions, I floated my hands over her upper body, applied light touch below the waist, and avoided her back. After about 30 minutes during the first session, I noticed that Mary became calmer, began breathing deeper, and drifted into sleep, a typical response to Reiki. At the end of the session, I left without waking her up. Her husband told me the following evening during her second session that she woke up around 6:00 AM and said that her pain was not as "horrible" and she was not as "panicky." She rated her pain as 10 again at the second session, and she fell asleep halfway into the session. She often drifted in and out of sleep during the sessions. At the end of the second session, Mary rated her pain to be 7. She slept on the recliner for 4 nights and was able to sleep in the bed on the fifth night. At the end of the 11th session, Mary rated her pain as 3 and she was sleeping through the night in her bed. Mary did not take any medication, but did take supplements, such as curcumin, bromelain, vitamin D, acetyl-L-carnitine, and magnesium. She also took whole-food multivitamins and applied Arnica gel on the back of her neck and shoulders. Her incision was in the front of her neck.

With each session, Mary became more comfortable and experienced less pain. At the end of the first week, her appetite returned and she laughed about things that happened at the hospital and during the first couple of days after coming home. Her painful experience of trying to lie down in the bed became an amusing story as she related it to others a couple of weeks after surgery. Her sore throat and swallowing also improved. Her 2-week visit with the doctor was good, and her doctor commented about her bravery for tolerating pain without taking any medication. She chose not to tell him about her experience with Reiki, but she said that she had a lot of prayers. We always began the Reiki sessions with a prayer.

At the 2-month checkup, her doctor said that her neck was healing as expected and that everything looked good. She was back to work and did not report any pain. At the 3-month follow-up session with me, Mary said that she was free from most of the pre- and post-surgery symptoms and that she experienced "very little" pain occasionally. I asked her to rate her pain at this visit and she rated it as 1. We had one last 30-minute Reiki session. It has been over 2 years since Mary had surgery. At a recent encounter in the mall, she said that she was doing well with her health and work, and that her neck had healed well. She made no reference to pain.

CONCLUSION

Reiki represents an ancient art of self-healing and healing others. It is a simple modality that can be learned by anyone, regardless of their nationality, creed, culture, sex, age, and wellness level. One does not need to go beyond the first degree, because it provides all that one needs to facilitate healing oneself or others. However, all 3 Reiki degrees can be achieved by anyone who has a continued desire of experiencing Reiki at deeper levels. Reiki is believed to facilitate relaxation, reduce pain and anxiety, promote healing, improve fatigue and depression, and strengthen overall well-being. Although there are many anecdotal stories of positive physical, mental, and spiritual changes in people after receiving Reiki therapy, the scientific evidence to support these claims is scant. More well-designed and controlled studies on the efficacy of Reiki are needed for it to be accepted within the mainstream health care system. Because Reiki is so easy to learn, a time may come when health care professionals may advise it to be included in the preventive care program in addition to balanced diet and exercise. However, there is some evidence of the overcommercialization of Reiki, which seems to give ammunition to those who are critical of this modality. In his book on spiritual healing research, Benor[16] listed 3 limitations of Reiki. Besides inadequate preparation of later generations of masters and lack of formal structure for supervision/certification, he assessed high fees (up to several thousand dollars) for master-level training as a limitation. Therefore, it bears great responsibility on those who are committed to preserving the integrity of Reiki practice that they work toward keeping the practice free of internal bickering, competition, outrageous profit schemes, power struggle, gimmicky commercialization, and other such evils of modern materialism.

REFERENCES

1. Baginski BJ, Sharamon S. *Reiki: Universal Life Energy*. Mendocino, CA: Life Rhythm; 1988.
2. Haberly HJ. *Reiki: Hawayo Takata's Story*. Garrett Park, MD: Archedigm Publications; 1990.
3. Jarrell DG. *Reiki Plus Natural Healing*. Celina, TN: Hibernia West; 1991.
4. Rand WL. *Reiki, The Healing Touch: First & Second Degree Manual*. 3rd ed. Southfield, MI: Vision Publications; 2000.

5. Dressen LJ, Singg S. Effects of Reiki on pain and selected affective and personality variables of chronically ill patients. *Subtle Energies & Energy Medicine.* 1998;9(1):51-82.
6. Singg S, Dressen LJ. Desirable self-perceived psychophysiological changes in chronically ill patients: an experimental study of Reiki. Presented at: Ninth Annual Conference of the International Society for the Study of Subtle Energies and Energy Medicine; June 1999. Boulder, CO.
7. Baldwin AL, Vitale A, Brownell E, Scicinski J, Kearns M, Rand W. The Touchstone Process: an ongoing critical evaluation of Reiki in the scientific literature. *Holist Nurs Pract.* 2010;24(5):260-276.
8. Barnett L, Chambers M. *Reiki Energy Medicine: Bringing Healing Touch Into Home, Hospital, and Hospice.* Rochester, VT: Healing Arts Press; 1996.
9. Gerber R. *Vibrational Medicine: New Choices for Healing Ourselves.* Santa Fe, NM: Bear & Company; 1988.
10. International Society for Study of Subtle Energies and Energy Medicine. Intentionality and consciousness. *Bridges.* 1999;10(3):1-20.
11. International Society for the Study of Subtle Energies and Energy Medicine. Intentionality and consciousness: expanding horizons in energy medicine. *Bridges.* 1999;10(4):1-20.
12. Horan P. *Empowerment Through Reiki: The Path to Personal and Global Transformation.* Wilmot, WI: Lotus Light Publications; 1989.
13. The International Association of Reiki Professionals (IARP). www.iarp.org. Accessed February 13, 2016.
14. The Reiki Page. www.thereikipage.com/directory/index.php. Accessed February 13, 2016.
15. van Sell SL. Reiki: an ancient touch therapy. *RN.* 1996;59(2):57-59.
16. Vitale AT. An integrative review of Reiki touch therapy research. *Holist Nurs Pract.* 2007;21(4):167-179.
17. Lee MS, Pittler MH, Ernst E. Effects of Reiki in clinical practice: a systematic review of randomized clinical trials. *Int J Clin Pract.* 2008;62(6):947-954.
18. van der Vaart S, Gijsen VM, de Wildt SN, et al. A systematic review of the therapeutic effects of Reiki. *J Altern Complement Med.* 2009;15(11):1157-1169.
19. Thrane S, Cohen SM. Effect of Reiki therapy on pain and anxiety in adults: an in-depth literature review of randomized trials with effect size calculations. *Pain Manag Nurs.* 2014;15(4):897-908.
20. The Center for Reiki Research. www.centerforreikiresearch.org. Accessed February 13, 2016.
21. Baldwin AL, Schwartz GE. Personal interaction with a Reiki practitioner decreases noise-induced microvascular damage in an animal model. *J Altern Complement Med.* 2006;12(1):15-22.
22. Vitale A. Nurses' lived experience of Reiki for self-care. *Holist Nurs Pract.* 2009;23(3):129-145.
23. Whelan KM, Wishnia GS. Reiki therapy: the benefits to a nurse/Reiki practitioner. *Holist Nurs Pract.* 2003;17(4):209-217.
24. Assefi N, Bogart A, Goldberg J, Buchwald D. Reiki for the treatment of fibromyalgia: a randomized controlled trial. *J Altern Complement Med.* 2008;14(9):1115-1122.
25. Baldwin AL, Wagers C, Schwartz GE. Reiki improves heart rate homeostasis in laboratory rats. *J Altern Complement Med.* 2008;14(4):417-422.
26. Vitale AT, O'Connor PC. The effect of Reiki on pain and anxiety in women with abdominal hysterectomies: a quasi-experimental pilot study. *Holist Nurs Pract.* 2006;20(6):263-272.
27. Crawford SE, Leaver VW, Mahoney SD. Using Reiki to decrease memory and behavior problems in mild cognitive impairment and mild Alzheimer's disease. *J Altern Complement Med.* 2006;12(9):911-913.
28. Shiflett SC, Nayak S, Bid C, et al. Effect of Reiki treatments on functional recovery in patients in poststroke rehabilitation: a pilot study. *J Altern Complement Med.* 2002;8(6):755-763.
29. Shore AG. Long-term effects of energetic healing on symptoms of psychological depression and self-perceived stress. *Altern Ther Health Med.* 2004;10(3):42-48.
30. Wirth DP, Brenlan DR, Levine RJ, Rodriguez CM. The effect of complementary healing therapy on postoperative pain after surgical removal of impacted third molar teeth. *Complement Ther Med.* 1993;1:133-138.
31. Witte D, Dundes L. Harnessing life energy or wishful thinking? Reiki, placebo Reiki, meditation, and music. *Altern Complement Ther.* 2001;7(5):304-309.
32. Thornton L. A study of Reiki, an energy field treatment, using Roger's science. *Rogerian Nurs Sci News.* 1996;8(3):14-15.
33. Wardell DW, Engebretson J. Biological correlates of Reiki Touch healing. *J Adv Nurs.* 2001;3(4):439-445.
34. Olson K, Hanson J. Using Reiki to manage pain: a preliminary report. *Cancer Prev Control.* 1997;1(2):108-113.
35. Schiller R. Reiki: a starting point for integrative medicine. *Altern Ther Health Med.* 2003;9:20-22.
36. Olson K, Hanson J, Michaud M. A phase II trial of Reiki for management of pain in advanced cancer patients. *J Pain Symptom Manage.* 2003;26(5):990-997.
37. Miles P, True G. Reiki—a review of biofield therapy history, theory, practice and research. *Altern Ther Health Med.* 2003;9:62-71.
38. Engebretson J, Wardell D. Experience of a Reiki session. *Altern Ther Health Med.* 2002;8:48-53.
39. Ray B. *The Reiki Factor.* St. Petersburg, FL: Radiance Associates; 1985.
40. Bullock M. Reiki: a complementary therapy for life. *Am J Hosp Palliat Care.* 1997;14(1):31-33.
41. Singg S. Use of Reiki, a biofield therapy for stress and pain management. Presentation at: Psychological Association of Greater West Texas; April 24, 2015. San Angelo, Texas.

42. Alandydy P, Alandydy K. Using Reiki to support surgical patients. *J Nurs Care Qual.* 1999;13(4):89-91.
43. Sawyer J. The first Reiki practitioner in our OR. *Association of Operating Room Nurses Journal.* 1998;67(3):674-677.
44. Wing J, Wolf A. How we got Reiki into the hospital. *Reiki News.* 2000;Sept:28-29.
45. Rand WL. Reiki News articles: the International Center for Reiki Training. *The International Center for Reiki Training.* www.reiki.org/reikinews/reiki_in_hospitals.html. Accessed February 13, 2016.
46. International Association of Reiki Professionals. IARP Code of Ethics. www.iarp.org/iarp-code-ethics. Accessed February 13, 2016.
47. Nield-Anderson L, Ameling A. The empowering nature of Reiki as a complementary therapy. *Holist Nurs Pract.* 2000;14(3):21-29.
48. Mansour AA, Beuche M, Laing G, Leis A, Nurse J. A study to test the effectiveness of placebo Reiki standardization procedure developed for a planned Reiki efficacy study. *J Altern Complement Med.* 1999;5(2):153-164.

17

Qi Gong for Health and Healing

Jennifer M. Bottomley, PhD, MS, PT

Qi gong is a therapeutic Chinese practice that has been used for thousands of years to optimize and restore energy (Qi) to the body, mind, and spirit. Elements of Taoist and Buddhist philosophies form the foundation of Qi gong, which promotes health and vitality through gentle exercises for the breath, body, mind, and voice.[1] Qi gong is an alternative therapy that recognizes the strong connection between the body and the mind. It is an ancient traditional form of a group of techniques referred to as energy medicine.[2] Energy medicine techniques derive from traditional Chinese medicine and are based on the concept that health and healing are dependent on a balance of vital energy, a still mind, and controlled emotions. Physical dysfunctions result from disordered patterns of energy of long standing. Reversal of the physical problems, according to Qi gong theories, requires a return to balance and ordered energy.[3] Qi gong is a system that teaches an individual to live in a state of energy equilibrium. Hypothetically, Qi gong relies on no external physical interventions, but rather, relies on one's mind control to prevent illness, heal existing physical and emotional problems, and promote health and happiness. This chapter will describe the use of these techniques with people who have long-term physical disabilities and other pathologies.

Qi gong is an exercise form, similar to T'ai Chi, that is particularly helpful in an elderly population because of its slow, controlled, non-impact-type movements and postures, which displace and thereby stimulate the cognizant control of the center of gravity. T'ai Chi was derived from Qi gong and has the same philosophical origins. Qi gong exercise form incorporates all of the motions that often become restricted with inactivity and aging. A distinguishing element of Qi gong is the use of static postures, which, from a therapeutic perspective, are particularly helpful in individuals with movement limitations and in those who are frail. Qi gong integrates deep breathing, meditation, self-massage, movements, and postures. Qi gong improves respiration, stresses trunk control, expands the base of support, improves rotation of the trunk and coordination of isolated extremity motions, and helps to facilitate awareness of movement and position. Self-massage techniques stimulate circulation and affect nutritional absorption, flexibility, and sensory awareness. The meditative component of Qi gong serves to make an individual more aware of his or her body; enhance his or her ability to control muscle tension, posturing, and movement; and facilitate a peacefulness of mind that leads to an overall sense of well-being.[4,5]

Davis CM.
Integrative Therapies in Rehabilitation: Evidence for Efficacy in Therapy, Prevention, and Wellness, Fourth Edition (pp 259-282).
© 2017 Taylor & Francis Group.

DEFINITION

Qi gong (pronounced chee-gong) translates as *breathing exercise* or *energy skill*. It has a long history in China[6,7]; in fact, it has been recorded in the medical literature since ancient times and is an important component of traditional Chinese medicine. It has been practiced by the Chinese people for thousands of years, both to improve and maintain health and to develop greater power for the martial arts. *Qi* is the energy that circulates within the body, and *gong* means work or exercise, so *Qi gong* means the cultivation of the body's energy to increase and control its work capacity through the increase of circulation and energy flow.[1-7]

Qi gong exercise includes different methods of practice, breathing, self-massage, movement, postures, and meditation. In theory, by adopting various postures of the body and regulating breathing and mind, a person can cultivate vital energy to cure illness and maintain health.[7,8]

PRINCIPLES

To fully understand Qi gong, there are several concepts that must be reviewed. The following section is a brief description of each of the principles of Chinese Qi gong.

Vital Energy (Chi or Qi): Concept of Chi and Energy Flow

The first concept is that of Qi, or chi. Qi is the foundation of all Chinese medical theory and Qi gong.[3] It corresponds to the Greek *pneuma* and the Sanskrit *prana*, and is considered to be the vital force and energy flow in all living things. Qi can be best explained as a type of energy very much like electricity, which flows through the human or animal body. It is a theory of traditional Chinese medicine that *vital energy*, or Qi, has profound effects on health and that breathing exercise can increase vital energy, thereby preventing illness. Vital energy is the material foundation of the movement of life, the essence of life. It activates the physiological functions of the internal organs. Qi, prana, pneuma, life force, or internal energy (also steam, vapor, air) describes the enhancement of energy flow though breathing exercise. When life stops, the circulation of vital energy disappears. A strong vital energy gives good health and a weak vital energy gives poor health.[1,3,7,8]

Qi can also be explained as a medium of sensing or feeling. For example, if an individual injures an extremity, the Qi flow in the nerves of the extremity is disturbed and stimulated to a higher energy state. This higher energy state causes a sensational feeling that is interpreted as pain by the brain. The difference in energy potential causes an increased flow of Qi and blood to that area to begin repairing the damage. Complete healing occurs when the energy is once again balanced. If the damage is not completely repaired, the energy remains unbalanced and pain will persist.

Yin and Yang Energy = Chi

Qi gong is also based on the principle of *Yin* and *Yang*, which describes the relationship of complementary qualities, such as soft and hard, female and male, dark and light, or slow and fast. Yin and Yang are often described as the unity of opposites (eg, sympathetic and parasympathetic, north and south, positive and negative, heavy and light, life and death, day and night). One cannot exist without the other. They are 2 opposing but complementary forces exerting universal influence. Yin is heavy and tends to sink downward. Yang is light and tends to float upward. Yin is the black, or negative, while Yang is the white, or positive. Yin is passive and Yang is active. Yin represents quiet and rest, whereas Yang represents movement.

Figure 11-1 in Chapter 11 represents the universally accepted concept of Yin and Yang energy pictorially. Yin (greater) always contains some Yang (lesser), Yang (greater) always contains some Yin (lesser). The purpose of Qi gong exercises is to achieve a balance of Yin and Yang. Refer to Chapter 11 for a more comprehensive discussion of the concept of Yin and Yang.

Meridians and Channels

Qi channels, or meridians, refer to the pathways that create the relationship between vital energy and nature.[1-4] A channel or meridian is a major connector of each internal organ with the rest of the body. Imbalance in the energy levels of any organ will affect all of the other organs of the body. These channels frequently follow the major nerves and arteries.[3-7]

Another concept of Qi gong is the acupuncture points. Along each channel are the "cavities," points where electrical conductivity is higher than the surrounding area, commonly known as *acupuncture points*, which are used to stimulate the entire Qi system. Figure 17-1 displays the commonly accepted energy channels as represented in acupuncture points. Energy channels throughout the body regulate chi (Qi) flow. The body is hypothetically composed of 8 energy channels (thought of as *Qi reservoirs*) and has 12 meridians (thought of as *Qi rivers*) that run throughout the body. The meridians and channels systematically include all parts of the trunk and extremities. When Qi is stagnant in one channel, the corresponding organ will be affected.[1,3]

The Five Elements

Another principle in Qi gong is that of the 5 elements (water, wood, fire, earth, and metal). The 5 elements are understood better as forces, energy, and agents rather than as material elements. The emphasis is on principles and laws of nature, the outlook is dynamic and not static. The emphasis of this philosophy is placed on the harmony and balance of these elements. The concept is one of unity in multiplicity. Table 17-1 provides a summary of how each of the 5 elements is associated with particular organs, colors, flavors, emotions, and the like.

No element is superior to the others. Each interacts with the other 4 differently and yet a balance is maintained in nature. For instance, we might say that water can dowse a fire, but fire can boil water and change it to steam. It is hypothesized that the circulation of Qi is governed by the time of day and the season of the year. Qi circulates within the body from conception to death, but the part of the body where the Qi is strongest changes around the clock.

Qi gong is interwoven with the 5-element theory and the movements are connected to different organs, sounds, and emotions, to name a few. For instance, the bear posture in Qi gong is felt to be useful when there is an imbalance of energy flow in the area of the kidneys. The bird posture stimulates the heart channel and allows for opening the chest and reduction of pressure in the back and chest area. Yawning, scratching, rubbing, stretching, groaning, and even crying are activities that are considered to bring the body into a more comfortable state. The practice of Qi gong recognizes that the internal and external are connected. Energy flowing through the internal organs, for instance, will express itself through an external posture or movement or emotion. Movements such as neck stretching, face rubbing, and laughing, all movements that we often practice involuntarily, can be said to have behind them a Qi gong theory based on the flow of energy through the channels and meridians. Every spontaneous posture or movement is thought to be a natural attempt to bring about balance and systemic homeostasis.

Hypothetical Relationship of Mind-Body Exercise to Health

Current research indicates that the practice of mind-body forms of exercise, such as Qi gong and T'ai Chi, can improve balance, reduce falls, and increase strength and flexibility. In addition, these exercise forms enhance cardiovascular, respiratory, and immune system function[8] and promote emotional and spiritual well-being. Qi gong and its derivative, T'ai Chi, have been found to lower blood pressure and the stress hormone cortisol levels. Hypothetically, Qi gong maintains the balance and homeostasis of the entire system. The practice of Qi gong helps to generate, channel, conserve, and direct energy.[9]

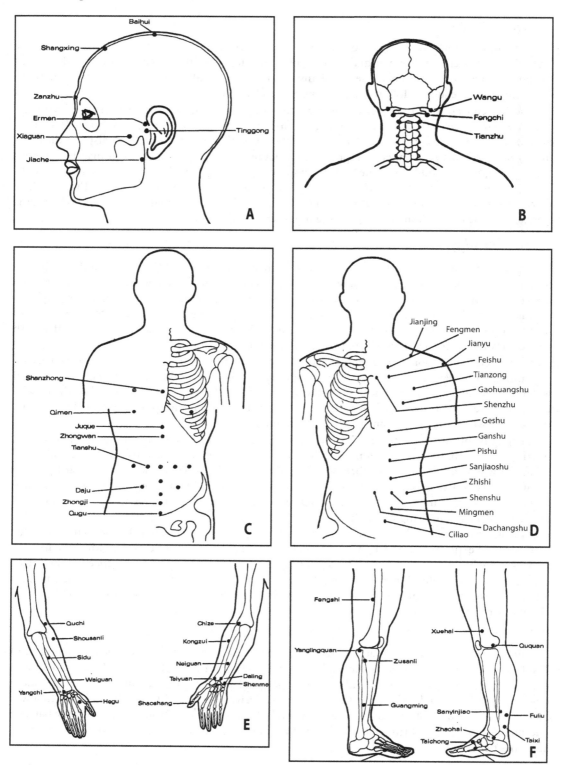

Figure 17-1. (A) Acupuncture points on the head. (B) Acupuncture points on the neck. (C) Acupuncture points on the front of the trunk. (D) Acupuncture points on the back of the trunk. (E) Acupuncture points on the arms. (F) Acupuncture points on the legs.

	WATER	WOOD	FIRE	EARTH	METAL
			TABLE 17-1 **THE FIVE ELEMENTS**		
Organs	Kidneys	Liver	Heart	Spleen	Lungs
Animal	Bear	Deer	Bird	Monkey	Tiger
Color	Blue/black	Green	Red	Yellow	White
Sound	Groaning	Shouting	Laughing	Singing	Weeping
Smell	Putrid	Rancid	Scorched	Fragrant	Rotten
Taste	Salty	Sour	Bitter	Sweet	Pungent
Emotion	Fear	Anger	Joy	Sympathy	Grief
Season	Winter	Spring	Summer	Late summer	Autumn
Time of Day	3 PM to 7 PM	11 PM to 1 AM	11 AM to 3 PM 1 PM to 11 PM	7 AM to 11 AM	3 AM to 7 AM

EVIDENCE OF EFFICACY

Electrical Activity and Energy Flow

Although a number of studies on traditional Chinese medicine, such as Qi gong, have explored physiologic changes associated with this intervention, few studies have evaluated human cerebral evoked potentials in relation to Qi gong. Xu and associates[10] examined the changes in evoked potentials and electroencephalogram (EEG) during Qi gong stimulation. These researchers found significant changes in evoked potential components originating from the cortex, suggesting both facilitating and inhibitory effects on the cortex during Qi gong. No significant changes occurred in these measures in the subcortex. Qi gong stimulation had an effect by increasing electrical activity of the somatosensory, visual, and auditory pathways up to the cortex, suggesting that this postural/exercise modality has the potential of stimulating and balancing the energy flow in the neurological tracts.[10]

Neuroendocrine and Hormone Levels

Omura and coworkers[11,12] evaluated hormone and neuroendocrine activity associated with Qi gong stimulation and found enhanced neurotransmission in organs related to the meridians involved during the posture or movement of the exercise. These studies found that within the boundary of most acupuncture points and meridian lines were high concentrations of neurotransmitters and hormones, including acetylcholine, methionine-enkephalin, beta-endorphin, adrenocorticotropic hormone, secretin, cholecystokinin, norepinephrine, serotonin, gammaaminobutyric acid, dopamine, dynorphin,[1-13] prostaglandin E1, estrogen (especially estriol and estradiol), testosterone, and progesterone.[11] No significant amounts of these neurotransmitters and hormones were found at the surrounding area outside of meridian and acupuncture points.[11]

Stress hormones, as measured by salivary cortisol levels, have been found to significantly drop during and after exercise practice.[13,14] This is not only important in managing stress and tension-related pathologies, but also in improving the immune system's overall ability to maintain homeostasis.

Omura et al[11] observed the response of plasma growth hormone, insulin-like growth factor I, and testosterone to a period of Qi training with Qi gong exercise and relaxation techniques. They found that plasma growth hormone increased greater than sevenfold in elderly trainees compared with close to twofold in younger subjects. Insulin-like growth factor I showed a significant increase in young subjects, but no response in the elderly.[11] Conversely, testosterone showed a significant increase in elderly subjects and no response in the young. These results suggest that Qi gong is a potential method for modulating the secretion of growth hormone in the young and elderly, and possibly affect disorders, such as growth hormone deficiency in children and osteoporosis in the elderly.[11]

Campo and colleagues[15] showed an improvement in neuroendocrine and energy production in patients with prostate cancer. Energy production was significantly improved with 3 to 5 weeks of Qi gong practice daily.[15] In another endocrine study by Li and associates,[16] the effects of Qi gong training on the secretion of thyroid and parathyroid hormones in elderly subjects was investigated. Qi gong induced a slight increase in thyroid-stimulating hormone. Triiodothyronine (T3) and thyroxine (T4) were shown to significantly increase and be closely correlated. An increase in the plasma level of T3 was associated with the secretion of T4. The plasma concentrations of calcitonin and parathyroid hormone were also increased; however, there was a slight decrease in ionized calcium. These results suggest that Qi gong training modulates the secretion of thyroid hormones, calcium metabolism, and parathyroid hormones in the elderly.[16] They also suggest an influence on bone health and reduction of osteoporotic problems often associated with radiation and chemotherapy for cancer care.

Cancer

Although definitive studies demonstrating significant changes in outcomes with cancer interventions and Qi gong specifically have not been undertaken, alternative exercise forms have been shown to enhance the immune system, provide pain relief, and result in relief of symptoms often accompanying radiation, chemotherapy, and surgery.[15-19] Qi gong exercise, postures, meditation, self-massage, and breathing have been found to positively affect mood, outlook, and quality-of-life measure; enhance overall strength, flexibility, and functional capabilities; and result in greater relaxation and pain management.[18,19]

With the practice of Qi gong therapy, patients with breast cancer demonstrated an improvement of the side effects of chemotherapy. The white blood cell count also decreased during the first course of chemotherapy in these individuals.[20] Clearly, further research is warranted in determining whether there is a relationship between cancer prevention and treatment and Qi gong.

Immunological Function

Qi gong is a type of psychosomatic exercise that integrates meditation, slow physical movement, and breath, to which numerous physical and mental benefits have been classically ascribed. Research indicates that Qi gong also has a beneficial effect on immunological function. One month of practicing Qi gong resulted in significant immunological changes that enhanced leukocyte, immunoglobulin, and other immune system components in older individuals whose immune system function had been deemed to be suppressed.[21] These findings are important in frailer older individuals who succumb to simple infection due to an unresponsive or sluggish immune system function.

Cardiovascular and Cardiopulmonary Measures

Cardiovascular endurance improves with Qi gong and T'ai Chi exercises. These movement therapies have been found to increase the resistance to cardiovascular diseases and may actually delay the decline of cardiorespiratory function in older adults.[22] Qi gong improves the ability to maintain activity levels and allows for a high energy return for daily activities. Although the observation of

Qi gong exercise would not lend to the thought that it was an aerobic activity, research has found that it is, in fact, a low-to-moderate–intensity exercise with a significant aerobic effect.[23,24] Further, it has also been found to be a safe exercise for individuals at high risk for cardiovascular disease.[25]

Qi gong may be prescribed as a suitable aerobic exercise for older adults[26] and is the most recommended aerobic exercise for individuals with coronary artery disease. An additional benefit to Qi gong and T'ai Chi exercise has been realized by a significant reduction in both systolic and diastolic blood pressure.[27]

To investigate the physiologic effects of Qi gong training, Lee and associates[28] investigated changes in blood pressure, heart rate, and respiratory rate before, during, and after Qi training (meditative/relaxation postures in Qi gong training). Heart rate, respiratory rate, systolic blood pressure, and rate-pressure product were significantly decreased during Qi gong postures, suggesting that Qi gong training has physiological effects that indicate stabilization of the cardiovascular system.[29] In addition, progressive relaxation and Qi gong exercise improved the quality of life for cardiac patients with reference to physiologic and psychological measures in a 2006 study.[30] The calming effect of Qi gong is one very notable outcome of routine participation in this exercise mode in cardiac patients.[30,31]

Respiratory function has also been shown to improve with enhanced ventilatory capacity without cardiovascular stress.[25,26] Research indicates that one of the primary benefits is the efficient use of ventilatory volume and extremely efficient breathing patterns.

Diabetes

Tsujiuchi and associates[32] studied the effect of Qi gong relaxation exercise on the control of type 2 diabetes mellitus. They found a reduction in daily insulin needs as a result of daily practice of Qi gong meditation and postures. Further studies are indicated to determine whether Qi gong exercise has a long-term effect on the progression of diabetes.

Flexibility and Muscle Strength

Flexibility is improved through the stretching and eccentric/concentric contraction of the muscles. Qi gong provides increased resistance to muscle and joint injury and prevents mild muscle soreness if performed before and after vigorous activity. Further, muscle strength has been shown to improve through daily Qi gong activities. Movement patterns become less strenuous as muscles become stronger. Strong abdominal and lower back muscles prevent lower back problems. Stronger postural muscles improve posture. The appearance of muscle fitness improves as muscles become firmer. Generally, Qi gong practitioners have a higher level of endurance because of the improvement in muscle strength and flexibility.[33]

Omura,[34] in the process of evaluating the external effects of Qi gong, showed that Qi gong energy has a polarity that influences the strength of muscles. A positive polarity enhanced muscle strength and velocity measures, whereas a negative polarity resulted in a decrease in muscle force production and a slowing of contraction velocity. The polarity changes depending on how Qi gong exercises are done (eccentric/concentric contractions or relaxation phases) and from which part of the body movement and energy emanate. In general, it was found that when a positive polarity is facilitated during active contraction and movement involving painful areas, spastic muscles, or extremities with arteries in vasoconstriction, it results in a subsequent reversal of polarity (negative) and relief of symptoms associated with these disturbances. It was also found that Qi gong not only improved the microcirculatory disturbance and relaxed spastic muscles and vasoconstrictive arteries, but also reduced or eliminated the pain and selectively enhanced drug uptake in these areas.[36]

Balance and Posture

Balance is substantially better in individuals practicing Qi gong and T'ai Chi exercises. Leung and Tsang's study[35] comparing different T'ai Chi forms and Qi gong demonstrated improvement in strength, mobility, balance, and endurance, and a Cochrane review showed a significant improvement in balance capabilities through gentle movement exercises, specifically T'ai Chi and Qi gong.[36] As a result, there have been studies that indicate a significant reduction in falls. For instance, Wolf and associates[37] found that daily practice of T'ai Chi exercises reduced falls by 47%. Significantly, there was a concomitant reduction in the fear of falling.

Bone Mass and Joint Integrity

As Qi gong is an inherently weight-bearing exercise that improves muscle strength, intuitively it can be stated that it would also increase bone mass. This could be a future research study in relation to the use of Qi gong or T'ai Chi in the presence of osteoporosis. Posadzki et al[38] found that these exercise forms were very effective in individuals with inflammatory joint diseases. No exacerbation in joint symptoms of individuals with rheumatoid arthritis or other joint problems were experienced by exercise participants, and exercising participants were observed to have more efficient biomechanical function as a result of improved strength, joint mobility, and muscle/tendon flexibility.[38] Additional benefits of improved endurance of muscle was realized in those who regularly performed Qi gong exercise 3 to 5 days/week.

Pain

Wu and associates[39] studied the effects of Qi gong on treatment-resistant patients with late-stage complex regional pain syndromes. The experimental group received instructions in directing Qi energy flow and instructions in Qi gong exercise (including home exercise) by a Qi gong master. The control group received similar instructions by a sham master. Exercises were performed in 6 40-minute Qi gong sessions over a 3-week period with daily home exercises. Outcome measures included thermography, swelling, discoloration, muscle wasting, range of motion, pain intensity rating, medication usage, behavior assessment (activity level and domestic disability), and frequency of pain awakening, mood assessment, and anxiety assessment. The authors reported that the genuine Qi gong group experienced 82% less pain by the end of the first training session compared with 45% less pain among the control group. By the sixth session, 91% of the experimental group reported pain relief compared with 36% of the control group. The researchers concluded that Qi gong training results in pain reduction and long-term reduction of anxiety.[39]

In elderly individuals with chronic pain syndromes, research indicates that Qi gong is a non-medication approach to managing pain without the significant side effects often experienced by older adults.[40] Older individuals with fibromyalgia, an otherwise functionally debilitating condition, have also been found to experience substantial pain relief after short-term Qi gong therapy.[41] This has significant ramifications for the treatment of pain and the quality of life in frailer older individuals.

Parkinson's Disease

Irrespective of limited evidence, traditional physical therapy and an array of complementary methods have been applied in the treatment of patients with Parkinson's disease. An investigation from 2006 found immediate and sustained effects of Qi gong on motor and non-motor symptoms of Parkinson's disease.[42] Immediate outcomes were a decrease in rigidity, improved initiation of movement, control and coordination, and greater endurance. These motor symptoms were sustained as long as Qi gong exercise continued. Additionally, depression scores decreased in Parkinson's patients participating in regular Qi gong exercise over a 6-month period.[42]

Psychophysiological Reactions and Mood

Based on the self-reports of Qi gong exercisers, the practice has a significant positive effect on mood states. An improved sense of well-being has been documented by reported reduction in tension, anxiety, fatigue, depression, and confusion.[1,3,5,12-14,43] Additional benefits were improved mental attitude toward work, self, and life in general; a greater ability to cope with stress; better, regular, and restful sleep patterns; healthier eating habits; a greater ability to avoid or control mild depression; and a sense of harmony reported by a better communication pathway among body, mind, and spirit (eg, a sense of well-being).

The physiologic effects of Qi gong linked with psychophysiological reactions include changes in EEG, electromyography, respiratory movement, heart rate, skin potential, skin temperature, sympathetic nerve function, function in the stomach and intestine, metabolism, and endocrine and immune systems.[44] Some of the psychological effects reported during Qi gong exercise related to motor phenomena and perceptual changes include a sensation of warmness, chilliness, itching in the skin, numbness, soreness, bloating, relaxation, tenseness, floating, dropping, circulation of the intrinsic Qi, and electric shock. These phenomena appear to be transient and associated with the actual exercise period or latent effects for brief periods following the termination of exercise.[44]

Psychological effects of Qi gong therapy have also been demonstrated in the treatment of depression. One study showed that regular Qi gong practice could relieve depression and improve self-efficacy and personal well-being among elderly persons with chronic physical illness and depression.[45]

Identifying alternative exercise modalities in an effort to stimulate and promote participation in physical activity, especially among older adults, is a critical health consideration and challenge. Medical Qi gong has been shown to be a moderate-intensity physical activity that demonstrates both physiological and psychological benefits for older individuals. Additionally, it is a form of exercise that results in better patient compliance than more traditional exercise forms.[46] In other words, older individuals are much more likely to enjoy Qi gong exercise and to be motivated to participate in this alternative exercise modality on a regular and ongoing basis.

Addiction

Smelson et al[47] explored the effectiveness of Qi gong therapy on the detoxification of cocaine addicts compared with medical and non-medical treatment. The interventions were as follows: a Qi gong group practiced Qi gong exercise and received Qi adjustments from a Qi gong master daily; a medication group received a detoxification drug by a 10-day gradual reduction method; and a control group received only basic care and medications to treat severe withdrawal symptoms. A reduction of withdrawal symptoms and drug cravings in the Qi gong group occurred more rapidly than in the other groups. From the first day of intervention, the Qi gong group had significantly lower mean symptom scores than did the other groups. The Qi gong and medication groups both had significantly lower anxiety scores compared with the control group; however, the Qi gong group had significantly lower scores on this measure than did the medication group. By the fifth day of treatment, all subjects in the Qi gong group had negative urinalysis results. It took the medication group 9 days and the non-medical group 11 days to clear the drug from urine tests. These results suggest that Qi gong may be an effective alternative for cocaine detoxification without side effects. Although research in other areas of addiction has not included the use of Qi gong, the results of this study by Smelson et al[47] surely warrants evaluation in other addictive groups.

Overall Mind-Body Fitness and Well-Being

Mind-body fitness is associated with integration and balance in muscular strength, flexibility, balance, coordination, and, perhaps most importantly from a health promotion viewpoint, improved mental development and self-efficacy. Qi gong combines mindfulness with physical activity and generates a temporary self-state or inwardly focused contemplative state: *mindful exercise*. It incorporates a focus on the present moment, in contrast to conventional exercise performance that emphasizes fat burning, body sculpting, or heart rate elevation.[1-3,7,48]

In addition, research has found a significant participant recidivism.[48] In other words, as mentioned previously, because an individual enjoys the exercise form, he or she is more likely to stick with it. Qi gong teaches the patient/participant to be mindful of the intrinsic energy from which he or she may ultimately perceive greater self-control and empowerment by becoming intentionally aware of breathing and specific proprioceptive sensations while performing gentle, fluid movements. It is an authentic mastery experience—self-mastery is the hallmark of mind-body fitness conditioning.

Thoughts, behaviors, attitudes, proprioceptive awareness, and pain perception affect bodily functions.[48] Body-mind functions and kinesthetic sensations evoke changes in perception, attitude, or behavior. There is a strong basis in neuroscience for this. Neurons, neurotransmitters, and associated receptor proteins are activated. More than 80 billion neurons exist in the adult human brain. Each receives input from 5 to 40,000 other neuronal axons. The perception of self or an environmental event (eg, exercise, anger, joy) is directly related to the number of neurons, neurotransmitters, and associated receptor proteins that are activated.

This slow, controlled movement involves the limbic system (thalamus, hypothalamus, and hippocampus). The electrochemical information from active neuronal circuits is ultimately transduced by the various structures of the limbic system into the hormones of behavior.[49-51] Much of this transduction is accomplished by the putative hypothalamic-pituitary-adrenal (HPA) axis. There is a reduction in catecholamine and glucocorticoid production. This axis can be viewed as one neuroendocrine pathway for mind-body interventions that focuses on reducing stress-related catecholamine and glucocorticoid production. One principle in molecular biology is that the synthesis and function of neuroactive substances are dictated by a range of genetic and environmental influences. Mind-body therapies, such as hypnosis, T'ai Chi, Qi gong, and meditation, alter the neurophysiology of this process by increasing parasympathetic tone.

The following is a list of theoretical differences in mechanisms responsible for exercise-associated affective states comparing conventional vs mindful exercise:

- The "endorphin high" is a consequence of aerobic exercise: endorphins are a class of endogenous neuroactive substances with morphine-like actions.

- Considerable evidence shows that to elicit an endorphin-mediated response, one must stress the musculoskeletal system to some critical duration of exercise-intensity threshold.

- Alternatively, evidence shows that much of the reduction in tension with aerobic exercise is somatic (eg, muscular), whereas meditative activity instills more of a central relaxation response.

Meditative states have long been associated with changes in EEG activity.[50-52] Analysis of the EEG activity indicates that the meditative state is a unique state of consciousness and is separate from wakefulness, drowsiness, or sleep.[50] There appears to be a significant difference between EEG activity during meditative states of Qi gong compared with rest states with eyes closed. Zhang and associates[50] found a clear difference in EEG waves during the Qi gong state compared with the resting state. The EEG alpha activity during the Qi gong state occurs predominantly in the anterior regions. The peak frequency of EEG alpha rhythm is slower than the resting state during Qi gong, and the change of EEG during Qi gong between anterior and posterior half is negatively correlated.[51,52] Changes of the EEGs of Qi gong masters during the Qi gong state were different from those recorded during the resting state with their closed eyes.[52]

Liu and colleagues[53] found that Qi gong training caused an enhancement of brainstem auditory–evoked response with a concomitant depression of cortical (stress) responses. These observations may be related to healing and other health benefits of Qi gong.

To generate the greatest potential for affective beneficence, some combination of muscular exercise and mindful activity should be incorporated into the individual's exercise program. The response to mind-body exercise hypothetically falls in a range between meditation and vigorous aerobic exercise. Activity with a meditative component is less prone to activating the hypothalmic-pituitary-adrenal (HPA) axis and associated increases in tension and anxiety.

Table 17-2 presents a summary of the comparative physiological responses to acute meditative activity and aerobic exercise assimilated through this author's study of mind-body exercise.

TABLE 17-2

COMPARATIVE PHYSIOLOGIC RESPONSES TO ACUTE MEDITATIVE ACTIVITY AND AEROBIC EXERCISE

	MEDITATION	MUSCULAR EXERCISE (70% TO 80% VO$_2$MAX)
Neurobiological	Increased alpha EEG activity	Decreased alpha EEG activity
	Right hemisphere activation	Left hemisphere activation
	Decreased SNS arousal	Increased SNS arousal
	Decreased HPA activation	Increased HPA activation
Cardiorespiratory	Decreased heart rate and BP	Increased heart rate, BP, and Q
	Increased HRV	Decreased HRV
	Decreased VO$_2$	Increased VO$_2$
Metabolic	Neutral RQ (eg, 0.85)	Increased RQ (CHO)
	Decreased blood lactate	Increased blood lactate
Musculoskeletal	Relaxation	Contraction
	Decreased EMG activity	Increased EMG activity
Endocrine	Decreased EPI, cortisol	Increased EPI, cortisol
	Decreased serum GH, TSH	Increased serum GH, TSH
	Decreased serum prolactin	Increased serum prolactin
	Decreased ACTH	Increased ACTH
	Decreased beta-endorphin	Increased beta-endorphin
Cognitive	Decreased arousal	Increased arousal

SNS = sympathetic nervous system; BP = blood pressure; Q = cardiac output; HRV = heart rate variability; VO$_2$ = oxygen consumption; RQ = respiratory quotient; CHO = ratio of carbohydrate to fat oxidation; EMG = electromyographic activity; muscular tension EPI = epinephrine; GH = growth hormone; TSH = thyroid-stimulating hormone; ACTH = adrenocorticotrophic hormone

TECHNIQUES USED IN QI GONG

Self-Massage

This method of exercise is said to calm the mind and stimulate the internal organs. Self-massage is a "wake-up" exercise practiced before Qi gong postures, movement, and meditation. People have always instinctively rubbed or massaged sore muscles and other painful areas to ease their pain and to help the sore muscles recover more quickly. The therapeutic effects of massage are known worldwide. The Japanese have used acupressure-based massage, which is derived from Chinese massage, for centuries. The Greeks have used slapping the skin (a form of massage) to treat various disorders. The Qi gong system of self-massage fully systemizes massage to harmonize with the theory of Qi circulation. Primarily, self-massage in Qi gong follows the pathways of the channels and meridians.

Figures 17-2 through 17-12 demonstrate the methods of self-massage use to calm the mind and stimulate the internal organs. Self-massage has been said to benefit many chronic problems, including insomnia, anxiety, stomach and intestinal problems, cardiac diseases, pulmonary disorders, and high blood pressure.

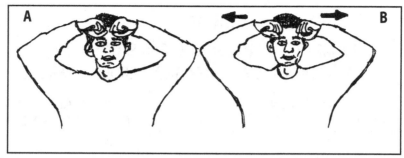

Figure 17-2. Rubbing the forehead. (A) Place both fists in the center of your forehead with the knuckles together, then (B) gently slide the fist across the forehead toward the temple in a smoothing action.

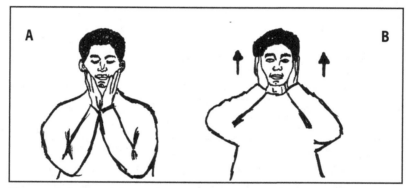

Figure 17-3. Stroking the sides of the face upward. (A) Place the hands on the side of the face, palms inward, with the finger tips just below the ear. (B) Stroke the face with the hands in an upward motion.

Movement and Postures

Movement and postures are major components of Qi gong exercise. The theory of combining postures and movement is based on the principle of Yin and Yang, passive and active, still and moving. In the postures, specific muscle groups are stressed, but they are not tensed. For example, in one posture, the arms are extended in front of the body as if they were hugging a tree. This position is held and what is experienced is that the nerves, muscles, and circulation in the areas of the shoulder and arm become "excited." The muscles holding the posture might fatigue and fasciculate, and there may be a sense of warmth or tingling in the areas of the arms, shoulders, and trunk that are being challenged. This is considered to be the generation of Qi or energy. When the arms are relaxed and dropped, the kinetic Qi seems to flow into the areas of lower potential much like an electric battery circulates electricity when a circuit is made. These postures not only improve strength and flexibility, but have also been shown to significantly improve endurance and aerobic capacity. Figures 17-13 through 17-16 are examples of static meditative Qi gong postures.

With practice of the individual standing postures, there is typically a progression to sequencing of mixed standing postures. These are invigorating and more physically demanding. Due to the length of this chapter, these postures will not be discussed here. The reader is referred to the list of additional reading materials for instructional materials on these postures. Mixing standing postures is a means of focusing the energy in each of the 12 channels (meridians).

In moving, the mind concentrates on the breath and at the same time imagines guiding energy to a specific area. With concentration on the movement, the control of Qi is more efficient and the muscles can exert maximal power. Emphasis during movement is placed on a calm, relaxed, and

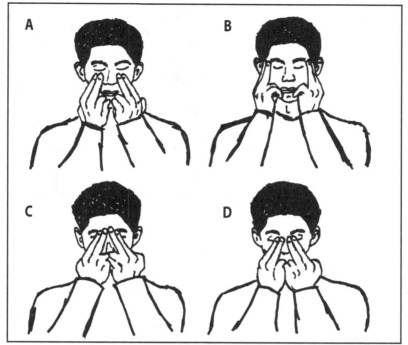

Figure 17-4. Massaging the orbit of the eye. (A) Place the index and middle fingers below the lower lid of the eye, starting in the inner corner. (B) Gently rub the eyes in a circular direction moving to the outside, (C) over the eyes, under the eyebrows, (D) down on the inside of the orbit completing the circle. Repeat 3 times.

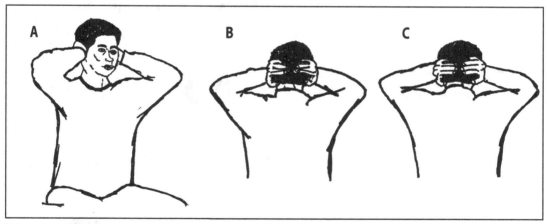

Figure 17-5. Sounding the drum. (A) Place the palm of the hands over the ears, covering the area just over the most forward area of the ears (laogong point) with the fingers behind the head. (B) Place the index finger across the middle finger, then (C) slide the index finger off and back alongside into its natural position. Repeat 6 times.

natural movement pattern. Strongly tensed muscles are felt to narrow the Qi channels. Repeated movements away from the center of the body and then back in a slow and controlled fashion have been shown to build strength and flexibility. More importantly, because movement always challenges the center of gravity, awareness of kinesthetic and proprioceptive stimuli become acute.

There are many exercise routines practiced by Qi gong practitioners. A popular routine is called the *Eight Pieces of Brocade* (or *Silk*). There are several varieties and distinct styles of this exercise

Figure 17-6. Opening the sinus. (A) Make a fist, then, using both hands, place the first joint of the thumb on the bridge of the nose, then (B) gently draw both fists away in a smooth action across each check.

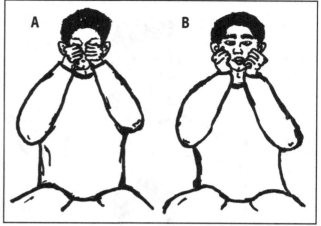

Figure 17-7. Washing the mouth with Qi. (A) Purse the lips and draw in air. Hold the air at the back of the mouth and then (B) push to the front of the mouth, without exhaling. Swallow the saliva and exhale. Repeat 10 times.

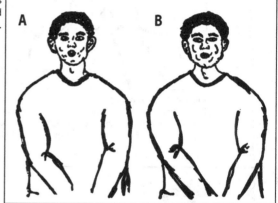

Figure 17-8. Rolling the arms while stroking the neck. (A) Place the hands on the back of the neck, interlocking the fingers. (B) Slide the hands from side, (C) back to the center, and (D) to the opposite side. Repeat 10 times.

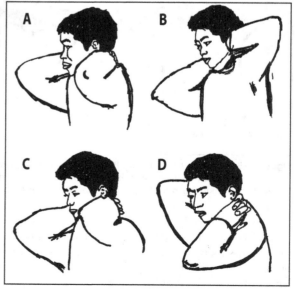

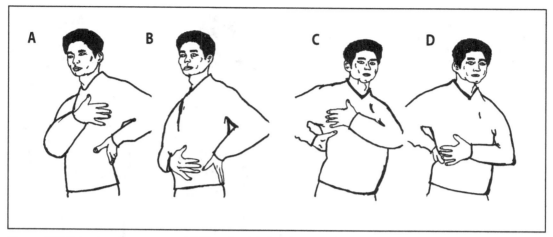

Figure 17-9. Releasing chest pressure. (A) Place the right hand on the left side of the chest, at the same time taking the left hand behind and placing it on the back. (B) Move the hands in a downward stroke finishing at the waist. Breathe out slowly when the hands reach the finishing point. (C and D) Repeat this on the right. Repeat 3 times, alternating sides.

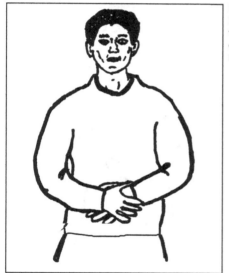

Figure 17-10. Stroking the dantian in a circular motion. Place the right hand under the left hand, placing them on the dantian, 2 inches below the navel. Rotate the hands in small circles going from right to left, gradually making the circles larger, before decreasing to small again. Repeat 10 times.

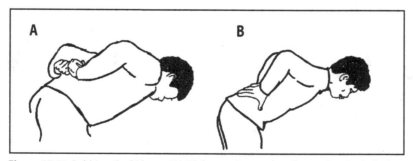

Figure 17-11. Rubbing the kidneys. (A) While standing up, lean forward and rub the low back with the inside of your fist. (B) Alternate this with a downward stroking motion. Repeat 10 times.

Figure 17-12. Circling the knees. (A) Standing up, lean forward with your hands on your knees, and the knees bent slightly. (B) Open and close the knees in an outward circling motion, then in an inward circling motion. Repeat 10 times in each direction.

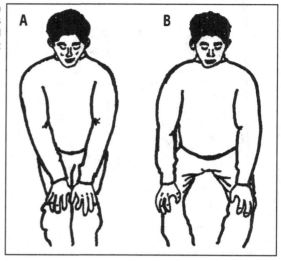

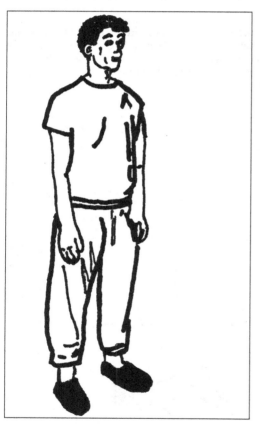

Figure 17-13. Simple standing posture. Stand upright naturally, raising the crown of the head. Close the mouth, relax the shoulders, concentrate on the dantian (2 inches below the navel), half close your eyes to avoid visual distractions.

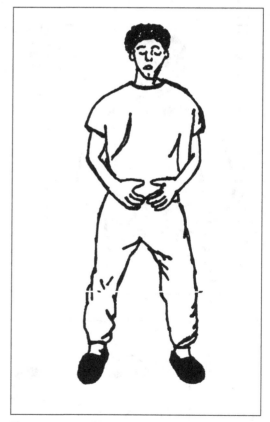

Figure 17-14. Holding the Qi in the dantian. Stand, slightly bending the legs, hold both hands as shown in front of the dantian. Keep the mind on the dantian and, while keeping the shoulders and chest relaxed, let your stomach move out when you breathe.

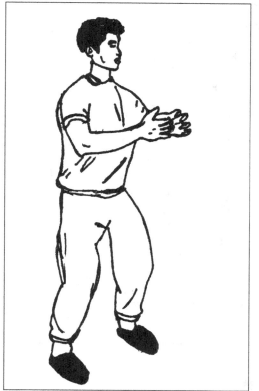

Figure 17-15. Hugging the tree. Stand erect, with shoulders relaxed and legs slightly bent, creating a circle in front of the body with your arms. This posture is one of the oldest Qi gong methods of practice handed down known for strengthening all systems.

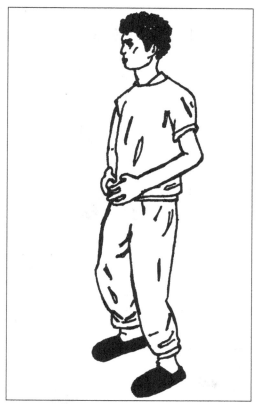

Figure 17-16. Small circle standing position. Half closing the eyes without focusing, bend your knees and concentrate on the dantian. Relax the shoulders and the back and hold the hands over the dantian region without touching the abdominal area.

form, all of them effective. The name comes from brocade or silk cloth, which was originally used when doing the exercises. Today, the exercises are typically done without pieces of silk. Figures 17-17 through 17-24 depict a commonly used exercise routine.

Breathing

Breathing techniques are employed with postures and movement. During postures, it is believed that Qi can be accumulated with breathing and concentration (meditation), and that it is possible to guide the flow or circulation of Qi by directing the breath. Movement patterns also lend well to facilitating breathing techniques and directing the flow of energy. When the movement opens up an area, such as in the arm movement away from the chest, inspiration accompanies the motion. Deep breathing can be directed toward the fingertips and the breath held momentarily at the completion of the movement. Upon return to the resting posture, exhalation relaxes the individual back to the starting position. Self-massage also utilizes breathing during massage techniques. Meditatively, awareness of the areas being massaged and directing the Qi (the breath) to that area further enhance the beneficial effects on circulation, oxygenation, and the flow of energy.

Meditation

The key to successful practice of Qi gong exercises is concentration on the area being moved or postured and concentration on the breath as described previously. This is meditation. *Meditation* is defined as close or continued thought, serious contemplation, or mental reflection.

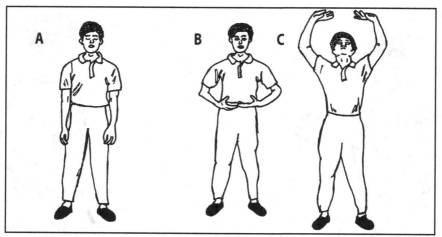

Figure 17-17. Supporting the sky with 2 hands. (A) Stand in a relaxed position with feet under hips. Look straight ahead and breathe through nose. Relax all joints and meditate for a few moments to gain concentration. (B) Slowly raise arms in a circle in front of your body while inhaling, turn palms over and stretch up as though holding up the sky. (C) At the same time, lift heels off ground. Exhale while lowering arms and heels returning to the starting position. Health benefits: relaxes the muscles and stretches the arms, legs, and torso. Accompanied by deep breathing, it affects the chest, abdomen, and pelvis. It also helps to correct poor posture.

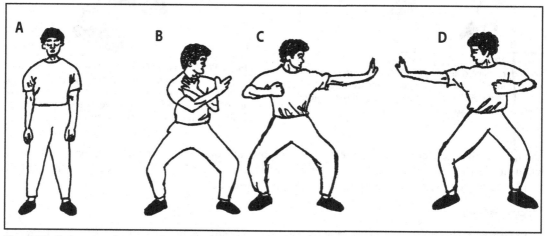

Figure 17-18. Drawing the bow to the left and right. (A) Stand in a relaxed position. (B) Step to left and bend knees to assume a horse-riding position. Cross arms in front of chest, right arm outside, left arm inside. Then with thumb and forefinger of left hand extended and other three fingers curled, stretch left arm out to left, eyes following, breathing in. (C) At the same time, clench right hand and stretch to right as though pulling a bow. Return to preparation position while exhaling. (D) Repeat to opposite direction. Health benefits: movement concentrates on the chest, shoulder, and arm muscles; provides weight shifting; helps circulation.

The concentration on movements and sensations of the Qi gong movements focuses the mind on movement patterns and postures. This moving meditation is of great importance in gaining the full benefits of this exercise form.

Three Primary Methods of Qi Gong

Of interest are the different forms and applications of the techniques described in the previous sections. There are 3 primary philosophies in the practice of Qi gong. The Taoist philosophy strives for the balance between Yin and Yang, and so Qi gong methods include postures and movements in

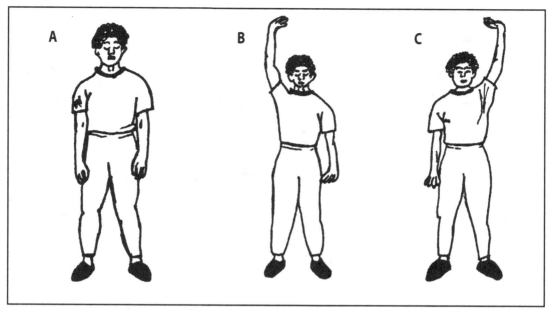

Figure 17-19. Lifting one arm. (A) Stand straight, feet shoulder width apart and arms at side. (B) Raise right arm over head, palm up, fingers together and pointing to left; at the same time press left hand down, palm down, fingers together and pointing straight ahead. Breathe in while doing this. Return to preparation position while exhaling. (C) Repeat to opposite side. Health benefits: stretches arms and trunk; affects liver, gall bladder, spleen, and stomach; strengthens the digestive system.

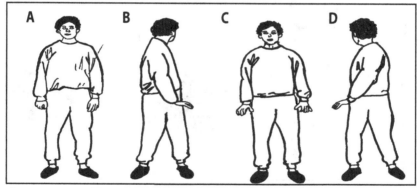

Figure 17-20. Looking backward. (A) Stand straight with palms lightly touching thighs, extend wrist with palms down and fingers forward. (B) Turn head to the left slowly while inhaling and looking over your shoulder (keeping pelvis forward). (C) Return to starting position while exhaling. (D) Turn head to the right slowly while inhaling and leading movement with eyes looking backward. Return to preparation position while exhaling. Health benefits: involves turning the head, rolling the eyeballs, challenging balance, and stretching trunk; strengthens neck and trunk muscles; revitalizes the nervous system.

addition to breathing and meditation. The Buddhist philosophy of Qi gong is primarily one on Yin. They seek calm through maintaining postures and incorporating the components of respiration and meditation. Moving meditation is primarily the philosophy used in medical or martial arts. This philosophy incorporates Yang and is directed toward dynamic movement, such as that experienced in T'ai Chi. Although this latter philosophy is more commonly practiced by health practitioners, this author is finding that the combination of movement and postures is substantially more efficacious

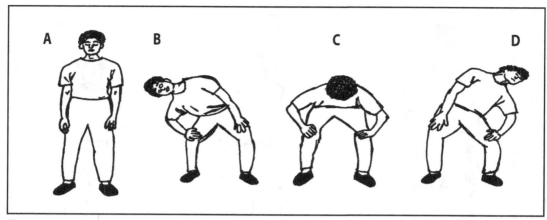

Figure 17-21. Killing heart fire by rotating head and body. (A) Stand straight with arms at side, bend knees to assume a horse-riding position with legs wide apart, placing hands on thighs with thumbs pointing outward. (B) Bend forward from waist and rotate body toward left while inhaling; at the same time, sway buttocks toward right. (C) Return to start position while exhaling. (D) Repeat in opposite direction. Health benefits: involves using the whole body and is excellent for relaxation.

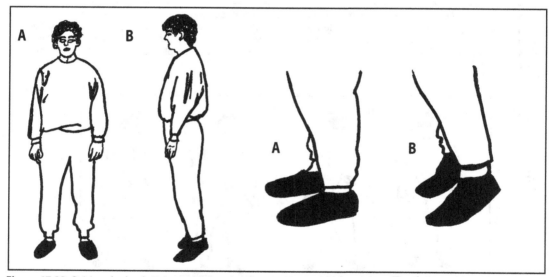

Figure 17-22. Raising the heels 7 times. (A) Stand naturally with your feet shoulder width apart. (B) Keeping both legs straight, raise heels off the floor while inhaling. While exhaling let go and lower heels to the ground. Do this 7 times in succession in time with your breathing. Health benefits: beneficial for the spine, posture, circulation, and the internal organs.

from a clinical perspective when working with an older adult population. This is certainly an area that should lead to some significant research projects in the future.

CONCLUSION

There is so much to Qi gong that it is impossible to cover all of the theory and training in a short chapter. It is recommended that if a clinician is interested in studying and acquiring skills in Qi gong, he or she should seek out a Qi gong master. A Qi gong teacher will instruct you in the proper forms and techniques; however, serious study of this movement form requires the understanding

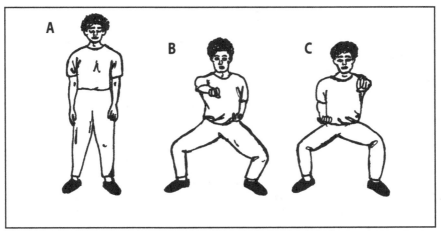

Figure 17-23. Punching with tiger eyes. (A) Stand with legs wide apart, fists at waist, and palms up. (B) Bend knees to assume a horse-riding position. Inhale. With palms turning down and glaring eyes following movement, stretch right fist slowly forward as in a punching movement while exhaling. Return to starting position while inhaling. (C) Repeat on left. Health benefits: the emphasis here is on glaring eyes; exercise with eyes following thrusting fist helps concentration; movement builds up energy and strength.

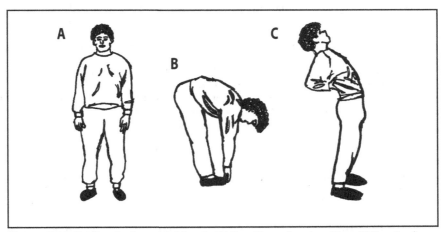

Figure 17-24. Holding the feet with 2 hands. (A) Stand in a relaxed position. (B) Keeping knees straight and head slightly raised, bend forward slowly and hold toes or ankles while exhaling. (C) Return to starting position and, with hands holding back at waist level, bend slowing backward while inhaling. Repeat. Health benefits: good for kidneys and other internal organs; challenges balance and vestibular system; stretches and strengthens trunk muscles, which, in turn, affects internal organs.

of the philosophy behind the movements and principles underlying the application of each movement, posture, breathing technique, self-massaging technique, and the very important component of meditation. There are also numerous videotapes that are available to guide you in this exercise form for the therapeutic use of this movement modality with your older patients.

It is well known that Qi gong practice is beneficial to human health,[54] but it is less known that Qi gong may also be effective therapy to treat many otherwise "untreatable" conditions. The use of Qi gong has been identified by the National Institutes of Health as one of a list of alternative therapies that has been targeted for research funding. The increasing body of research related to the use of Qi gong as a valuable therapeutic intervention substantiates our need as professionals to evaluate the merits of this exercise form.

REFERENCES

1. de Sa Ferreira A. Evidence-based practice of Chinese medicine in physical rehabilitation science. *Chin J Integr Med.* 2013;19(10):723-729.
2. Hankey A, McCrum S. Qigong: life energy and a new science of life. *J Altern Complement Med.* 2006;12(9):841-842.
3. Sancier KM, Holman D. Commentary: multifaceted health benefits of medical qigong. *J Altern Complement Med.* 2004;10(1):163-165.
4. Witt C, Becker M, Bandelin K, Soellner R, Willich SN. Qigong for school children: a pilot study. *J Altern Complement Med.* 2005;11(1):41-47.
5. Wagner B. Chinese meditation pattern. Qi Gong: to learn from tigers and bears. Series: relaxation technique 1. Centers of vital energy [article in German]. *Fortschr Med.* 1999;117(8):55.
6. Jouper J, Hassmen P, Johansson M. Qigong exercise with concentration predicts increased health. *Am J Chin Med.* 2006;34(6):949-957.
7. Staud R. Effectiveness of CAM therapy: understanding the evidence. *Rheum Dis Clin North Am.* 2011;37(1):9-17.
8. Li TY, Yeh ML. The application of qi-gong therapy to health care. *Hu Li Za Zhi.* 2005;52(3):65-70.
9. Lee MS, Kim MK, Ryu H. Qi-training (Qi gong) enhanced immune functions: what is the underlying mechanism? *Int J Neurosci.* 2005;115(8):1099-1104.
10. Xu M, Tomotake M, Ikuta T, Ishimoto Y, Okura M. The effect of Qi-gong and acupuncture on human cerebral evoked potentials and electroencephalogram. *J Med Invest.* 1998;44(3-4):163-171.
11. Omura Y, Lin TL, Debreceni L, et al. Unique changes found on the Qi Gong (Chi Gong) Master's and patient's body during Qi Gong treatment; their relationships to certain meridians & acupuncture points and the re-creation of therapeutic Qi Gong states by children & adults. *Acupunct Electrother Res.* 1989;14(1):61-89.
12. Omura Y. Connections found between each meridian (heart, stomach, triple burner, etc.) & organ representation area of corresponding internal organs in each side of the cerebral cortex; release of common neurotransmitters and hormones unique to each meridian and corresponding acupuncture point & internal organ after acupuncture, electrical stimulation, mechanical stimulation (including shiatsu), soft laser stimulation or QI Gong. *Acupunct Electrother Res.* 1989;14(2):155-186.
13. Abbott R, Lavretsky H. Tai Chi and Qigong for the treatment and prevention of mental disorders. *Psychiatr Clin North Am.* 2013;36(1):109-119.
14. Chan ES, Koh D, Teo YC, Hj Tamin R, Lim A, Gredericks S. Biochemical psychometric evaluation of self-healing qigong as a stress reduction tool. *Complement Ther Clin Pract.* 2013;19(4):179-183.
15. Campo RA, Agarwal N, Lastayo PC, et al. Levels of fatigue and distress in senior prostate cancer survivors enrolled in a 12-week randomized controlled trial of Qigong. *J Cancer Surviv.* 2014;8(1):60-69.
16. Li DT, Wang J, Jiang HY, et al. Quantitative evaluation of Qi Gong effects on syndromes of osteoporosis. *Zhong Xi Yi Jie He Xue Bao.* 2012;10(11):1254-1262.
17. Lee MS, Yang SH, Lee KK, Moon SR. Effects of Qi therapy (external Qigong) on symptoms of advanced cancer: a single case study. *Eur J Cancer Care (Engl).* 2005;14(5):457-462.
18. Fong SS, Ng SS, Luk WS, et al. Effects of qigong exercise on limb lymphedema and blood flow in survivors of breast cancer: a pilot study. *Integr Cancer Ther.* 2014;13(1):54-61.
19. Overcash J, Will KM, Lipetz DW. The benefits of medical qigong in patients with cancer: a descriptive pilot study. *Clin J Oncol Nurs.* 2013;17(6):654-658.
20. Yeh ML, Lee TI, Chen HH, Chao TY. The influence of Chan-Chuang Qi-Gong therapy on complete blood cell counts in breast cancer patients treated with chemotherapy. *Cancer Nurs.* 2006;29(2):149-157.
21. Manzaneque JM, Vera FM, Maldonado EF, et al. Assessment of immunological parameters following a Qi gong training program. *Med Sci Monit.* 2004;10(6):CR264-CR270.
22. Chan AW, Lee A, Lee DT, et al. The sustaining effects of Tai Chi & Qigong of physiological health for COPD patients: a randomized controlled trail. *Complement Ther Med.* 2013;21(6):585-594.
23. Lee MS, Kim MK, Lee YH. Effects of Qi-therapy (external Qi gong) on cardiac autonomic tone: a randomized placebo controlled study. *Int J Neurosci.* 2005;115(9):1345-1350.
24. Kim SH, Schneider SM, Kravitz L, Mermier C, Burge MR. Mind-body practices for posttraumatic stress-disorder. *J Investig Med.* 2013;61(5):827-834.
25. Ding M, Zhang W, Li K, Chen X. Effectiveness of t'ai chi and qigong on chronic obstructive pulmonary disease: a systematic review and meta-analysis. *J Altern Complement Med.* 2014; 20(2):79-86.
26. Lorenc AB, Wang Y, Madge SL, Hu X, Mian AM, Robinson N. Meditative movement for respiratory function: a systematic review. *Respir Care.* 2014;59(3):427-440.
27. Wang T. Analysis and comparison of theories of circulation of blood and qui in both eastern and western ancient medicines. *Zhonggue Zhong Xi Yi Jie He Za Zhi.* 2014;34(9):1035-1041.
28. Lee MS, Lim HJ, Lee MS. Impact of Qi gong exercise on self-efficacy and other cognitive perceptual variables in patients with essential hypertension. *J Altern Complement Med.* 2004;10(4):675-680.
29. Freeman SR, Hanik SA, Littlejohn ML, et al. Sit, breathe, smile: effects of single and weekly seated Qigong on blood pressure and quality of long-term-care. *Complement Ther Clin Pract.* 2014;20(1):48-53.

30. Hui PN, Wan M, Chan WK, Yung PM. An evaluation of two behavioral rehabilitation programs, qigong versus progressive relaxation, in improving the quality of life in cardiac patients. *J Altern Complementy Med.* 2006;12(4):373-378.

31. Stenlund T, Lindstrom B, Granlund, Burell G. Cardiac rehabilitation for the elderly: Qi Gong and group discussions. *Eur J Cardiovasc Prev Rehabil.* 2005;12(1):5-11.

32. Tsujiuchi T, Kumano H, Yoshiuchi K, et al. The effect of Qi-gong relaxation exercise on the control of type 2 diabetes mellitus: a randomized controlled trial. *Diabetes Care.* 2002;25(1):241-242.

33. Bottomley JM. The use of T'ai Chi as a movement modality in orthopedics. *Orthop Phys Ther Clin N Am.* 2000;9(3):361-373.

34. Omura Y. Storing of Qi gong energy in various materials and drugs (Qi gongnization): its clinical application for treatment of pain, circulatory disturbance, bacterial or viral infections, heavy metal deposits, and related intractable medical problems by selectively enhancing circulation and drug uptake. *Acupunct Electrother Res.* 1990;15(2):137-157.

35. Leung ES, Tsang WW. Comparison of the kinetic characteristics of standing and sitting Tai Chi forms. *Disabil Rehabil.* 2008;30(25):1891-1900.

36. Howe TE, Rochester L, Neil F, Skelton DA, Ballinger C. Exercise for improving balance in older people. *Cochrane Database Syst Rev.* 2011;(11):CD004963.

37. Wolf SL, Barnhart HX, Kutner NG, et al. Reducing frailty and falls in older persons: an investigation of T'ai Chi and computerized balance training. *J Am Geriatr Soc.* 1996;44:599-600.

38. Posadzki P, Parekh S, O'Driscoll ML, Mucha D. Qi Gong's relationship to educational kinesiology: a qualitative approach. *J Bodyw Mov Ther.* 2010;14(1):73-79.

39. Wu WH, Bandilla E, Ciccone DS, et al. Effects of Qi gong on late-stage complex regional pain syndrome. *Altern Ther Health Med.* 1999;5(1):45-54.

40. Yang KH, Kim YH, Lee MS. Efficacy of Qi-therapy (external Qi gong) for elderly people with chronic pain. *Int J Neurosci.* 2005;115(7):949-963.

41. Astin JA, Berman BM, Bausell B, Lee WL, Hochberg M, Forys KL. The efficacy of mindfulness meditation plus Qi gong movement therapy in the treatment of fibromyalgia. *J Rheumatol.* 2003;30(10):2257-2262.

42. Schmitz-Hubsch T, Pyfer D, Kielwein K, et al. Qi gong exercise for the symptoms of Parkinson's disease: a randomized, controlled pilot study. *Mov Disord.* 2006;21(4):543-548.

43. Shneerson C, Taskila T, Gale N, Greenfield S, Chen YF. The effect of complementary and alternative medicine on the quality of life of cancer survivors: a systematic review and meta-analyses. *Complement Ther Med.* 2013;21(4):417-429.

44. Wang CW, Chan CH, Ho RT, Chan JS, Ng SM, Chan CL. Managing stress and anxiety through qigong exercise in healthy adults: a systematic review and meta-analysis of randomized controlled trials. *BMC Complement Altern Med.* 2014;14:8.

45. Tsung HW, Fung KM, Chan AS, Lee G, Chan F. Effect of a Qi gong exercise programme on elderly with depression. *Int J Geriatr Psychiatry.* 2006;21(9):890-897.

46. Kjos V, Etnier JL. Pilot study comparing physical and psychological responses in medical Qi gong and walking. *J Aging Phys Act.* 2006;14(3):241-251.

47. Smelson D, Chen KW, Ziedonis D, et al. A pilot study of Qigong for reducing cocaine craving in early recovery. *J Altern Complement Med.* 2013;19(2):97-101.

48. Chen AC. Higher cortical modulation of pain perception in the human brain: psychological determinant. *Neurosci Bull.* 2009;25(5):267-276.

49. Bloom FE, Lazerson A. *Brain, Mind, and Behavior.* 2nd ed. New York, NY: WH Freeman & Co; 1988.

50. Zhang JZ, Zhoa J, He QN. EEG findings during special physical state (Qi gong state) by means of compressed spectral array and topographic mapping. *Comput Biol Med.* 1988;18(6):455-463.

51. He QN, Zhang JZ, Li JZ. The effects of long-term Qi gong exercise on brain function as manifested by computer analysis. 1988;8(3):177-182.

52. Zhang JZ, Li JZ, He QN. Statistical brain topographic mapping analysis for EEGs recorded during Qi gong states. *Int J Neurosci.* 1988;38(3-4):415-425.

53. Liu GL, Cui RQ, Li GZ, Huang CM. Changes in brainstem and cortical auditory potentials during Qi gong meditation. *Am J Chin Med.* 1990;18(3-4):95-103.

54. Chen KW, Turner FD. A case study of simultaneous recovery from multiple physical symptoms with medical Qi gong therapy. *J Altern Complement Med.* 2004;10(1):159-162.

ADDITIONAL RESOURCES

Chen NN. *Breathing Spaces: Qigong, Psychiatry, and Healing in China.* New York, NY: Columbia University Press; 2003.

Clark A. *Secrets of Qigong.* Evergreen; 2003.

Cohen KS. *The Way of Qigong: The Art and Science of Chinese Energy Healing.* Toronto, Ontario, Canada: Random House of Canada; 1999.

Fick F. *Five Animal Frolics Qi Gong: Crane and Bear Exercises.* Taipei, Taiwan: Shen Long Publishing; 2005.

Garripoli G. *Qigong: Essence of the Healing Dance.* Deerfield, FL: Health Communications, Inc; 1999.

Ho PY. *Li, Qi, and Shu: An Introduction to Science and Civilization in China.* Mineloa, NY: Dover Publications; 2000.

Holland A. *Voices of Qi: An Introductory Guide to Traditional Chinese Medicine.* Berkley, CA: North Atlantic Books; 2000.

Karchmer E. Magic, science and qigong in contemporary china. In: Blum SD, Jensen LM. *China Off Center: Mapping the Margins of the Middle Kingdom.* Honolulu, HI: University of Hawaii Press; 2002: 311–22.

Lee MS, Oh B, Ernst E. Qigong for healthcare: an overview of systematic reviews. *JRSM Short Rep.* 2011;2(2):7.

Liang S-Y, Wu W-C, Breiter-Wu D. *Qigong Empowerment: A Guide to Medical, Taoist, Buddhist, and Wushu Energy Cultivation.* East Providence, RI: Way of the Dragon Pub; 1997.

Liu TJ, Qiang XM, eds. *Chinese Medical Qigong,* 3rd ed. Philadelphia, PA: Singing Dragon; 2013.

Micozzi MS. *Fundamentals of Complementary and Alternative Medicine,* Kindle Edition. Philadelphia, PA: Elsevier Health Sciences; 2010.

Miura K. The revival of qi. In: Kohl L, ed. *Taoist Meditation and Longevity Techniques.* Ann Arbor, MI: Center For Chinese Studies: University of Michigan, Ann Arbor; 1989.

Otehode U. The creation and reemergence of qigong in china. In: Ashiwa Y, Wank, DL. *Making Religion, Making the State: The Politics of Religion in Modern China.* Stanford, CA: Stanford University Press; 2009: 941–265.

Palmer DA. *Qigong Fever: Body, Science, and Utopia in China.* New York, NY: Columbia University Press; 2007.

Patterson J. Use of Sound in Qigong. Portland Tai Chi Academy. http://portlandtaichiacademy.com. Accessed May 31, 2016.

Penny B. Qigong, daoism and science: some contexts for the qigong boom. In: Lee M, Syrokomla-Stefanowska AD. *Modernisation of the Chinese Past.* Sydney, Australia: Wild Peony; 1993: 166–179.

Voigt J. The man who invented "qigong." Qi. *The Journal of Traditional Eastern Health & Fitness.* 2013;23(3):28–33.

Wushu Association, Chinese. *Liu Zi Jue: Six Sounds Approach to Qigong Breathing Exercises (Chinese Health Qigong).* Philadelphia, PA: Singing Dragon; 2008.

Xu X. *Qigong for Treating Common Ailments.* Wolfeboro, NH: YMAA Publication Center; 2000.

Yang J-M. *Qigong for Health and Martial Arts: Exercises and Meditation.* Wolfeboro, NH: YMAA Publication Center; 1998.

Yang J-M. *Qigong, The Secret of Youth.* Wolfeboro, NH: YMAA Publication Center; 2000.

Yang J-M.. *Eight Simple Qigong Exercises for Health: The Eight Pieces of Brocade.* Wolfeboro, NH: YMAA Publication Center; 2007.

YeYoung B. Lineage Transmission of Qi Gong. *YeYoung Culture Studies.* http://literati-tradition.com. Accessed May 31, 2016.

YeYoung B. Origins of Qi Gong. *YeYoung Culture Studies.* http://literati-tradition.com. Accessed May 31, 2016.

Zhang H-C. *Wild Goose Qigong: Natural Movement for Healthy Living.* Wolfeboro, NH: YMAA Publication Center;2000.

Acupuncture Theory and Acupuncture-Like Therapeutics in Physical Therapy

*Patrick J. LaRiccia, MD, MSCE; Kerri Sowers, PT, DPT, NCS;
Lynn B. Littman, MA, MAc, LAc, DiplAc; and Mary Lou
Galantino, PT, MS, PhD*

TRADITIONAL CHINESE ACUPUNCTURE CONCEPTS

Acupuncture has been in existence for at least 2000 years. It is a part of traditional Chinese medicine (TCM), which contains concepts of Yin and Yang, Qi (pronounced chee), and meridians, among others. TCM has undergone change and evolution.[1,2] The concept of Qi is very important in acupuncture. Qi is considered "vital energy" that courses through pathways of the body called *meridians* (Figure 18-1). Qi moving through the meridians is analogous to blood moving through blood vessels. Disease results if there is a hindrance or obstruction of blood flow (eg, peripheral vascular disease, coronary artery disease), if there is a deficiency of blood volume (eg, anemia), or if there is hindrance or obstruction of the flow of Qi through the meridians. A deficiency in the amount of Qi is signaled in the symptom of fatigue. In acupuncture, the goal of therapy is to restore the proper circulation of Qi. Acupuncture points, also called *acupoints* (Figure 18-2), are locations where the Qi coursing through the meridians is transported to the surface of the body.[3] There are 361 "regular points" that fall on the 14 most-frequently utilized meridians; there are 40 extrameridian (EM) points that are not on the 14 meridians; and there are Ashi points, which are tender spots. "Tender spots can be used as acupoints, and this was the primary method for point selection in early acupuncture and moxibustion treatments. Without specific names and definite locations, Ashi points are considered to represent the earliest stage of acupoint evolution. Clinically, they are mostly used for pain syndromes."[3] The 14 frequently-used meridians travel essentially longitudinally along the body (see Figure 18-1); however, there are interconnections with each other. Also, most of the meridians have a connection to a specific visceral organ (eg, heart, gallbladder, liver).

The acupuncturist must first make a decision as to which acupuncture points to stimulate, followed by decisions regarding the stimulation technique itself (ie, needle, needle plus moxibustion, moxibustion alone, needles with electrical stimulation through the needles). Moxibustion involves burning the herb artemisia vulgaris near the acupuncture points in one of a number of specific

Davis CM.
*Integrative Therapies in Rehabilitation: Evidence for Efficacy in Therapy,
Prevention, and Wellness, Fourth Edition* (pp 283-304).
© 2017 Taylor & Francis Group.

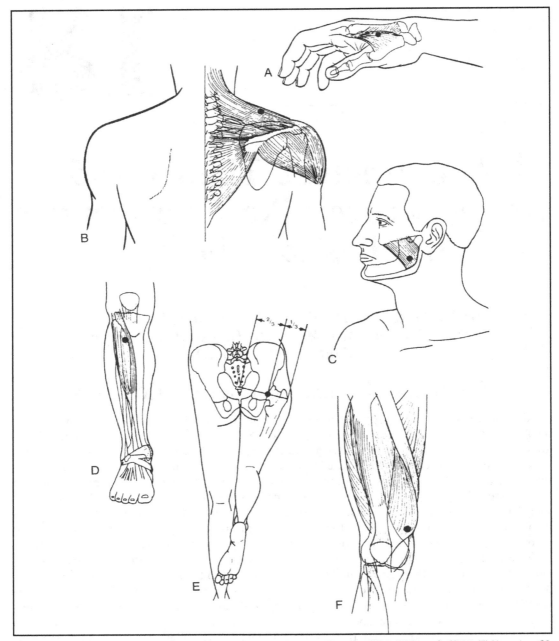

Figure 18-1. Acupuncture points. (A) Hegu, LI 4. (B) Jianjing, GB 21. (C) Jiache, ST 6. (D) Zusanli, ST 36. (E) Huantiao, GB 30. (F) Xuehai, SP 10. (Reprinted from *Orthopadeic Physical Therapy Clinics of North America*, 9(3), LaRiccia PJ, Acupuncture and physical therapy, 432, ©2000 with permission from Elsevier.)

manners. Decisions must also be made about the depth of insertion, direction of insertion, type of needle manipulation, duration needles are left in place, frequency of treatments, and number of treatments. One can see that there is an enormous number of ways a treatment can be performed. Different schools of thought will address the various dimensions of acupuncture treatment, including point selection, depth of insertion, and needle manipulation, in different ways. In mainland China where the TCM style is dominant, the depth of insertion and needle manipulation will result in a

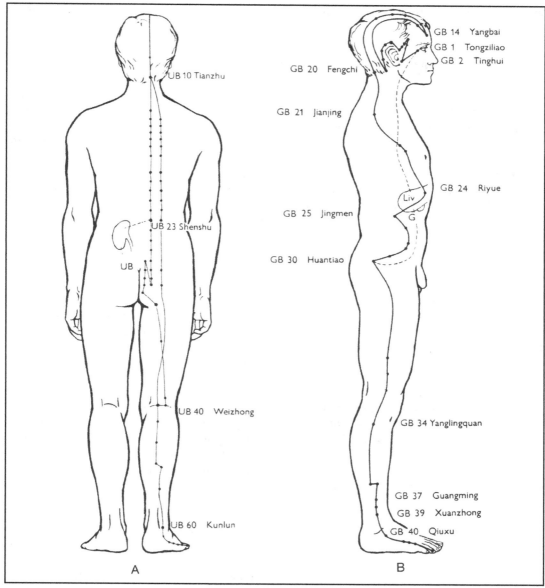

Figure 18-2. (A) Bladder meridian and (B) gallbladder meridian. GB=gallbladder; Liv=liver; UB=urinary bladder. (Reprinted from *Orthopaedic Physical Therapy Clinics of North America,* 9(3), LaRiccia PJ, Acupuncture and physical therapy, 430, ©2000 with permission from Elsevier.)

feeling of "de qi" (a temporary feeling of numbness, fullness, or heaviness), while certain Japanese acupuncture styles cause no discomfort at all. Some of the various schools of thought include TCM, Japanese, Korean, French Energetic, Worsley Five-Element, and modern neuroanatomical methods.

An important point selection method for musculoskeletal pain will be described. This point selection method is a method used for what TCM practitioners call *Bi syndromes*. Bi syndromes are manifested by soreness, pain, numbness, and heavy sensation of the limbs and joints, as well as limitation of movement. Acupuncture points located in the area of pain (local points) and distal to the involved area but on meridians running through the involved area are chosen; Ashi points are also used.[4] Randomized controlled clinical trials comparing different acupuncture styles are needed to refine acupuncture treatment by guiding point selection, stimulation method, and other dimensions of acupuncture treatment.

MODERN PHYSIOLOGICAL FINDINGS

In this section, we will discuss the following: (1) a spinal cord and brain model of acupuncture analgesia as described by Pomeranz[5]; (2) support for the endorphin explanation of acupuncture analgesia; (3) the autonomic nervous system effects of acupuncture; (4) the relationship of acupuncture to hypnosis; (5) the characteristics of acupuncture points; and (6) the neuroimaging of acupuncture effects.

Among the most notable researchers in the modern physiology of acupuncture are Han[6] of Beijing and Pomeranz[5,7] of Toronto. Both have completed enormous amounts of basic laboratory work and have published numerous empirical research reports and reviews. Liao et al[2] have also written an extensive review of the physiological aspects of acupuncture and human acupuncture research issues.

Spinal Cord and Brain Model of Acupuncture Analgesia

The following is a simplified version of the model proposed by Pomeranz[5] (Figure 18-3). Type II, III, and IV afferents from muscle transmit the acupuncture stimulus to the spinal cord, while A delta afferents transmit the acupuncture stimulus from the skin. In the spinal cord, ascending pain transmission is blocked in a segmental fashion via enkephalin and dynorphin. When the acupuncture stimulus reaches the midbrain, enkephalin activates a descending pain inhibition system that utilizes serotonin and norepinephrine. After the acupuncture stimulus reaches the hypothalamus, the arcuate nucleus releases ß-endorphin into the midbrain, resulting in further activation of the descending pain inhibition pathway. Hypothalamic activity also induces the pituitary to release ß-endorphin. ß-endorphin reaches the brain via a retrograde passage in the pituitary-portal system and reinforces activation of the descending pain inhibition system. The pituitary co-releases ß-endorphin and adrenocorticotropic hormone into the systemic circulation. This helps explain the anti-inflammatory effects of acupuncture. In addition to the core description presented earlier, studies suggest the involvement of the limbic system in acupuncture analgesia, including the amygdala, hippocampus, cingulate, and cerebellar vermis, which may relate to the emotional component of pain.[8,9]

Support for the Endorphin Explanation of Acupuncture Analgesia

Converging lines of evidence are powerful arguments in science for validating theories. The endorphin hypothesis as a major mechanism for the analgesic effect of acupuncture has at least 17 lines of converging evidence. Of these, we will focus on the following 9 lines:

1. Naloxone, naltrexone, cyclazocine, and diprenorphine are all opioid antagonists that can block acupuncture analgesia.[5,10]

2. Blockage of acupuncture analgesia by naloxone is stereospecific for the L-isomer. This implicates a receptor mechanism rather than a side effect, such as membrane fluidization.[5,10]

3. Macroinjections of naloxone via the systemic circulation can block acupuncture analgesia. However, microinjections are only successful if the injection is into areas of the nervous system where there is endorphin activity. Microinjections of antibodies to ß-endorphin, enkephalin, and dynorphin must also be site specific to block acupuncture analgesia. Thus, the microinjection of antisera to dynorphin is effective if given intrathecally, but not if given in the midbrain.[5,11]

4. Mice with endorphin receptor deficiency do less well with acupuncture.[5,12]

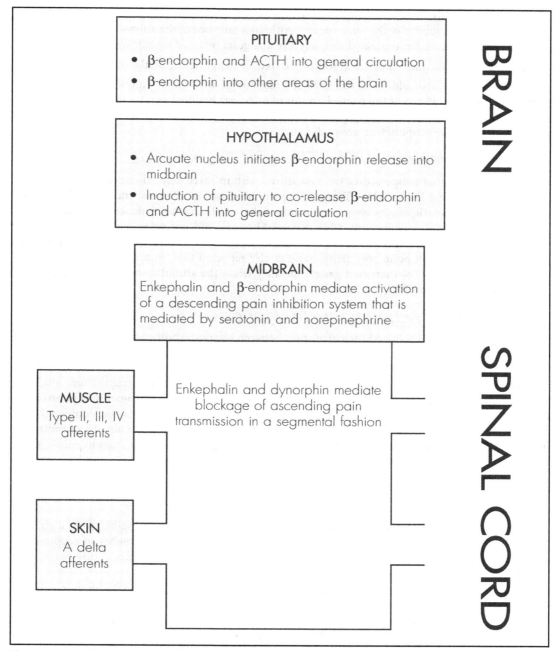

Figure 18-3. Spinal cord and brain model by Pomeranz.

5. Endorphin-deficient rats respond less well to acupuncture.[5,13]

6. There is an increase in cerebrospinal fluid endorphins and a decrease in brain endorphins after acupuncture.[5,14]

7. Enzyme blockers that retard the breakdown of the endorphins enhance acupuncture analgesia.[5,15]

8. Experiments have been performed in which the circulation of one animal subject is crossed into another animal subject of the same species. Although only one of the animals received acupuncture, both animals demonstrated acupuncture analgesia reversed by naloxone.[5,16]

9. Pituitary ablation and suppression techniques reduce acupuncture analgesia.[5,17]

Pomeranz[5,18] has also addressed the issue of stress analgesia in detail. In one of the studies performed by his group,[19] one of the control groups of mice was handled exactly the same throughout an experiment that included the application of painful stimuli. This group did not exhibit an analgesic effect, while the acupuncture group did.

Autonomic Nervous System Effects of Acupuncture

Face, hand, and foot temperatures were measured with infrared color thermographs before and after acupuncture in a 1989 study.[20] Temperature was increased in all areas, and these diffuse nonsegmental sympatholytic effects were long lasting. Sakai et al[21] found evidence for sympatholytic activity resulting from acupuncture, while Knardahl et al[22] did not using a different methodology. Further, Longhurst[23] and Yang et al[24] addressed sympathetic and parasympathetic effects of acupuncture, along with point specificity. Yang et al[24] reported that, in a rat model, the stimulation of Pericardium 6 (P6) increased gastric motility while the stimulation of Conception Vessel 12 decreased gastric motility.

Relationship of Acupuncture to Hypnosis

Several studies have evaluated the correlation between hypnotizability and acupuncture results, with Liao and Wen,[25] Peng et al,[26] and Ulett[27] reporting no correlation. Other studies have reported on the failure of naloxone to modify hypnotic analgesia.[28-30] As noted previously, naloxone blocks acupuncture analgesia. Successful veterinary acupuncture and the fact that acupuncture analgesia has been produced across different species of animals[5] provide an argument against hypnosis as an explanation for the effects of acupuncture. In a study by Lu et al,[31] hypnosis was compared with acupuncture in a quasi-experimental design of subjects with head and neck pain. The results suggested that patients with psychogenic pain of nonorganic origin benefit most from hypnosis, those with acute pain have greater pain relief from acupuncture, and those with chronic pain have variable results.

Characteristics of Acupuncture Points

Anatomically, the most notable characteristics of acupoints (acupuncture points) from a physical therapy perspective are frequency of coincidence with trigger points,[5,32] frequency of acupuncture points near motor points of neuromuscular attachments, and frequency of acupuncture points near blood vessels in the vicinity of neuromuscular attachments.[5,33]

Soh[34] in Korea has successfully visualized the Bonghan duct, which may be the anatomical basis of the acupuncture meridian system, which in biophysical terms is a system of optical channels of biophotons.[34] In addition, a pilot study by Moncayo et al[35] used in vivo localization of anatomical structures with magnetic resonance imaging (MRI) sequences to show the relationship of acupuncture points to tendino-fascial and muscular structures. Hsiu et al[36] used Doppler laser flowmetry to demonstrate that there is a larger blood supply in microvascular beds at acupoints than at non-acupoints.

An additional notable characteristic of acupuncture points is that dermatomes at least partially determine the therapeutic efficacy of acupuncture.[37] Acupuncture points within certain spinal segments of the trunk affect the functioning of the organs that receive autonomic innervation from the same spinal segments. However, there appears to be no relationship between the myotome level of acupuncture points in the extremities and nonmuscular clinical indications.[38]

Finally, Langevin and Yandow[39] suggest that the network of acupuncture points and meridians can be viewed as a representation of the network formed by interstitial connective tissue, which is supported by ultrasound imaging that shows connective tissue cleavage planes at acupuncture points. They found an 80% correspondence between sites of acupuncture points and intermuscular or intramuscular planes in post-mortem tissue sections.[39]

Physiologically, acupuncture points sometimes have decreased electrical resistance as compared to the surrounding skin.[5] Konofagou and Langevin[40] imaged the tissue displacements recurring before and after needle rotation and suggest that tissue displacement caused by needle movements pull and deform the connective tissue, effectively sending a mechanical signal into the subcutaneous tissue, affecting the neural, vascular, and lymphatic elements present within the connective tissue. Fox et al[41] used ultrasound elastography to demonstrate that the acupuncture needling of intramuscular connective tissue results in an enhanced longitudinal displacement and strain pattern as compared with needling over a muscle where the displacement or strain pattern is predominantly transverse. Langevin[42] further suggests that the mechanical stimulation of connective tissue during acupuncture needling has direct effects on restoring the health of connective tissue in addition to analgesic effects.

Ahn et al[43] suggest that collagenous bands are associated with decreased electrical impedance and therefore may be the basis for the reduced electrical impedance reported at certain acupuncture meridians at subcutaneous and intramuscular depths. Shang[44] investigated the neurobiology of acupuncture points, which suggests that acupuncture points and meridians have higher electrical conductance associated with a higher density of gap junctions.

Additionally, acupuncture points have been found to have higher temperatures, higher metabolic rates, and increased carbon dioxide release.[44] The findings from Hsiu et al[36] of increased blood supply at acupoints suggests that stimulation of an acupoint may change microcirculatory perfusion, vessel elasticity, the number of blood vessels in the microvascular bed, and/or perfusion resistance.

A study by Li et al[45] using a rat model showed that acupuncture points may be excitable muscle/skin-nerve complexes with an increased density of peripheral nerve endings and receptive fields. Alternatively, Wick et al[46] performed immunohistochemistry on biopsies of fresh cadaver skin and found that human acupuncture points are associated with a significantly decreased number and density of subcutaneous nerve structures compared with non-acupuncture points. This pilot study contradicts several animal studies that suggest that acupuncture points have a higher density of nerve endings, and points out the need for more research.

Another study compared the force required to remove the needle from selected acupuncture points where the de qi sensation was present with non-acupuncture locations.[47] Researchers found that the force necessary to remove the needle from an acupuncture point was significantly greater than the nonacupuncture point, suggesting that there may be biomechanical differences at those locations.[47]

Neuroimaging of Acupuncture Effects

Various brain imaging techniques have been used to study the effects of acupuncture. The imaging techniques include electroencephalography, functional MRI, magnetoencephalography, positron emission tomography, somatosensory evoked potential, and single-photon emission computed tomography (SPECT).[48] Newberg et al[49] reported a series of SPECT studies in subjects with chronic pain who were treated with acupuncture. The report suggested that there is asymmetrical blood flow to the right and left thalami in patients with chronic pain and that acupuncture improved the blood flow symmetry.

Dhond et al[48] summarized the findings of imagining studies and reported that acupuncture modulates corticolimbic and brainstem networks supporting endogenous antinociception, alters somatomotor cortex processing and cortical somatotopy in patients with chronic pain and stroke, may modulate autonomic nervous system function, and may modulate activity within brain networks supporting attention and higher cognition.

SAFETY OF ACUPUNCTURE

The 1998 National Institutes of Health (NIH) Consensus Development Panel on Acupuncture[50] and the United States Food and Drug Administration (FDA)[51] consider acupuncture safe when done by qualified practitioners using sterile needles. Acupuncture is safer than many of our standard therapies. One study calculated that an acupuncturist might cause less than one serious event per 100 years of full-time practice.[51] Another study published in 2001 in the United Kingdom surveyed 34,407 treatments and found no report of serious adverse events that would lead to hospital admission, permanent disability, or death.[53] Additionally, only 43 minor adverse events (1.3/1000 treatments) were reported, including severe nausea, fainting, mild bruising, site pain, and bleeding. In a systematic review of acupuncture safety, the authors concluded that minor complications may be more common than previously thought; the chance of a serious event continues to be rare.[54] Minor complications in this review included bleeding, aggravation of pain (often followed by increased relief after additional sessions), bruising, nausea, vomiting, burns, or failure to have needles removed following treatment.

Several more recent reviews have confirmed that acupuncture treatment performed by qualified practitioners continues to be a relatively safe and effective therapy with a low risk of adverse experiences in clinical practice. A prospective survey conducted in 2004 reported 7.1% minor adverse experiences and only 5 serious adverse experiences in 97,733 acupuncture patients.[55] A 2008 study reported one serious adverse experience in 1865 treatments, which is a risk of 5.361/10,000 treatments.[56] A subsequent prospective observational study conducted in 2009 surveyed 229,230 patients who had approximately 10 treatments each; 8.6% reported one or more adverse experience and 2.29% reported an adverse experience that required treatment.[57] The authors concluded that most of the complications, which included bleeding/hematoma, pain, and vegetative symptoms, were minor in nature. Finally, a 2011 study from China evaluated 1968 patients; while 74 patients had at least one adverse experience during the treatment period, there were no serious adverse experiences reported.[58] Minor conditions reported included hematoma, bleeding, bruising, and needle-site pain.

CLINICAL STUDIES

The authors (KS and MLG) reviewed 136 publications covering acupuncture without electricity (conventional acupuncture), acupuncture with electricity (electroacupuncture), surface electrode acupuncture point stimulation (SEAPS or acupuncture-like transcutaneous electrical nerve stimulation [TENS]), and laser acupuncture (stimulation of acupuncture points with a cold laser).[59-194] The study types were empirical, narrative reviews, systematic reviews, and meta-analyses. The conclusions of the authors were tabulated with the following results: 90 out of 136 (66%) were favorable, 18 out of 136 (13%) were inconclusive, and 28 out of 136 (21%) were unfavorable.

In addition to the usual design and statistical considerations, there are 5 research-critical appraisal issues of importance that are often overlooked by editors, researchers, peer reviewers, and health care providers regarding journal publications. These issues are as follows:

1. Use of the Standards for Reporting Interventions in Controlled Trials of Acupuncture (STRICTA) guidelines

2. Respect for the paradigm; simply stated, if method A is reported effective in daily practice, did the researchers evaluate method A or a different method?

3. Generalizability of research study results across different acupuncture methods

4. Sham acupuncture controls

5. The application of acupuncture research results to everyday practice

Use of the STRICTA Guidelines

As described in the first section of this chapter, there are many ways of performing acupuncture. Different schools of thought (eg, TCM, Japanese, Korean) will address the various dimensions of acupuncture treatment, such as point selection, depth of insertion, and needle manipulation, among others, in different ways. Also, the experience and training of the acupuncturist may influence the treatment outcome. To critically appraise a publication of an acupuncture study, the reader must be apprised of each dimension of the study. This is best accomplished by use of a standardized method of reporting acupuncture studies with the acronym STRICTA.[195] Unfortunately, studies are published that do not follow the STRICTA guidelines, thus hindering their proper interpretation.

Respect for the Paradigm

Hammerslag[196] notes that a considerable proportion of acupuncture trials used acupuncture methods that did not respect the paradigm. Many of these used fixed acupuncture points and did not individualize sessions as is usual in an Asian medical model. An example of evaluating method B instead of method A follows.

In 1997, a negative controlled trial of acupuncture was reported.[197] The study was prompted by a retrospective analysis of 27 patients with psoriasis who had an excellent response to classical Chinese acupuncture, complemented with topical needling of the psoriatic lesions, ear acupuncture, and a Chinese herbal remedy. However, for standardization purposes, needling of the psoriatic lesions was left out during the conduct of the study, thus changing the method of acupuncture that was observed to be effective.

To allow the reader of a research article to determine whether the paradigm has been respected, studies must clearly describe and reference their treatment method. The references can include standard acupuncture texts, acupuncture research literature, and acupuncture experts. The background of the acupuncture expert should be stated. There should be a clear statement as to the opinion of the expert regarding whether the study method accurately represents the acupuncture technique being tested. At minimum, published studies should follow the STRICTA guidelines.[195]

Generalizability of Research Study Results Across Different Acupuncture Methods

The previously mentioned 1998 NIH acupuncture panel[50] touches on this issue, which is difficult because there are so many different acupuncture methods. This issue applies to both negative and positive results. Shlay et al[198] reported that a standardized acupuncture regimen was no better than sham acupuncture for the pain of HIV peripheral neuropathy. This article also reported that amitriptyline 75 mg was no better than placebo capsules. In both the acupuncture arm and the amitriptyline arm, one cannot generalize to another acupuncture method or to a higher dosage of amitriptyline. In 1999, Berman et al[199] reported positive results for the adjunctive use of acupuncture in the treatment of knee osteoarthritis. They used a specific method derived from TCM theory regarding Bi syndromes. However, one cannot readily generalize from this that other acupuncture methods derived from Japanese, Korean, or French Energetics will also be effective. Since acupuncture is a group of methods, we are not able to test all methods in a single study.

Sham Acupuncture Controls

A major concern about sham needling is the possibility that piercing the skin may activate alternative pain modulation systems; there may also be local effects on healing, a release of vasoactive substances, or trigger point effects.[200] Lund et al[201] investigated whether minimal, superficial, or sham acupuncture could be considered an inert placebo. The authors outlined how light touch on the skin stimulates mechanoreceptors linked to unmyelinated C afferents, which may lead to both emotional and hormonal reactions. This may be how sham interventions seem to be as effective as true acupuncture in some conditions, especially those with an increased sensory component.

A study by Kong et al[202] investigated brain activity through functional MRI associated with placebo analgesia via sham acupuncture treatment. The authors concluded that the right anterior insula, bilateral rostral anterior cingulate cortex, dorsolateral prefrontal cortex, and parietal cortex play an important role in placebo modulation of pain perception.[202] In light of Lund et al's study,[201] did Kong's study[202] brain map a placebo response or did it brain map the response associated with a treatment that uses light touch instead of needle piercing? A systematic review by Dincer and Linde[203] analyzed 47 randomized controlled trials that compared true acupuncture to various types of sham acupuncture, including trials that used blunt-tipped placebo needles that do not penetrate the skin. The authors concluded that there is no single adequate sham intervention for acupuncture trials. Lundeberg et al[204] and Birch[205] point out the consequences of falsely assuming that sham procedures are inert. There are negative consequences for the interpretation of individual trials, meta-analyses, and clinical guidelines. Birch[205] calls for researchers to present evidence that their sham procedure is truly inert.

Interestingly, *sham acupuncture* is defined in the laboratory as needling at non-acupuncture points. Sham acupuncture fails in acute laboratory pain studies. Placebo pills bring about analgesia in only 3% of cases[5,206,207] of acute laboratory pain. Sham acupuncture in the context of chronic pain in humans is problematic. In clinical human studies, placebo analgesia works in 30% to 35% of patients, sham acupuncture works in 33% to 50% of patients, and true points are effective in approximately 55% to 85% of patients. Therefore, to show statistical significance in studies that incorporate sham acupuncture control groups, a minimum of 122 subjects must be included in the study.[5,208] Systematic reviews and meta-analyses looking at neck pain[209] and back pain[210,211] have been published in which none of the studies using sham controls had a large enough study population.

Sham controls may be less problematic in areas of study that do not look at pain. For instance, a study of acupuncture for stroke recovery[212] using sham controls was positive for acupuncture, as was a study of chemotherapy-associated nausea and vomiting.[213] Multiple acupuncture points can turn on the endorphin mechanism. Clinical observation indicates that the effective area of an acupuncture point is increased during chronic processes. Studies that utilize sham points should describe in detail their locations and cite evidence that the sham points are inactive as per the previously mentioned recommendations of Birch.[205]

Application of Acupuncture Research Results to Everyday Practice

In 1997, deaths from nonsteroidal anti-inflammatory drug toxicity in the United States was almost equal to the number of deaths from AIDS that year.[214] In 1998, the *Journal of the American Medical Association* published an article indicating that deaths from adverse reactions to properly administered prescription drugs ranked between the fourth and sixth leading cause of death in United States hospitals.[215] A number of randomized controlled trials have indicated that acupuncture and acupuncture-like treatments are effective adjunctive treatments to standard treatment regimens (eg, stroke rehabilitation[216,217]). Acupuncture has also appeared as effective as standard treatments for temporomandibular joint disorders in some randomized controlled studies.[218]

In light of this information, is it unreasonable to consider acupuncture or acupuncture-like modalities more often in our physical therapy treatment plans? Few would disagree that it is imperative for health care providers to present patients with safe and effective treatment options, including those safe and effective options that health care providers would select for themselves and their families. Naturally, the strength of evidence for and against effectiveness and safety would be presented along with the frequencies or absolute probabilities (absolute risk reduction, number needed to treat, number needed to harm) of success and each type of possible adverse event.

APPLICATION OF ACUPUNCTURE CONCEPTS AND ACUPUNCTURE-LIKE MODALITIES TO PHYSICAL THERAPY

Accessing the Acupuncture Point and Meridian System

To access the acupuncture point and meridian system, one must have a knowledge of the location of the acupuncture points and their meridians (see Figures 18-1 and 18-2). A detailed exposition of traditional Chinese anatomy is beyond the scope of this chapter. Liao,[2] Stux and Pomeranz,[219] and Xinnong[220] are excellent authors with which to begin. Once the anatomy is known, there are multiple ways to access the system. Access is not restricted to acupuncture needles, but can be obtained additionally through manual pressure, surface electrical stimulation, piezoelectric devices, moxibustion, infrared lamps, low-energy (cold) lasers, and other direct methods. The system can also be accessed by T'ai Chi movements, Qi gong postures, breathing techniques, mental practices, and yoga. Sharma et al[221] noted an increase and balance of acumeridian energies after 3 weeks of yoga-lifestyle practice and suggest that improvement in health is due to increased prana levels and improved physiological regulation.

Before proceeding further, one must note that some confusion has arisen in the literature regarding the term *electrical acupuncture* (also known as *electroacupuncture*). One must differentiate between electrical stimulation applied to acupuncture needles and electrical stimulation applied to surface electrodes resting on acupuncture points. Originally, electrical acupuncture referred only to electrical stimulation applied to acupuncture needles. This original definition should be maintained. When one stimulates acupuncture points via surface electrodes, one could consider using the acronym SEAPS or use the more-common term *acupuncture-like TENS*.

There are a number of studies in which the acupuncture system was accessed without needles. In KS and MLG's review of 136 articles (see the Clinical Studies section) there were 10 empirical studies in which SEAPS was evaluated in a separate treatment arm.[84,98,111,120,132,151,176,180,204] There were also 7 empirical studies in which laser acupuncture was evaluated in a separate treatment arm.[103,104,109,114,135,136,139] Regarding the SEAPS studies, 7 out of 10 (70%) were favorable, 2 out of 10 (20%) were unfavorable, and 1 out of 10 (10%) was inconclusive. Regarding the laser acupuncture studies, 5 out of 7 (71%) were favorable, 1 out of 7 (14%) was unfavorable, and 1 out of 7 (14%) was inconclusive. Ballegaard et al[222] incorporated shiatsu, which involves manual pressure to acupuncture points, in a treatment package that also included acupuncture and lifestyle adjustment. A series of 69 patients were treated with this package for angina pectoris. The results were positive.

Dundee and McMillan[223] report successfully using a portable-operated square wave stimulator fixed at 10 Hz with a large electrocardiogram surface electrode on acupuncture point P6 to control nausea and vomiting. Milne et al[224] conducted a systematic review of 5 randomized controlled trials of TENS for chronic low back pain. Active TENS treatment included both conventional and acupuncture-like modes. The variability of the outcome measures across studies and the small number of studies reviewed pointed to a clear need for more and better designed studies. Osiri et al[225] reported positive support for TENS in a systematic review, which included acupuncture-like TENS for knee osteoarthritis. However, here again was a need for better-designed studies. Chao et al[226] used TENS over acupuncture points for pain relief in women during the first stage of labor. Their results showed that TENS over acupuncture points provided significantly increased pain relief compared with placebo TENS (very low stimulation; sensory setting). Fargas-Babjak et al[121] used a surface electrical stimulation device designed by Pomeranz called the Codetron (EHM Rehabilitation Technologies) to stimulate acupuncture points in patients with chronic pain. This randomized controlled, double-blind study showed benefit to patients. Galantino et al[227] demonstrated in a pilot study that surface electrical stimulation of acupuncture points ST36, LIV3, K1, and BL60 decreased pain in HIV patients with peripheral neuropathy. The source of electrical stimulation was an H-wave machine from Electronic Waveform Lab Inc. Ng et al[140] conducted a randomized controlled trial with participants with knee osteoarthritis using electroacupuncture (2 Hz) or TENS (2 Hz, pulse width of 200) compared to an education-based control group. This study showed both electroacupuncture and TENS (at acupuncture points) to be effective in significantly reducing osteoarthritis-based knee pain after 8 treatment sessions. Wong[169] showed enhanced stroke rehabilitation using electrical stimulation of acupuncture points through surface electrodes. The HANS device (Wearnes Technology) was used in the study

In a randomized controlled, double-blind study, Naeser et al[228] showed improvement in patients with carpal tunnel syndrome with the use of a combination of cold laser acupuncture point stimulation and microamps TENS. (The laser device was Dynatronics model 1620 and the microamps TENS device was Microstim model 100 [Microstim Inc].) Pontinen[229] has discussed cold laser stimulation of acupuncture points and trigger points for musculoskeletal disorders, along with cold laser therapy for other medical disorders.

In a literature review, Gur[230] discusses the potential mechanisms of pain relief through laser therapy. These include collagen proliferation, anti-inflammatory effects, circulation enhancement, peripheral nerve stimulation, and analgesic effects. In a study by Allais et al,[231] acupuncture, TENS, and infrared laser therapy at acupuncture points were used for the treatment of transformed migraines. The results showed that all 3 treatment groups showed a significant decrease in migraine frequency, but the acupuncture group demonstrated the longest-lasting beneficial effects. All 3 treatment groups utilized the same 6 acupuncture point locations (with additional points selected on an individual basis). Finally, Tsuruoka et al[232] suggest that the use of ultrasound to deliver vibration energy allows patients to avoid the potential pain and skin damage relating to needle insertion. The study noted that noninvasive, focal ultrasound is as effective as standard acupuncture for increase in blood flow volume.

These studies point to the need for more randomized clinical trials to further determine optimal parameters for use in physical therapy clinical practice. If one keeps in mind these examples and remembers the long-established practices of acupressure or shiatsu, one can easily imagine potential application of traditional acupuncture concepts to physical therapy.

Research Possibilities

In addition to randomized controlled trials with double blinding as some of the acupuncture system modalities might allow, individual physical therapists and small group physical therapy facilities might consider well-documented case studies and case series to improve their practices. These smaller studies would contribute to the field by stimulating new ideas and setting the stage for larger studies at university centers. Ottenbacher[233] has written a useful book for doing such research.

Some of the acupuncture system modalities, including acupressure, can also be utilized at home by patients. After initial training by a physical therapist, the physical therapist would act as a coach for setting goals and monitoring adherence to the home acupressure program. Research exploring methods of promoting home therapy adherence for acupuncture system modalities may contribute to improved quality of life for our aging population. While this chapter review did not investigate the utilization of acupuncture in patients with cognitive disorders, acupressure techniques have been used in elderly patients with dementia as an alternative treatment intervention for caregivers. Yang,[234] for instance, reported the results of a pilot study that suggests acupressure is an effective and noninvasive intervention for agitation in patients with dementia.

Delivery of Care Issues

To perform needle acupuncture requires a program of study followed by licensure or registration. To access the acupuncture system without needles may or may not require licensure or registration, depending on the modality and individual state laws. However, further training in traditional Chinese anatomy and physiology is a requisite. The use of cold lasers and electrical stimulation of the acupuncture system requires training and/or supervision or collaboration with a physician acupuncturist or a licensed acupuncturist who is knowledgeable about the use of cold lasers and electrical stimulation in the acupuncture system. One must be aware of any applicable FDA regulations.

To move the profession of physical therapy forward, collaboration across borders is essential. The International Acupuncture Association of Physical Therapists, founded in 1991, is a network of physical therapy associations and persons with interest in the practice of acupuncture. It became a subgroup of the World Confederation for Physical Therapy in 1999. According to its website, it was formed by a core group of physiotherapists from Australia, South Africa, New Zealand, Sweden, and United Kingdom, where physiotherapists had been practicing acupuncture since the early 1980s. Standards of practice for basic safety have been established and accepted by member countries (www.iaapt.org).

For further information on training in TCM for non-physicians, the reader can contact organizations listed in the Additional Resources section at the end of this chapter.

CONCLUSION

Acupuncture and its system of acupuncture points and meridians holds exciting promise for more effective physical therapy and presents opportunities for physical therapy research aimed at greater availability of care utilizing this Asian system of medicine. Although in the United States physical therapists are unable to insert needles for treatment, a number of acupuncture points are incorporated into clinical practice through electrical stimulation interventions and cold laser applications. Therefore, greater knowledge of specific points relevant to optimizing treatment for various conditions may be on the horizon for standardizing SEAPS and cold laser stimulation in clinical practice. Future clinical research is needed to determine dose-effect relationships, treatment frequency, treatment duration, optimum number of treatments, optimal timing to integrate acupuncture and/or physical therapy, and the best time to initiate each therapy.

ACKNOWLEDGMENTS

Dr. LaRiccia wishes to express his gratitude to the Won Sook Chung Foundation in Moorestown, New Jersey, for allowing him to take substantial time from his daily work projects to participate in the updating of this chapter.

REFERENCES

1. Kaptchuk T. *The Web That Has No Weaver: Understanding Chinese Medicine.* New York, NY: Congdon & Weed; 1993.
2. Liao SJ, Lee MHM, Ng LK. *Principles and Practice of Contemporary Acupuncture.* New York, NY: Marcel Dekker; 1994.
3. Xinnong C. Introduction to acupoints. In: *Chinese Acupuncture and Moxibustion.* Beijing, China: Foreign Languages Press; 1987: 108-109.
4. Xinnong C. Internal diseases. In: *Chinese Acupuncture and Moxibustion.* Beijing, China: Foreign Languages Press; 1987: 439-441.
5. Pomeranz B. Scientific basis of acupuncture. In: Stux G, Pomeranz B, eds. *Acupuncture: Textbook and Atlas.* Berlin, Germany: Springer-Verlag; 1987: 1-34.
6. Han J. Central neurotransmitters and acupuncture analgesia. In: Stux G, Pomeranz B, eds. *Scientific Basis of Acupuncture.* Berlin, Germany: Springer-Verlag; 1989: 7-34.
7. Pomeranz B. Acupuncture research related to pain, drug addiction and nerve regeneration. In: Stux G, Pomeranz B, eds. *Scientific Basis of Acupuncture.* Berlin, Germany: Springer-Verlag; 1989: 35-52.
8. Napadow V, Webb JM, Pearson N, et al. Neurobiological correlates of acupuncture: November 17-18, 2005 conference report. *J Altern Complement Med.* 2006;12(9):931-935.

9. Wu M-T, Hsieh J-C, Xiong J, et al. Central nervous pathway for acupuncture stimulation: localization of processing with functional MR imaging of the brain—preliminary experience. *Neuroradiology.* 1999;212:133-141.

10. Cheng RS, Pomeranz BH. Electroacupuncture analgesia is mediated by stereospecific opiate receptors and is reversed by antagonists of type I receptors. *Life Sci.* 1979;26:631-639.

11. Han JS, Xic GX. Dynorphin: important mediator for electroacupuncture analgesia in the spinal cord of the rabbit. *Pain.* 1984;18:367-377.

12. Peets J, Pomeranz B. CXBX mice deficient in opiate receptors show poor electroacupuncture analgesia. *Nature.* 1978;273:675-676.

13. Murai M, Takeshige C, Hishida F, et al. Correlation between individual variations in effectiveness of acupuncture analgesia and that in contents of brain endogenous morphine-like factors. In: Takeshige C, ed. *Studies on the Mechanism of Acupuncture Analgesia Based on Animal Experiments.* Tokyo, Japan: Showa University Press; 1986: 542.

14. Pert A, Dionne R, Ng L, et al. Alterations in rat central nervous system endorphins following transauricular electroacupuncture. *Brain Res.* 1981;224:83-98.

15. Ehrenpreis S. Analgesic properties of enkephalinase inhibitors: animal and human studies. *Prog Clin Biol Res.* 1985;192:363-370.

16. Lee Peng CH, Yang MMP, Kok SH, et al. Endorphin release: a possible mechanism of AA. *Comp Med East West.* 1978;6:57-60.

17. Cheng R, Pomeranz B, Yu G. Dexamethasone partially reduces and 2% saline treatment abolishes electroacupuncture analgesia: these findings implicate pituitary endorphins. *Life Sci.* 1979;24:1481-1486.

18. Pomeranz B. Relation of stress-induced analgesia to acupuncture analgesia. *Ann N Y Acad Sci.* 1986;467(1):444-447.

19. Pomeranz B, Chiu D. Naloxone blocks acupuncture analgesia and causes hyperalgesia: endorphin is implicated. *Life Sci.* 1976;19:1757-1762.

20. Lee MHM, Ernst M. Clinical and research observations on acupuncture analgesia and thermography. In: Stux G, Pomeranz B, eds. *Scientific Basis of Acupuncture.* Berlin, Germany: Springer-Verlag; 1989: 157-176.

21. Sakai S, Hori E, Umeno K, et al. Specific acupuncture sensation correlates with EEGs and autonomic changes in human subjects. *Auton Neurosci.* 2007;133:158-169.

22. Knardahl S, Elam M, Olausson B, et al. Sympathetic nerve activity after acupuncture in humans. *Pain.* 1998;75:19-25.

23. Longhurst J. Acupuncture's cardiovascular actions: a mechanistic perspective. *Medical Acupuncture.* 2013;25(2):101-113.

24. Yang ZK, Wu ML Xin JJ, et al. Manual acupuncture and laser acupuncture for autonomic regulations in rats: observation on heart rate variability and gastric motility. *Evid Based Complement Alternat Med.* 2013;2013:276320.

25. Liao SJ, Wen K. Patient's hypnotizability and their responses to acupuncture treatments for pain relief. A preliminary statistical study. *Am J Acupuncture.* 1976;4:263-268.

26. Peng ATC, Behar S, Yu SJ. Long term therapeutic effects of electroacupuncture for chronic neck and shoulder pain—a double blind study. *Acupunct Electrother Res.* 1987;12:37-44.

27. Ulett G. Studies supporting the concept of physiological acupuncture. In: Stux G, Pomeranz B, eds. *Scientific Basis of Acupuncture.* Berlin, Germany: Springer-Verlag; 1989: 177-196.

28. Barber J, Mayer DJ. Evaluation of the efficacy and neural mechanism of a hypnotic analgesia procedure in experimental and clinical dental pain. *Pain.* 1977;4:41-48.

29. Goldstein A, Hilgard ER. Failure of opiate antagonist naloxone to modify hypnotic analgesia. *Proc Nat Acad Sci.* 1975;72:2041-2043.

30. Nasrallah HA, Holley TY, Janowsky DS. Opiate antagonism fails to reverse hypnotic-induced analgesia. *Lancet.* 1979;1(8130):1355.

31. Lu DP, Lu GP, Kleinman L. Acupuncture and clinical hypnosis for facial and neck pain: a single crossover comparison. *Am J Clin Hypn.* 2001;44(2):141-148.

32. Melzack R, Stillwell DM, Fox EJ. Trigger points and acupuncture points for pain: correlations and implications. *Pain.* 1987;3:3-23.

33. Dung H. Anatomical features contributing to the formation of acupuncture points. *Am J Acupunct.* 1984;12:139-143.

34. Soh K-S. Bonghan duct and acupuncture meridian as optical channel of biophoton. *J Kor Phys Soc.* 2004;45:1196-1198.

35. Moncayo R, Rudisch A, Diemling M, et al. In-vivo visualization of the anatomical structures related to the acupuncture points Dai mai and Shen mai by MRI: a single-case pilot study. *BMC Med Imaging.* 2007;7:4.

36. Hsiu H, Huang SM, Chao PT, et al. Microcirculatory characteristics of acupuncture points obtained by laser Doppler flowmetry. *Physiol Meas.* 2007;28(10):N77-N86.

37. Ferreira AS, Luiz AB. Role of dermatomes in the determination of therapeutic characteristics of channel acupoints: a similarity-based analysis of data compiled from literature. *Chin Med.* 2013;8:24.

38. Cheng KJ. Neuroanatomical characteristics of acupuncture points: relationship between their anatomical locations and traditional clinical indications. *Acupunct Med.* 2011;29(4):289-294.

39. Langevin HM, Yandow JA. Relationship of acupuncture points and meridians to connective tissue planes. *Anat Rec.* 2002;269(6):257-265.

40. Konofagou EE, Langevin HM. Using ultrasound to understand acupuncture. Acupuncture needle manipulation and its effect on connective tissue. *IEEE Eng Med Biol Mag.* 2005;24(2):41-46.

41. Fox JR, Gray W, Koptiuch C, et al. Anisotropic tissue motion induced by acupuncture needling along intermuscular connective tissue planes. *J Altern Complement Med.* 2014;20(4):290-294.

42. Langevin HM. Acupuncture, connective tissue, and peripheral sensory modulation. *Crit Rev Eukaryot Gene Expr.* 2014;24(3):249-253.

43. Ahn AC, Park M, Shaw JR, et al. Electrical impedance of acupuncture meridians: the relevance of subcutaneous collagenous bands. *PLoS One.* 2010;5(7):e11907.

44. Shang C. The past, present and future of meridian system research. *Clinical Acupuncture and Oriental Medicine.* 2000;1:115-124.

45. Li AH, Zhang JM, Xie YK. Human acupuncture points mapped in rats are associated with excitable muscle/skin-nerve complexes with enriched nerve endings. *Brain Res.* 2004;1012:154-159.

46. Wick F, Wick N, Wick MC. Morphological analysis of human acupuncture points through immunohistochemistry. *Am J Phys Med Rehab.* 2007;86(1):7-11.

47. Langevin HM, Churchill DL, Fox JR, et al. Biomechanical response to acupuncture needling in humans. *J Applied Physiol.* 2001;91:2471-2478.

48. Dhond RP, Kettner N, Napadow V. Neuroimagining acupuncture effects in the brain. *J Altern Complement Med.* 2007;13:603-616.

49. Newberg AB, LaRiccia PJ, Lee BY, et al. Cerebral blood flow effects of pain and acupuncture: a preliminary single-photon emission computed tomography imagining study. *J Neuroimaging.* 2005;15:43-49.

50. NIH Consensus Conference. Acupuncture. *JAMA.* 1998;280(17):1518-1524.

51. Lyte CD. Safety and regulation of acupuncture needles and other devices. In: *Program and Abstracts NIH Consensus Development Conference on Acupuncture, November 3-5, 1997.* Bethesda, MD: 51-54.

52. Norheim AJ, Fønnebø V. Acupuncture adverse effects are more than occasional case reports: results from questionnaires among 1,135 randomly selected doctors and 197 acupuncturists. *Compl Therap Med.* 1996;4:8-13.

53. MacPherson H, Thomas K, Walters S, et al. The York acupuncture safety study: prospective survey of 34,000 treatments by traditional acupuncturists. *BMJ.* 2001;323:486-487.

54. Ernst E, White A. Prospective studies of the safety of acupuncture: a systematic review. *Am J Med.* 2001;110:481-485.

55. Melchart D, Weidenhammer W, Streng A, et al. Investigation of adverse effects of acupuncture in 97733 patients. *Arch Intern Med.* 2004;164(1):104-105.

56. Jindal V, Ge A, Mansky PJ. Safety and efficiency of acupuncture in children: a review of the evidence. *Pediatr Hematol Oncol.* 2008;30(6):431-442.

57. Witt CM, Pach D, Brinkhaus B, et al. Safety of acupuncture: results of a prospective observational study with 229,230 patients and introduction of a medical information and consent form. *Forsch Komplementmed.* 2009;16(2):91-97.

58. Zhao L, Zhang FW, Li Y, et al. Adverse events associated with acupuncture: three multicenter randomized controlled trials of 1968 cases in China. *Trials.* 2011;12:87.

59. Chao LF, Zhang AL, Liu HE, et al. The efficacy of acupoint stimulation for the management of therapy-related adverse events in patients with breast cancer: a systematic review. *Breast Cancer Res Treat.* 2009;118(2):255-267. doi:10.1007/s10549-009-0533-8.

60. Mao JJ, Xie SX, Farrar JT, et al. A randomized trial of electro-acupuncture for arthralgia related to aromatase inhibitor use. *EBM Reviews—Cochrane Central Register of Controlled Trials: European Journal of Cancer.* 2014;50(2):267-276.

61. Chen H, Liu T-Y, Zhu J, et al. Electroacupuncture treatment for pancreatic cancer pain: a randomized controlled trial. *EBM Reviews—Cochrane Central Register of Controlled Trials: Pancreatology.* 2013;13(6):594-597.

62. Yu H, Schröder S, Liu Y, et al. Hemiparesis after operation of astrocytoma grade II in adults: effects of acupuncture on sensory-motor behavior and quality of life. *Evid Based Complement Altern Med.* 2013;2013:1-13.

63. Mao JJ, Bruner DW, Stricker C, et al. Feasibility trial of electroacupuncture for aromatase inhibitor-related arthralgia in breast cancer survivors. *Integr Cancer Ther.* 2009;8(2):123-129.

64. Deare JC, Zheng Z, Xue CC, et al. Acupuncture for treating fibromyalgia. *Cochrane Database Syst Rev.* 2013;5:CD007070.

65. Hadianfard MJ, Pairizi PH. A randomized clinical trial of fibromyalgia treatment with acupuncture compared with fluoxetine. *Iran Red Crescent Med J.* 2012;14(10):631-640.

66. Lam M, Galvin R, Curry P. Effectiveness of acupuncture for nonspecific chronic low back pain: a systematic review and meta-analysis. *Spine.* 2013;38(24):2124-2138.

67. Weiss J, Quante S, Xue F, et al. Effectiveness and acceptance of acupuncture in patients with chronic low back pain: results of a prospective, randomized, controlled trial. *J Altern Complement Med.* 2013;19(12):935-941.

68. Inoue M, Nakajima M, Hojo T, et al. Spinal nerve root electroacupuncture for symptomatic treatment of lumbar spinal canal stenosis unresponsive to standard acupuncture: a prospective case series. *Acupunct Med.* 2012;30(2):103-108.

69. DiCesare A, Giombini A, DiCesare M, et al. Comparison between the effects of trigger point mesotherapy versus acupuncture points mesotherapy in the treatment of chronic low back pain: a short term randomized controlled trial. *Complement Ther Med.* 2011;19(1):19-26.

70. Fiore P, Panza F, Cassatella G, et al. Short-term effects of high-intensity laser therapy versus ultrasound therapy in the treatment of low back pain: a randomized controlled trial. *Eur J Phys Rehabil Med.* 2011;47(3):367-373.

71. Furlan AD, van Tulder M, Cherkin D, et al. Acupuncture and dry-needling for low back pain. *Cochrane Database Syst Rev.* 2005;1:CD001351.

72. Shanker N, Thakur M, Tandon OP, et al. Autonomic status and pain profile in patients of chronic low back pain and following electroacupuncture therapy: a randomized control trial. *Indian J Physiol Pharmacol.* 2011;55(1):25-36.

73. Yeh ML, Chung YC, Chen KM, et al. Pain reduction of acupoint electrical stimulation for patients with spinal surgery: a placebo-controlled study. *Int J Nurs Stud.* 2011;48(6):703-709.

74. Furlan AD, Imamura M, Dryden T, et al. Massage for low back pain: an updated systemic review within the framework of the Cochrane Back Review Group. *Spine.* 2009;34:1669-1684.

75. Lin ML, Lin MH, Fen JJ, et al. A comparison between pulsed radiofrequency and electro-acupuncture for relieving pain in patients with chronic low back pain. *Acupunct Electrother Resh.* 2010;35(3-4):133-146.

76. Kumnerddee W. Effectiveness comparison between Thai traditional massage and Chinese acupuncture for myofascial back pain in Thai military personnel: a preliminary report. *Chotmaihet Thangphaet (J of the Medical Association of Thailand).* 2009;92(1): S117-123.

77. Zhao BX, Wang KZ, Zhao JX, et al. Clinical effects of acupuncture after surgical operation in patients with prolapse of the lumbar intervertebral disc. *J Tradit Chin Med.* 2008;28(4):250-254.

78. Chu J, Yuen KF, Wang BH, et al. Electrical twitch-obtaining intramuscular stimulation in lower back pain: a pilot study. *Am J Phys Med Rehab.* 2004;83(2):104-111.

79. Yeung CK, Leung MC, Chow DH. The use of electro-acupuncture in conjunction with exercise for the treatment of chronic low-back pain. *J Altern Complement Med.* 2003;9(4):479-490.

80. Molsberger AF, Mau J, Pawelec DB, et al. Does acupuncture improve the orthopedic management of chronic low back pain—a randomized, blinded, controlled trial with 3 months follow up. *Pain.* 2002;99(3):579-587.

81. Carlsson CP, Sjolund BH. Acupuncture for chronic low back pain: a randomized placebo-controlled study with long-term follow-up. *Clin J Pain.* 2001;17(4):296-305.

82. Uemoto L, Nascimento de Azevedo R, Almeida Alfaya T, et al. Myofascial trigger point therapy: laser therapy and dry needling. *Curr Pain Headache Rep.* 2013;17(9):357.

83. Simma I, Gleditsch JM, Simma L, et al. Immediate effects of microsystem acupuncture in patients with oromyofacial pain and craniomandibular disorders (CMD): a double-blind, placebo-controlled trial. *Br Dent J.* 2009;207(12):E26.

84. Huang L-J, Luo W-J, Zhang K-B, et al. Efficacy observation on cervical spondylosis of vertebral artery type treated with warm needling and rehabilitation physiotherapy. *World Journal of Acupuncture-Moxibustion.* 2012;22(2):12-16.

85. Sahin N, Ozcan E, Sezen K, et al. Efficacy of acupuncture in patients with chronic neck pain—a randomized, sham controlled trial. *Acupunct Electrother Res.* 2010;35(1-2):17-27.

86. Trinh K, Graham N, Gross AR, et al. Acupuncture for neck disorders. *Cochrane Database Syst Rev.* 2010;3:CD004870.

87. Chan DK, Johnson MI, Sun KO, et al. Electrical acustimulation of the wrist for chronic neck pain: a randomized, sham-controlled trial using wrist-ankle acustimulation device. *Clin J Pain.* 2009;25(4):320-326.

88. Chiu TT, Hui-Chan CW, Chein G. A randomized clinical trial of TENS and exercise for patients with chronic neck pain. *Clin Rehabil.* 2005;19(8):850-860.

89. Windmill J, Fisher E, Eccleston C, et al. Interventions for the reduction of prescribed opioid use in chronic noncancer pain. *Cochrane Database Syst Rev.* 2013;9:CD010323.

90. Barlas P, Ting SL, Chesterton LS, et al. Effects of intensity of electroacupuncture upon experimental pain in healthy human volunteers: a randomized, double-blind, placebo-controlled study. *Pain.* 2006;122(1-2):81-89.

91. Smith MJ, Tong HC. Manual acupuncture for analgesia during electromyography: a pilot study. *Arch Phys Med Rehabil.* 2005;86(9):1741-1744.

92. Ferreira LA, de Oliveira RG, Guimaraes JP, et al. Laser acupuncture in patients with temporomandibular dysfunction: a randomized controlled trial. *Lasers Med Sci.* 2013;28(6):1549-1558.

93. Hotta PT, Hotta TH, Bataglion C, et al. EMG analysis after laser acupuncture in patients with temporomandibular dysfunction (TMD): implications for practice. *Complement Ther Clin Pract.* 2010;16(3):158-160.

94. Raustia AM, Pohjola RT. Acupuncture compared with stomatognathic treatment for TMJ dysfunction. Part III: effect of treatment on mobility. *J Prosthet Dent.* 1986;56(5):616-623.

95. Oh B, Kimble B, Costa DS, et al. Acupuncture for treatment of arthralgia secondary to aromatase inhibitor therapy in women with early breast cancer: pilot study. *Acupunct Med.* 2013;31(3):264-271.

96. Hurlow A, Bennett MI, Robb KA, et al. Transcutaneous electric nerve stimulation (TENS) for cancer pain in adults. *Cochrane Database Syst Rev.* 2012;3:CD006276.

97. Kerr DP, Walsh DM, Baxter D. Acupuncture in the management of chronic low back pain: a blinded randomized controlled trial. *Clin J Pain.* 2003;19(6):364-370.

98. Katsoulis J, Ausfeld-Hafter B, Windecker-Getaz I, et al. Laser acupuncture for myofascial pain of the masticatory muscles: a controlled pilot study. *Schweiz Monatsschr Zahnmed.* 2010;120(3):213-225.

99. Franca DL, Senna-Fernandes V, Cortez CM, et al. Tension neck syndrome treated by acupuncture combined with physiotherapy: a comparative clinical trial (pilot study). *Complement Ther Med.* 2008;16(5):268-277.

100. Claydon LS, Chesterton LS, Barlas P, et al. Dose-specific effects of transcutaneous electrical nerve stimulation (TENS) on experimental pain: a systematic review. *Clin J Pain.* 2011;27(7):635-647.

101. Lehmann TR, Russell DW, Spratt KF. The impact of patients with nonorganic physical findings on a controlled trial of transcutaneous electrical nerve stimulation and electroacupuncture. *Spine.* 1983;8(6):625-634.

102. Waseem Z, Boulias C, Gordon A, et al. Botulinum toxin injections for low-back pain and sciatica. *Cochrane Database Syst Rev.* 2011;1:CD008257.

103. Glazov G, Schattner P, Lopez D, et al. Laser acupuncture for chronic non-specific low back pain: a controlled clinical trial. *Acupunct Med.* 2009;27(3):94-100.

104. Kennedy S, Baxter GD, Kerr DP, et al. Acupuncture for acute non-specific low back pain: a pilot randomized non-penetrating sham controlled trial. *Complement Ther Med.* 2008;16(3):139-146.

105. Khadilkar A, Odebiyi DO, Brosseau L, et al. Transcutaneous electrical nerve stimulation (TENS) versus placebo for chronic low-back pain. *Cochrane Database Syst Rev.* 2008;4:CD003008.

106. Milne S, Welch V, Brosseau L, et al. Review: transcutaneous electrical nerve stimulation is not effective for chronic low-back pain. *ACP Journal Club.* 2001;135(3):99.

107. Lehman TR, Russell DW, Spratt KF, et al. Efficacy of electroacupuncture and TENS in the rehabilitation of chronic low back pain patients. *Pain.* 1986;26(3):277-290.

108. Ma C, Wu S, Li G, et al. Comparison of miniscalpel-needle release, acupuncture needling, and stretching exercise to trigger point in myofascial pain syndrome. *Clin J Pain.* 2010;26(3):251-257.

109. Sahin N, Albayrak I, Ugurlu H. Effect of different transcutaneous electrical stimulation modalities on cervical myofascial pain syndrome. *J Musculoskeletal Pain.* 2011;19(1):18-23.

110. Cameron ID, Wang E, Sindhusake D. A randomized trial comparing acupuncture and simulated acupuncture for subacute and chronic whiplash. *Spine.* 2011;36(26):E1659-E1665.

111. Korpan MI, Dezu Y, Schneider B, et al. Acupuncture in the treatment of posttraumatic pain syndrome. *Acta Orthop Belg.* 1999;65(2):197-201.

112. Chang WD, Wu JH, Yang WJ, et al. Therapeutic effects of low-level laser on lateral epicondylitis from differential interventions of Chinese-Western medicine: systematic review. *Photomed Laser Surg.* 2010;28(3):327-336.

113. Fink M, Wolkenstein E, Luennemann M, et al. Chronic epicondylitis: effects of real and sham acupuncture treatment: a randomized controlled patient- and examiner-blinded long-term trial. *Forsch Komplementarmed Klass Naturheilkd.* 2002;9(4):210-215.

114. Fink M, Wolkenstein E, Karst M, et al. Acupuncture in chronic epicondylitis: a randomized controlled trial. *Rheumatology.* 2002;41(2):205-209.

115. Tsui P, Leung MC. Comparison of the effectiveness between manual acupuncture and electro-acupuncture on patients with tennis elbow. *Acupunct Electrother Res.* 2002;27(2):107-117.

116. Weiner DK, Moore CG, Morone NE, et al. Efficacy of periosteal stimulation for chronic pain associated with advanced knee osteoarthritis: a randomized, controlled clinical trial. *Clin Ther.* 2013;35(11):1703-1720.

117. De Luigi AJ. Complementary and alternative medicine in osteoarthritis. *Phys Med Rehabil.* 2012;4(5 suppl):S122-S133.

118. Ye L, Kalichman L, Spittle A, et al. Effects of rehabilitative interventions on pain, function and physical impairments in people with hand osteoarthritis: a systematic review. *Arthritis Res Ther.* 2011;13(1):R28.

119. Manheimer E, Cheng K, Linde K, et al. Acupuncture for peripheral joint osteoarthritis. *Cochrane Database Syst Rev.* 2010;1:CD001977.

120. Ahsin S, Saleem S, Bhatti AM, et al. Clinical and endocrinological changes after electro-acupuncture treatment in patients with osteoarthritis of the knee. *Pain.* 2009;147(1-3):60-66.

121. Fargas-Babjak AM, Pomeranz B, Rooney PJ. Acupuncture like stimulation with codetron for rehabilitation of patients with chronic pain syndrome and osteoarthritis. *Acupunct Electrother Res Int J.* 1992;17:95-105.

122. Fink MG, Kunsebeck H, Wipperman B, et al. Non-specific effects of traditional Chinese acupuncture in osteoarthritis of the hip. *Complement Ther Med.* 2001;9(2):82-89.

123. Ashraf A, Zarei F, Hadianfard MJ, et al. Comparison of the effect of lateral wedge insole and acupuncture in medial compartment knee osteoarthritis: a randomized controlled trial. *Knee.* 2014;21(2):439-444.

124. Zhao L, Shen X, Cheng K, et al. Validating a nonacupoint sham control for laser treatment of knee osteoarthritis. *Photomed Laser Surg.* 2010;28(3):351-356.

125. Shen X, Zhao L, Ding G, et al. Effect of combined laser acupuncture on knee osteoarthritis: a pilot study. *Lasers Med Sci.* 2009;24(2):129-136.

126. Taechaarpornkul W, Suvapan D, Theppanom C, et al. Comparison of the effectiveness of six and two acupuncture point regimens in osteoarthritis of the knee: a randomized trial. *Acupunct Med.* 2009;27(1):3-8.

127. Lu Y, He Z. Rehabilitative treatment for knee osteoarthritis in 28 hemiplegic patients after stroke. *Neural Regeneration Research.* 2007;2(11):702-704.

128. Yurtkuran M, Alp A, Konur S, et al. Laser acupuncture in knee osteoarthritis: a double-blind randomized controlled study. *Photomed Laser Surg.* 2007;25(1):14-20.

129. Arichi A, Arichi H, Toda S. Acupuncture and rehabilitation (III) effects of acupuncture applied to the normal side on osteoarthritis deformans and rheumatoid arthritis of the knee and on disorders in motility of the knee joint after cerebral hemorrhage and thrombosis. *Am J Chin Med.* 1983;11(1-4):146-149.

130. Kumnerddee W, Pattapong N. Efficacy of electro-acupuncture in chronic plantar fasciitis: a randomized controlled trial. *Am J Chin Med.* 2012;40(6):1167-1176.

131. Carey TS. Adding single-point acupuncture to physiotherapy for painful shoulder improved function and reduced pain. *ACP Journal Club.* 2008;149(4):12.

132. Vas J, Ortega C, Olmo V, et al. Single-point acupuncture and physiotherapy for the treatment of painful shoulder: a multicenter randomized controlled trial. *Rheumatology.* 2008;47(6):887-893.

133. Dyson-Hudson TA, Kadar P, LaFountaine M, et al. Acupuncture for chronic shoulder pain in persons with spinal cord injury: a small-scale clinical trial. *Arch Phys Med Rehabil.* 2007;88(10):1276-1283.

134. Dyson-Hudson TA, Shiflett SC, Kirshblum SC, et al. Acupuncture and Trager psychophysical integration in the treatment of wheelchair user's shoulder pain in individuals with spinal cord injury. *Arch Phys Med Rehabil.* 2001;82(8):1038-1046.

135. Felson D. Some nondrug therapies improve pain and function in osteoarthritis. *ACP Journal Club.* 1995;122(1):7.

136. Green S, Buchbinder R, Hetrick S. Acupuncture for shoulder pain. *Cochrane Database Syst Rev.* 2005;2:CD005319.

137. Kim TH, Lee MS, Kim KH, et al. Acupuncture for treating acute ankle sprains in adults. *Cochrane Database Syst Rev.* 2014;6:CD009065.

138. Green S, Buchbinder R, Barnsley L, et al. Acupuncture for lateral elbow pain. *Cochrane Database Syst Rev.* 2002;1:CD003527.

139. Suarez-Almazor ME, Looney C, Liu Y, et al. A randomized controlled trial of acupuncture for osteoarthritis of the knee: effects of patient-provider communication. *Arthritis Care Res.* 2010;62(9):1229-1236.

140. Ng MM, Leung MC, Poon DM. The effects of electro-acupuncture and transcutaneous electrical nerve stimulation on patients with painful osteoarthritic knees: a randomized controlled trial with follow-up evaluation. *J Altern Complement Med.* 2003;9(5):641-649.

141. Du L-Z. Observation on the therapeutic effect of time-oriented points opening of Linggui Bafa for Bell's palsy. *World J Acupuncture-Moxibusion.* 2013;23(3):42-45.

142. Liu ZH, Qi YC, Pan PG, et al. Clinical observation on treatment of clearing the Governor Vessel and refreshing the mind needling in neural development and remediation of children with cerebral palsy. *Chin J Integr Med.* 2013;19(7):505-509.

143. Zhang P-Y, Hu F-F. Influence of cluster needling at scalp acupoints combined with rehabilitation training on balance functions of children with cerebral palsy. *World J Acupuncture-Moxibustion.* 2012;22(4):23-26,31.

144. Wang XF, Hu XL. Therapeutic effects on spastic cerebral palsy in children: acupuncture and massage at the Shu and He acupoints versus routine acupoints. *Neural Regeneration Res.* 2008;3(1):53-56.

145. Wu Y, Zou LP, Han TL, et al. Randomized controlled trial of traditional Chinese medicine (acupuncture and tuina) in cerebral palsy: part 1—any increase in seizure in integrated acupuncture and rehabilitation group versus rehabilitation group? *J Altern Complement Med.* 2008;14(8):1005-1009.

146. Zhang LH, Du JJ, Li XJ, et al. Serum level changes of insulin-like growth factor-1 and amino acids in children with cerebral palsy following functional exercise plus head acupuncture therapy. *Neural Regeneration Res.* 2006;1(6):525-528.

147. Khosrawi S, Moghtaderi A, Haghighat S. Acupuncture in treatment of carpal tunnel syndrome: a randomized controlled trial study. *J Res Med Sci.* 2012;17(1):1-7.

148. Kumnerddee W, Kaewtong A. Efficacy of acupuncture versus night splinting for carpal tunnel syndrome: a randomized clinical trial. *J Med Assoc Thai.* 2010;93(12):1463-1469.

149. Hauer K, Wendt I, Schwenk M, et al. Stimulation of acupoint ST-34 acutely improves gait performance in geriatric patients during rehabilitation: a randomized controlled trial. *Arch Phys Med Rehabil.* 2011;92(1):7-14.

150. Yu H, Schröder S, Liu Y, et al. Hemiparesis after operation of astrocytoma grad II in adults: effects of acupuncture on sensory-motor behavior and quality of life. *Evid Based Complement Altern Med.* 2013;2013:859763.

151. He X-Z, Dai S-Q, Su L. Controlled observation of posthemiplegic omalgia treated by acupuncture-moxibustion and rehabilitation. *World J of Acupuncture-Moxibustion.* 2012;22(4):18-22.

152. Li N, Tian F, Wang C, et al. Therapeutic effect of acupuncture and massage for shoulder-hand syndrome in hemiplegia patients: a clinical two-center randomized controlled trial. *J Tradit Chin Med.* 2012;32(3):343-349.

153. Mao M, Chen X, Chen Y, et al. Stage-oriented comprehensive acupuncture treatment plus rehabilitation training for apoplectic hemiplegia. *J Tradit Chin Med.* 2008;28(2):90-93.

154. Donnellan CP, Shanley J. Comparison of the effect of two types of acupuncture on quality of life in secondary progressive multiple sclerosis: a preliminary single-blind randomized controlled trial. *Clin Rehabil.* 2008;22(3):195-205.

155. Deng Z, Su J, Cai L, et al. Evidence-based treatment for acute spinal cord injury. *Neural Regeneration Res.* 2011;6(23):1791-1795.

156. Wong AM, Leong CP, Su TY, et al. Clinical trial of acupuncture for patients with spinal cord injuries. *Am J Phys Med Rehabil.* 2003;82(1):21-27.

157. Cheng PT, Wong MK, Chang PL. A therapeutic trial of acupuncture in neurogenic bladder of spinal cord injured patients—a preliminary report. *Spinal Cord.* 1998;36(7):476-480.

158. Wang BH, Lin CL, Li TM, et al. Selection of acupoints for managing upper-extremity spasticity in chronic stroke patients. *Clin Interv Aging.* 2014;9:147-156.

159. Liu S, Shi Z-Y. Observation on the therapeutic effect of scalp acupuncture and body acupuncture in combination with rehabilitation exercise for hemiplegia and shoulder pain after stroke. *World J of Acupuncture-Moxibustion.* 2013;23(1):21-26.

160. Zhang Y, Jin H, Ma D, et al. Efficacy of integrated rehabilitation techniques of traditional Chinese medicine for ischemic stroke: a randomized controlled trial. *Am J Chin Med.* 2013;41(5):971-981.

161. Gao H, Gao X, Liang G, et al. Contra-lateral needling in the treatment of hemiplegia due to acute ischemic stroke. *Acupunct Electrother Res.* 2012;37(1):1-12.

162. Hegyi G, Szigeti GP. Rehabilitation of stroke patients using Yamamoto New Scalp Acupuncture: a pilot study. *J Altern Complement Med.* 2012;18(10):971-977.

163. Gong W, Zhang T, Cui L, et al. Electro-acupuncture at Zusanli (ST 36) to improve lower extremity motor function in sensory disturbance patients with cerebral stroke: a randomized controlled study of 240 cases. *Neural Regeneration Res.* 2009;11:935-940.

164. Liu SY, Hsieh CL, Wei TS, et al. Acupuncture stimulation improves balance function in stroke patients: a single-blinded controlled, randomized study. *Am J Chin Med.* 2009;37(3):483-494.

165. Yan T, Hui-Chan CW. Transcutaneous electrical stimulation on acupuncture points improves muscle function in subjects after acute stroke: a randomized controlled trial. *J Rehabil Med.* 2009;41(5):312-316.

166. Liu W, Mukherjee M, Sun C, et al. Electroacupuncture may help motor recovery in chronic stroke survivors: a pilot study. *J Rehabil Res Dev.* 2008;45(4):587-595.

167. Mukherjee M, McPeak LK, Redford JB, et al. The effect of electro-acupuncture on spasticity of the wrist joint in chronic stroke survivors. *Arch Phys Med Rehabil.* 2007;88(2):159-166.

168. Alexander DN, Cen S, Sullivan KJ, et al. Effects of acupuncture treatment on poststroke motor recovery and physical function: a pilot study. *Neurorehabil Neural Repair.* 2004;18(4):259-267.

169. Wong AM, Su TY, Tang FT, et al. Clinical trial of electrical acupuncture on hemiplegic stroke patients. *Am J Phys Med Rehabil.* 1999;78(2):117-122.

170. Kjendahl A, Sällström S, Osten PE, et al. A one year follow-up study on the effects of acupuncture in the treatment of stroke patients in the subacute stage: a randomized, controlled study. *Clin Rehabil.* 1997;11(3):192-200.

171. Sällström S, Kjendahl A, Osten PE, et al. Acupuncture in the treatment of stroke patients in the subacute stage: a randomized, controlled study. *Complement Ther Med.* 1996;4(3):193-197.

172. Teixeira LJ, Valbuza JS, Prado GF. Physical therapy for Bell's palsy (idiopathic facial paralysis). *Cochrane Database Syst Rev.* 2011;12:CD006283.

173. Chen N, Zhou M, He L, et al. Acupuncture for Bell's palsy. *Cochrane Database Sys Rev.* 2010;8:CD002914.

174. Duncan B, Shen K, Zou LP, et al. Evaluating intense rehabilitative therapies with and without acupuncture for children with cerebral palsy: a randomized controlled trial. *Arch Phys Med Rehabil.* 2012;93(5):808-815.

175. Chau ACM, Cheung RTF, Jiang X, et al. Acupuncture of motor-implicated acupoints on subacute stroke patients: an fMRI evaluation study. *Med Acupunct.* 2009;21(4):233-241.

176. Wu H. Acupuncture and stroke rehabilitation. *CMAJ.* 2010;182(16):1711-1712.

177. Xie Y, Wang L, He J, et al. Acupuncture for dysphagia in acute stroke. *Cochrane Database Syst Rev.* 2008;3:CD006076.

178. Zhang SH, Liu M, Asplund K, et al. Acupuncture for acute stroke. *Cochrane Database Syst Rev.* 2005;2:CD003317.

179. Li G, Jack CR Jr, Yang ES. An fMRI study of somatosensory-implicated acupuncture points in stable somatosensory stroke patients. *J Magn Reson Imaging.* 2006;24(5):1018-1024.

180. Wong V, Cheuk DK, Lee S, et al. Acupuncture for acute management and rehabilitation of traumatic brain injury. *Cochrane Database Syst Rev.* 2013;3:CD007700.

181. O'Connor D, Marshall S, Massy-Westropp N. Non-surgical treatment (other than steroid injection) for carpal tunnel syndrome. *Cochrane Database Syst Rev.* 2003;1:CD003219.

182. Penza P, Bricchi M, Scola A, et al. Electroacupuncture is not effective in chronic painful neuropathies. *Pain Med.* 2011;12(12):1819-1823.

183. Cristian A, Katz M, Cutrone E, et al. Evaluation of acupuncture in the treatment of Parkinson's disease: a double-blind pilot study. *Mov Disord.* 2005;20(9):1185-1188.

184. Park SW, Yi SH, Lee JA, et al. Acupuncture for the treatment of spasticity after stroke: a meta-analysis of randomized controlled trials. *J Altern Complement Med.* 2014;20(9):672-682.

185. Bai YL, Li L, Hu YS, et al. Prospective, randomized controlled trial of physiotherapy and acupuncture on motor function and daily activities in patients with ischemic stroke. *J Altern Complement Med.* 2013;19(8):684-689.

186. Zhu Y, Zhang L, Ouyang G, et al. Acupuncture in subacute stroke: no benefits detected. *Phys Ther.* 2013;93(11):1447-1455.

187. Zhuangl LX, Xu SF, D'Adamo CR, et al. An effectiveness study comparing acupuncture, physiotherapy, and their combination in poststroke rehabilitation: a multicentered, randomized, controlled clinical trial. *Altern Ther Health Med.* 2012;18(3):8-14.

188. Hopwood V, Lewith G, Prescott P, et al. Evaluating the efficacy of acupuncture in defined aspects of stroke recover: a randomized, placebo controlled single blind study. *J Neruol.* 2008;255(6):858-866.

189. Park J, White AR, James MA, et al. Acupuncture for subacute stroke rehabilitation: a sham-controlled, subject- and assessor-blind, randomized trial. *Arch Intern Med.* 2005;165(17):2026-2031.

190. Wayne PM, Krebs DE, Macklin EA, et al. Acupuncture for upper-extremity rehabilitation in chronic stroke: a randomized sham-controlled study. *Arch Phys Med Rehabil.* 2005;86(12):2248-2255.

191. Fink M, Rollnik JD, Bijak M, et al. Needle acupuncture in chronic poststroke leg spasticity. *Arch Phys Med Rehabil.* 2004;85(4):667-672.

192. Sze FK, Wong, E, Yi X, et al. Does acupuncture have additional value to standard poststroke motor rehabilitation? *Stroke.* 2002;33(1):186-194.

193. Johansson BB, Haker E, von Arbin M, et al. Acupuncture and transcutaneous nerve stimulation in stroke rehabilitation: a randomized, controlled trial. *Stroke.* 2001;32(3):707-713.

194. Gosman-Hedström G, Claesson L, Klingenstierna U, et al. Effects of acupuncture treatment on daily life activities and quality of life: a controlled, prospective, and randomized study of acute stroke patients. *Stroke.* 1998;29(10):2100-2108.

195. MacPherson H, White A, Cummings M, et al. Standards for reporting interventions in controlled trials of acupuncture: the STRICTA recommendations. *J Altern Complement Med.* 2002;8:85-89.

196. Hammerslag R. Methodological and ethical issues in acupuncture research. In: *Programs and Abstracts NIH Consensus Development Conference on Acupuncture, November 3-5, 1997.* Bethesda, MD: 45-49.

197. Jerner B, Skogh M, Vahlquist A. A controlled trial of acupuncture in psoriasis: no convincing effect. *Acta Dermato-Venereologica.* 1997;77:154-156.

198. Shlay JC, Chaloner K, Max MB, et al. Acupuncture and amitriptyline for pain due to HIV-related peripheral neuropathy: a randomized controlled trial. *JAMA.* 1998;280:1590-1595.

199. Berman BM, Singh B, Lao L, et al. A randomized trial of acupuncture as an adjunctive therapy in osteoarthritis of the knee. *Rheumatology.* 1999;38:346-354.

200. Kleinhenz J, Streitberger K, Windeler J, et al. Randomized clinical trial comparing the effects of acupuncture and a newly designed placebo needle in rotator cuff tendinitis. *Pain.* 1999;83:235-241.

201. Lund I, Lundeberg T. Are minimal, superficial or sham acupuncture procedures acceptable as inert placebo controls? *Acupunct Med.* 2006;24(1):13-15.

202. Kong J, Gollub R, Rosman IS, et al. Brain activity associated with expectancy-enhanced placebo analgesia as measured by functional magnetic resonance imaging. *J Neurosci.* 2006;26(2):381-388.

203. Dincer F, Linde K. Sham interventions in randomized clinical trials of acupuncture—a review. *Compl Ther Med.* 2003;11:235-242.

204. Lundeberg T, Lind I, Naslund J, et al. The emperor's sham-wrong assumption that sham needling is sham. *Acupunt Med.* 2008;26(4):239-242.

205. Birch A. A review and analysis of placebo treatments, placebo effects and placebo controls in trials of medical procedures when sham is not inert. *J Altern Complement Med.* 2006;12(3):303-310.

206. Chapman CR, Chen AC, Bonica JJ. Effects of intrasegmental electrical acupuncture on dental pain: evaluation by threshold estimation and sensory decision theory. *Pain.* 1977;3:213-227.

207. Stacher G, Wancura I, Bauer P, et al. Effect of acupuncture on pain threshold and pain tolerance determined by electrical stimulation of the skin: a controlled study. *Am J Chin Med.* 1975;3(2):143-146.

208. Vincent CA, Richardson PH. The evaluation of therapeutic acupuncture: concepts and methods. *Pain.* 1986;24(1):1-13.

209. White AR, Ernst E. A systematic review of randomized controlled trials of acupuncture for neck pain. *Rheumatology.* 1999;38(2):143-147.

210. van Tulder MW, Cherkin DC, Berman B, et al. The effectiveness of acupuncture in the management of acute and chronic low back pain: a systematic review within the framework of the Cochrane Collaboration back review group. *Spine.* 1999;24:1113-1123.

211. Ernst E, White A. Acupuncture for back pain: a meta-analysis of randomized controlled trials. *Arch Intern Med.* 1998;158:2235-2241.

212. Naeser MA, Alexander MP, Stiassny-Eder DGV, et al. Real vs. sham acupuncture in the treatment of paralysis in acute stroke patients—a CT scan lesion site study. *J Neurol Rehab.* 1992;6:163-173.

213. Shen J. Adjunct antiemesis electroacupuncture in stem cell transplantation. *Proc Amer Soc Clin Oncol.* 1997;148:2a.

214. Wolfe MM, Lichtenstein DR, Singh G. Gastrointestinal toxicity of nonsteroidal anti-inflammatory drugs. *N Engl J Med.* 1999;340:1888-1899.

215. Lazarou J, Pomeranz B, Corey PN. Incidence of adverse drug reactions in hospitalized patients: a meta-analysis of prospective studies. *JAMA.* 1998;279:1200-1205.

216. Johansson K, Lindgren I, Widner H, et al. Can sensory stimulation improve functional outcome in stroke patients? *Neurology.* 1993;43:2189-2192.

217. Wong AM, Su TY, Tang FT, et al. Clinical trial of electrical acupuncture on hemiplegic stroke patients. *Am J Phys Med Rehab.* 1999;78:117-122.

218. Ernst E, White A. Acupuncture as a treatment for temporomandibular joint dysfunction: a systematic review of randomized trials. *Arch Otolaryngol Head Neck Surg.* 1999;125:269-272.

219. Stux G, Pomeranz BE. *Acupuncture: Textbook and Atlas.* Berlin, Germany: Springer-Verlag; 1987.

220. Xinnong C. *Chinese Acupuncture and Moxibusion.* Beijing, China: Foreign Languages Press; 1987.

221. Sharma B, Hankey A, Nagilla N, et al. Can yoga practices benefit health by improving organism regulation? Evidence from electrodermal measures of acupuncture meridians. *Int J Yoga.* 2014;7(1):32-40.

222. Ballegaard S, Norrelund S, Smith DF. Cost-benefit use of acupuncture, Shiatsu and lifestyle adjustment for treatment of patients with severe angina pectoris. *Acupunct Electrother Res Int J.* 1966;21:187-197.

223. Dundee JW, McMillan C. Clinical uses of P6 acupuncture antiemesis. *Acupunct Electrother Res Int J.* 1990;15:211-215.

224. Milne S, Welch V, Brosseau L, et al. Transcutaneous electrical nerve stimulation (TENS) for chronic low back pain. *Cochrane Database Syst Rev.* 2001;2:CD003008.

225. Osiri M, Welch V, Brosseau L, et al. Transcutaneous electrical nerve stimulation for knee osteoarthritis. *Cochrane Database Syst Rev.* 2000;4:CD002328.

226. Chao AS, Chao A, Wang TH, et al. Pain relief by applying transcutaneous electrical nerve stimulation (TENS) on acupuncture points during the first stage of labor: a randomized double-blind placebo-controlled trial. *Pain.* 2007;127:214.

227. Galantino MLA, Eke-Oro S, Findley TW, et al. Use of noninvasive electroacupuncture for the treatment of HOV-related peripheral neuropathy: a pilot study. *J Altern Complement Med.* 1999;3:135-142.

228. Naeser MA, Hahn K, Lieberman B. Real vs sham laser acupuncture and microamp TENS to treat carpal tunnel syndrome and work-site wrist pain: a pilot study. *Lasers Surg Med.* 1996;8(suppl):7.

229. Pontinen P. *Low Level Laser Therapy as a Medical Treatment Modality.* Jarmpere, Finland: Art Urpo Ltd; 1992.

230. Gur A. Physical therapy modalities in management of fibromyalgia. *Curr Pharm Des.* 2006;12(1):29-35.

231. Allais G, De Lorenzo C, Quirico PE, et al. Non-pharmacological approaches to chronic headaches: transcutaneous electrical nerve stimulation, laser therapy and acupuncture in transformed migraine treatment. *Neurol Sci.* 2003;24:S138-S142.

232. Tsuruoka N, Watanabe M, Takayama S, et al. Brief effect of acupoint stimulation using focused ultrasound. *J Altern Complement Med.* 2013;19(5):416-419.

233. Ottenbacher K. *Evaluating Clinical Change: Strategies for Occupational and Physical Therapists.* Baltimore, MD: Williams and Wilkins; 1986.

234. Yang MH, Wu SC, Lin JG, et al. The efficacy of acupressure for decreasing agitated behavior in dementia: a pilot study. *J Clin Nurs.* 2007;16(2):308-315.

Additional Resources

- Accreditation Commission for Acupuncture and Oriental Medicine

  (ACAOM)

  8941 Aztec Drive

  Eden Prairie, MN 55347

  Phone: (952) 212-2434

  www.acaom.org

- American Organization for Bodywork Therapies of Asia (AOBTA)

  1010 County Route 561

  Voorhees, NJ 08043

  Phone (856) 782-1616

  www.aobta.org

Medical doctors and doctors of osteopathy can contact the following:

- American Academy of Medical Acupuncture (AAMA)

  1970 East Grand Avenue, Suite 330

  El Segundo, CA 90245

  Phone: (310) 364-0193

  www.medicalacupuncture.org

- American College of Acupuncture

  1021 Park Avenue

  New York, NY 10028

  Phone: (212) 876-9781

  www.acupuncturesociety.com

19

Dry Needling

Jan Dommerholt, PT, DPT, MPS, DAAPM

Dry needling (DN) is becoming increasingly used in physical therapy practice in many countries around the world. Judging by the number of DN continuing education course offerings throughout the United States, there were fewer than 10 DN courses nationwide in 2004, while in 2014 there were nearly 20 DN course providers, each offering many DN courses! Other countries have experienced a similar growth in course offerings and exponential interest in DN. The initial focus of most continuing education programs was primarily on trigger point (TrP)-DN, but DN is increasingly being used to address other indications as well, such as tendinopathies and enthesopathies.[1,2] The main objectives of DN are to decrease pain, increase local circulation and range of motion, and improve muscle strength and tissue mobility in conjunction with other physical therapy approaches. In addition to physical therapists, other health care providers, including occupational therapists, dentists, physicians, veterinarians, myotherapists, and athletic trainers, have started integrating DN into clinical practice, depending on the local jurisdiction. Professional and amateur athletes are employing the technique to enhance athletic performance and speed up recovery after injury. In veterinary medicine, DN is applied to improve canine and equine athletic performance in addition to more common medical applications.[3,4]

In 1984, Maryland was the first United States state to approve DN to be within the scope of physical therapy practice. Currently, DN is within the scope of physical therapy practice in most states in the United States and in a growing number of countries, such as Australia, Canada, Dubai, Ireland, the Netherlands, New Zealand, Norway, South Africa, Spain, Sweden, and Switzerland, among many others. National physical therapy associations in Australia, Ireland, New Zealand, Switzerland, and the United States have developed DN guidelines and educational resources.

HISTORY

The first mention of a DN technique appeared in 1821 when Churchill[5] reported using ladies' hat pins for the treatment of lumbago. The term *dry needling* was not used until 1947 in an article about low back pain.[6] Paulett[6] emphasized that DN was most effective when the muscle would exhibit a reflex spasm, which later became known as a *local twitch response* (LTR).[7] Although DN can be used for a variety of indications, the vast majority of published research focuses on myofascial pain and TrPs.[8]

Historically, TrP phenomena have been described for many centuries going back as far as the 16th century.[9] In 1816, Balfour described "nodular tumours and thickenings which were painful to

Davis CM.
Integrative Therapies in Rehabilitation: Evidence for Efficacy in Therapy, Prevention, and Wellness, Fourth Edition (pp 305-323).
© 2017 Taylor & Francis Group.

the touch, and from which pains shot to neighbouring parts," which is the first description in history that resembles the current definition.[10] Myofascial pain is a common musculoskeletal pain condition characterized by the presence of TrPs with local and referred pain. Of interest is that pain management specialists have a greater appreciation of myofascial pain than general practitioners.[11,12] Myofascial pain, TrPs, and DN are only marginally accepted in mainstream medicine in spite of an emerging and growing body of scientific evidence.[13] The first TrP book was published in 1931 in Germany,[14] more than 50 years before Travell and Simons[15] released their TrP manual. Travell and Simons did not routinely use DN in their clinical practices, but employed TrP injections with 0.5% procaine in combination with the spray and stretch technique and moist heat.[16]

The use of an anesthetic for the treatment of tender spots in muscles was first explored by Harman and Young[17] in 1940, but soon thereafter, others suggested that pain relief could be achieved by needling without an injectate.[18,19] It was not until 1979 that Lewit[2] explored this concept further. He described needling 312 pain sites in 241 patients, including TrPs, scar tissue, insertion points of ligaments, muscle spasms, tendons, entheses, periosteum, and joints. Immediate analgesia without hypesthesia, referred to as "the needle effect," was noted in nearly 87% of subjects, with permanent relief of tenderness for 92 targets.[2] In 1980, Gunn and coworkers[20] published the first scientific study on the successful use of DN of motor points in the treatment of individuals with low back pain. Since these early publications, multiple other papers have followed including case reports,[21-24] reviews,[25-28] papers exploring DN techniques and mechanisms,[29-31] clinical studies,[32-35] and papers about the safety of DN,[36,37] among others. Dunning and colleagues[1] argued that physical therapists should consider high-quality acupuncture studies and suggested that ignoring randomized clinical acupuncture trials would limit the ability to optimally use DN in clinical practice.

From a medical and physical therapy perspective, DN has evolved out of the use of TrP injections in the United States.[38] In some other countries, physical therapists incorporated aspects of acupuncture practice especially for pain management and orthopedic and sport-related injuries.[39-41] Within the context of physical therapy, however, DN is more closely related to manual physical therapy than to acupuncture, even though DN is performed with the same solid filament needle.[38] In the most recent edition of the *Guide to Physical Therapist Practice*, the American Physical Therapy Association (APTA) includes DN as part of the practice of manual physical therapy.[42]

CONTROVERSIES

The use of DN by physical therapists is not without controversy, especially in the United States, where primarily non-medical acupuncturists and acupuncture boards and societies continue to attempt to ban DN by physical therapists and chiropractors.[43] They maintain that DN has always been a part of acupuncture and therefore, they feel that physical therapists and chiropractors who are using DN are, in fact, practicing acupuncture without a license.[44] As an example, after 25 years of the use of DN by Maryland-based physical therapists, the Maryland Board of Acupuncture and the state's acupuncture society claimed that DN by physical therapists would constitute a public health hazard, even though not a single adverse event had ever been reported to any state board. They even convinced legislators to introduce new laws that would have prohibited DN by physical therapists. Because of strong physical therapy lobbying, DN remained within the scope of PT practice in Maryland. Similar efforts have been attempted in several other states. In some jurisdictions, medical doctors and chiropractors have raised concerns about DN by physical therapists. In addition to suggesting that physical therapists would put patients at increased risk, acupuncturists often argue that physical therapists could potentially needle so-called "forbidden points," which they believe to be abortifacient in spite of an overwhelming lack of evidence to the contrary.[45-47] Acupuncturist Amaro[48] recommended that practitioners of acupuncture "absorb the philosophy and procedure of DN as an adjunct for musculoskeletal pain control," while acupuncturists Matsumoto and Birch[49] suggested to consider acupuncture as a myofascial therapy.

According to some acupuncture sources, TrPs have been recognized as so-called ashi points as far back as 652 CE,[44] but others maintain that there is less than a 20% overlap between acupuncture and TrPs.[50,51] Melzack et al[52] erroneously assumed a 71% overlap between acupuncture point and TrP locations, which reflects a serious misunderstanding of the nature and characteristics of both kinds of points.[50] Although Travell and Simons indicated common TrP locations in their textbooks, they never suggested that these points should be used as definitive TrP maps that can be compared to other "point systems," such as acupuncture points.[53] The TrP locations by Travell and Simons are also not all inclusive. In other words, when examining a patient for the presence of TrPs, the examination should not be limited to just the points mentioned in Travell's publications. Travell marked 7 common locations for TrPs in the trapezius muscles, for example, but in clinical practice it is not uncommon to identify many more TrPs in this muscle, especially in a patient with tension-type headaches, migraines, or whiplash-associated disorders.[54-56] The concepts of acupuncture and DN are sometimes poorly distinguished and occasionally, the terms are used interchangeably (ie, when authors refer to DN as "trigger point acupuncture").[8,57] Dorsher[58] considers referred pain patterns associated with TrPs as a confirmation of acupuncture meridians. Most United States-based DN continuing education programs have not incorporated the acupuncture literature into their DN approach,[59] but physical therapists in some other countries have adopted Western and more traditional acupuncture concepts.[60,61]

An entirely different controversy relates to the construct of myofascial pain itself and whether TrPs even exist.[62] Quintner and colleagues[63] claimed to have refuted the entire TrP construct, but Dommerholt and Gerwin[64] disputed their observations as a biased review of the literature replete with unsupported opinions and accusations. Meakins[65] also expressed his doubts in a recent commentary and concluded that the theory of myofascial pain "has never been adequately explained." He dismissed the current TrP hypotheses as an example of pareidolia, which he described as a "vague and obscure stimulus that is perceived as something clear and distinct."[65] According to Meakins, when clinicians locate TrPs, they are palpating perfectly normal anatomy, which they interpret as TrPs based on their belief or expectations.[65] Others maintain that TrPs cannot be reliably identified and therefore nearly all TrP studies would necessarily be flawed,[66,67] even though several studies demonstrated that experienced clinicians can easily identify TrPs with evidence of acceptable intra- and interrater reliability.[68-71] Contrary to the assumptions and opinions of these authors, there is much recent research in support of DN and myofascial pain.

MYOFASCIAL PAIN

To comprehend why clinicians would consider using DN in clinical practice, a basic appreciation of the current thinking about myofascial pain is necessary. TrPs are the hallmark feature of myofascial pain, but they occur with most, if not all, other musculoskeletal pain diagnoses, such as osteoarthritis of the hip or knee,[72] epicondylalgia,[73] low back pain,[27] tension-type headaches,[55] migraines,[74] chronic shoulder pain,[75] post-mastectomy surgery,[76] post-lumpectomy surgery,[77] or with visceral conditions, such as interstitial cystitis,[78] irritable bowel syndrome,[79] endometriosis,[80] dysmenorrhea,[81] or prostatitis,[82] among others. TrPs may be associated with psychological, visceral, endocrine, infectious, and metabolic conditions. Because of the common presence of TrPs with painful conditions, there is some debate whether myofascial pain is a disease, a process, or a syndrome.[13] Infants do not have TrPs,[83] but TrPs become more common by 3 to 4 years of age and this trend continues with advancing age.[84,85] This suggests that TrPs are not necessarily a pathological entity,[86] unless they lead to persistent pain or motor dysfunctions, such as muscle weakness or inhibition, muscle cramps, or altered motor recruitment patterns.[87]

Although Travell expressed her initial thoughts about myofascial pain over 60 years ago, high-quality research of myofascial pain and TrPs is still in its infancy, which partially explains why there are multiple hypotheses of the etiology and pathophysiology of myofascial pain, including the Central Modulation Hypothesis,[88,89] the Neurogenic Hypothesis,[90] the Neurophysiologic

Hypothesis,[91] the Radiculopathy Hypothesis,[40] the Neuritis Hypothesis,[63] the Mechanistic Hypothesis,[92] the Integrated Trigger Point Hypothesis,[53] and the Integrated Hypothesis (IH).[93] It is beyond the scope of this chapter to review all different perspectives other than the IH, which is the most accepted and best-supported model.[93]

Since its introduction in 1999, the IH has been developed further and expanded significantly.[94-96] The current thinking proposes that an excessive nonquantal release of acetylcholine from motor endplates depolarizes the post-junctional membrane, leading to sustained contractures known as *taut bands*. The increased release of acetylcholine is supported objectively by the presence of spontaneous electrical activity or endplate noise,[97] which has been confirmed in humans and animals.[98-100] The prevalence of endplate noise is directly correlated with the degree of irritability of a TrP.[101] Ballyns and colleagues[102] demonstrated that these bands commonly block major arteries, causing a retrograde blood flow, hypoxia, and ischemia.[103,104] The ischemia causes a significant drop in the pH with values well below 5,[105,106] which can fully activate nociceptive acid sensing ion channels, transient receptor potential vanilloid channels, and several other receptors, such as transient and short transient receptor potential cation channels.[107,108] Activation of acid-sensing ion channels initiates myalgia and causes mechanical hyperalgesia,[109,110] partially because of the release of multiple sensitizing substances, such as bradykinin, calcitonin gene-related peptide, substance P, tumor necrosis-factor peptide of multiple sensitizing substances, and su, which have been confirmed in the immediate milieu of active TrPs.[105,106] Glutamate has not yet been identified specifically in the close environment of TrPs, but it has been confirmed in myofascial pain conditions.[111] In mice, the onset of hypoxia led to an immediate increased acetylcholine release at the motor endplate.[112] TrPs are located in close proximity to dysfunctional motor endplates in well-defined innervation muscle zones.[113]

CHARACTERISTICS OF A TRIGGER POINT

A TrP is a hyperirritable spot in a taut band of a skeletal muscle that is painful on compression, stretch, and overload or contraction of the muscle, and usually features a distinct referred pain pattern.[53] Using magnetic resonance imaging elastography and ultrasound elastography, researchers were able to demonstrate that these taut bands feature increased stiffness, reduced vibration amplitude, higher peak systolic velocities, and negative diastolic velocities compared with normal muscle sites.[102,114,115] There is general agreement that any kind of muscle overuse or direct trauma to the muscle can lead to the development of TrPs, particularly with sustained or repetitive low-level muscle contractions, unaccustomed eccentric muscle contractions, and submaximal or maximal concentric muscle contractions.[96,116]

Clinically, TrPs are divided into active and latent TrPs. Both types of TrPs feature local and referred pain, but only active TrPs reproduce the symptoms experienced by patients as their usual or familiar pain. Clinicians can distinguish persons with active TrPs from those without by using a systematic musculoskeletal evaluation with distinct differences in physical findings and self-reports of pain, sleep disturbance, disability, health status, and mood.[117] Using sonography, TrPs can be visualized[118,119]; active TrPs are larger than latent TrPs, have greater referred pain areas,[102] and feature more endplate noise.[101] The local pain at TrPs is due to sensitization of muscle nociceptors and, to a lesser degree, to non-nociceptor activation.[120-122] It is known that muscle pain can impair descending inhibitory pathways, which is another aspect of central sensitization.[123] Referred pain, also known as *secondary hyperalgesia*, is a feature of central sensitization. Rubin et al[124,125] confirmed that the maintenance of referred pain depends on ongoing nociceptive input from the site of primary muscle pain. Although he did not consider TrPs, there is much evidence that TrPs function as peripheral sources of ongoing nociceptive input contributing to the propagation of central sensitization and widespread pain,[93,97,126] including fibromyalgia,[127-129] but also of whiplash-associated pain,[56,130] migraines,[74] tension-type headaches,[131] post-mastectomy surgery,[132] and temporomandibular disorders,[133] among others. Of great clinical interest is that the treatment of TrPs can reverse and eliminate referred pain.[134]

INTRODUCTION TO TRIGGER POINT-DRY NEEDLING

To practice TrP-DN requires training and excellent palpation skills. Clinicians need to develop a high degree of kinesthetic perception to visualize a 3-dimensional image of the pathway the needle takes within the patient's body based on excellent anatomical knowledge. TrPs are identified with manual palpation using either a flat or pincer palpation technique and can be palpated accurately in most muscles with only a few exceptions, such as the lateral pterygoid and iliacus muscles. In those cases, the needle can be used as a palpation tool.[59] TrP-DN is divided into superficial and deep DN based on the depth of needling.

Superficial Trigger Point-Dry Needling

With superficial TrP-DN, the needle is placed into the superficial tissues overlying a TrP without going deep enough to actually target the TrP directly.[135] Baldry recommends inserting an acupuncture needle into the tissues overlying a TrP at a depth of approximately 5 to 10 mm for 30 seconds. In case of any residual pain, the needle is inserted for another 2 to 3 minutes. The patient's response determines the intensity and duration of the stimulus.[9]

Deep Trigger Point-Dry Needling

With deep TrP-DN, the needle is placed into the TrP with the objective of eliciting a so-called LTR. Different authors have recommended variations of deep DN approaches, such as Hong's fast-in-fast-out technique,[7] or Chow's screw-in-screw-out technique.[136] Several electromyography and sonography studies have shown that eliciting LTRs significantly increases the effectiveness of TrP-DN.[7,137,138] An LTR is an involuntary spinal cord reflex contraction of muscle fibers within a taut band, which can be elicited by manually strumming or needling a taut band or TrP.[137,139,140] LTRs can be observed visually, recorded electromyographically, or visualized with sonography.[59] An LTR is correlated with an immediate decrease of the concentrations of many noxious chemicals found in the close environment of active TrPs,[59,105,106,141] which may explain why patients commonly experience a sudden decrease in their pain perception after DN. Other potential mechanisms of DN may include the release of endogenous opioids and the activation of the autonomous nervous system.[142,143]

IMPLEMENTATION OF TRIGGER POINT-DRY NEEDLING

TrP-DN must be dosed properly. Eliciting only one LTR is usually not therapeutic and can be quite aggravating. On the other hand, excessive DN in the same location may cause significant tissue damage, resulting in an inflammatory response with notable swelling and an increase in the concentration of many of the observed chemical substances.[141] In a mouse model, the needle punctures from DN healed completely within a week after treatment.[144] Rotating the needle during DN may increase its effectiveness by simultaneously stretching fibroblasts, which can trigger a cascade of cellular and molecular events, including cytoskeletal reorganization, cell contraction, a release of growth factors, the stimulation of intracellular signaling pathways, variations in gene expression and extracellular matrix composition, and, eventually, a reduction of pain.[145,146] Rotating the needle can be uncomfortable due to activation of A-δ fibers, but it may also trigger enkephalinergic, serotonergic, and noradrenergic inhibitory systems.[147] It is not recommended for all patients.

Some authors and clinicians have proposed to leave needles in place for 10 to 30 minutes,[1] which is based primarily on acupuncture practice and guidelines. There is no convincing evidence that leaving needles in place would result in better outcomes than TrP-DN with eliciting LTRs. There is also limited evidence that adding electrical currents to the filament needles would improve therapeutic outcomes significantly.[59,148] Furthermore, there is no consensus about the optimal parameters for electrical stimulation with needle electrodes.[59,148-151] For nociceptive pain, frequencies between 2 and 4 Hz with high intensity are commonly used, which may trigger the release of endorphins and enkephalins. For neuropathic pain, higher frequencies of 80 to 100 Hz are used to facilitate the release of dynorphin, gamma-aminobutyric acid, and galanin.[152]

There are different perspectives on the need for post-needling treatments. Travell and Simons[15] and Simons et al[53] advocated stretching the treated muscles following TrP injections, but they never used DN in their practices. Applying a vapocoolant spray following DN, known as the *spray and stretch technique*, only had a short-term (6-hour) effect on post-needling soreness and may be useful to comfort patients immediately following DN[153]; however, applying manual pressure over the TrP region did reduce its intensity and duration for 48 hours.[154] Many clinicians consider post-needling soreness as a negative experience that should be prevented or treated. They may recommend either hot or cold applications or perhaps over-the-counter analgesic medications.

An interesting research question is, however, whether post-needling soreness is, in fact, something that should be avoided. When athletes experience moderate post-exercise soreness, how many consider it to be a negative experience? Post-exercise soreness can range from tenderness to severe debilitating pain. Most instances of post-needling soreness are not experienced as debilitating pain, but as moderate discomfort lasting less than 72 hours. It would be interesting to explore whether soreness following DN would still be considered as a negative phenomenon if its occurrence would be presented as a positive sign rather than a negative experience that requires special care.

SAFETY OF TRIGGER POINT-DRY NEEDLING

Many studies, case reports, and reviews have shown that DN is a safe and effective technique in the hands of properly trained physical therapists and other health care providers. The most severe adverse events associated with DN include pneumothorax,[37] spinal cord injuries,[155,156] and cardiac tamponade, although the latter has only been described with TrP injections and not with TrP-DN.[157] A report from New Zealand showed that DN was associated with 18% of major adverse events of acupuncture vs 76% for sustained acupuncture.[158] An analysis of signs and symptoms revealed that 81% of adverse events were considered minor. As a side note, in New Zealand, DN by physiotherapists is considered part of the practice of physical therapy acupuncture.

A recent study of the risk of adverse events of DN by trained physical therapists showed that the risk of a significant adverse event was less than 0.04% compared with almost 14% for ibuprofen and 19% for aspirin.[36] In addition, the underwriting company for the physical therapy professional liability insurance endorsed by the APTA has not observed any increase in claims related to DN by licensed physical therapists.

EFFICACY EVIDENCE OF TRIGGER POINT-DRY NEEDLING

The efficacy of DN is well established.[159,160] A major issue with studies of invasive procedures, such as DN and acupuncture, is that it is difficult to include a true placebo group. It is questionable whether sham needling procedures, for example, by using a placebo needle or by applying superficial needling are appropriate control groups for studies examining the efficacy of deep DN.[161] Any needling is likely to have some physiological effect, such as a change in pain thresholds, an expectancy of a positive outcome, or a release of endorphins.[162-164]

At this point in time, there is only one truly double-blind controlled study in the scientific literature demonstrating the efficacy of TrP-DN.[33] Researchers in Spain examined the effect of TrP-DN on preventing post-surgical pain following a total knee arthroscopy. What makes this study unique is that the DN procedures were administered while the subjects were under general or partial anesthesia, which means that they were truly blinded to the procedure. Forty individuals were randomly assigned to a DN group or to a no-needling group. Approximately 4 to 5 hours before the surgery, all subjects were examined for the presence of TrPs in the hip adductors, the hamstrings and quadriceps, the tensor fasciae latae, the gastrocnemius, and the popliteal muscles. Immediately after the subjects were anesthetized, they received either TrP-DN to the previously identified TrPs or no treatment. Assessments were performed pre-surgically and at 1, 3, and 6 months post-surgery by an independent examiner. The examiner and subjects were blinded to the group allocation. The DN group experienced a level of pain reduction during the first month following the surgery, which the control group did not reach until 6 months.[33] This study is one of the most important DN outcome studies given the unique placebo design and dramatic outcome. TrP-DN clearly made a very significant difference for the subjects in the intervention group compared with the subjects in the control group.

Several TrP-DN studies include multiple variables, which makes it difficult to determine the contributions of DN to the final outcome. In an Italian study of 101 subjects with hemiparetic shoulder pain, DN was the only variable, making it an excellent example of the effects of TrP-DN in this patient population.[35] The subjects were randomly assigned to 1 of 2 groups. Both groups participated in the same comprehensive rehabilitation program, but only one group received TrP-DN to several shoulder muscles. The study showed that the addition of DN to the standard rehabilitation program reduced the severity and frequency of pain, reduced analgesic medication intake, and restored normal sleep patterns.[35] This is also an important study because TrP-DN was, indeed, the only variable. Unfortunately, the subjects were not blinded to the procedure, which could have influenced the outcome.

Even the awareness of potentially getting needled in a particular study can already influence its outcome.[164] Patients' expectations and beliefs about a positive outcome can activate the dorsolateral prefrontal cortex and the anterior cingulate cortex, irrespective of whether they received real needling, sham needling with a placebo needle, or just a skin prick.[164] In a recent study, Tekin and associates[165] found that DN significantly reduced pain and improved the quality of life; the authors used a superficial needling technique as the sham DN procedure. Although the authors considered their study to be a double-blinded, randomized trial, it is likely that they compared the effects of deep DN with superficial DN, although that was probably not their intent.

Cagnie and colleagues[29] demonstrated that DN improves the local circulation in the upper trapezius muscle even when TrPs are not being targeted. Another study involving 50 patients with subacute sciatica and associated TrPs in the gluteus minimus muscle showed that DN of these TrPs combined with a 5-minute/TrP application of infrared thermography caused significant vasodilation in the region of referred pain.[166,167] Considering that TrPs feature decreased perfusion and ischemia, these studies suggests that DN can indeed play a significant role in reversing ischemia and lowered pH, and as such reduce peripheral nociceptive input from TrPs. Multiple case reports illustrated that DN is effective in the treatment of acute neck pain,[21] thoracic spine pain,[22] and adhesive capsulitis,[168] while several other reports demonstrated the effectiveness of DN in athletes[23,24,169] and ballet dancers.[170]

Several meta-review articles have confirmed that DN is an effective modality, but controversy remains whether DN is as effective as TrP injections. Ong and Claydon[28] concluded that DN is cheaper and has fewer side effects than injection therapy or laser, but another meta-review showed that DN was equally as effective as standard care.[26] In an older review, Cummings and White[25] observed that DN was equally effective as TrP injections, but whether needling therapies were more efficacious than placebo was neither supported nor refuted by the evidence. Another study confirmed that the effect of TrP injections was similar to DN, but the effects of DN were longer lasting.[171]

TRIGGER POINT-DRY NEEDLING
FOR HEAD, NECK, AND SHOULDER PAIN

Several studies looked at the effectiveness of DN for head, neck, and shoulder pain. A Spanish study, for example, showed that even a single session of TrP-DN in the upper trapezius muscle decreased pain in the neck and improved pressure thresholds and cervical range of motion.[172] A similar study suggested that including a single session of TrP-DN in the first week of a multimodal physical therapy approach may facilitate faster increases in function in individuals with postoperative shoulder pain.[173] Calvo-Lobo and colleagues[174] examined the efficacy of a single session of DN of one active and one latent TrP in the infraspinatus muscle of elderly patients with nonspecific shoulder pain. The outcome measures included numerical pain rating scale, pressure pain threshold measurements over the anterior deltoid and extensor carpi radialis brevis muscles, and grip strength. The authors concluded that DN reduced the shoulder pain, but also the mechanosensitivity of the extensor muscle. The reduction in shoulder pain did not reach statistical significance, which the authors attributed to the small sample size of only 20 participants for the total study.[174]

A more extensive study confirmed that DN significantly improved pain scores, pressure thresholds, and outcome measures using the Disabilities of the Arm, Shoulder and Hand test.[175] DN of latent TrPs combined with stretching restored normal muscle activation patterns in the shoulder.[176,177] Liu and colleagues[160] performed a meta-analysis of the effectiveness of DN for neck and shoulder pain and concluded that, compared with a control group, DN was effective in the short term, but TrP injections were found to be superior to DN. This contradicts the findings of Couto and associates,[178] who showed that DN and TrP injections were more effective than a sham procedure, but DN was more effective in improving pain, the quality of sleep, and the overall well-being of the patient compared with TrP injections.

When comparing the effects of TrP-DN to TrP manual therapy, the 2 approaches resulted in similar outcomes for pain, disability, and cervical range of motion, but the DN group experienced greater improvements in pressure pain thresholds over the cervical spine.[179] Rayegani and colleagues[180] measured comparable outcomes for DN and other physical therapy modalities in patients with myofascial pain involving the upper trapezius muscles, whereas Sukumar and Mathias[181] found that DN was more effective than conventional physical therapy for the treatment of patients with adhesive capsulitis. Further, Kietrys et al[182,183] found that DN performed better than sham or placebo procedures for upper-quarter myofascial pain.

DN of the lateral pterygoid muscle showed better efficacy in reducing pain and improving maximum mouth opening, laterality, and protrusion movements than a combination of methocarbamol and paracetamol.[184] Although the lateral pterygoid cannot be palpated manually, TrPs in this muscle can be treated using a solid filament needle,[31,185]; however, it is unlikely that DN of this muscle can accurately target TrPs.

TRIGGER POINT-DRY NEEDLING
FOR LOW BACK AND LOWER-EXTREMITY PAIN

A few studies considered DN for the low back and lower-extremity disorders. According to a 2005 Cochrane review, DN can be a useful adjunct to other therapies for patients with chronic low back pain.[27] As already mentioned, a placebo-controlled, double blind study of the effectiveness of TrP-DN on the prevention of post-total-knee-arthroscopy pain demonstrated that subjects who were needled right before the surgery while they were under anesthesia demanded significantly less pain medication and reached comfortable levels of pain in approximately 1 month compared with 6 months for the subjects in the control groups.[33] DN provided a significant reduction in plantar heel pain in an Australian study by Cotchett and associates.[32] Another study demonstrated that the pain associated with hip and knee arthritis can be successfully treated by addressing TrPs in the muscles overlying these joints.[72] Spanish researchers concluded that TrP-DN in the fibularis muscle contributed significantly to better outcomes in pain and function in patients with chronic ankle instability.[186] Subjects in the experimental and control groups received the same proprioceptive and strengthening training. Subjects in the experimental group also received TrP-DN, making DN the only variable. The between-group effect sizes were large for all outcome measures in favor the DN group.[186]

TRIGGER POINT-DRY NEEDLING FOR SPASTICITY AND CHRONIC PAIN

DN can reduce spasticity in patients with cerebrovascular accident (CVA).[187] A study of 101 subjects with hemiparetic shoulder pain showed that DN reduced the severity and frequency of pain, reduced analgesic medication intake, and restored normal sleep patterns.[35] This study is of particular interest, as the only variable was the use of DN. A recent case report of a 53-year-old man with a 13-year history of spasticity related to a CVA showed that his spasticity scores improved and he had slightly improved shoulder and hand function following DN.[188] Further, a Spanish study of 120 patients diagnosed with fibromyalgia reported that subjects in a superficial DN group experienced significant improvements in pain, sleep, pressure pain thresholds, functional scores using the 36-item Short-Form Survey, and global subjective improvement. The authors did not look specifically for TrPs but needled over tender points.[189]

TENDINOPATHY

Tendinopathy, previously known as *tendinitis* or *tendinosis*,[190] is a painful condition of tendons commonly seen in sports and occupational injuries.[191-193] Common tendinopathies include Achilles tendinopathy,[194] supraspinatus tendinopathy,[195] biceps tendinopathy,[196] patellar tendinopathy or jumper's knee,[197] and lateral and medial epicondylopathy,[198] among others. Thirty percent of musculoskeletal ailments seen by general practitioners and at least 30% to 50% of sports injuries are attributed to tendinopathies.[199,200] Runners experience a 10-fold increase in Achilles tendinopathy compared to age-matched controls.[201]

The term *tendinitis* has been abandoned, as it does not reflect the nature of the condition accurately, since inflammation is not a characteristic of tendinopathy. The term *tendinosis* describes the condition more accurately with consideration for the histopathology, collagen degeneration and disorganization, and increased cellularity following tendon injury.[202,203] Nevertheless, the term *tendinopathy* is preferred, mostly because it does not make any assumptions about the etiology or pathology.[204] Several changes occur with the overuse of tendons, such as chondroid metaplasia of the tendon, an expression of nitric oxide and insulin-like growth factor, the release of matrix metalloproteinases, and even tendon cell apoptosis.[203] The pain of tendinopathies is associated with an increase in the number of mast cells, which release histamine and tryptase, and an activation of protease-activated receptors[205]; however, pro-inflammatory mediators, such as prostaglandins, cytokines, and neuropeptides, also play a significant role.[206]

Although tendinopathies are very common, there is little solid evidence for any of the therapeutic interventions currently used by physical therapists, chiropractors, and other health care providers, such as ultrasound,[207] eccentric loading,[208] friction massage,[209] manipulations and mobilizations,[204] fascial manipulation,[210] orthotics,[211] laser therapy,[204] or anti-inflammatories and glucocorticoid injections.[203] Eccentric strengthening and low-level laser therapy may be helpful, but larger multicenter studies are needed.[203,212]

ENTHESOPATHY

Enthesopathies are commonly observed with myofascial pain,[213] yet little is known about the underlying mechanisms within a myofascial context. An enthesis is the location of the insertion of a tendon, fascia, or ligament into bone.[214,215] A fibrocartilaginous enthesis attaches directly to bone due to an absence of periosteum, while a fibrous enthesis features dense fibrous connective tissue that connects the tendon to periosteum.[216] Similar to the differences between tendinopathy and tendinitis, an *enthesitis* is an inflammation of the enthesis, while an enthesopathy describes a much broader concept. An *enthesopathy* is commonly defined as a pathological change at an enthesis due to an inflammatory, metabolic, degenerative, or traumatic condition.[216] Enthesopathy-related pain is usually not due to an inflammatory process; however, the etiology and underlying pathology are not yet known. Enthesopathies can be part of systemic conditions or local processes, such as overuse or injury.[214] Many rheumatological conditions feature enthesopathies, including rheumatoid arthritis, diffuse idiopathic skeletal hyperostosis, and chondrocalcinosis. Enthesopathies associated with myofascial pain are likely due to local mechanical overload. In sports, the most common anatomical sites for enthesopathies include the rotator cuff, the Achilles tendon insertion, the lateral epicondyle of the humerus, the lower pole of the patella, and the plantar fascia of the heel.[216]

Entheses feature many A-δ fibers, and may, as such, become sources of nociceptive input, especially since entheses are prone to local mechanical overuse and resulting microtrauma.[216,217] The presence of sensory nerves also suggests that entheses may have a proprioceptive function.[216] Most tendons and ligaments have an oblique orientation relative to the bone, which can create direct connections to the bone prior to its true attachment and can impact stress dissipation. The tendon can also connect to other adjacent structures, including fibrocartilage, adipose tissue, bursae, and even sensory nerve endings, which collectively have been referred to as the "enthesis organ."[214,217,218]

A study of the prevalence of enthesopathies among children showed that 68 of 234 children had at least one painful enthesis.[219] Some studies of athletes suggest that up to 50% of their injuries involve tendons, their sheaths, and insertions.[216] Enthesopathies are quite common, but the optimal treatment approach is not known. Most currently used interventions are empirically based without sound scientific evidence.

DRY NEEDLING FOR TENDINOPATHY AND ENTHESOPATHY

The research on DN for tendinopathies is promising, but is still in its infancy.[220,221] Little is known, for example, about optimal dosage and preferred needling technique, indications and contraindications, whether some tendons are more susceptible to DN, and whether DN can be used as a stand-alone therapy or should be combined with the administration of blood products, such as autologous platelet-rich plasma, or other physical therapy interventions. Jayaseelan and colleagues[222] described 2 case reports using a multimodal approach consisting of eccentric training, TrP-DN, and core stabilization for the treatment of individuals with proximal hamstrings tendinopathy, but they did not include any actual tendon DN. Ultrasound-guided tendon needling for the treatment of tennis elbow was reported to be effective in breaking up calcifications when combined with prednisone injections,[223] but the report did not include a control group and did not assess whether the effects could have been the result of the injections. Another study of the effect of needling on calcifying supraspinatus tendinopathy demonstrated that puncturing calcified deposits was effective.[224] A Czech study showed that DN of calcareous rotator cuff tendinopathy was as effective as arthroscopic surgery and much less expensive.[225]

The question remains what the mechanisms are of tendinopathy DN. It appears that the needle can break up calcifications, which would suggest a mechanical mechanism. DN can increase the local blood flow, especially when the clinician uses a pecking or peppering technique causing multiple fenestrations, which can be advantageous as many tendons are poorly vascularized.[226] Stenhouse and colleagues[227] described directing the needle 40 to 50 times through the long axis of the tendon in a time span of only 2 minutes. In contrast, needling a tendon only 5 times was effective in the majority of subjects with epicondylalgia based on scores on a visual analog scale.[228] In addition to the increased circulation, there is some evidence that DN can facilitate an increase in the concentration of platelet-derived growth factor and transforming growth factor beta and activate local fibroblasts, which will promote tendon healing.[220]

Little, if anything, is known about DN for enthesopathies. There is anecdotal evidence that needling painful entheses of the posterior neck muscles may be beneficial for patients with migraine or tension-type headaches. To treat entheses, a solid filament needle is placed directly into the tight tendon-bone junction. Next, the needle is rotated to provide a mechanical stretch to the tissue, which likely will lengthen fibroblasts[229] and reduce their nociceptive input.[146]

CASE EXAMPLE

Ms. H.V. was a 36-year-old patient with a long-standing history of chronic tension-type headaches. She reported suffering from left-sided retroorbital headaches and vertex pain at least 3 to 5 times per week. She would resort to over-the-counter nonsteroidal anti-inflammatories, but they only provided temporary and incomplete relief. She rated the pain intensity as between 4 and 8 on a visual analog scale from 0 to 10. She worked as a systems analyst, which involved long hours of computer work. Ms. H.V. had bifocal glasses. The patient presented with moderate forward head posture and a loss of the normal cervical lordosis, limited cervical rotation to the left, and limited side-bending to the right. The C3-C5 spinal segments were hypomobile. The evaluation for the presence of myofascial TrPs revealed active TrPs in the left sternocleidomastoid, upper trapezius, temporalis, and splenius capitis muscles. The attachments of the posterior cervical muscles at the cranium were very tender with palpation. Ms. H.V.'s treatment plan included DN of TrPs initially of the sternocleidomastoid and upper trapezius muscles, DN of the entheses, spinal manipulation, and postural corrections.

During the first treatment session, DN of TrPs in the sternocleidomastoid and upper trapezius muscles triggered her familiar headache. The DN was combined with cervical manipulations of the hypomobile segments. The therapist reviewed postural correction exercises with her and requested photographs from the patient while at her workstation. When she returned to physical therapy 2 weeks later, she reported a reduction in the frequency of her headaches to twice/week and decreased pain levels of 3 to 4 on a visual analog scale. During her second treatment session, TrPs in the sternocleidomastoid, upper trapezius, and splenius capitis were treated with DN. This time, the entheses were also treated with rotation of the needles. The therapist reviewed the pictures of Ms. H.V. at her workstation, and recommended that she obtain computer glasses with a focal distance of 16 to 22 inches. It was clear that the bifocal glasses increased her forward head posture. The patient was treated for a total of 6 sessions combining TrP-DN, DN of the entheses, spinal manipulations, and posture corrections.

The treatment plan was based on the current available scientific evidence. TrPs in the sternocleidomastoid, trapezius, and temporalis muscles feature referred pain into the retroorbital region[53] and are frequently involved in tension-type headaches.[131,230,231] DN of TrPs is an effective treatment approach.[34] Spinal dysfunction is common in patients with tension-type headaches.[232] Manipulation of the C3 spinal segment can decrease the pressure pain threshold of TrPs in the trapezius muscle.[233] Forward head posture is also commonly seen in patients with tension-type headaches[55,231] and a gradual correction of forward head posture is instrumental in normalizing muscle activation patterns.[234]

CONCLUSION

This chapter discussed the current state of affairs of DN for a variety of clinical conditions. While there is much evidence to use DN in the treatment of TrPs, the evidence is still lacking for DN of tendinopathies and even more for enthesopathies. DN is usually part of a multimodal physical therapy approach. To learn DN, specific training is required since DN is an invasive procedure. The safety of DN by physical therapists has been established, contrary to inaccurate assumptions made by select groups of health care providers. DN is a valid evidence-informed treatment technique.

REFERENCES

1. Dunning J, Butts R, Mourad F, Young I, Flannagan S, Perreault T. Dry needling: a literature review with implications for clinical practice guidelines. *Phys Ther Rev.* 2014;19(4):252-265.
2. Lewit K. The needle effect in the relief of myofascial pain. *Pain.* 1979;6:83-90.
3. Wall R. Introduction to myofascial trigger points in dogs. *Topics in Companion Animal Medicine.* 2014;29(2):43-48.
4. Frank EM. Myofascial trigger point diagnostic criteria in the dog. *J Musculoskelet Pain.* 1999;7(1-2):231-237.
5. Churchill JM. A treatise on acupuncturation being a description of a surgical operation originally peculiar to the Japanese and Chinese, and by them denominated zin—king, now introduced into European practice, with directions for its performance and cases illustrating its success. London, United Kingdom: Simpkins & Marshall; 1821.
6. Paulett JD. Low back pain. *Lancet.* 1947;2:272-276.
7. Hong CZ. Lidocaine injection versus dry needling to myofascial trigger point. The importance of the local twitch response. *Am J Phys Med Rehabil.* 1994;73(4):256-263.
8. Legge D. A history of dry needling. *J Musculoskelet Pain.* 2014;23(3):301-307.
9. Baldry PE. *Acupuncture, Trigger Points and Musculoskeletal Pain.* Edinburgh, Scotland: Churchill Livingstone; 2005.
10. Stockman R. The causes, pathology, and treatment of chronic rheumatism. *Edinburgh Med J.* 1904;15:107-116.
11. Fleckenstein J, Zaps D, Rüger LJ, et al. Discrepancy between prevalence and perceived effectiveness of treatment methods in myofascial pain syndrome: results of a cross-sectional, nationwide survey. *BMC Musculoskelet Disord.* 2010;11(1):32.
12. Harden RN, Bruehl SP, Gass S, Niemiec C, Barbick B. Signs and symptoms of the myofascial pain syndrome: a national survey of pain management providers. *Clin J Pain.* 2000;16(1):64-72.
13. Shah JP, Thaker N, Heimur J, Aredo JV, Sikdar S, Gerber LH. Myofascial trigger points then and now: a historical and scientific perspective. *Phys Med Rehab.* 2015;7(7):746-761.
14. Lange M. *Die Muskelhärten (Myogelosen).* München, Germany: J.F. Lehmann's Verlag; 1931.
15. Travell JG, Simons DG. *Myofascial Pain and Dysfunction: The Trigger Point Manual.* Baltimore, MD: Williams & Wilkins; 1983.
16. Travell J. Basis for the multiple uses of local block of somatic trigger areas (procaine infiltration and ethyl chloride spray). *Miss Valley Med.* 1949;71:13-22.
17. Harman JB, Young RH. Muscle lesions simulating visceral disease. *Lancet.* 1940;235:1111-1113.
18. Brav EA, Sigmond H. The local and regional injection treatment of low back pain and sciatica. *Ann Intern Med.* 1941;15:840-852.
19. Steinbrocker O. Therapeutic injections in painful musculoskeletal disorders. *JAMA.* 1944;125:397-401.
20. Gunn CC, Milbrandt WE, Little AS, Mason KE. Dry needling of muscle motor points for chronic low-back pain: a randomized clinical trial with long-term follow-up. *Spine.* 1980;5(3):279-291.
21. Pavkovich R. The use of dry needling for a subject with acute onset of neck pain: a case report. *Int J Sports Phys Ther.* 2015;10(1):104-113.
22. Rock JM, Rainey CE. Treatment of nonspecific thoracic spine pain with trigger point dry needling and intramuscular electrical stimulation: a case series. *Int J Sports Phys Ther.* 2014;9(5):699-711.
23. Dembowski SC, Westrick RB, Zylstra E, Johnson MR. Treatment of hamstring strain in a collegiate pole-vaulter integrating dry needling with an eccentric training program: a resident's case report. *Int J Sports Phys Ther.* 2013;8(3):328-339.
24. Paantjens MA. Dry needling en adductorenmanipulatie voor de behandeling van een voetballer met adductorgerelateerde liespijn. *Ned Mil Genees Tijdschr.* 2013;66-61-68:64-70.
25. Cummings TM, White AR. Needling therapies in the management of myofascial trigger point pain: a systematic review. *Arch Phys Med Rehabil.* 2001;82(7):986-992.
26. Tough EA, White AR, Cummings TM, Richards SH, Campbell JL. Acupuncture and dry needling in the management of myofascial trigger point pain: a systematic review and meta-analysis of randomised controlled trials. *Eur J Pain.* 2009;13(1):3-10.

27. Furlan A, Tulder M, Cherkin D, et al. Acupuncture and dry-needling for low back pain: an updated systematic review within the framework of the Cochrane Collaboration. *Spine.* 2005;30(8):944-963.
28. Ong J, Claydon LS. The effect of dry needling for myofascial trigger points in the neck and shoulders: a systematic review and meta-analysis. *J Bodyw Mov Ther.* 2014;18(3):390-398.
29. Cagnie B, Barbe T, De Ridder E, Van Oosterwijck J, Cools A, Danneels L. The influence of dry needling of the trapezius muscle on muscle blood flow and oxygenation. *J Manipulative Physiol Ther.* 2012;35(9):685-691.
30. Bubnov RV. The use of trigger point "dry" needling under ultrasound guidance for the treatment of myofascial pain (technological innovation and literature review). *Lik Sprava.* 2010;(5-6):56-64.
31. Mesa-Jimenez JA, Sanchez-Gutierrez J, de-la-Hoz-Aizpurua JL, Fernández-de-las-Peñas C. Cadaveric validation of dry needle placement in the lateral pterygoid muscle. *J Manipulative Physiol Ther.* 2015;38(2):145-150.
32. Cotchett MP, Munteanu SE, Landorf KB. Effectiveness of trigger point dry needling for plantar heel pain: a randomized controlled trial. *Phys Ther.* 2014;94(8):1083-1094.
33. Mayoral O, Salvat I, Martin MT, et al. Efficacy of myofascial trigger point dry needling in the prevention of pain after total knee arthroplasty: a randomized, double-blinded, placebo-controlled trial. *Evid Based Complement Alternat Med.* 2013;2013:694941.
34. France S, Bown J, Nowosilskyj M, Mott M, Rand S, Walters J. Evidence for the use of dry needling and physiotherapy in the management of cervicogenic or tension-type headache: a systematic review. *Cephalalgia.* 2014;34(12):994-1003.
35. Dilorenzo L, Traballesi M, Morelli D, et al. Hemiparetic shoulder pain syndrome treated with deep dry needling during early rehabilitation: a prospective, open-label, randomized investigation. *J Musculoskelet Pain.* 2004;12(2):25-34.
36. Brady S, McEvoy J, Dommerholt J, Doody C. Adverse events following dry needling: a prospective survey of chartered physiotherapists. *J Manual Manipul Ther.* 2014;22(3):134-140.
37. Cummings M, Ross-Marrs R, Gerwin R. Pneumothorax complication of deep dry needling demonstration. *Acupunct Med.* 2014;32(6):517-519.
38. Dommerholt J. Dry needling—peripheral and central considerations. *J Manual Manipul Ther.* 2011;19(4):223-237.
39. Australian Physiotherapy Association. Australian Physiotherapy Association Position Statement: Scope of Practice. Camberwell, Victoria, Australia; 2009.
40. Gunn CC. *The Gunn Approach to the Treatment of Chronic Pain.* 2nd ed. New York, NY: Churchill Livingstone; 1997.
41. Physiotherapy Acupuncture Association of New Zealand (PAANZ). *Guidelines for Safe Acupuncture and Dry Needling Practice.* Wellington, New Zealand: PAANZ; 2014.
42. American Physical Therapy Association. *Guide to Physical Therapist Practice 3.0.* Alexandria, VA: American Physical Therapy Association; 2014.
43. Hobbs V. Dry needling and acupuncture emergin professional issues. In: *Qi Unity Report.* Sacramento, CA: American Association of Acupuncture and Oriental Medicine; 2007.
44. Janz S, Adams JH. Acupuncture by another name: dry needling in Australia. *Aust J Acupunct Chin Med.* 2011;6(2):3-11.
45. Cummings M. 'Forbidden points' in pregnancy: no plausible mechanism for risk. *Acupunct Med.* 2011;29:140-142.
46. Smith CA, Crowther CA, Collins CT, Coyle ME. Acupuncture to induce labor: a randomized controlled trial. *Obstet Gynecol.* 2008;112(5):1067-1074.
47. Tsuei JJ, Lai Y, Sharma SD. The influence of acupuncture stimulation during pregnancy: the induction and inhibition of labor. *Obstet Gynecol.* 1977;50(4):479-498.
48. Amaro JA. When acupuncture becomes "dry needling." *Acupunct Today.* 2007;8(11):33,43.
49. Matsumoto K, Birch S. *Hara Diagnosis: Regelctions on the Sea.* Brookline, MA: Paradigm Publications; 1988.
50. Birch S. Trigger point—acupuncture point correlations revisited. *J Altern Complement Med.* 2003;9(1):91-103.
51. Birch S. On the impossibility of trigger point-acupoint equivalence: a commentary on Peter Dorsher's analysis. *J Altern Complement Med.* 2008;14(4):343-345.
52. Melzack R, Stillwell DM, Fox EJ. Trigger points and acupuncture points for pain: correlations and implications. *Pain.* 1977;3(1):3-23.
53. Simons DG, Travell JG, Simons LS. *Travell and Simons' Myofascial Pain and Dysfunction: The Trigger Point Manual.* 2nd ed. Baltimore, MD: Williams & Wilkins; 1999.
54. Calandre EP, Hidalgo J, Garcia-Leiva JM, Rico-Villademoros F. Trigger point evaluation in migraine patients: an indication of peripheral sensitization linked to migraine predisposition? *Eur J Neurol.* 2006;13(3):244-249.
55. Fernández de las Peñas C, Cuadrado ML, Pareja JA. Myofascial trigger points, neck mobility, and forward head posture in episodic tension-type headache. *Headache.* 2007;47(5):662-672.
56. Freeman MD, Nystrom A, Centeno C. Chronic whiplash and central sensitization; an evaluation of the role of a myofascial trigger points in pain modulation. *J Brachial Plex Peripher Nerve Inj.* 2009;4:2.
57. Itoh K, Hirota S, Katsumi Y, Ochi H, Kitakoji H. Trigger point acupuncture for treatment of knee osteoarthritis—a preliminary RCT for a pragmatic trial. *Acupunct Med.* 2008;26(1):17-26.
58. Dorsher PT. Myofascial referred-pain data provide physiologic evidence of acupuncture meridians. *J Pain.* 2009;10(7):723-731.

59. Dommerholt J, Mayoral O, Gröbli C. Trigger point dry needling. *J Manual Manipulative Ther.* 2006;14(4):E70-E87.

60. Bradnam L. A proposed clinical reasoning model for western acupuncture. *NZ J Physiotherapy.* 2003;31(1):40-45.

61. White A, Cummings M, Filshie J. *An Introduction to Western Medical Acupuncture.* Edinburgh, Scotland: Churchill Livingstone; 2008.

62. Bohr T. Problems with myofascial pain syndrome and fibromyalgia syndrome. *Neurology.* 1996;46(3):593-597.

63. Quintner JL, Bove GM, Cohen ML. A critical evaluation of the trigger point phenomenon. *Rheumatology (Oxford).* 2015;54(3):392-399.

64. Dommerholt J, Gerwin RD. A critical evaluation of Quintner et al: missing the point. *J Bodyw Mov Ther.* 2015;19:193-204.

65. Meakins A. Soft tissue sore spots of an unknown origin. *Br J Sports Med.* 2015;49:348.

66. Lucas N, Macaskill P, Irwig L, Moran R, Bogduk N. Reliability of physical examination for diagnosis of myofascial trigger points: a systematic review of the literature. *Clin J Pain.* 2009;25(1):80-89.

67. Myburgh C, Larsen AH, Hartvigsen J. A systematic, critical review of manual palpation for identifying myofascial trigger points: evidence and clinical significance. *Arch Phys Med Rehabil.* 2008;89(6):1169-1176.

68. Bron C, Franssen J, Wensing M, Oostendorp RAB. Interrater reliability of palpation of myofascial trigger points in three shoulder muscles. *J Man Manipulative Ther.* 2007;15(4):203-215.

69. Gerwin RD, Shannon S, Hong CZ, Hubbard D, Gevirtz R. Interrater reliability in myofascial trigger point examination. *Pain.* 1997;69(1-2):65-73.

70. Al-Shenqiti AM, Oldham JA. Test-retest reliability of myofascial trigger point detection in patients with rotator cuff tendonitis. *Clin Rehabil.* 2005;19(5):482-487.

71. Barbero M, Bertoli P, Cescon C, Macmillan F, Coutts F, Gatti R. Intra-rater reliability of an experienced physiotherapist in locating myofascial trigger points in upper trapezius muscle. *J Manual Manipul Ther.* 2012;20(4):171-177.

72. Bajaj P, Bajaj P, Graven-Nielsen T, Arendt-Nielsen L. Trigger points in patients with lower limb osteoarthritis. *J Musculoskelet Pain.* 2001;9(3):17-33.

73. Fernández-Carnero J, Fernández de las Peñas CF, de la Llave-Rincón AI, Ge HY, Arendt-Nielsen L. Prevalence of and referred pain from myofascial trigger points in the forearm muscles in patients with lateral epicondylalgia. *Clin J Pain.* 2007;23(4):353-360.

74. Giamberardino MA, Tafuri E, Savini A, et al. Contribution of myofascial trigger points to migraine symptoms. *J Pain.* 2007;8(11):869-878.

75. Bron C, Dommerholt J, Stegenga B, Wensing M, Oostendorp RA. High prevalence of shoulder girdle muscles with myofascial trigger points in patients with shoulder pain. *BMC Musculoskelet Disord.* 2011;12(1):139.

76. Torres Lacomba M, Mayoral del Moral O, Coperias Zazo JL, Gerwin RD, Goni AZ. Incidence of myofascial pain syndrome in breast cancer surgery: a prospective study. *Clin J Pain.* 2010;26(4):320-325.

77. Fernandez-Lao C, Cantarero-Villanueva I, Fernández-de-las-Peñas C, Del-Moral-Avila R, Menjon-Beltran S, Arroyo-Morales M. Widespread mechanical pain hypersensitivity as a sign of central sensitization after breast cancer surgery: comparison between mastectomy and lumpectomy. *Pain Medicine.* 2011;12(1):72-78.

78. Weiss JM. Pelvic floor myofascial trigger points: manual therapy for interstitial cystitis and the urgency-frequency syndrome. *J Urol.* 2001;166(6):2226-2231.

79. Doggweiler-Wiygul R. Urologic myofascial pain syndromes. *Curr Pain Headache Rep.* 2004;8(6):445-451.

80. Jarrell J. Endometriosis and abdominal myofascial pain in adults and adolescents. *Curr Pain Headache Rep.* 2011;15(5):368-376.

81. Huang Q-M, Liu L. Wet needling of myofascial trigger points in abdominal muscles for treatment of primary dysmenorrhoea. *Acupunct Med.* 2014;32:346-349.

82. Zermann DH, Ishigooka M, Doggweiler R, Schmidt RA. Chronic prostatitis: a myofascial pain syndrome? *Infect Urol.* 1999;12(3):84-92.

83. Kao MJ, Han TI, Kuan TS, Hsieh YL, Su BH, Hong CZ. Myofascial trigger points in early life. *Arch Phys Med Rehabil.* 2007;88(2):251-254.

84. Vecchiet L. Muscle pain and aging. *J Musculoskelet Pain.* 2002;10(1/2):5-22.

85. Han TI, Hong CZ, Kuo FC, Hsieh YL, Chou LW, Kao MJ. Mechanical pain sensitivity of deep tissues in children—possible development of myofascial trigger points in children. *BMC Musculoskelet Disord.* 2012;13:13.

86. Chaitow L, Delany JW. *Clinical Application of Neuromuscular Techniques: The Upper Body.* Edinburgh, Scotland: Churchill Livingstone; 2008.

87. Dommerholt J, Bron C, Franssen JLM. Myofascial trigger points; an evidence-informed review. *J Manual Manipulative Ther.* 2006;14(4):203-221.

88. Hocking MJ. Exploring the central modulation hypothesis: do ancient memory mechanisms underlie the pathophysiology of trigger points? *Curr Pain Headache Rep.* 2013;17(7):347.

89. Hocking MJL. Trigger points and central modulation—a new hypothesis. *J Musculoskelet Pain.* 2010;18(2):186-203.

90. Srbely JZ. New trends in the treatment and management of myofascial pain syndrome. *Curr Pain Headache Rep.* 2010;14(5):346-352.

91. Partanen JV, Ojala TA, Arokoski JPA. Myofascial syndrome and pain: a neurophysiological approach. *Pathophysiology.* 2010;17(1):19-28.

92. Jafri MS. Mechanisms of Myofascial Pain. International scholarly research notices. 2014;14. doi:10.1155/2014/523924.

93. Fernández-de-Las-Peñas C, Dommerholt J. Myofascial trigger points: peripheral or central phenomenon? *Curr Rheumatol Rep.* 2014;16(1):395.

94. Simons DG. Review of enigmatic MTrPs as a common cause of enigmatic musculoskeletal pain and dysfunction. *J Electromyogr Kinesiol.* 2004;14:95-107.

95. McPartland JM, Simons DG. Myofascial trigger points: translating molecular theory into manual therapy. *J Man Manipulative Ther.* 2006;14(4):232-239.

96. Gerwin RD, Dommerholt J, Shah JP. An expansion of Simons' integrated hypothesis of trigger point formation. *Curr Pain Headache Rep.* 2004;8(6):468-475.

97. Ge HY, Fernández-de-Las-Peñas C, Yue SW. Myofascial trigger points: spontaneous electrical activity and its consequences for pain induction and propagation. *Chinese Medicine.* 2011;6:13.

98. Macgregor J, Graf von Schweinitz D. Needle electromyographic activity of myofascial trigger points and control sites in equine cleidobrachialis muscle—an observational study. *Acupunct Med.* 2006;24(2):61-70.

99. Hong C-Z, Yu J. Spontaneous electrical activity of rabbit trigger spot after transection of spinal cord and peripheral nerve. *J Musculoskelet Pain.* 1998;6(4):45-58.

100. Couppé C, Midttun A, Hilden J, Jørgensen U, Oxholm P, Fuglsang-Frederiksen A. Spontaneous needle electromyographic activity in myofascial trigger points in the infraspinatus muscle: a blinded assessment. *J Musculoskelet Pain.* 2001;9(3):7-17.

101. Kuan TS, Hsieh YL, Chen SM, Chen JT, Yen WC, Hong CZ. The myofascial trigger point region: correlation between the degree of irritability and the prevalence of endplate noise. *Am J Phys Med Rehabil.* 2007;86(3):183-189.

102. Ballyns JJ, Shah JP, Hammond J, Gebreab T, Gerber LH, Sikdar S. Objective sonographic measures for characterizing myofascial trigger points associated with cervical pain. *J Ultrasound Med.* 2011;30(10):1331-1340.

103. Brückle W, Sückfull M, Fleckenstein W, Weiss C, Müller W. Gewebe-pO2-Messung in der verspannten Rückenmuskulatur (m. erector spinae). *Z Rheumatol.* 1990;49:208-216.

104. Sikdar S, Ortiz R, Gebreab T, Gerber LH, Shah JP. Understanding the vascular environment of myofascial trigger points using ultrasonic imaging and computational modeling. *Conf Proc IEEE Eng Med Biol Soc.* 2010;2010:5302-5305.

105. Shah J, Phillips T, Danoff JV, Gerber LH. A novel microanalytical technique for assaying soft tissue demonstrates significant quantitative biomechanical differences in 3 clinically distinct groups: normal, latent and active. *Arch Phys Med Rehabil.* 2003;84:A4.

106. Shah JP, Danoff JV, Desai MJ, et al. Biochemicals associated with pain and inflammation are elevated in sites near to and remote from active myofascial trigger points. *Arch Phys Med Rehabil.* 2008;89(1):16-23.

107. Hagberg H. Intracellular pH during ischemia in skeletal muscle: relationship to membrane potential, extracellular pH, tissue lactic acid and ATP. *Pflugers Arch.* 1985;404(4):342-347.

108. Gerdle B, Ghafouri B, Ernberg M, Larsson B. Chronic musculoskeletal pain: review of mechanisms and biochemical biomarkers as assessed by the microdialysis technique. *J Pain Res.* 2014;7:313-326.

109. Sluka KA, Gregory NS. The dichotomized role for acid sensing ion channels in musculoskeletal pain and inflammation. *Neuropharmacology.* 2015;94:58-63.

110. Sluka KA, Radhakrishnan R, Benson CJ, et al. ASIC3 in muscle mediates mechanical, but not heat, hyperalgesia associated with muscle inflammation. *Pain.* 2007;129(1-2):102-112.

111. Castrillon EE, Ernberg M, Cairns BE, et al. Interstitial glutamate concentration is elevated in the masseter muscle of myofascial temporomandibular disorder patients. *J Orofac Pain.* 2010;24(4):350-360.

112. Bukharaeva EA, Salakhutdinov RI, Vyskocil F, Nikolsky EE. Spontaneous quantal and non-quantal release of acetylcholine at mouse endplate during onset of hypoxia. *Physiol Res.* 2005;54(2):251-255.

113. Barbero M, Cescon C, Tettamanti A, et al. Myofascial trigger points and innervation zone locations in upper trapezius muscles. *BMC Musculoskelet Disord.* 2013;14:179.

114. Chen Q, Basford J, An KN. Ability of magnetic resonance elastography to assess taut bands. *Clin Biomech (Bristol, Avon).* 2008;23(5):623-629.

115. Chen Q, Bensamoun S, Basford JR, Thompson JM, An KN. Identification and quantification of myofascial taut bands with magnetic resonance elastography. *Arch Phys Med Rehabil.* 2007;88(12):1658-1661.

116. Bron C, Dommerholt J. Etiology of myofascial trigger points. *Curr Pain Headache Rep.* 2012;16(5):439-444.

117. Gerber LH, Sikdar S, Armstrong K, et al. A systematic comparison between subjects with no pain and pain associated with active myofascial trigger points. *PM & R.* 2013;5(11):931-938.

118. Sikdar S, Shah JP, Gebreab T, et al. Novel applications of ultrasound technology to visualize and characterize myofascial trigger points and surrounding soft tissue. *Arch Phys Med Rehabil.* 2009;90(11):1829-1838.

119. Turo D, Otto P, Shah JP, et al. Ultrasonic characterization of the upper trapezius muscle in patients with chronic neck pain. *Ultrason Imaging.* 2013;35(2):173-187.

120. Ge HY, Serrao M, Andersen OK, Graven-Nielsen T, Arendt-Nielsen L. Increased H-reflex response induced by intramuscular electrical stimulation of latent myofascial trigger points. *Acupunct Med.* 2009;27(4):150-154.

121. Mense S. How do muscle lesions such as latent and active trigger points influence central nociceptive neurons? *J Musculokelet Pain.* 2010;18(4):348-353.

122. Wang Y-H, Ding X-L, Zhang Y, et al. Ischemic compression block attenuates mechanical hyperalgesia evoked from latent myofascial trigger points. *Exp Brain Res.* 2009;202(2):265-270.

123. Arendt-Nielsen L, Sluka KA, Nie HL. Experimental muscle pain impairs descending inhibition. *Pain.* 2008;140(3):465-471.

124. Rubin TK, Gandevia SC, Henderson LA, Macefield VG. Effects of intramuscular anesthesia on the expression of primary and referred pain induced by intramuscular injection of hypertonic saline. *J Pain.* 2009;10(8):829-835.

125. Rubin TK, Henderson LA, Macefield VG. Changes in the spatiotemporal expression of local and referred pain following repeated intramuscular injections of hypertonic saline: a longitudinal study. *J Pain.* 2010;11(8):737-745.

126. Arendt-Nielsen L, Castaldo M. MTPs are a peripheral source of nociception. *Pain Med.* 2015;16(4):625-627.

127. Staud R, Nagel S, Robinson ME, Price DD. Enhanced central pain processing of fibromyalgia patients is maintained by muscle afferent input: a randomized, double-blind, placebo-controlled study. *Pain.* 2009;145(1-2):96-104.

128. Affaitati G, Costantini R, Fabrizio A, Lapenna D, Tafuri E, Giamberardino MA. Effects of treatment of peripheral pain generators in fibromyalgia patients. *Eur J Pain.* 2011;15(1):61-69.

129. Ge HY, Nie H, Madeleine P, Danneskiold-Samsoe B, Graven-Nielsen T, Arendt-Nielsen L. Contribution of the local and referred pain from active myofascial trigger points in fibromyalgia syndrome. *Pain.* 2009;147(1-3):233-240.

130. Dommerholt J. Whiplash injury, muscle pain & motor dysfunction. In: Mense S, Gerwin RD, eds. *Muscle Pain—An Update: Mechanisms, Diagnosis and Treatment.* Heidelberg, Germany: Springer; 2010: 247-288.

131. Fernández-de-las-Peñas C, Ge HY, Alonso-Blanco C, González-Iglesias J, Arendt-Nielsen L. Referred pain areas of active myofascial trigger points in head, neck, and shoulder muscles, in chronic tension type headache. *J Bodyw Mov Ther.* 2010;14(4):391-396.

132. Fernandez-Lao C, Cantarero-Villanueva I, Fernández-de-Las-Peñas C, Del-Moral-Avila R, Arendt-Nielsen L, Arroyo-Morales M. Myofascial trigger points in neck and shoulder muscles and widespread pressure pain hypersensitivity in patients with postmastectomy pain: evidence of peripheral and central sensitization. *Clin J Pain.* 2010;26(9):798-806.

133. Fernandez-de-Las-Peñas C, Galan-Del-Rio F, Alonso-Blanco C, Jimenez-Garcia R, Arendt-Nielsen L, Svensson P. Referred pain from muscle trigger points in the masticatory and neck-shoulder musculature in women with temporomandibular disorders. *J Pain.* 2010;11(12):1295-1304.

134. Arendt-Nielsen L, Laursen RJ, Drewes AM. Referred pain as an indicator for neural plasticity. *Prog Brain Res.* 2000;129:343-356.

135. Baldry P. Superficial versus deep dry needling. *Acupunct Med.* 2002;20(2-3):78-81.

136. Chou L-W, Hong JY, Hong C-Z. A new technique for acupuncture therapy and its effectiveness in treating fibromyalgia syndrome: a case report. *J Musculoskelet Pain.* 2008;16(3):193-198.

137. Hong CZ, Torigoe Y, Yu J. The localized twitch responses in responsive bands of rabbit skeletal muscle are related to the reflexes at spinal cord level. *J Musculoskelet Pain.* 1995;3:15-33.

138. Rha DW, Shin JC, Kim YK, Jung JH, Kim YU, Lee SC. Detecting local twitch responses of myofascial trigger points in the lower-back muscles using ultrasonography. *Arch Phys Med Rehabil.* 2011;92(10):1576-1580.e1.

139. Hong CZ. Persistence of local twitch response with loss of conduction to and from the spinal cord. *Arch Phys Med Rehabil.* 1994;75(1):12-16.

140. Kuan TS, Hong CZ, Chen JT, Chen SM, Chien CH. The spinal cord connections of the myofascial trigger spots. *Eur J Pain.* 2007;11(6):624-634.

141. Hsieh Y-L, Yang S-A, Yang C-C, Chou L-W. Dry needling at myofascial trigger spots of rabbit skeletal muscles modulates the biochemicals associated with pain, inflammation, and hypoxia. *Evid Based Complement Alternat Med.* 2012;2012:342165.

142. Peng CH, Yang MM, Kok SH, Woo YK. Endorphin release: a possible mechanism of acupuncture analgesia. *Comp Med East West.* 1978;6(1):57-60.

143. Oke SL, Tracey KJ. The inflammatory reflex and the role of complementary and alternative medical therapies. *Ann N Y Acad Sci.* 2009;1172:172-180.

144. Domingo A, Mayoral O, Monterde S, Santafe MM. Neuromuscular damage and repair after dry needling in mice. *Evid Based Complement Alternat Med.* 2013;2013:260806.

145. Langevin HM, Bouffard NA, Badger GJ, Churchill DL, Howe AK. Subcutaneous tissue fibroblast cytoskeletal remodeling induced by acupuncture: evidence for a mechanotransduction-based mechanism. *J Cell Physiol.* 2006;207(3):767-774.

146. Chiquet M, Renedo AS, Huber F, Fluck M. How do fibroblasts translate mechanical signals into changes in extracellular matrix production? *Matrix Biol.* 2003;22(1):73-80.

147. Bowsher D. Mechanisms of acupuncture. In: Filshie J, White A, eds. *Western Acupuncture: A Western Scientific Approach.* Edinburgh, Scotland: Churchill Livingstone; 1998: 69-82.

148. Mayoral del Moral O. Fisioterapia invasiva del síndrome de dolor miofascial. *Fisioterapia.* 2005;27(2):69-75.

149. Lee SH, Chen CC, Lee CS, Lin TC, Chan RC. Effects of needle electrical intramuscular stimulation on shoulder and cervical myofascial pain syndrome and microcirculation. *J Chin Med Assoc.* 2008;71(4):200-206.

150. Lee SH, Lee BC. Electroacupuncture relieves pain in men with chronic prostatitis/chronic pelvic pain syndrome: three-arm randomized trial. *Urology.* 2009;73(5):1036-1041.

151. Lee SW, Liong ML, Yuen KH, et al. Acupuncture versus sham acupuncture for chronic prostatitis/chronic pelvic pain. *Am J Med.* 2008;121(1):79.e1-7.

152. Lundeberg T, Stener-Victorin E. Is there a physiological basis for the use of acupuncture in pain? *Int Congress Series*. 2002;1238:3-10.

153. Martin-Pintado Zugasti A, Rodriguez-Fernandez AL, Garcia-Muro F, et al. Effects of spray and stretch on post-needling soreness and sensitivity after dry needling of a latent myofascial trigger point. *Arch Phys Med Rehabil*. 2014;95(10):1925-1932.

154. Martin-Pintado-Zugasti A, Pecos-Martin D, Rodriguez-Fernandez AL, et al. Ischemic compression after dry needling of a latent myofascial trigger point reduces postneedling soreness intensity and duration. *PM & R*. 2015;7(10):1026-1034.

155. Lee JH, Lee H, Jo DJ. An acute cervical epidural hematoma as a complication of dry needling. *Spine (Phila Pa 1976)*. 2011;36(13):E891-E893.

156. Ji GY, Oh CH, Choi WS, Lee JB. Three cases of hemiplegia after cervical paraspinal muscle needling. *Spine J*. 2015;15(3):e9-e13.

157. Jung JW, Kim SR, Jeon SY, Bang SR, Kim YH, Lee SE. Cardiac tamponade following ultrasonography-guided trigger point injection. *J Musculoskelet Pain*. 2014;22(4):389-391.

158. McDowell JM, Johnson GM. Acupuncture needling styles and reports of associated adverse reactions to acupuncture. *Medical Acupuncture*. 2014;26:271-278.

159. Gerber LH, Shah J, Rosenberger W, et al. Dry needling alters trigger points in the upper trapezius muscle and reduces pain in subjects with chronic myofascial pain. *PM & R*. 2015;7(7):11-18.

160. Liu L, Huang QM, Liu QG, et al. Effectiveness of dry needling for myofascial trigger points associated with neck and shoulder pain: a systematic review and meta-analysis. *Arch Phys Med Rehabil*. 2015;96(5):944-955.

161. White P, Lewith G, Hopwood V, Prescott P. The placebo needle, is it a valid and convincing placebo for use in acupuncture trials? A randomised, single-blind, cross-over pilot trial. *Pain*. 2003;106(3):401-409.

162. Birch S. A review and analysis of placebo treatments, placebo effects, and placebo controls in trials of medical procedures when sham is not inert. *J Altern Complement Med*. 2006;12(3):303-310.

163. Lund I, Naslund J, Lundeberg T. Minimal acupuncture is not a valid placebo control in randomised controlled trials of acupuncture: a physiologist's perspective. *Chinese Medicine*. 2009;4:1.

164. Pariente J, White P, Frackowiak RS, Lewith G. Expectancy and belief modulate the neuronal substrates of pain treated by acupuncture. *Neuroimage*. 2005;25(4):1161-1167.

165. Tekin L, Akarsu S, Durmus O, Cakar E, Dincer U, Kiralp MZ. The effect of dry needling in the treatment of myofascial pain syndrome: a randomized double-blinded placebo-controlled trial. *Clin Rheumatol*. 2013;32(3):309-315.

166. Skorupska E, Rychlik M, Pawelec W, Samborski W. Dry needling related short-term vasodilation in chronic sciatica under infrared thermovision. *Evid Based Complement Alternat Med*. 2015;2015:214374.

167. Skorupska E, Rychlik M, Samborski W. Intensive vasodilatation in the sciatic pain area after dry needling. *BMC Complement Altern Med*. 2015;15(1):72.

168. Clewley D, Flynn TW, Koppenhaver S. Trigger point dry needling as an adjunct treatment for a patient with adhesive capsulitis of the shoulder. *J Orthop Sports Phys Ther*. 2014;44(2):92-101.

169. Osborne NJ, Gatt IT. Management of shoulder injuries using dry needling in elite volleyball players. *Acupuncture in Medicine*. 2010;28(1):42-45.

170. Mason JS, Tansey KA, Westrick RB. Treatment of subacute posterior knee pain in an adolescent ballet dancer utilizing trigger point dry needling: a case report. *Int J Sports Phys Ther*. 2014;9(1):116-124.

171. Ga H, Koh HJ, Choi JH, Kim CH. Intramuscular and nerve root stimulation vs lidocaine injection to trigger points in myofascial pain syndrome. *J Rehabil Med*. 2007;39(5):374-378.

172. Mejuto-Vazquez MJ, Salom-Moreno J, Ortega-Santiago R, Truyols-Dominguez S, Fernández-de-Las-Peñas C. Short-term changes in neck pain, widespread pressure pain sensitivity, and cervical range of motion after the application of trigger point dry needling in patients with acute mechanical neck pain: a randomized clinical trial. *J Orthop Sports Phys Ther*. 2014;44(4):252-260.

173. Arias-Buria JL, Valero-Alcaide R, Cleland JA, et al. Inclusion of trigger point dry needling in a multimodal physical therapy program for postoperative shoulder pain: a randomized clinical trial. *J Manipulative Physiol Ther*. 2015;38(3):179-187.

174. Calvo-Lobo C, Pacheco-da-Costa S, Hita-Herranz E. Efficacy of deep dry needling on latent myofascial trigger points in older adults with nonspecific shoulder pain: a randomized, controlled clinical trial pilot study. *J Geriatr Phys Ther*. 2015;epub ahead of print.

175. Ziaeifar M, Arab AM, Karimi N, Nourbakhsh MR. The effect of dry needling on pain, pressure pain threshold and disability in patients with a myofascial trigger point in the upper trapezius muscle. *J Bodyw Mov Ther*. 2014;18(2):298-305.

176. Lucas KR, Polus BI, Rich PS. Latent myofascial trigger points: their effects on muscle activation and movement efficiency. *J Bodyw Mov Ther*. 2004;8:160-166.

177. Lucas KR, Rich PA, Polus BI. Muscle activation patterns in the scapular positioning muscles during loaded scapular plane elevation: the effects of latent myofascial trigger points. *Clin Biomechanics*. 2010;25(8):765-770.

178. Couto C, de Souza IC, Torres IL, Fregni F, Caumo W. Paraspinal stimulation combined with trigger point needling and needle rotation for the treatment of myofascial pain: a randomized sham-controlled clinical trial. *Clin J Pain*. 2014;30(3):214-223.

179. Llamas-Ramos R, Pecos-Martin D, Gallego-Izquierdo T, et al. Comparison of the short-term outcomes between trigger point dry needling and trigger point manual therapy for the management of chronic mechanical neck pain: a randomized clinical trial. *J Orthop Sports Phys Ther.* 2014;44(11):852-861.

180. Rayegani SM, Bayat M, Bahrami MH, Raeissadat SA, Kargozar E. Comparison of dry needling and physiotherapy in treatment of myofascial pain syndrome. *Clin Rheumatol.* 2014;33(6):859-864.

181. Sukumar S, Mathias L. Effects of intramuscular manual therapy on improving shoulder abduction in adhesive capsulitis—a single blinded RCT. *Global J Multidisciplinary Studies.* 2014;3(12):41-50.

182. Kietrys DM, Palombaro KM, Azzaretto E, et al. Effectiveness of dry needling for upper-quarter myofascial pain: a systematic review and meta-analysis. *J Orthop Sports Phys Ther.* 2013;43(9):620-634.

183. Kietrys DM, Palombaro KM, Mannheimer JS. Dry needling for management of pain in the upper quarter and craniofacial region. *Curr Pain Headache Rep.* 2014;18(8):437.

184. Gonzalez-Perez LM, Infante-Cossio P, Granados-Nunez M, Urresti-Lopez FJ, Lopez-Martos R, Ruiz-Canela-Mendez P. Deep dry needling of trigger points located in the lateral pterygoid muscle: efficacy and safety of treatment for management of myofascial pain and temporomandibular dysfunction. *Medicina oral, patologia oral y cirugia bucal.* 2015;20(3):e326-e333.

185. Gonzalez-Perez LM, Infante-Cossio P, Granados-Nunez M, Urresti-Lopez FJ. Treatment of temporomandibular myofascial pain with deep dry needling. *Medicina oral, patologia oral y cirugia bucal.* 2012;17(5):e781-e785.

186. Salom-Moreno J, Ayuso-Casado B, Tamaral-Costa B, Sánchez-Milá Z, Fernández-de-las-Peñas C, Alburquerque-Sendi F. Trigger point dry needling and proprioceptive exercises for the management of chronic ankle instability: a randomized clinical trial. *Evid Based Complement Alternat Med.* 2015;2015. doi: 10.1155/2015/790209.

187. Salom-Moreno J, Sanchez-Mila Z, Ortega-Santiago R, Palacios-Cena M, Truyol-Dominguez S, Fernández-de-las-Peñas C. Changes in spasticity, widespread pressure pain sensitivity, and baropodometry after the application of dry needling in patients who have had a stroke: a randomized controlled trial. *J Manipulative Physiol Ther.* 2014;37(8):569-579.

188. Ansari NN, Naghdi S, Fakhari Z, Radinmehr H, Hasson S. Dry needling for the treatment of poststroke muscle spasticity: a prospective case report. *Neuro Rehabilitation.* 2015;36(1):61-65.

189. Casanueva B, Rivas P, Rodero B, Quintial C, Llorca J, Gonzalez-Gay MA. Short-term improvement following dry needle stimulation of tender points in fibromyalgia. *Rheumatol Int.* 2014;34(6):861-866.

190. Fredberg U. Tendinopathy—tendinitis or tendinosis? The question is still open. *Scand J Med Sci Sports.* 2004;14(4):270-272.

191. Scott A, Docking S, Vicenzino B, et al. Sports and exercise-related tendinopathies: a review of selected topical issues by participants of the second International Scientific Tendinopathy Symposium (ISTS) Vancouver 2012. *Br J Sports Med.* 2013;47(9):536-544.

192. Biundo JJ Jr, Irwin RW, Umpierre E. Sports and other soft tissue injuries, tendinitis, bursitis, and occupation-related syndromes. *Curr Opin Rheumatol.* 2001;13(2):146-149.

193. Reinking M. Tendinopathy in athletes. *Phys Ther Sport.* 2012;13(1):3-10.

194. Jarvinen TA, Kannus P, Maffulli N, Khan KM. Achilles tendon disorders: etiology and epidemiology. *Foot Ankle Clin.* 2005;10(2):255-266.

195. Redondo-Alonso L, Chamorro-Moriana G, Jimenez-Rejano JJ, Lopez-Tarrida P, Ridao-Fernandez C. Relationship between chronic pathologies of the supraspinatus tendon and the long head of the biceps tendon: systematic review. *BMC Musculoskelet Disord.* 2014;15:377.

196. Mellano CR, Shin JJ, Yanke AB, Verma NN. Disorders of the long head of the biceps tendon. *Instr Course Lect.* 2015;64:567-576.

197. Christian RA, Rossy WH, Sherman OH. Patellar tendinopathy—recent developments toward treatment. *Bull Hosp Jt Dis (2013).* 2014;72(3):217-224.

198. Long L, Briscoe S, Cooper C, Hyde C, Crathorne L. What is the clinical effectiveness and cost-effectiveness of conservative interventions for tendinopathy? An overview of systematic reviews of clinical effectiveness and systematic review of economic evaluations. *Health Technol Assess.* 2015;19(8):1-134.

199. Jarvinen M. Epidemiology of tendon injuries in sports. *Clin Sports Med.* 1992;11(3):493-504.

200. Kaux JF, Forthomme B, Goff CL, Crielaard JM, Croisier JL. Current opinions on tendinopathy. *J Sports Sci Med.* 2011;10(2):238-253.

201. Sorosky B, Press J, Plastaras C, Rittenberg J. The practical management of Achilles tendinopathy. *Clin J Sport Med.* 2004;14(1):40-44.

202. Morrey ME, Dean BJF, Carr AJ, Morrey BF. Tendinopathy: same disease different results—why? *Oper Tech Orthop.* 2013;23:39-49.

203. Andres BM, Murrell GA. Treatment of tendinopathy: what works, what does not, and what is on the horizon. *Clin Orthop Relat Res.* 2008;466(7):1539-1554.

204. Pfefer MT, Cooper SR, Uhl NL. Chiropractic management of tendinopathy: a literature synthesis. *J Manipulative Physiol Ther.* 2009;32(1):41-52.

205. Christensen J, Alfredson H, Andersson G. Protease-activated receptors in the Achilles tendon—a potential explanation for the excessive pain signalling in tendinopathy. *Molecular Pain.* 2015;11(1):13.

206. Fredberg U, Stengaard-Pedersen K. Chronic tendinopathy tissue pathology, pain mechanisms, and etiology with a special focus on inflammation. *Scand J Med Sci Sports.* 2008;18(1):3-15.
207. Desmeules F, Boudreault J, Roy JS, Dionne C, Fremont P, MacDermid JC. The efficacy of therapeutic ultrasound for rotator cuff tendinopathy: a systematic review and meta-analysis. *Phys Ther Sport.* 2014;16(3):276-284.
208. Camargo PR, Alburquerque-Sendin F, Salvini TF. Eccentric training as a new approach for rotator cuff tendinopathy: review and perspectives. *World J Orthop.* 2014;5(5):634-644.
209. Joseph MF, Taft K, Moskwa M, Denegar CR. Deep friction massage to treat tendinopathy: a systematic review of a classic treatment in the face of a new paradigm of understanding. *J Sport Rehabil.* 2012;21(4):343-353.
210. Pedrelli A, Stecco C, Day JA. Treating patellar tendinopathy with fascial manipulation. *J Bodyw Mov Ther.* 2009;13(1):73-80.
211. Simpson MR, Howard TM. Tendinopathies of the foot and ankle. *Am Fam Physician.* 2009;80(10):1107-1114.
212. Haslerud S, Magnussen LH, Joensen J, Lopes-Martins RA, Bjordal JM. The efficacy of low-level laser therapy for shoulder tendinopathy: a systematic review and meta-analysis of randomized controlled trials. *Physiother Res Int.* 2014;20(2):108-125.
213. Bismil Q, Bismil M. Myofascial-entheseal dysfunction in chronic whiplash injury: an observational study. *JRSM Short Reports.* 2012;3(8):57.
214. Slobodin G, Rozenbaum M, Boulman N, Rosner I. Varied presentations of enthesopathy. *Semin Arthritis Rheum.* 2007;37(2):119-126.
215. Freemont AJ. Enthesopathies. *Curr Diagnostic Pathol.* 2002;8:1-10.
216. Benjamin M, Toumi H, Ralphs JR, Bydder G, Best TM, Milz S. Where tendons and ligaments meet bone: attachment sites ('entheses') in relation to exercise and/or mechanical load. *J Anat.* 2006;208(4):471-490.
217. Benjamin M, McGonagle D. The anatomical basis for disease localisation in seronegative spondyloarthropathy at entheses and related sites. *J Anat.* 2001;199(Pt 5):503-526.
218. Benjamin M, Ralphs JR. Entheses—the bony attachments of tendons and ligaments. *Ital J Anat Embryol.* 2001;106(2 Suppl 1):151-157.
219. Sherry DD, Sapp LR. Enthesalgia in childhood: site-specific tenderness in healthy subjects and in patients with seronegative enthesopathic arthropathy. *J Rheumatol.* 2003;30(6):1335-1340.
220. Nagraba L, Tuchalska J, Mitek T, Stolarczyk A, Deszczynski J. Dry needling as a method of tendinopathy treatment. *Ortop Traumatol Rehabil.* 2013;15(2):109-116.
221. Krey D, Borchers J, McCamey K. Tendon needling for treatment of tendinopathy: a systematic review. *Phys Sportsmed.* 2015;43(1):80-86.
222. Jayaseelan DJ, Moats N, Ricardo CR. Rehabilitation of proximal hamstring tendinopathy utilizing eccentric training, lumbopelvic stabilization, and trigger point dry needling: 2 case reports. *J Orthop Sports Phys Ther.* 2014;44(3):198-205.
223. Zhu J, Hu B, Xing C, Li J. Ultrasound-guided, minimally invasive, percutaneous needle puncture treatment for tennis elbow. *Adv Ther.* 2008;25(10):1031-1036.
224. Zhu J, Jiang Y, Hu Y, Xing C, Hu B. Evaluating the long-term effect of ultrasound-guided needle puncture without aspiration on calcifying supraspinatus tendinitis. *Adv Ther.* 2008;25(11):1229-1234.
225. Lubojacky J. [Calcareous tendinitis of the shoulder. Treatment by needling]. *Acta Chir Orthop Traumatol Cech.* 2009;76(3):225-231.
226. Kubo K, Yajima H, Takayama M, Ikebukuro T, Mizoguchi H, Takakura N. Effects of acupuncture and heating on blood volume and oxygen saturation of human Achilles tendon in vivo. *Eur J Appl Physiol.* 2010;109(3):545-550.
227. Stenhouse G, Sookur P, Watson M. Do blood growth factors offer additional benefit in refractory lateral epicondylitis? A prospective, randomized pilot trial of dry needling as a stand-alone procedure versus dry needling and autologous conditioned plasma. *Skeletal Radiol.* 2013;42(11):1515-1520.
228. Mishra AK, Skrepnik NV, Edwards SG, et al. Efficacy of platelet-rich plasma for chronic tennis elbow: a double-blind, prospective, multicenter, randomized controlled trial of 230 patients. *Am J Sports Med.* 2014;42(2):463-471.
229. Langevin HM, Bouffard NA, Badger GJ, Iatridis JC, Howe AK. Dynamic fibroblast cytoskeletal response to subcutaneous tissue stretch ex vivo and in vivo. *Am J Physiol Cell Physiol.* 2005;288(3):C747-C756.
230. Alonso-Blanco C, de-la-Llave-Rincon AI, Fernández-de-las-Peñas C. Muscle trigger point therapy in tension-type headache. *Expert Rev Neurother.* 2012;12(3):315-322.
231. Fricton JR, Kroening R, Haley D, Siegert R. Myofascial pain syndrome of the head and neck: a review of clinical characteristics of 164 patients. *Oral Surg Oral Med Oral Pathol.* 1985;60(6):615-623.
232. Graff-Radford SB, Newman AC. The role of temporomandibular disorders and cervical dysfunction in tension-type headache. *Curr Pain Headache Rep.* 2002;6(5):387-391.
233. Ruiz-Saez M, Fernández-de-las-Peñas C, Blanco CR, Martinez-Segura R, Garcia-Leon R. Changes in pressure pain sensitivity in latent myofascial trigger points in the upper trapezius muscle after a cervical spine manipulation in pain-free subjects. *J Manipulative Physiol Ther.* 2007;30(8):578-583.
234. McLean L. The effect of postural correction on muscle activation amplitudes recorded from the cervicobrachial region. *J Electromyogr Kinesiol.* 2005;15(6):527-535.

20

Therapeutic Touch

Ellen Zambo Anderson, PT, PhD, GCS

Therapeutic touch (TT) is a complementary therapy used to promote health and healing. A modern interpretation of the "laying of hands" but without a religious context, TT is offered as an intervention for reducing pain and anxiety, accelerating the healing process, and promoting a sense of well-being.[1] TT was developed in the 1970s by Dolores Krieger, RN, PhD, and Dora Kunz, and follows a protocol of assessment and intervention that is different from similar-sounding approaches, such as *Healing Touch*, *Touch for Health*, or *therapeutic massage*. The name *therapeutic touch* is, nevertheless, misleading because the practitioner does not always need to touch the client or patient to provide a therapeutic intervention. TT is considered by many to be a nursing intervention and is taught in many nursing school curricula across the country. Krieger, herself a nurse, and Kunz, however, believe that any person who wants to facilitate health and healing can become a TT practitioner.[2] Specific medical or psychological training is not required to become a TT practitioner.

HISTORY

The work of Krieger and Kunz began in the 1960s when Krieger was studying at the New York University (NYU) College of Nursing. Krieger, who has since been named Professor Emeritus at NYU, and Kunz, a psychic healer, set out to investigate the phenomenon and the characteristics of people known as *healers*. Their observations of healers and research into ancient medical systems led them to the conclusion that healers are not "chosen" by a higher entity. Rather, healers merely possess a heightened sensitivity to their patient's state of health and being and are able to effect change through intention and energy. Krieger's belief that others are capable of developing this heightened sensitivity motivated her to develop a process in which a patient's status could be assessed and enhanced through intention and modulation of energy. Krieger points out, however, that TT does not "cure" diseases or other medical conditions. Rather, TT facilitates an improvement in energy flow, thereby creating an environment in which the body's own healing powers can be maximized.

THERAPEUTIC TOUCH AND ENERGY FIELDS

The concept of internal and external subtle energies and their relationship to health has been promoted in many ancient medical systems, such as Ayurveda and traditional Chinese medicine.[3,4] Contemporary scientists and philosophers have also suggested theoretical frameworks pertaining

Davis CM.
*Integrative Therapies in Rehabilitation: Evidence for Efficacy in Therapy,
Prevention, and Wellness, Fourth Edition*(pp 325-335).
© 2017 Taylor & Francis Group.

to the existence and interaction of biological, environmental, and spiritual energy. Weber[5,6] has integrated ideas from ancient Eastern philosophies of energy with concepts of quantum physics and the work of theoretical physicist David Bohm.[7,8] He suggests that the universe is a unitary flow of energy and that all matter and life are inextricably linked. Similarly, Rogers[9,10] has proposed that humans are multidimensional energy fields indivisible from energy fields of the environment and all matter. Furthermore, Rogers suggests that energy fields are distinguishable by their patterns and that energy fields are infinite, open, and in continuous motion. Defined according to Rogers' framework, TT is a plausible intervention in which the practitioner is able to detect the energy fields and patterns of a client and modulate, if necessary, the energy fields with the intention of promoting health and wellness.

THERAPEUTIC TOUCH AND CHAKRAS

Writings by Krieger[1,2,11] reflect a close alignment with the assumptions and teachings of *Ayurveda*, a medical system that has been practiced in India for more than 5000 years.[3] Ayurveda assumes that all life is based on vital life energy known as *prana* and that mind, body, spirit, and environment are inextricably linked. Disease is the end result of energetic imbalance among these domains and disharmony with the environment. Ayurveda holds that vital energy is centered in 7 major and several lesser chakras located throughout the body. The 7 major *chakras*, which means "wheels" in Sanskrit, are described as "whirling vortices of energy."[12] They are located within the body's core and are aligned vertically from the base of the coccyx to the crown. Each chakra is associated with a major endocrine gland and nerve plexus and is responsible for receiving, transforming, and releasing vital life energy. Lesser chakras are located in the palms and feet, in addition to other areas. Krieger proposes that TT practitioners utilize the hand chakras to perceive and modulate the energy of their clients.

FOUNDATIONAL PREMISES OF THERAPEUTIC TOUCH

Krieger offers 4 premises that underpin TT's process and approach to healing.[2] The first assumption is that the body is an open energy system that allows for the transfer of energy between people and the environment. The second assumption is that the body is bilaterally symmetrical, inferring that there is a pattern to the underlying human energy field. The third and fourth are that illness is the result of energy imbalance and the body can often initiate self-healing.[2]

PRACTICE OF THERAPEUTIC TOUCH

A TT session is always individualized and typically runs approximately 20 to 30 minutes. TT is not contraindicated for any specific conditions, yet practitioners are encouraged to limit the time of their intervention for persons who are elderly, young, or very weak. It is usually performed with the client fully dressed and sitting in a chair or standing; however, TT can be applied with client lying down. A TT practitioner begins the process by centering his or her consciousness.[1] *Centering* is the process of bringing the mind into a quiet, focused state of consciousness. During centering, breath, imagery, meditation, and/or visualizations can be used to establish an inner-sense equilibrium and stillness.[2] From this state of centeredness, the practitioner is able to initiate an assessment of the client's subtle energy fields. In the *assessment* phase of TT, the practitioner places his or her palms 2 to 3 inches from the client's head, using the spine as a reference for bilateral symmetry. The practitioner then moves his or her hands down the client's body, carefully noting characteristics of the client's energy field and acknowledging the energy flow that is perceived. During this assessment phase, the TT practitioner will make note of how the client's energy feels and will begin to determine which centers or areas can benefit from intervention. A practitioner, for example, may describe a client's energy as feeling tingly, vibratory, or cold, or the practitioner may perceive a client's energy flow to be sluggish or blocked in a certain area and will make a mental note to return to that area with the intention of improving that energy flow.

Krieger[2] describes the next step in the TT process to be "unruffling the field," which she explains as a sweeping away of bound up or congested energy. This activity can also be used to reestablish rhythm in the client's energy field and set the stage for the practitioner to begin directing and modulating the transfer and flow of human energy. During the balancing stage of the TT intervention, the practitioner can direct his or her own energy to the client and/or direct the client's own energy. Directing and modulating is performed with the intention of balancing the flow and amount of energy so that the client's energy field is perceived to be symmetrical. Lastly, TT practitioners assess the client's energy field to determine when the intervention is complete. Krieger suggests that improving energy flow and balance is critical in creating an environment in which healing can occur.[2]

TRAINING IN THERAPEUTIC TOUCH

The Therapeutic Touch International Association (TTIA) was established as Nurse Healers-Professional Associates International, Inc (NH-PAI) in 1979 under the leadership of Krieger and Kunz.[13] NH-PAI is the body that sets the standards and offers credentials to practitioners and teachers of TT, while TTIA is the membership arm of the organization.

To apply TT in a health care or private practice setting, practitioners should have completed a 12 contact-hour basic level workshop, taught by a qualified therapeutic touch teacher (QTTT) and have made a commitment of at least 1 year of mentoring with a QTTT. An intermediate class can be taken approximately 6 months later, after which the TT practitioner can practice without a mentor. Those wanting to be recognized by the TTIA as being a qualified TT practitioner must adhere to the TTIA Code of Ethics, demonstrate compassion or the desire to help another person, and regularly participate in meditation, mindfulness, or centering practices. To become a QTTT, practitioners should have maintained a consistent practice of TT for 5 years and practice daily meditation or equivalent mindfulness/centering exercises. In addition, the practitioner must complete 2 advanced-level workshops and participated in a teaching mentorship for a minimum of 1 year with a qualified QTTT. All QTTTs must adhere to an approved TTIA Teaching Curriculum.

EVIDENCE OF EFFICACY

TT has received a fair amount of attention in the scientific literature. As with most emerging approaches in health and medicine, descriptive articles and anecdotal reports dominated the early literature. Since the 1980s, however, numerous researchers have investigated TT, and several review articles have been written since 1997 on the state of research on TT.[14-23] Perhaps the most well-known, controversial research with TT was published in the April 1, 1998 issue of the *Journal of the American Medical Association* wherein a sixth-grade student conducted an experiment in which TT practitioners were asked to detect whether the experimenter's hand was closer to the practitioner's left or right hand.[24] Of the 280 trials conducted, the practitioners identified the correct hand 44% of the time. The results were written in part by the young student's mother, a member of the Questionable Nurse Practices Task Force and the National Council Against Health Fraud Inc, and the cofounder of Quackwatch Inc, a website dedicated to identifying health fraud and quackery. The authors concluded that failure to accurately detect human energy fields is "...unrefuted evidence that the claims of TT are groundless and that further professional use is unjustified."[20] Critics of the study were quick to identify serious flaws in the study's design[25-27] and improper statistical analysis.[27] In addition, Leskowitz[26] suggested that the only logical conclusion of this study is that, given the described set of experimental conditions, a human energy field could not be reliably detected. The leap to refuting TT is unsubstantiated because the intervention of TT as described by Krieger[2] was never administered.

Reduction of Anxiety

Much research in TT has focused on its effectiveness for the reduction of pain and anxiety, and enhancement of healing processes Although several researchers have investigated the effectiveness of TT in reducing anxiety, Robinson et al[23] were unable to identify any studies that included subjects with an anxiety disorder as defined by the *Diagnostic and Statistical Manual of Mental Disorders,*[28] *Fourth Edition, the International Classification of Diseases, 10th revision*, or any other validated diagnostic instruments. Instead, anxiety has been associated with stress and mood and has not been identified as a specific diagnosis for subjects in TT research. In fact, comparing the results of the studies that have included anxiety as an outcome measure is often difficult due to subject variability and/or differences in how anxiety is measured. Ireland,[29] for example, demonstrated that children ages 6 to 12 years who were HIV positive and received TT experienced a significant reduction in anxiety compared with control subjects who received sham, or mock, TT. Anxiety was measured using a subscale of the Spielberger State-Trait Anxiety Inventory (STAI) for Children. Kramer[30] also investigated the use of TT in children, but her subjects were 2 weeks to 2 years of age and were not HIV positive. The patients in Kramer's study were hospitalized for either an acute illness, injury, or surgery; stress or anxiety reduction was determined by measuring heart rate, skin temperature, and galvanic skin response.[30]

Hospitalized patients have been the subjects in several studies investigating TT and reduction in anxiety. Quinn and Strelkauskas,[31] Heidt,[32] and Zolfaghari et al[33] studied patients admitted to a hospital with cardiovascular diagnoses. Quinn and Strelkauskas[31] and Heidt[32] found that subjects who received TT experienced significant reductions in state-anxiety on the STAI compared to control groups, who received mock or placebo TT. Zolfaghar et al[33] studied women who had been scheduled for cardiac catheterization and were randomized to receive either 10 to 15 minutes of usual care, TT, or mock TT 1 hour before the catheterization. Just before surgery, women who received TT were found to have a significant reduction in state-anxiety on the STAI, whereas women in the control and mock TT groups were found to have a significant increase in state-anxiety. During the catheterization, women who received TT were also found to have lower vital signs and fewer cardiac arrhythmias during the catheterization compared with women in the other groups.[33]

The application of TT for managing anxiety in persons with severe burns has also been investigated. Turner and colleagues[34] measured anxiety using the visual analogue scale (VAS) for anxiety and found that TT was associated with a reduction in anxiety of patients hospitalized for severe burns. However, Busch and colleagues,[35] who used the Burn Specific Pain Anxiety Scale to measure anxiety, found no differences in mean anxiety scores between the TT group and the nursing presence (NP) control group, although within group analysis revealed that subjects in the TT group had a decrease in their mean anxiety scores whereas those in the NP group demonstrated a slight increase.

In addition to inpatients with cardiac conditions and burns, researchers have investigated the usefulness for managing anxiety with TT in other patient populations. Gagne and Toye[36] compared TT with relaxation therapy and sham TT for inpatients with psychiatric diagnoses and found that TT was more effective than sham TT in reducing anxiety, but that relaxation therapy was just as effective as TT. In a study of hospitalized pregnant women known to have chemical dependency, daily TT sessions were found to help reduce anxiety and withdrawal symptoms when compared with women who received either standard ward care or a shared activity period with a registered nurse.[37] Patients in a long-term care facility were studied by Simington and Laing[38] and were found to have significantly reduced state-anxiety following a back rub with TT intervention compared to patients in the control group, who only received a back rub. In a study of older adults in which the subjects were recruited from inpatient and outpatient facilities, Lin and Taylor[39] found that subjects who received TT had significant reductions of anxiety as measured by Form Y-1 of the STAI compared to subjects who received mock TT.

Investigators have also sought to determine the effectiveness for decreasing anxiety in persons with cancer. Jackson and colleagues[40] conducted a review of the literature in which they used the search words *healing touch, therapeutic touch, cancer, pain,* and *anxiety* and rated the articles they found from level I (highest) to level VII (lowest) based on the rating system described by Melnyk and Fineout-Overholdt.[41] They found one study by Samarel and colleagues,[42] which was given a level III rating because the subjects were not randomized to either the experimental or control group. In that study, investigators analyzed the use of dialogue and TT with patients who had to undergo surgery for breast cancer. Treatment was administered in subject's home within 7 days of surgery and 24 hours after hospital discharge. The experimental group received 10 minutes of TT and 20 minutes of dialogue. The control group received 10 minutes of sitting quietly and 20 minutes of dialogue. The experimental group had significantly lower preoperative anxiety scores than the control group, but no difference was found in postoperative measures. The other study identified by Melnyk and Fineout-Overholdt[41] and written by Kelley and colleagues[43] was given a level IV rating because it was a cohort study and was based on the data obtained by Samarel.[42] Similar results were reported by Frank and colleagues.[44] In this experiment, 82 women received either TT (n = 42) or sham TT (n = 40) as they underwent a stereotactic core biopsy (SCB) of a breast lesion. Using a VAS, all subjects were found to have less fear and feelings of restlessness and nervousness post-SCB as compared to pre-SCB scores, but no differences were seen between the TT and sham TT groups.

Applying TT with healthy subjects for the purposes of reducing anxiety has also been investigated. Olson and Sneed[45] administered TT to professional caregiver/health care students who were grouped as either having high anxiety or low-moderate anxiety according to the results of 3 self-report measures of anxiety: Profile of Mood States, STAI, and VAS. Both groups were then split, with half of the subjects receiving TT and the other half sitting quietly for 15 minutes. No statistically significant reduction of anxiety was found between groups, but reduction of anxiety for the high-anxiety group was greater with TT compared to the high-anxiety group who sat quietly. The authors suggested that a larger sample size would be necessary to determine statistically significant differences. Small sample size is also concern in a study by Engle and Graney[46] in which 11 healthy subjects received one session of either TT or sham TT. Pulse rate and amplitude, blood pressure, skin temperature, anxiety, perceived health status, and time perception were measured pre- and post-intervention. No differences were noted except for significant decreases in total pulse amplitude and perceived duration of time. A reduction of total pulse amplitude may indicate vasoconstriction and a potential adverse effect of TT, whereas the clinical importance of a decreased perceived duration of time is unclear. Lafreniere and colleagues[47] investigated TT in healthy subjects and reported that participants who were randomly assigned to receive TT showed a significantly greater reduction in mood disturbance and anxiety compared to subjects who did not receive TT. Although the design of this study included random assignment, the control group did not receive sham TT and thus subjects were aware whether they did or did not receive TT. This design flaw seriously limits the conclusions that can be made from this experiment.

A review of the literature suggests that TT's usefulness in reducing anxiety is unclear. Although a number of researchers have reported benefits of TT, others have found no effects when compared to control groups that received sham TT. In particular, it appears that TT is not particularly effective for reducing anxiety in young, healthy subjects.

Reduction of Pain

Several researchers have investigated the potential of TT to reduce pain in a variety of patient populations. In 2 previously cited studies measuring anxiety, Samarel et al[42] and Turner et al[34] also included pain measures in their assessment of TT. Samarel and colleagues[42] found a reduction of pain in patients with breast cancer who received TT, but the amount of pain relief did not reach statistical significance. Turner, on the other hand, reported a significant reduction in pain on the McGill Pain Questionnaire with patients who were admitted to the hospital with serious burns. Researchers have also found that TT appears to be helpful in reducing pain in other patient populations. Leskowitz[48] presented a case report in which a 62-year-old male with a 4-year history of phantom limb pain was successfully treated with TT. Prior to the application of TT, the subject's pain ranged from an 8 to 10 on a self-reported VAS with 10 being the maximum intensity. Previous interventions, such as medication, stress management, hypnosis, transcutaneous nervous stimulation, and ultrasound, reduced his pain to between 6 and 8, but long-term pain management with all of these techniques were inadequate. In contrast, the subject reported 0 pain on the VAS with the first TT session; and with self-administered TT, the subject has been able to maintain his pain at a 0 to 1 on a VAS.

Two studies were conducted to assess the potential for TT to decrease pain in patients with osteoarthritis (OA).[49,50] In the study by Eckes Peck,[49] a 2-group longitudinal design was used in which subjects served as their own controls and repeated VAS scores were used to measure pain and distress. Subjects in one group received TT, whereas subjects in the other group received progressive muscular relaxation (PMR). A statistically significant decrease in pain was recorded in the TT group from baseline to the first TT session, with further decreases noted in subsequent treatments. Similarly, the mean score for pain decreased progressively with each session of PMR. However, when TT and PMR were compared using multivariate analysis of variance, PMR was found to be more effective for decreasing pain than TT.

In a single-blind, randomized, control experiment, Gordon et al[50] also investigated the effect TT might have on reducing pain in patients with OA. Subjects were proportionately randomized based on OA severity into 1 of 3 subject groups. Pain was measured using a VAS and the West Haven-Yale Multidimensional Pain Inventory (MPI). The treatment group received TT, the placebo group received mock TT (MTT), and the control group received no intervention. In comparing pain reduction across the groups, the group who received TT had significantly decreased pain when compared to both the placebo and control groups.

Lin and Taylor[39] conducted a single-blind randomized experiment to assess whether TT was helpful in reducing chronic pain in older adults. Subjects either received TT, MTT, or standard care. Similar to Gordon's findings,[50] subjects who received TT were found to have significantly less pain when compared to both the placebo and control groups, although the investigators measured pain using an 11-point numeric rating scale rather than a VAS or the MPI. Gregory and Verdouw[51] have also reported that older adults living in a care facility have benefited from TT, including a 40% reduction of pain. The researchers, however, "...sought to be as inclusive as possible in the context of a range of behavioral and physiological conditions," did not seek to control for any confounding variables, and did not include a control group in their design.[51]

Giasson and Bouchard[52] did have a control group when they investigated the effect of TT on the well-being of 20 persons with terminal cancer and found that after each of 3 TT sessions subjects reported improvement in their appetite and sense of inner peace and a reduction of pain. TT was also investigated with subjects who had chronic pain associated with fibromyalgia syndrome.[53] Subjects either received TT (n = 10) or listened to tapes about complementary therapies (n = 5) once a week for 6 weeks. No statistically significant improvement was noted on the Short-form McGill Pain Questionnaire, VAS, or Fibromyalgia Health Assessment Questionnaire. In a single-blinded cross-over study by Blankfield and colleagues,[54] persons with chronic pain associated with carpal tunnel syndrome received either 6 sessions of TT or 6 sessions of sham TT. Although there were no significant differences between the 2 groups in terms of changes in median motor nerve distal latencies, pain scores, and relaxation scores, both groups demonstrated significant immediate changes from baseline for all 3 dependent variables. The researchers have identified several limitations of the study, including small sample size and potential bias of the TT practitioners who also collected the electroneurometer data. They have also offered several interpretations of their findings. One interpretation that seems to warrant further investigation is the possibility that both TT and sham TT facilitated a relaxation response that may have influenced physiologic processes and contributed to the observed improvements in median nerve conduction velocities.

The effect of TT on acute pain rather than chronic pain has also been explored. Keller and Bzdek[55] demonstrated that subjects who received TT experienced a reduction of their tension headaches by an average of 70% on the McGill-Melzack Pain Questionnaire. This reduction was significant when compared to subjects who received MTT and reported an average 35% decline in their headaches. Meehan[56] assessed pain reduction in subjects who had postoperative pain from abdominal or pelvic surgery. Using a single-blind, randomized, single trial design, Meehan randomly assigned subjects to 1 of 3 groups: TT group, MTT group, and standard intervention (narcotic analgesic group). Subjects who received TT reported a reduction in pain of 13%, whereas subjects who received MTT did not report any pain control. Subjects who received standard intervention, however, experienced a 42% reduction in pain, indicating that analgesics were the intervention of choice for pain management in this patient population.[56]

In a study of pain due to vascular surgery and TT, Coakley and Duffy[57] not only measured pain using a VAS, they also measured levels of cortisol and natural killer cells (NKC), before and after surgery. Compared to a usual care control group and after controlling for age and number of days post-surgery, patients who received TT had a significant reduction in postoperative pain and cortisol levels and significantly higher NKC levels. These findings suggest that TT may have a positive effect on biologic or biobehavioral markers known to be affected by physiologic and psychological stress. Johnson and colleagues[58] also measured pain and cortisol along with heart rate variability (HRV) but did not find that TT had a positive effect on these outcome measures. In their study, preterm neonates were given either TT or sham TT before and after they received a heel lance procedure. The Premature Infant Pain Profile, which includes both behavioral and physiological components and has well-established reliability, validity, and clinical utility, was used to measure pain. HRV, used to determine a measure of sympathetic-parasympathetic balance, was measured through an infrared oximeter, and stress levels were measured through salivary cortisol. Compared to a group of preterm neonates who received sham TT, those who received TT did not demonstrate a significant reduction in pain or cortisol, nor did they show any changes in HRV.[58]

Several researchers have investigated the use of TT for pain reduction in subjects across a wide range of diagnoses and conditions. The literature provides some preliminary evidence to support the use of TT with older adults and persons with OA. Other research suggests that TT may be helpful in managing phantom limb pain, headaches, and pain associated with burns, although many studies have been of limited quality with issues related to the studies' design and methods. Inclusion of a control group, use of sham or MTT, duration and frequency of TT, and type of outcome measures are fairly inconsistent across the studies, limiting the ability to draw firm conclusions about the efficacy of TT for reducing pain. Most investigators have also identified small sample size as a factor that challenges the measurement of TT's effect and the studies' external validity.

Wound Healing

Most of the experimental studies in TT have assessed its efficacy for the reduction of anxiety and pain; however, several studies have been conducted to assess TT's capacity to facilitate wound healing. The Cochrane Collaboration published in 2014 an updated review of TT for healing acute wounds. In their review O'Mathuna and Ashford[22] reported that no new trials were identified since their last review in 2004. They reiterated their conclusion, based on 4 studies by Wirth,[59-62] that there is no robust evidence that TT promotes healing of acute wounds.

PROPOSED MECHANISM OF THERAPEUTIC TOUCH

In addition to Coakley and Duffy,[57] who measured cortisol and NKCs, and Johnson et al,[58] who measured cortisol and HRV, other researchers have considered the interdisciplinary field of psychoneuroimmunology as a potential way of explaining the mechanism by which TT may act on the body and whether measurable physiologic changes are associated with the commonly used self-report outcome measures, such as the VAS and STAI. Quinn and Strelkauskas[31] investigated the effects of TT on both bereaved subjects and the TT practitioners providing the intervention. Psychological measures included the STAI and Affect Balance Scale. A profile of immune functioning was established for practitioners and recipients by measuring lymphocyte subset composition, mixed lymphocyte reactivity, cell-mediated toxicity, lymphocyte stimulation (mitogen responsiveness), and NKCs. In general, changes identified in each participant's immunological profile were extremely varied from person to person, except in percentage of T8 cells. T8 or suppressor T cells were identified in terms of lymphocyte subset composition using cytoflurographic analysis. The percentage of suppressor T cells was found to be dramatically reduced in subjects following TT and at very low levels for the practitioners at all times. The authors concluded that TT appears to have an impact on lymphocyte subset composition through a diminution of T8 cells. From this conclusion, the researchers hypothesized that TT might enhance immune function by reducing immune suppression.[31]

Olson et al[63] also sought to determine whether TT would have an effect on the immunological profile of highly stressed subjects. Subjects were randomly assigned to either the experimental group, who received 3 sessions of TT, or to the control group, who did not receive any intervention. In addition to measuring stress, anxiety, and mood, the researchers obtained blood from each subject to measure 3 immunoglobulin classes (IgG, IgA, IgM), the IgG subclasses, and lymphocyte subpopulations. (Serum immunoglobulin levels and quantification of lymphocyte subpopulations are frequently used as indicators for immune system functioning.) Subjects who received TT did not have significantly different levels of IgA, IgM, IgG, or lymphocyte levels when compared to the control subjects, although the authors noted that the direction of change in the immunoglobulin and lymphocyte levels was supportive of their hypothesis.[63]

Other researchers have investigated potential mechanisms of action of TT by studying its effect on DNA synthesis and proliferation of human cells in culture. In a study by Gronowicz and colleagues[64] fibroblasts, tenocytes, and osteoblasts received 10-minute sessions of TT or sham TT. Two 10-minute TT/per week were found to significantly stimulate proliferation in the fibroblasts and tenocytes compared to the control groups. TT appeared to stimulate proliferation in osteoblasts with a significant difference observed when compared to the nonintervention group, but there was no difference in proliferation when compared to the sham TT group. In addition, the researchers observed a significant increase in [3H]-thymidine incorporation into the DNA of fibroblasts and tenocytes, but not in osteoblasts.

From the same laboratory, Jhaveri and colleagues[65] found that TT not only stimulated proliferation in human osteoblasts, but also significantly increased mineralization in the osteoblasts, decreased mineralization in an osteosarcoma-derived cell line, and stimulated an increase in mRNA expression for Type I collagen, compared to a control group of osteoblasts. The authors suggest the possibility that, similar to pulsed electromagnetic fields, which have been shown to stimulate bone formation, TT may affect biological changes through altering biomagnetic fields.

Wirth and Cram[66] also sought a physiologic explanation for the therapeutic effects of TT. They measured physiologic variables, including surface electromagnetic (EMG) activity at 4 different muscle groups, heart rate, hand temperature, head temperature, and end tidal CO_2 levels. This study also differed from others in that the authors utilized subjects who were daily meditators and, for the most part, had no acute or chronic health or psychological abnormalities. Several issues regarding the experimental design, subject selection, and independent variables raise concern for the reliability of the results, but subjects who received TT had a significant reduction in EMG activity at the C4, T6, and L3 paraspinals. The autonomic indicators showed a general trend toward lower arousal; however, the decline was not significant. These result suggest that TT may be helpful for local muscle relaxation, but a broader systemic effect on the autonomic nervous system may be limited.

The effect that TT may or may not have on bodily systems requires much more research. Links between stress, anxiety, and pain reduction with psychoneuroimmunological changes seem logical, but determining the appropriate dependent variables requires additional study. Researchers may need to consider a multitude of physiologic responses that together facilitate improvement in one's sense of well-being.

LIMITATIONS IN RESEARCH DESIGN OF MANY STUDIES

Several authors have written reviews of the TT literature and concluded that, despite preliminary research that supports the use of TT for pain, much more study and better research is required before clear recommendations about TT can be made.[14-21]

One methodological issue often discussed is the duration of the TT intervention. TT, as described by Krieger,[2] may be offered in sessions from 5 minutes to over 30 minutes, depending on the needs of the client. It is up to the practitioner to assess the client's energy field, intervene appropriately, and reassess. Some research studies, however, have required TT practitioners to administer TT for a designated period of time, regardless of what the practitioner determines to be the needs of the client. Supporters argue that this method allows for greater control of the independent variables. Opponents of this practice argue that limiting the duration of the TT intervention interferes with the potential for physiological and psychological changes to occur.

Another methodological concern is that all of the studies reviewed in this chapter and all of the studies included in the meta-analysis by Peters[21] were conducted with samples of convenience. Although several had 2 or more groups and reported random assignment to the groups, the assignment methods were not well described and drop-out rates were not adequately addressed. A few reviewers also raised issues related to potential bias of subjects and researchers.[16,21]

THERAPEUTIC TOUCH AND PLACEBO EFFECT

Meehan[18] raises the issue that controlled efficacy studies need to differentiate between the effects of TT and placebo effect. Several researchers[29,45,50,51] have attempted to use mock or sham TT in their studies as a way to control for placebo effect. Mock or sham TT has the appearance of TT, but is performed by a health care provider without TT training who engages in some form of mental activity to avoid a positive intention to help or heal. Debate and discussion continue as to whether mock TT is adequate for ensuring a single-blind control. One also needs to consider that double-blind control experiments will probably not be possible in TT research because the intent of the practitioner will always be subject to scrutiny.

Studies of mechanism and efficacy of TT have evolved from anecdotal reports to randomized control trials. However, the results have been mixed and the need to increase the scientific rigor of the study of TT continues to exist. Suggestions include improving the descriptions of the study sample, increasing the sample sizes, identifying appropriate biomarkers, and utilizing physiologic outcome measures in combination with the more commonly used self-report measures.

CONCLUSION

Therapists inclined to consider including complementary therapies into their plans of care will find support for TT as an intervention to reduce pain and, to a lesser extent, anxiety. As a noninvasive, nonpharmaceutical intervention, TT seems to have little potential for causing negative interactions with medications or other physiological conditions. Research that assesses the mechanism by which TT may alleviate pain will further advance the acceptance of TT into the medical and rehabilitation communities. In addition, assessment of the physiologic changes that occur with TT may further suggest patient diagnoses and conditions that might benefit the most from incorporating TT into a rehabilitation program. As experts in impairment, dysfunction, and pain management, physical and occupational therapists are well suited to collaborate with other scientists to conduct research in complementary therapies, such as TT.

REFERENCES

1. Krieger D. *Accepting Your Power to Heal: The Personal Practice of Therapeutic Touch.* Santa Fe, NM: Bear and Company; 1993.
2. Krieger D. *The Therapeutic Touch: How to Use Your Hands to Help or Heal.* New York, NY: Simon and Schuster; 1979.
3. Mishra L, Singh BB, Dagenais S. Ayurveda: a historical perspective and principles of the traditional. *Altern Ther Health Med.* 2001;7(2):36-42.
4. Veith I (trans). *The Yellow Emperor's Classic of Internal Medicine.* Berkeley, CA: University of California Press; 1970.
5. Weber R. Philosophical foundations and frameworks for healing. In: Borelli MD, Heidt P, eds. *Therapeutic Touch: A Book of Readings.* New York, NY: Springer; 1981.
6. Weber R. A philosophical perspective on touch. In: Barnard KE, Bazelton TB, eds. *Touch: The Foundation of Experience.* Madison, WI: International Universities Press; 1990.
7. Bohm D. *Wholeness and the Implicate Order.* Boston, MA: Routledge & Kegan Paul; 1980.
8. Bohm D. The implicate order and the super-implicate order. In: Weber E, ed. *Dialogues With Scientists and Sages: The Search for Unity.* New York, NY: Routledge & Kegan Paul; 1986.
9. Rogers ME. *Introduction to the Theoretical Basis of Nursing.* Philadelphia, PA: FA Davis; 1970.
10. Rogers ME. Science of unitary, irreducible human being: update 1990. In: Barrett E, ed. *Visions of Rogers' Science Based Nursing.* New York, NY: National League for Nursing; 1990.
11. Krieger D. *Therapeutic Touch Inner Workbook: Ventures in Transpersonal Healing.* Santa Fe, NM: Bear and Company, Inc; 1997.
12. Gerber R. *Vibrational Medicine: New Choices for Healing Ourselves.* Rev ed. Santa Fe, NM: Bear and Company, Inc; 1988.
13. Therapeutic Touch International Association. http://therapeutic-touch.org. Accessed February 15, 2016.
14. Ireland M, Olson O. Massage therapy and therapeutic touch in children: state of the science. *Altern Ther Health Med.* 2000;6(5):54-63.
15. Ramnarine-Singh S. The surgical significance of therapeutic touch. *Association of Operating Room Nurses.* 1999;69(2):358-369.
16. Winstead-Fry P, Kijek J. An integrative review and meta-analysis of therapeutic touch research. *Altern Ther Health Med.* 1999;5(6):58-67.
17. Easter A. The state of research on the effects of therapeutic touch. *J Holistic Nurs.* 1997;15(2):158-175.
18. Meehan TC. Therapeutic touch as a nursing intervention. *J Adv Nurs.* 1998;28(1):117-125.
19. Spence JE, Olsen MA. Quantitative research of therapeutic touch. An integrative review of the literature 1985-1995. *Scand J Caring Sci.* 1997;11(3):183-190.
20. Daley B. Therapeutic touch, nursing practice and contemporary cutaneous wound healing research. *J Adv Nurs.* 1997;25(6):1123-1132.
21. Peters RM. The effectiveness of therapeutic touch: a meta-analytic review. *Nurs Sci Q.* 1999;12(1):52-61.
22. O'Mathuna DP, Ashford RL. Therapeutic touch for healing acute wounds. *Cochrane Database Syst Rev.* 2014;7:CD002766.
23. Robinson J, Biley FC, Dolk H. Therapeutic touch for anxiety disorders. *Cochrane Database Syst Rev.* 2007;3:CD006240.
24. Rosa L, Rosa R, Sarner L, Barrett S. A close look at therapeutic touch. *JAMA.* 1998;279:1005-1010.
25. Achterberg J. Clearing the air in the therapeutic touch controversy. *Altern Ther Health Med.* 1998;4(4):100.
26. Leskowitz ED. Undebunking therapeutic touch. *Altern Ther Health Med.* 1998;4(4):101-102.
27. Cox T. A nurse-statistician reanalyzes data from the Rosa therapeutic touch study. *Altern Ther Health Med.* 2003;9(1):58-64.
28. American Psychiatric Association. *Diagnostic and statistical manual of mental disorders.* 4th ed. 2000. doi:10.1176/appi.books.9780890423349.
29. Ireland M. Therapeutic touch with HIV-infected children: a pilot study. *J Assoc Nursing AIDS Care.* 1998;9(4):68.
30. Kramer NA. Comparison of therapeutic touch and casual touch in stress reduction of hospitalized children. *Pediatr Nurs.* 1990;16(5):483-485.
31. Quinn JF, Strelkauskas AJ. Psychoimmunologic effects of therapeutic touch on practitioners and recently bereaved recipients: a pilot study. *Adv Nurs Sci.* 1993;15(4):13-26.
32. Heidt P. Effect of therapeutic touch on the anxiety level of hospitalized patients. *Nurs Res.* 1981;30(1):32-37.
33. Zolfaghari M, Eybpoosh S, Hazrati M. Effects of therapeutic touch on anxiety, vital signs, and cardiac dysrhythmia in a sample of Iranian women undergoing cardiac catheterization. *J Holistic Nurs.* 2012;30(4):225-234.
34. Turner JG, Clark AJ, Gauthier DK, Williams M. The effect of therapeutic touch on pain and anxiety in burn patients. *J Adv Nurs.* 1998;28(1):10-28.
35. Busch M, Visser A, Eybrechts M, et al. The implementation and evaluation of therapeutic touch in burn patients: an instructive experience of conducting a scientific study within a non-academic nursing setting. *Patient Educ Counseling.* 2012;89:439-446.

36. Gagne D, Toye RC. The effects of therapeutic touch and relaxation therapy in reducing anxiety. *Arch Psychiatr Nurs.* 1984;8(3):184-187.

37. Larden C, Palmer M, Lynne M, Janssen P. Efficacy of therapeutic touch in treating pregnant inpatients who have a chemical dependency. *J Holistic Nurs.* 2004;22(4):320-322.

38. Simington JA, Laing GP. Effects of therapeutic touch on anxiety in the institutionalized elderly. *Clin Nurs Res.* 1993;2(4):438-450.

39. Lin Y, Taylor AG. Effects of therapeutic touch in reducing pain and anxiety in an elderly population. *Integrative Medicine.* 1998;1(4):155-162.

40. Jackson E, Kellye M, McNeil P, Meyer E, Schlegel L, Eaton M. Does therapeutic touch help reduce pain and anxiety in patients with cancer? *Clin J Oncol Nsg.* 2008;12(1):113-120.

41. Melnyk B, Fineout-Overholt E. *Evidence-Based Practice in Nursing and Healthcare.* Philadelphia, PA: Lippincott Williams & Wilkins; 2005.

42. Samarel N, Fawcett J, Davis MM, Ryan FM. Effects of dialogue and therapeutic touch on preoperative and post-operative experiences of breast cancer surgery: an exploratory study. *Oncol Nurs Forum.* 1998;25(8):1369-1376.

43. Kelley AE, Sullivan P, Fawcett J, Samarel N. Therapeutic touch, quiet time, and dialogue: perceptions of women with breast cancer. *Once Nsg Forum.* 2004;31(3):625-631.

44. Frank LS, Frank JL, March D, Makari-Judson G, Barham RB, Mertens WC. Does therapeutic touch ease the discomfort or distress of patients undergoing stereotactic core breast biopsy? A randomized clinical trial. *Pain Med.* 2007;8(5):419-424.

45. Olson M, Sneed N. Anxiety and therapeutic touch. *Issues Ment Health Nurs.* 1995;16:97-108.

46. Engle VF, Graney MJ. Biobehavioral effects of therapeutic touch. *J Nurs Scholarsh.* 2003;32(3):287-293.

47. Lafreniere KD, Mutus B, Cameron S, et al. Effect of therapeutic touch on biochemical and mood indicators in women. *J Altern Complement Med.* 1999;5(4):367-370.

48. Leskowitz ED. Phantom limb pain treated with therapeutic touch: a case report. *Arch Phys Med Rehab.* 2000;81:552-524.

49. Eckes Peck SD. The effectiveness of therapeutic touch for decreasing pain in elders with degenerative arthritis. *J Holistic Nurs.* 1997;15(2):176-198.

50. Gordon A, Merenstein JH, D'Amico F, Hudgens D. The effects of therapeutic touch on patients with osteoarthritis of the knee. *J Fam Pract.* 1998;47(4):271-276.

51. Gregory S, Verdouw J. Therapeutic touch: its application for residents in aged care. *Aust Nurs J.* 2005;12(7):23-25.

52. Giasson M, Bouchard L. Effect of therapeutic touch on the well-being of persons with terminal cancer. *J Holistic Nurs.* 1998;16(3):383-398.

53. Denison B. Touch the pain away. New research on therapeutic touch and persons with fibromyalgia syndrome. *Holistic Nurs Pract.* 2004;12(3):142-151.

54. Blankfield RP, Sulzmann C, Fradle LG, Tapolyai AA, Zyzanski SJ. Therapeutic touch in the treatment of carpal tunnel syndrome. *J Am Board Fam Pract.* 2001;14(5):335-342.

55. Keller E, Bzdek VM. Effects of therapeutic touch on tension headache pain. *Nurs Res.* 1986;35(2):102-106.

56. Meehan TC. Therapeutic touch and postoperative pain: a Rogerian research study. *Nurs Sci Q.* 1993;6(2):69-78.

57. Coakley AM, Duffy ME. The effect of therapeutic touch on postoperative patients. *J Holistic Nsg.* 2010;28(3):193-200.

58. Johnson C, Campbell-Yeo M, Rich B, et al. Therapeutic touch is not therapeutic for procedural pain in very pre-term neonates. *Colin J Pain.* 2013;29(9):824-829.

59. Wirth DP. The effect of non-contact therapeutic touch on the healing rate of full thickness dermal wounds. *Subtle Energies.* 1992;1(1):1.

60. Wirth DP, Richardson JT, Eidleman WS, O'Malley AC. Full thickness dermal wounds treated with non-contact therapeutic touch: a replication and extension. *Complement Ther Med.* 1993;1(3):127-132.

61. Wirth DP, Barrett MJ, Eidleman WS. Non-contact therapeutic touch and wound re-epithelializational: an extension of previous research. *Complement Ther Med.* 1994;2(4):187-192.

62. Wirth DP, Richardson JT, Martinez RD, Eidelman WS, Lopez ME. Non-contact therapeutic touch intervention and full-thickness cutaneous wounds: a replication. *Complement Ther Med.* 1996;4(4):237-240.

63. Olson M, Sneed N, LaVia M, Virella G, Bonadonna R, Michel Y. Stress-induced immunosuppression and therapeutic touch. *Altern Ther Health Med.* 1997;3(2):68-74.

64. Gronowicz GA, Jhaveri A, Clarke, LW, Aronow, MS, Smith TA. Therapeutic touch stimulates the proliferation of human cells in culture. *J Altern Complement Ther.* 2008;14(3):233-239.

65. Jhavari A, Walsh SJ, Wang Y, McCarthy M, Gronowicz. Therapeutic touch affects DNA synthesis and mineralization of human osteoblasts in culture. *J Orthop Res.* 2008;26(11):1541-1546.

66. Wirth DP, Cram JR. Multi-site electromyographic analysis of non-contact therapeutic touch. *Int J Psychosom.* 1993;40(1-4):47-55.

Financial Disclosures

Dr. Brent Anderson has not disclosed any relevant financial relationships.

Dr. Ellen Zambo Anderson has no financial or proprietary interest in the materials presented herein.

John F. Barnes has no financial or proprietary interest in the materials presented herein.

Dr. Jennifer M. Bottomley has no financial or proprietary interest in the materials presented herein.

Dr. Carol M. Davis is a part-time teacher for J. F. Barnes Myofascial Release Seminars.

Dr. Judith E. Deutsch has no financial or proprietary interest in the materials presented herein.

Dr. Jan Dommerholt has no financial or proprietary interest in the materials presented herein.

Barbara Funk has no financial or proprietary interest in the materials presented herein.

Dr. Mary Lou Galantino has no financial or proprietary interest in the materials presented herein.

Deborah A. Giaquinto-Wahl has no financial or proprietary interest in the materials presented herein.

Dr. Janet Kahn has no financial or proprietary interest in the materials presented herein.

Dr. Kevin R. Kunkel has not disclosed any financial relationship.

Dr. Patrick J. LaRiccia has no financial or proprietary interest in the materials presented herein.

Lynn B. Littman has no financial or proprietary interest in the materials presented herein.

Dr. Teresa M. Miller has no financial or proprietary interest in the materials presented herein.

Dr. Sangeeta Singg has no financial or proprietary interest in the materials presented herein.

Dr. Kerri Sowers has no financial or proprietary interest in the materials presented herein.

Dr. James Stephens is an Independent Feldenkrais practitioner.

Dr. Matthew J. Taylor has no financial or proprietary interest in the materials presented herein.

Dr. Carolee Winstein has no financial or proprietary interest in the materials presented herein.

Index

Printed in the United States
by Baker & Taylor Publisher Services